THE CAESAREAN SECTION

THE CAESAREAN SECTION

Indications, Techniques, Complications and Alternatives with Notes on Obstetric Practice in the Tropics

Erik Domini MD FCOG (Padova)
Consultant Obstetrician and Gynaecologist (R)
Ospedale St. Spirito, Nizza Monferrato, Italy
Father Ambrosoli Memorial Hospital, Kalongo, Uganda
St Kizito Hospital, Matany, Uganda

Sara Guazzini MD FCOG (Florence)
Registrar
Department of Obstetrics and Gynaecology
Ospedale di Cittadella, Padova, Italy

Former Registrar
Department of Obstetrics
St Kizito Hospital, Matany, Uganda

Monica Guidi MD FCOG (Florence)
Registrar and Referee for Obstetrics
Department of Obstetrics and Gynaecology
Ospedale di Cittadella, Padova, Italy

Former Registrar
Department of Obstetrics
St Kizito Hospital, Matany, Uganda

Stefano Vicentini MD
Medical Superintendent (R)
St Kizito Hospital, Matany, Uganda

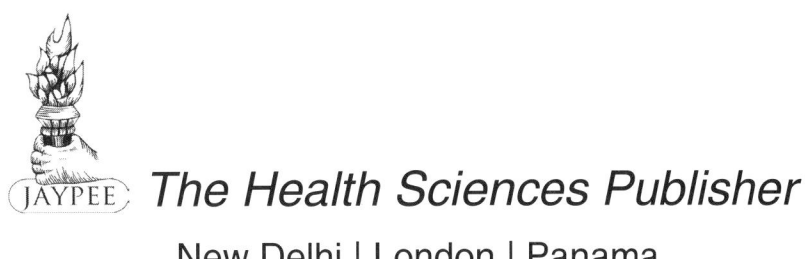

The Health Sciences Publisher
New Delhi | London | Panama

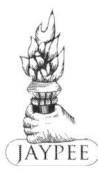
Jaypee Brothers Medical Publishers (P) Ltd

Headquarters
Jaypee Brothers Medical Publishers (P) Ltd
4838/24, Ansari Road, Daryaganj
New Delhi 110 002, India
Phone: +91-11-43574357
Fax: +91-11-43574314
Email: jaypee@jaypeebrothers.com

Overseas Offices

J.P. Medical Ltd
83 Victoria Street, London
SW1H 0HW (UK)
Phone: +44 20 3170 8910
Fax: +44 (0)20 3008 6180
Email: info@jpmedpub.com

Jaypee Brothers Medical Publishers (P) Ltd
17/1-B Babar Road, Block-B, Shaymali
Mohammadpur, Dhaka-1207
Bangladesh
Mobile: +08801912003485
Email: jaypeedhaka@gmail.com

Jaypee-Highlights Medical Publishers Inc
City of Knowledge, Bld. 235, 2nd Floor, Clayton
Panama City, Panama
Phone: +1 507-301-0496
Fax: +1 507-301-0499
Email: cservice@jphmedical.com

Jaypee Brothers Medical Publishers (P) Ltd
Bhotahity, Kathmandu, Nepal
Phone: +977-9741283608
Email: kathmandu@jaypeebrothers.com

Website: www.jaypeebrothers.com
Website: www.jaypeedigital.com

© 2017, Jaypee Brothers Medical Publishers

The views and opinions expressed in this book are solely those of the original contributor(s)/author(s) and do not necessarily represent those of editor(s) of the book.

All rights reserved. No part of this publication may be reproduced, stored or transmitted in any form or by any means, electronic, mechanical, photocopying, recording or otherwise, without the prior permission in writing of the publishers.

All brand names and product names used in this book are trade names, service marks, trademarks or registered trademarks of their respective owners. The publisher is not associated with any product or vendor mentioned in this book.

Medical knowledge and practice change constantly. This book is designed to provide accurate, authoritative information about the subject matter in question. However, readers are advised to check the most current information available on procedures included and check information from the manufacturer of each product to be administered, to verify the recommended dose, formula, method and duration of administration, adverse effects and contraindications. It is the responsibility of the practitioner to take all appropriate safety precautions. Neither the publisher nor the author(s)/editor(s) assume any liability for any injury and/or damage to persons or property arising from or related to use of material in this book.

This book is sold on the understanding that the publisher is not engaged in providing professional medical services. If such advice or services are required, the services of a competent medical professional should be sought.

Every effort has been made where necessary to contact holders of copyright to obtain permission to reproduce copyright material. If any have been inadvertently overlooked, the publisher will be pleased to make the necessary arrangements at the first opportunity.

Inquiries for bulk sales may be solicited at: jaypee@jaypeebrothers.com

The Caesarean Section

First Edition: **2017**

ISBN: 978-93-5270-019-6

Printed at Rajkamal Electric Press, Plot No. 2, Phase-IV, Kundli, Haryana.

Dedicated to

Our parents.
To the women of Uganda
we had the privilege to serve and admire

A Demetria, non infrequentemente nei miei pensieri,
sempre nel mio affetto e nella mia amicizia.

(To Demetria not infrequently in my thoughts,
always in my affection and love)

Preface

Experience comes from critical analysis of the therapeutic conducts and outcomes of the cases entrusted to our care. Some of these have a favourable outcomes, others do not have.

Events that develop in a positive way fade very soon from the memory; those with an ominous outcome leave the deepest trace, along with the nagging question: "*Should* I have managed it differently? *Could* it have been managed differently?"

These cases with unfavourable outcomes and the human suffering which we have witnessed and for which we were, perhaps, in part, responsible, albeit unwittingly, along with the wish that this suffering shall not have been in vain, have spurred us to write this book and the forthcoming *Treatise on Obstetric Surgery*.

In these two works, we have tried to make available to our younger colleagues what little we have learned over the course of our professional lives. Our aim is to reduce for them the number of nagging doubts that will inevitably accompany their professional lives, especially if conducted in the tropics.

There is a saying that "The first thing a doctor wants to be is rich, then famous, and lastly to be good at his job". We advise our youthful colleagues to stand this order on its head, and to strive first and foremost for mastery, which is attained through sacrifice and study, which brings to mind a favourite maxim of our teacher,

TNA Jeffcoate of Liverpool: *Presumption of knowledge is the major obstacle to knowledge.*

Wealth and fame will follow in due course.

Erik Domini
Sara Guazzini
Monica Guidi
Stefano Vicentini

Acknowledgements

Every acknowledgement closes with expressions of thanks and this one is no exception with the sole difference that there is nothing perfunctory about these words, as they express a need felt by the heart that I should acknowledge all those who have contributed either directly or indirectly to the present work.

To M/s Jaypee Brothers Medical Publishers (P) Ltd., New Delhi, India for publishing this monograph: It is a source of great pride to me that such a prestigious publishing house has accepted my text. Thank you!

To the co-authors of this book, who have accompanied me throughout and supported me with their enthusiasm and friendship. Thank you!

To my Ugandan colleagues, my partners during the years I spent in Uganda, goes all my admiration for their dedication to work and their technical skill.

The latter is the fruit of training provided by Uganda's faculties of medicine, among which the Medical Faculty at Makerere is the most outstanding. May I be permitted to mention here Eminton Odong, James Lemukol and Richard Edmund Sanya, John Bosco Nsubuga, Myango Patient?

I worked for years in close collaboration with Ugandan midwives, many of whom were trained at the Father Ambrosoli Midwifery School of Kalongo, one of the best in Uganda. The excellence of the training given there, and at other Schools of Obstetrics in Uganda, is well attested by the ability to resolve complex obstetric challenges, even when working in outlying medical centres.

I spent some intensive years in Kalongo and in Matany, and forged friendships there that remain in my memory and in my heart. I ask leave to call to mind the Sisters (Carmel et al.) and Tutors (Polly et al.) who run the Midwifery School of Kalongo, Sr. Paska, Alphonse Ayepa "Sir Alphonse" the anaesthetist who enabled me to operate on extremely complex cases in safety, Mary Annunciata Longole, Daniel Irusi, Betty Agan, Lilian Adwar and Hellen.

Two colleagues have left a deep mark on my professional life; even though they are of my generation, I consider them my masters: Thomas Raassen, President of the International Society of Obstetric Fistula Surgeons and Carlo Alberto Bonini, an extraordinary surgeon and gentleman.

I judge a publication, apart from by its conceptual content, also by its typographical attire, which facilitates both reading and understanding. My thanks for this are due to Giovanni Durando and to his wife, Ada Giaretto, for their skill, passion and patience.

The life of a physician, as that of any human being, is made up of more than just its professional side. I am privileged here to be able to thank Rita Prudenzano, my Ward Sister, Nizza Monferrato (Italy) Hospital, whose gifts of human understanding and professional ability have been indispensable for the proper running and harmony of the ward.

My memory and my friendship to: Adriana Platone, Giovanna Riva du Lac Capet, Lisa Corti Santini, Commander Giancarlo Basile and Crew of I.N. Training Ship "Stella Polare" Asti, 7th August 2016.

Erik Domini

Contents

SECTION 1: ANATOMY AND PHYSIOLOGY OF PARTURITION

1. **Parturition** — 3
2. **Birth Canal (Passageway)** — 4
   Bony pelvis 4
   Mixed types 23
3. **Uterus** — 25
   Mechanical functions 25
   Histology of the uterus 26
   Contractile activity 27
   Therapy 31
4. **Passenger (Foetus)** — 32
5. **Mechanism and Physiopathology of Parturition** — 33
   Mechanism of parturition 35
   Presentation 35
   Engagement 35
   Descent, rotation and progress 40
   Mechanism of parturition in various pelvic types 40

SECTION 2: DIAGNOSIS

6. **Diagnosis in Clinical Obstetrics** — 43
   Instruments 43
   Diagnosis in clinical obstetrics 43
   Pelvic inlet (superior pelvic strait) 61
7. **Partograph** — 75
   Structure of the partograph 78
   Progress of labour 78
   Uterine contractile activity 79
   Foetal well-being 79
   Treatment 81
   Maternal condition 81
   Filling in the partograph 81
   Matany partograph 86

SECTION 3: CAESAREAN SECTION AND MANAGEMENT

8. Indications for Caesarean Section Outside Labour — 91
Maternal indications   *91*
Foetal indications   *99*

9. Indications for Caesarean Section During Labour — 102
Preliminary considerations   *102*
Compromise of maternal–foetal gas exchange   *102*
Obstacles to the engagement and progress of labour   *103*
The two indications presented above in varying relations to each other   *105*

10. Trial of Labour — 106
Preliminary assessment of the gravid patient   *106*
Actual labour   *107*

11. Preparing for the Operation — 113
Preoperative fasting   *113*
Intravenous access   *113*
Venous cut down   *114*
Maternal intensive care   *115*

12. Anaesthesia — 121
Basic equipment   *121*
Basic medications   *121*
Patient's position   *121*
Types of anaesthesia   *123*
Fundamental rule   *123*
Premedication for anaesthesia   *123*
Monitoring anaesthesia   *123*
Spinal anaesthesia (isobaric subarachnoid)   *124*
General anaesthesia   *126*

13. Laparotomies — 128
Refresher of surgical anatomy of the abdominal wall   *128*
Laparotomy   *130*

14. The Various Types of Hysterotomy—Criteria of Choice — 144
Hysterotomy   *144*
Lower uterine segment   *144*
Criteria of hysterotomy choice   *146*

15. Transverse Hysterotomies — 147
Transverse transperitoneal hysterotomies   *147*
Technique used by the authors   *148*
High transverse hysterotomy   *152*
Method used by the authors   *154*
Extraperitoneal transverse hysterotomies   *157*

16. Vertical Hysterotomies — 162
Low vertical c-section *163*
Predominantly lower-segement c-section *164*
Vertical corpus/lower-segment c-section *165*

17. Management of Intraoperative Complications — 168
Control of haemorrhage *168*
Haemostatic procedures *169*
Uterine devascularisation *170*
Injury to the urinary tract *173*

18. Tubal Sterilization — 181
Indications *181*

19. Abdominal Wall Closure — 185
Physiological introduction of wound healing *185*
Repair of a vertical laparotomy wound *186*
Repair of a transverse laparotomy wound *191*

20. Perimortem and Postmortem Caesarean Delivery — 195
Physiopathology *195*
Indications *196*
Method *196*

21. Uterine Rupture — 198
Uterine rupture during pregnancy *198*
Uterine rupture during labour *199*

22. Monitoring Caesarean Section: Postoperative Recovery — 211
Ward doctor *211*
Observation *211*
Therapy *211*
Ward examination *214*
Abdominal compartment syndrome (ACS) *216*

23. Complications of the Laparotomic Wound Suture — 221
Wound dehiscence *221*
Aetiopathogenesis *221*
Enteric fistulas *225*
Symptomatology *225*

24. Postcaesarean Wound Dehiscence — 226
Early uterus and abdominal wall synchronous dehiscence *226*
Late dehiscence of hysterorrhaphy *227*

25. Obstructed Labour Injury Complex — 229
Vesicovaginal fistulas *229*
Anatomical functional classification of rectovaginal fistulas *231*

26. The Newborn — 236
Introductory remarks on physiopathology *236*
Meconium aspiration syndrome *237*
Labour assistance and assistance to the newborn *237*
Amniiotic fluid stained with meconium *243*

SECTION 4: ALTERNATIVES TO CAESAREAN SECTION

27. Version—Breech Presentation, Transverse and Oblique Lies — 249
Breech presentation *249*
Transverse lie *253*

28. Symphysiotomy–Vacuum Extraction (Foetus Alive–Head Engaged) — 257
Symphysiotomy *257*
Vacuum extraction *262*

29. Destructive Operations—A Vanishing Art in Modern Obstetrics (P Sikka, 2011) — 268
Craniotomy *269*
Evisceration *272*

Index *275*

SECTION 1

Anatomy and Physiology of Parturition

- Parturition
- Birth Canal (Passageway)
- Uterus
- Passenger (Foetus)
- Mechanism and Physiopathology of Parturition

CHAPTER 1

Parturition

Parturition is the transit of the product of conception (foetus, passenger) from the internal environment (the uterus) to the external one; the passageway is the birth canal; transit occurs under the action of a force developed by the container itself (the uterus).

Three structures, then, take part in the process of parturition: The passenger, the uterus—in its dual function of container and expulsive force (power) and the birth canal (passageway); we will therefore illustrate:

a. The birth canal (passage).
b. The uterus.
c. The passenger.

A substantial portion of the indications for caesarean section stem from a failure of these three components to interact harmoniously.

CHAPTER 2

Birth Canal (Passageway)

The birth canal, the passageway between the internal environment (uterus) and the external one, consists of a bony part (the bony pelvis) and of soft tissues.

BONY PELVIS

The bony pelvis (Fig. 2.1) is a ring of bones which rests upon the lower limbs and supports the spinal column. Shaped like a truncated cone with its base facing anterosuperiorly, it comprises two *innominate* or pelvic bones, one on each side, joined anteriorly and articulated with the sacrum posteriorly. At its inferior end, the sacrum articulates with the coccyx.

Pelvic Bone (OS Coxa)

Together with its paired contralateral bone, the pelvic bone defines the anterior and lateral boundaries of the pelvic girdle. Posteriorly, it articulates with the sacrum. A flat bone, the pelvic bone is composed of three parts: Ilium, ischium and pubis, forming an irregular quadrilateral with a twist along its longitudinal axis and a narrowing on its median portion. The pelvis presents external and internal surfaces, and four borders: Superior, inferior, anterior and posterior, with four angles where these four borders meet.

- The *external surface* (Fig. 2.2) has in its central portion a cavity: The *cotyloid cavity* (acetabulum), the cup-shaped hollow into which the head of the femur fits. Superior to this is the broad surface of the external iliac fossa, traversed by three ridges: The *posterior, anterior and inferior gluteal lines*. These lines divide it into three areas: Posterior, median and anterior, which respectively provide the insertions for the *gluteus maximus, gluteus medius* and *gluteus minimus muscles*. Caudal to the acetabulum is the obturator foramen
- The *internal or pelvic surface* (Fig. 2.3) is divided into a superior and an inferior portion by the *linea terminalis* (arcuate line of the ilium), an oblique line projecting in a superoinferior and posteroanterior direction.
  - The superior portion or *internal iliac fossa* is triangular in shape; from here much of the iliacus muscle originates
  - The inferior portion, situated inferiorly and posteriorly to the linea terminalis, presents:
    » A roughened, irregularly quadrilateral surface, the *iliac tuberosity*, which provides the insertions of the sturdy ligaments that join the pelvic bone to the sacrum
    » A joint surface, the *auricular part of the sacroiliac joint* (SIJ), which articulates with a similar, concave structure of the sacrum. This surface is C-shaped, with a short, almost horizontal, *inferior ramus* and a vertical *superior ramus*. The center of the C-curve contains an eminence called the *tubercle*; this corresponds to the concavity of the sacral auricular part of the SIJ, which is L-shaped. The tubercle acts as a pivot for *nutation* and *counternutation* movements of the sacrum during labor
    » A third flat, quadrilateral surface corresponds to the *cotyloid cavity*, which in its upper portion provides the origin of the external obturator muscle; distally and anterior to this we find the *obturator foramen*.

BIRTH CANAL (PASSAGEWAY)

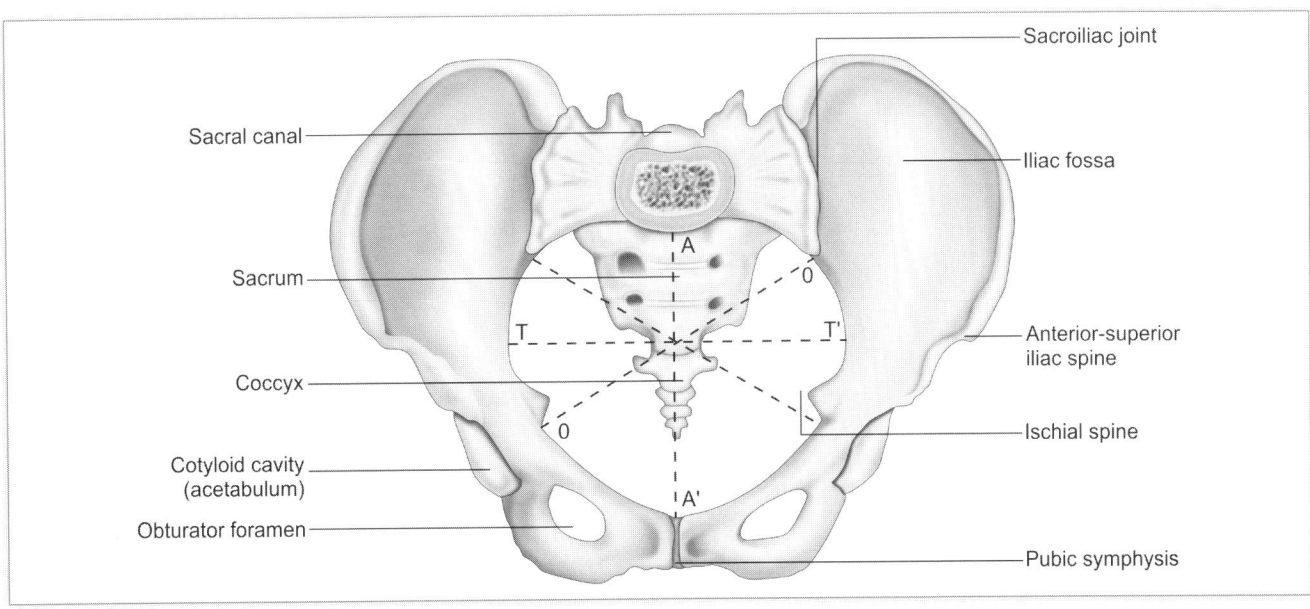

Fig. 2.1: Female pelvis, superior view. The dotted lines indicate the diameters of the pelvic inlet (superior pelvic strait). AA, anteroposterior diameter; TT, transverse diameter; OO oblique diameter
(From: Testut *Anatomia Umana*, Utet, Turin; by kind permission)

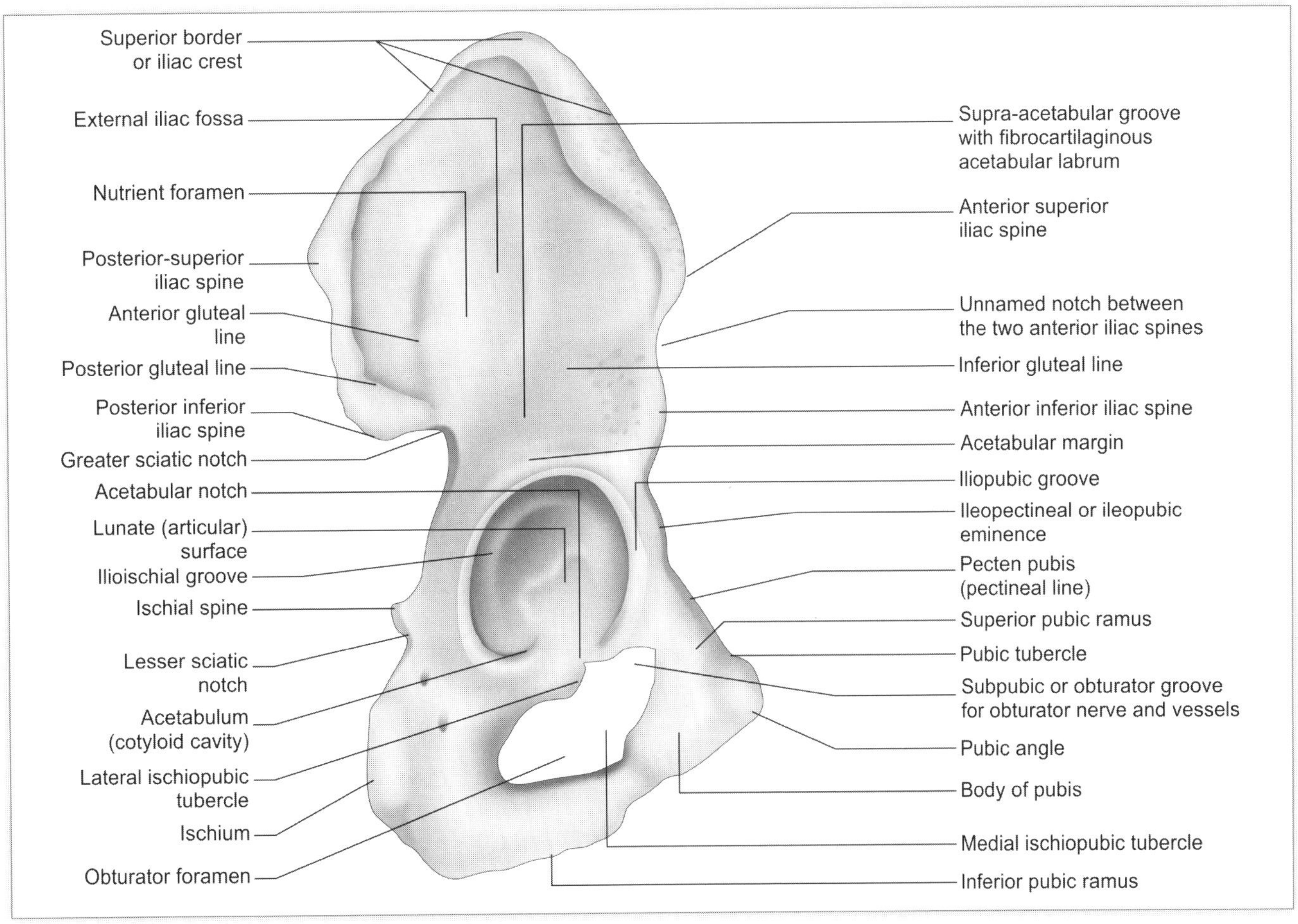

Fig. 2.2: Right pelvic bone (os coxa), external view
(From: Testut *Anatomia Umana*, Utet, Turin; by kind permission)

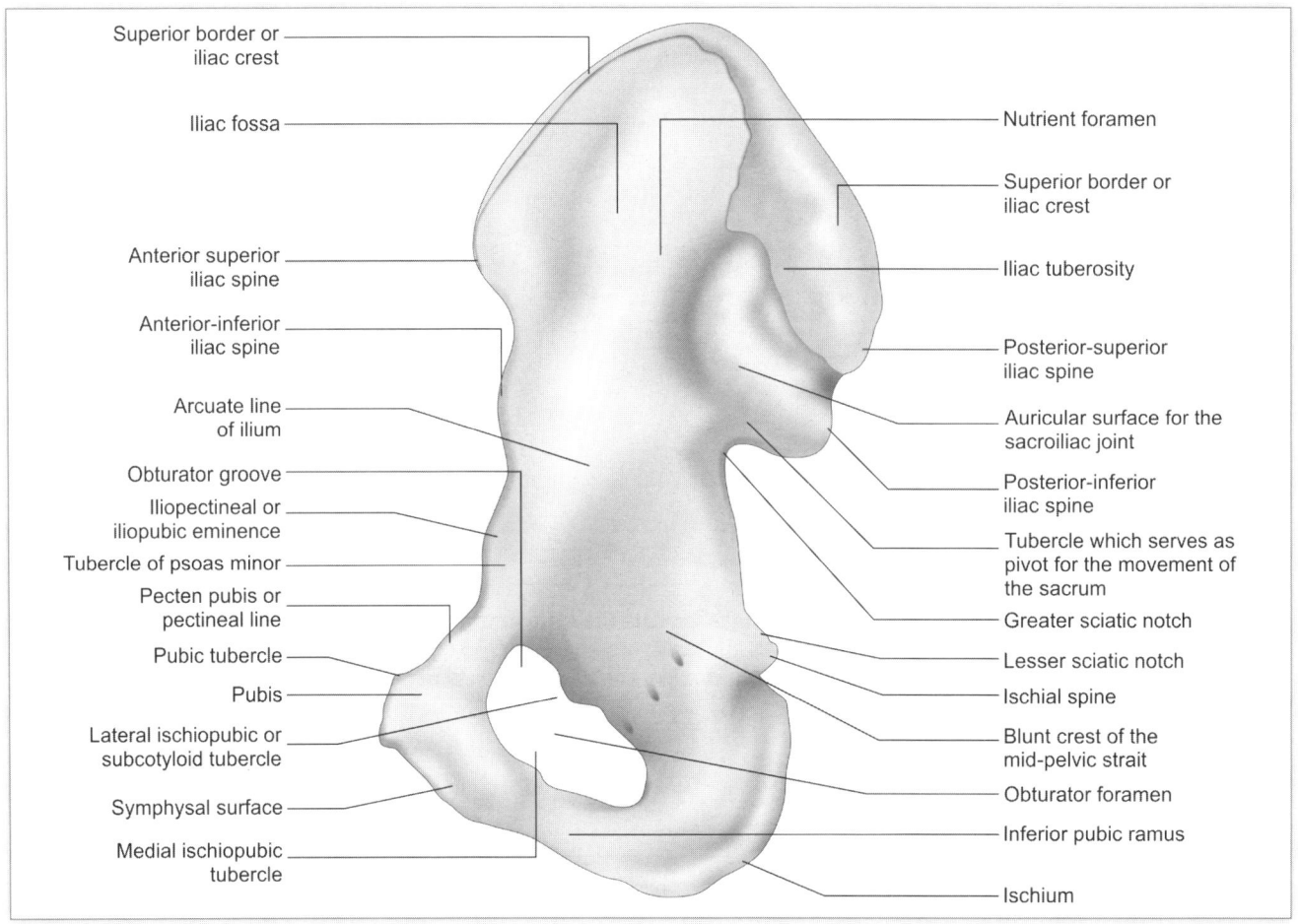

Fig. 2.3: Right pelvic bone, internal view
(From: Testut *Anatomia Umana*, Utet, Turin; by kind permission)

- The *anterior border* (Fig. 2.4) has an initially vertical stretch that abruptly changes direction and takes a horizontal course; the two portions form an angle of 140°. Proceeding caudally, we observe:
  - A rounded eminence: the *anterior superior iliac spine*, from which the inguinal ligament and the *sartorius and tensor fasciae latae muscles* originate
  - An unnamed notch, through which the lateral femoral cutaneous nerve passes
  - A second rounded eminence, the *anterior inferior iliac spine*, from which the straight head of the rectus femoris muscle (branch of quadriceps femoris muscle) originates
  - A grooved notch, 30–35 mm wide, through which the iliopsoas muscle passes
  - Rounded eminence, the *iliopubic eminence* in which the pectineal inguinal ligament inserts
  - A triangular surface, the *pectineal surface*, which corresponds to the pectineus muscle. This is bordered posteriorly by the pectineal line, the continuation of the *linea terminalis*. The *pectineal surface* has on its lateral margin a tubercle, the *tubercle of the psoas minor*, in which this muscle inserts. At its medial end, another tubercle is present, the *pubic tubercle*, in which the distal end of the inguinal ligament inserts. Medially to the pubic tubercle is a small ridged surface, extending for 1–2 cm, where the pyramidalis and the rectus abdominis muscles have their origins.

- The *posterior border* (Fig. 2.2) follows an almost vertical course and, proceeding caudally, it presents:
  - A first rounded eminence, the *posterior superior iliac spine*
  - A small notch
  - A second eminence, the *posterior inferior iliac spine* in which ligaments and muscles insert
  - A large, deep notch, the *greater sciatic notch*
  - A large, sturdy, transversely flattened triangular eminence, the *ischial spine*, on the top of which the

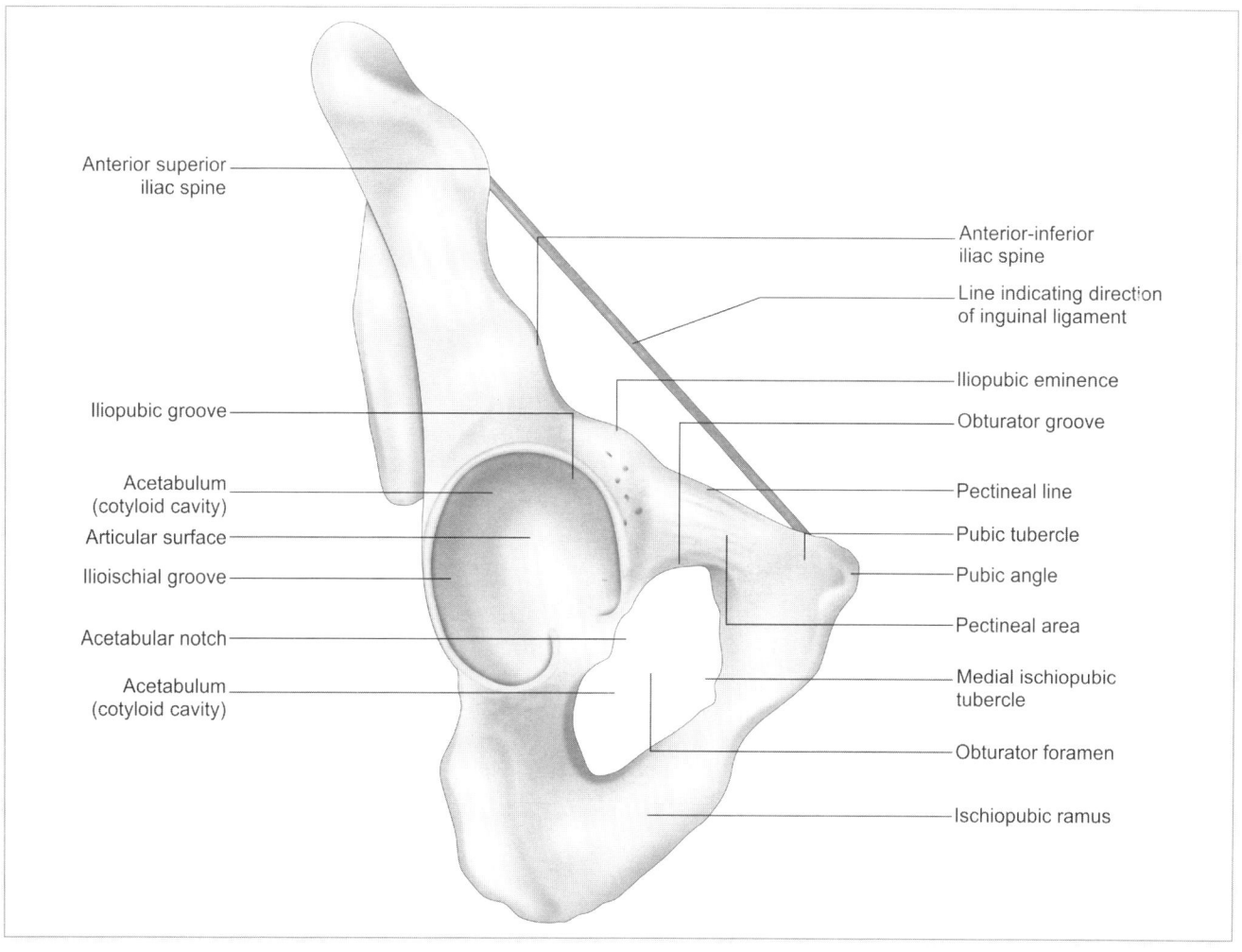

Fig. 2.4: Right pelvic bone, anterior view

sacrospinous ligament inserts. Posteriorly to this runs the *pudendal nerve*, which innervates the inferior third of the vagina and the perineum. On its internal face are the posterior fascicles of the *levator ani muscle*; inferiorly, the ischial spine:
» A small notch, the *lesser sciatic notch*, inferior to this
» A large protuberance, the *body of the ischium*.
- The superior border has the shape of an italic *S*; its anterior and posterior thirds are very thick.

Sacrum

The sacrum, an unpaired, median bone (Fig. 2.5), constitutes the base of the vertebral column and is situated beneath its lumbar section. Wedged between the two pelvic bones, it forms the posterosuperior wall of the pelvic cavity (Fig. 2.6) and articulates with the coccyx. Shaped like a four-cornered pyramid (Fig. 2.5) with its base facing upwards, the sacrum comprises a base, an apex and four surfaces: anterior or pelvic, posterior or dorsal and two lateral parts; the major axis describes a very pronounced curve that is concave on the anterior and convex on the posterior surface (Fig. 2.7).
- *Base* (Fig. 2.8) In standing alignment, this points forwards and upwards and presents:
  - on the midline proceeding anteroposteriorly, an oval or kidney-shaped articular surface with a transverse major axis, (Fig. 2.8, body of vertebra) which is the superior aspect of the body of the first sacral vertebra, Welker's *vertebra fulcralis*; posterior to this, a triangular opening, (Fig. 2.8, superior orifice of the sacral canal), the *superior orifice of the sacral canal*, and finally the orifice of the superior end of the median sacral crest
  - bilaterally to the midline, triangular surfaces with external bases, the *ala of the sacrum* and the two vertical protrusions or *superior articular processes* of the sacrum (Fig. 2.8, superior articular surface), which articulate at an angle of 45° with the *inferior*

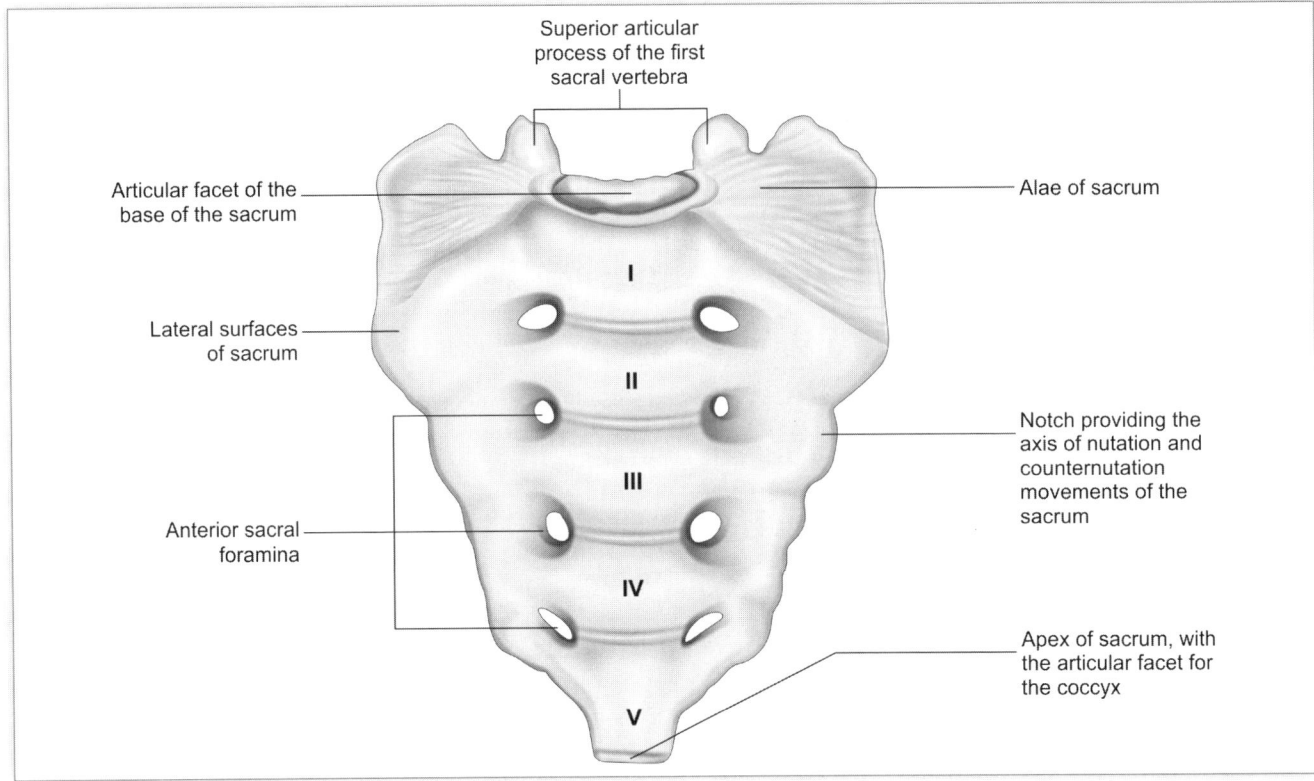

Fig. 2.5: Sacrum, anterior, or ventral or pelvic face. I, II, III, IV, V, five sacral vertebrae. (From Testut, Anatomia Umana, Utet, Turin; by kind permission)

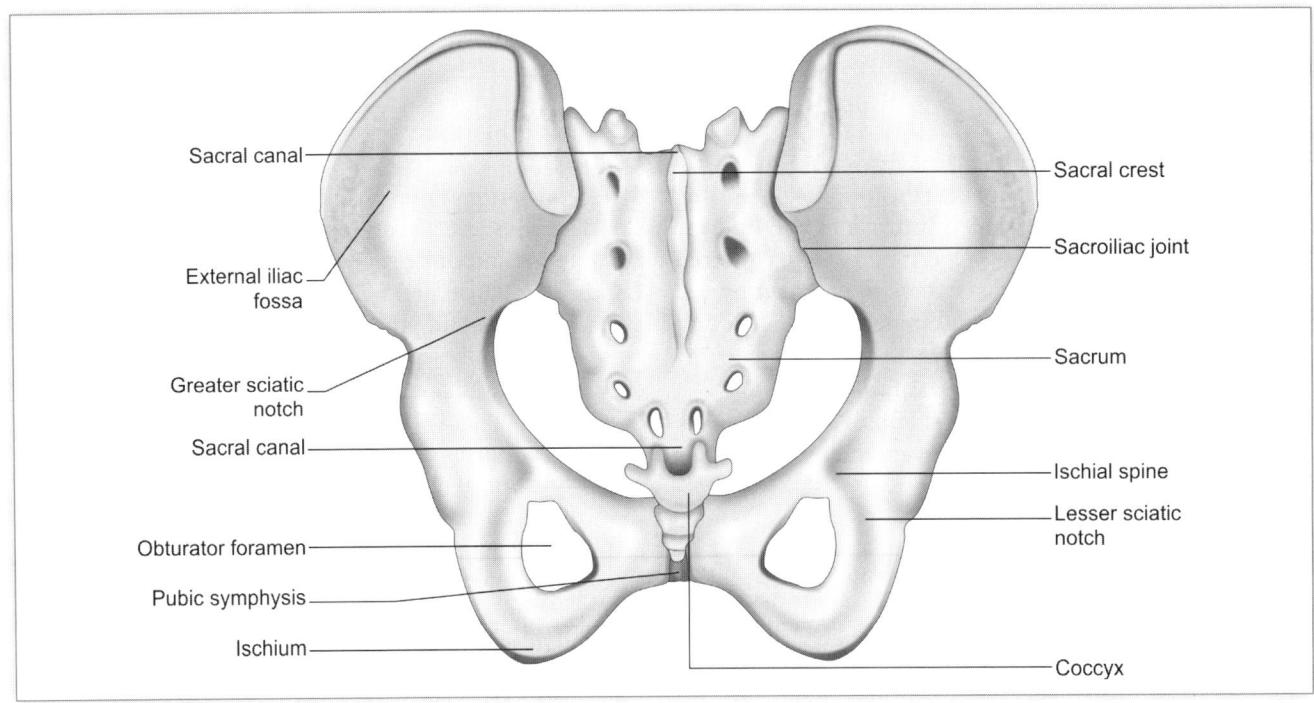

Fig. 2.6: Female pelvis, posterior or dorsal view (From Testut, Anatomia Umana, Utet, Turin; by kind permission)

BIRTH CANAL (PASSAGEWAY)

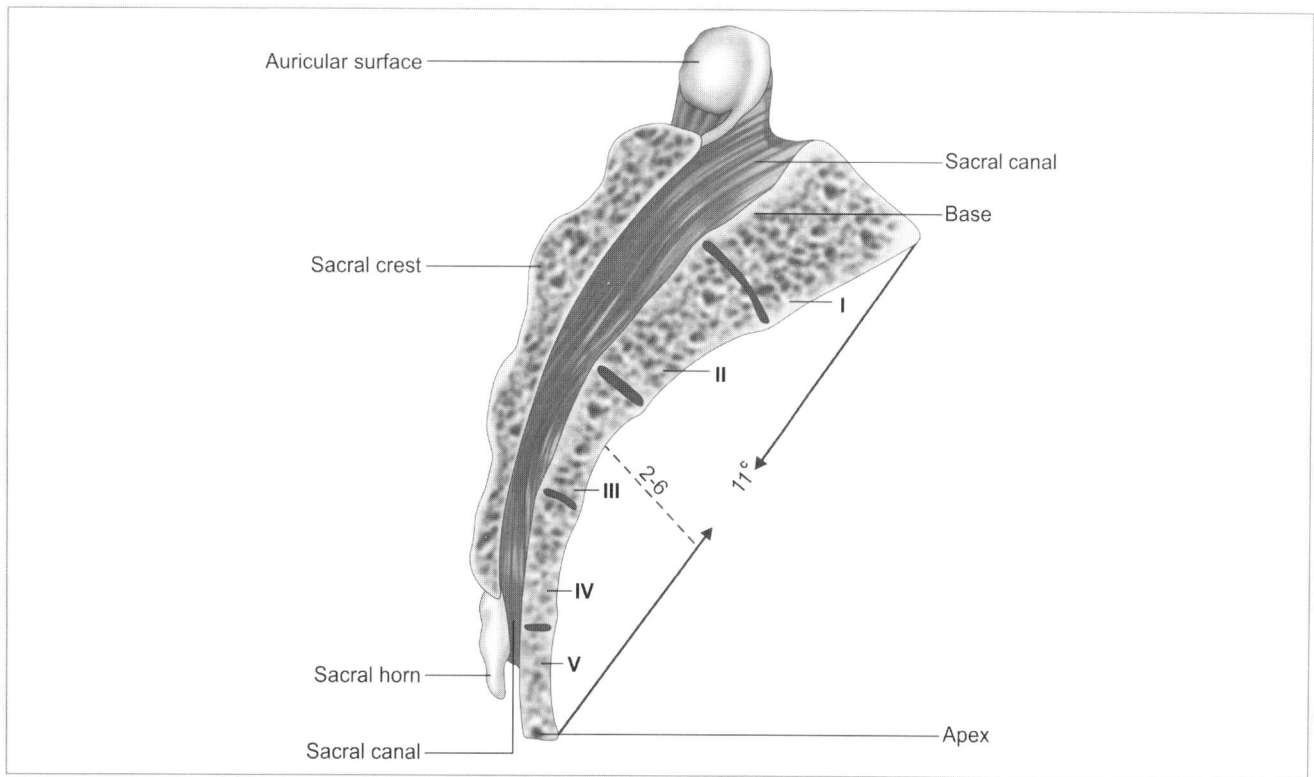

Fig. 2.7: Sagittal section of the sacrum showing the sacral canal. It can be seen how the major axis describes a very pronounced curve with the concavity facing downwards and ventrally. I, II, III, IV, V, the five sacral vertebrae (From Testut, *Anatomia Umana*, Utet, Turin; by kind permission)

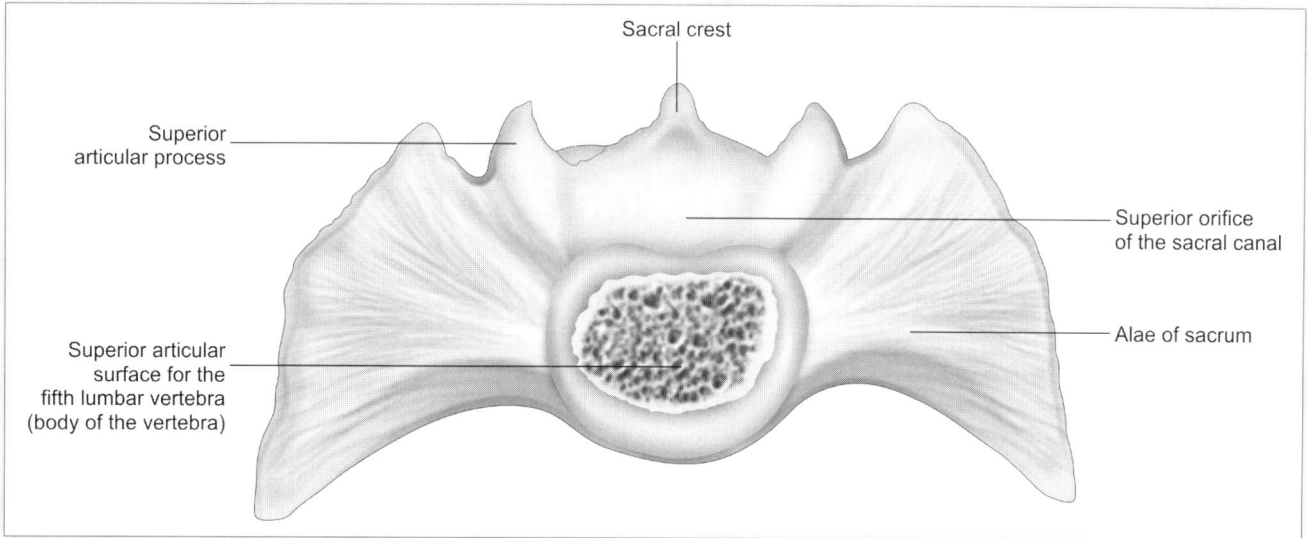

Fig. 2.8: Sacrum, superior view
(From Testut, *Anatomia Umana*, Utet, Turin; by kind permission)

articular process of the last lumbar vertebra. This joint is one of three mechanisms (see the paragraph on the lumbosacral joint) by which anterior slippage of L5 is prevented.

- *The anterior or pelvic surface* (Fig. 2.5): It is both vertically and transversely concave (Fig. 2.7); a bony column situated on the midline, it is constituted by the superimposition of the bodies of the sacral vertebrae (Fig. 2.5). At regular intervals, this is crossed by transverse protrusions, the *transverse ridges*, representing the area of fusion between the vertebrae. Four in number, these *transverse ridges* have an elliptical foramina at each end, the *pelvic or anterior sacral foramina*, through which the anterior rami of the spinal nerves pass
- *The dorsal surface* (Fig. 2.9), sharply convex both vertically and transversely, bears a raised, interrupted, *median sacral crest*, which continues the line of spinous processes of the vertebral column. This crest, corresponding with the third or sometimes the fourth sacral foramina, terminates in two divergent branches that circumscribe the lower portion of the sacral canal
- *The margins of the sacrum* (Fig. 2.10) could, at the cranial end, be better described as surfaces which, starting broad, narrow into simple edges. Their superior part has a wide articular surface, the *auricular surface of the sacro-iliac joint* (SIJ), a crescent-shaped concavity that articulates with a similar convex structure on the pelvic bone (Fig. 2.3, articular surface for the sacroiliac joint). These depressions and reliefs interlock to limit joint movement. Anteroposteriorly, the auricular surface is often bordered by a more or less pronounced groove, the *preauricular groove of the sacrum*, the insertion for the *anterior sacroiliac ligament*
- *Apex:* This is the inferior aspect of the fifth sacral vertebral body, with an oval surface with a long transverse diameter. It articulates with the coccyx and opens posteriorly to form the *sacral hiatus* (Fig. 2.9), which is the distal end of the sacral canal. This orifice, shaped like an inverted V, is bordered laterally by the sacral horns, which articulate with those of the coccyx
- *Sacral canal* (Fig. 2.7): The continuation of the vertebral canal of the lumbar spine, this runs through the entire length of the sacrum. Through the intervertebral foramina it communicates on each side with the four pairs of anterior and posterior sacral foramina. It contains the terminal dead-end of the spinal dura mater and the nerves which form the cauda equina.

These nerves enter the above-mentioned intervertebral foramina and divide into anterior and posterior branches, leading to the corresponding sacral foramina.

Coccyx (Fig. 2.1)

This is an unpaired, median bone situated inferior to the sacrum, of which it is a continuation; it consists of 4–5 atrophied vertebrae that are fused with each other.

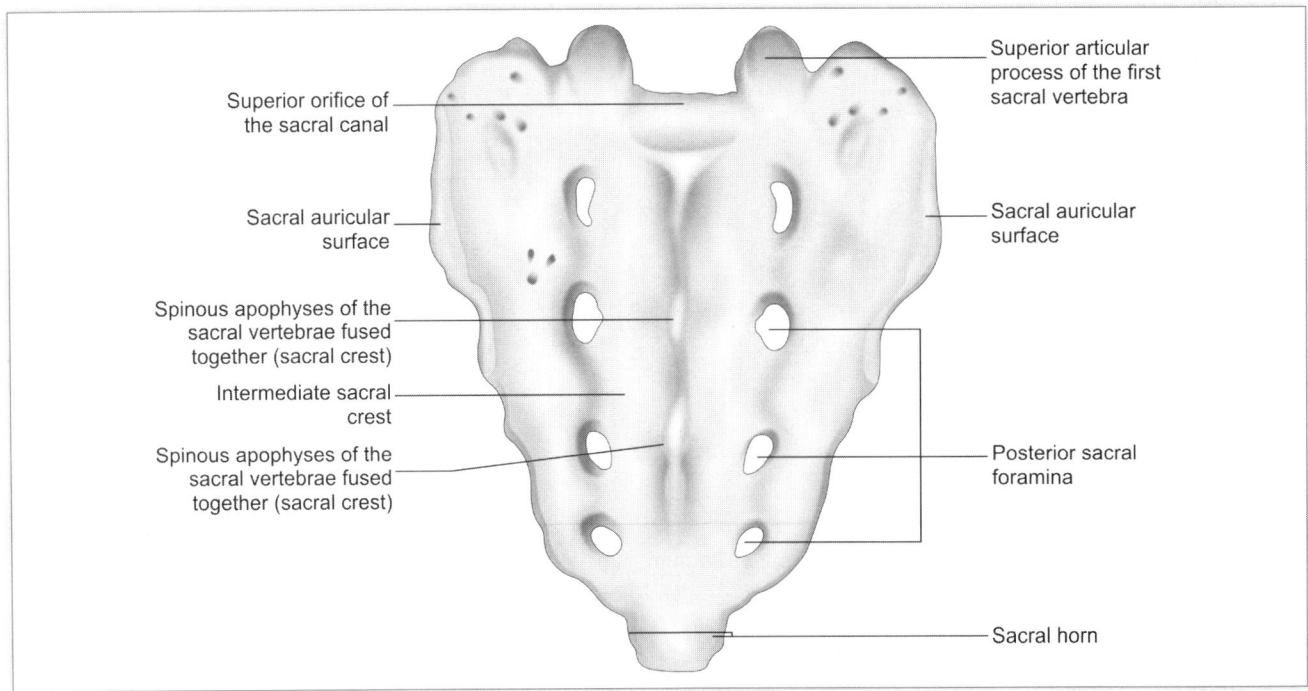

Fig. 2.9: Sacrum, posterior or dorsal aspect
(From Testut *Anatomia Umana*, Utet, Turin; by kind permission)

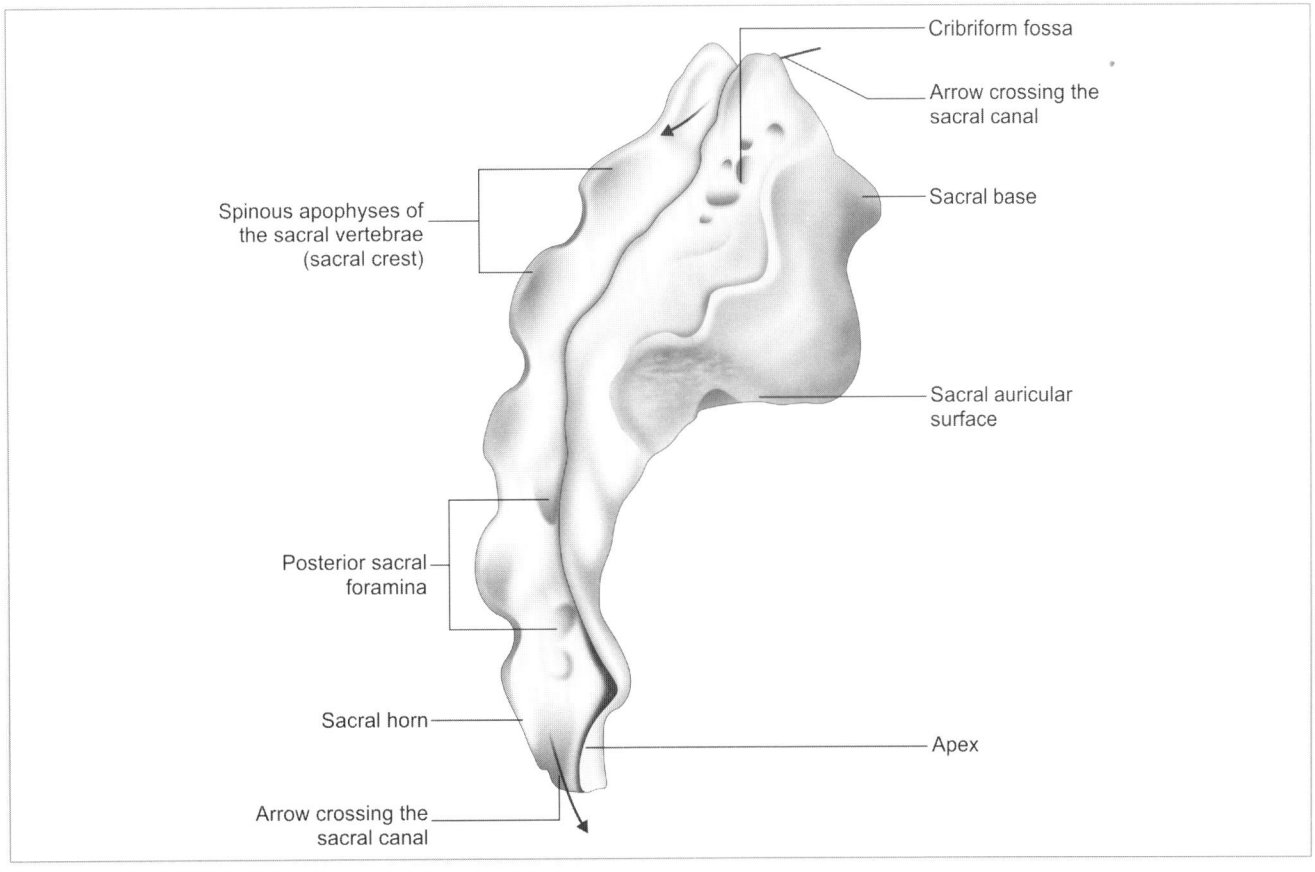

Fig. 2.10: Sacrum, left lateral aspect
(From Testut, *Anatomia Umana*, Utet, Turin; by kind permission)

Pelvic Joints

The pelvic girdle—the junction of the vertebral column and the femoral heads—is the structure within which pressure exerted by the trunk and counter-pressures coming up from the ground are manifested. The bones forming it respond to this dual stress by means of their highly effective interconnections, ensured by three joints: the pubic symphysis anteriorly and the two sacro-iliac joints posteriorly.

Pubic Symphysis (Fig. 2.11)

This is an amphiarthrosis (slightly mobile joint) which fuses the two pubic bones on the midline; its symphyseal surfaces are elliptical, 3–4 cm long and with a maximum width of 1–1.5 cm; the long axis, oblique posteriorly and downwards, has an inclination of about 30° to the horizontal plane.

The ligaments associated with the symphysis are divided into two groups:
- *Rigid structures*: The interpubic disc is a cone-shaped layer of fibrocartilage which, laterally, adheres intimately to the layer of hyaline cartilage covering the symphyseal surfaces and, at its margins, with the ligaments. This is the anatomical formation that is dissected during *symphysiotomy*
- *Elastic structures*: A fibrous periarticular sleeve, of which we can distinguish four ligaments:
  - *The anterior pubic ligament*, 5 mm thick, is closely connected with the fascial coverings of the muscles (pyramidalis, rectus abdominis, obliquus externus) arising from the conjoined rami of the pubis
  - *Posterior pubic ligament*, stretched between the two pubic bones; thin, membranous, it consists of the periosteum of the pelvis
  - *Superior pubic ligament:* This extends laterally along the crest of the pubis on each side to the pubic tubercle; it is a very thick fibrous mesh which, with the upper part of the anterior pubic ligament, limits the widening of the pubis and has, therefore, been defined as the "*frenum anatomicum chirurgicum superior*"!
  - *Inferior pubic or arcuate ligament:* This is a thick, crescent-shaped band of closely connected fibres that

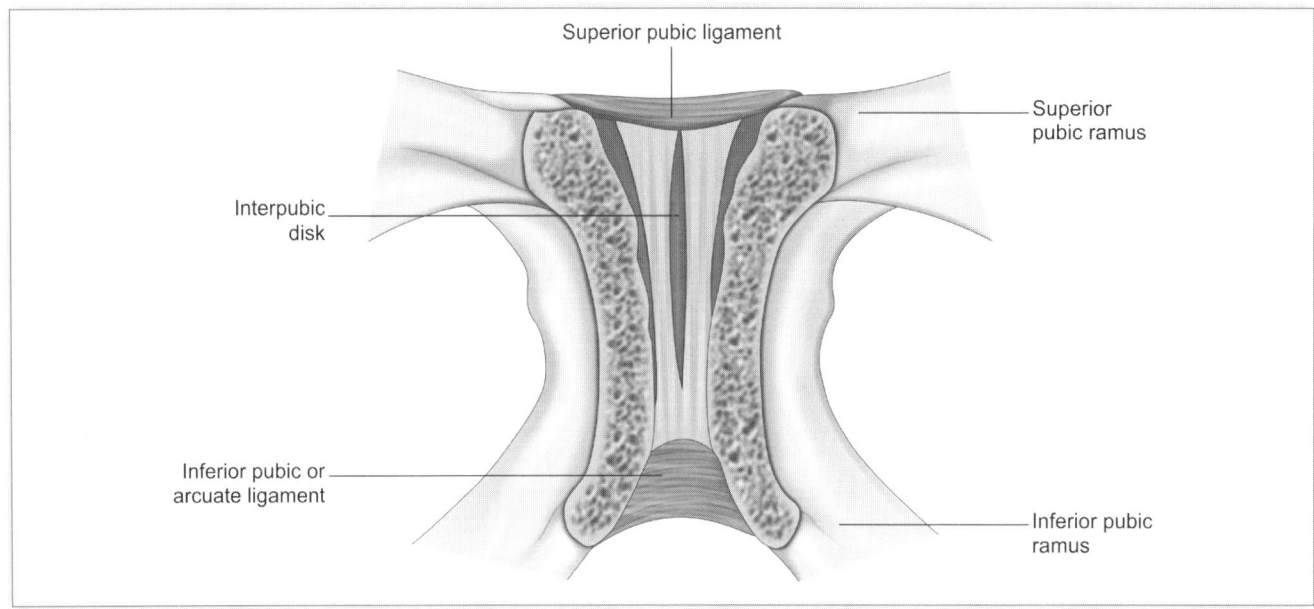

Fig. 2.11: Pubic symphysis, anterior view
(From P Kamina *Anatomia ginecologica ed ostetrica*, DEMI, Rome)

fills the angle between the pubic rami, it has a height of 10 mm on the midline, a border adhering to the uppermost portion of the pubic arch and a free, sharp, very tough edge, against which the foetal head fixes and rotates in the course of disengagement.

Sacroiliac Joint

The articular surfaces (Fig. 2.12) are called *auriculae* because of their crescent-like shape; each *auricula* has an inferior short branch, which is almost horizontal, and a superior, longer, almost vertical, branch. The articular surface of the sacrum corresponds to the first two sacral vertebrae and to the upper part of the third; overall, the joint is concave. The joint surface with the pelvic bone is situated on the internal face of the iliac ala, superior to the greater sciatic notch, and has the form of a filled-in letter L. These reliefs and depressions interlock with each other to limit the joint's movements while lending strength for its task of transmitting the weight of the body from the spinal column to the lower limb. A joint capsule attaches to the margins of the articular surfaces; the joint ligaments are distinguished between proximal and distal.

- **Core ligaments**: These are very strong and include: the anterior sacroiliac (Fig. 2.13) and *posterior long* and *short sacroiliac ligaments* (2.14); these cross the SIJ for its entire height from the top of the sacrum to the iliac ala.
  - The *anterior sacroiliac ligament* unites the base and lateral parts of the sacrum to the ilium and allows the pelvic bone to hinge against the sacrum without tearing. Following a symphysiotomy, this will allow the pubic symphysis to open by up to 6 cm (Farabeuf, 1894)
  - The *posterior sacroiliac ligament* (Fig. 2.14) consists essentially of two sets of fibres, deep and superficial, forming the *short and long posterior sacroiliac ligaments* respectively. The *short posterior sacroiliac ligament* passes from the iliac tuberosity to the back of the lateral portion of the sacrum and to the SIJ; the *long posterior sacroiliac ligament* passes inferiorly from the posterior superior iliac spine to the second, third and fourth articular tubercles of the sacrum (lateral sacral crest). The margins (superior and inferior) of both ligaments control and limit the *nutation* and *counternutation movements* of the sacrum
- *Distant ligaments:* These are the *large* and the *small sacro ischial ligaments* (Figs 2.13 and 2.14).
  - The fan-shaped *sacral tuberous ligament* is attached superiorly to the crest of the Ilium and posterior iliac spines and to the posterior aspect of the lower three sacral vertebrae. From this long concave surface fibers converge externally, posteriorly and inferiorly to form a narrow but very strong webbing. From here they expand fanwise once more to form an external bundle, one part of which inserts in the internal edge of the ischial tuberosity and another part internally and medially on of the internal aspect of the ischiopubic branch and on the aponeurosis of the obturator internus muscle

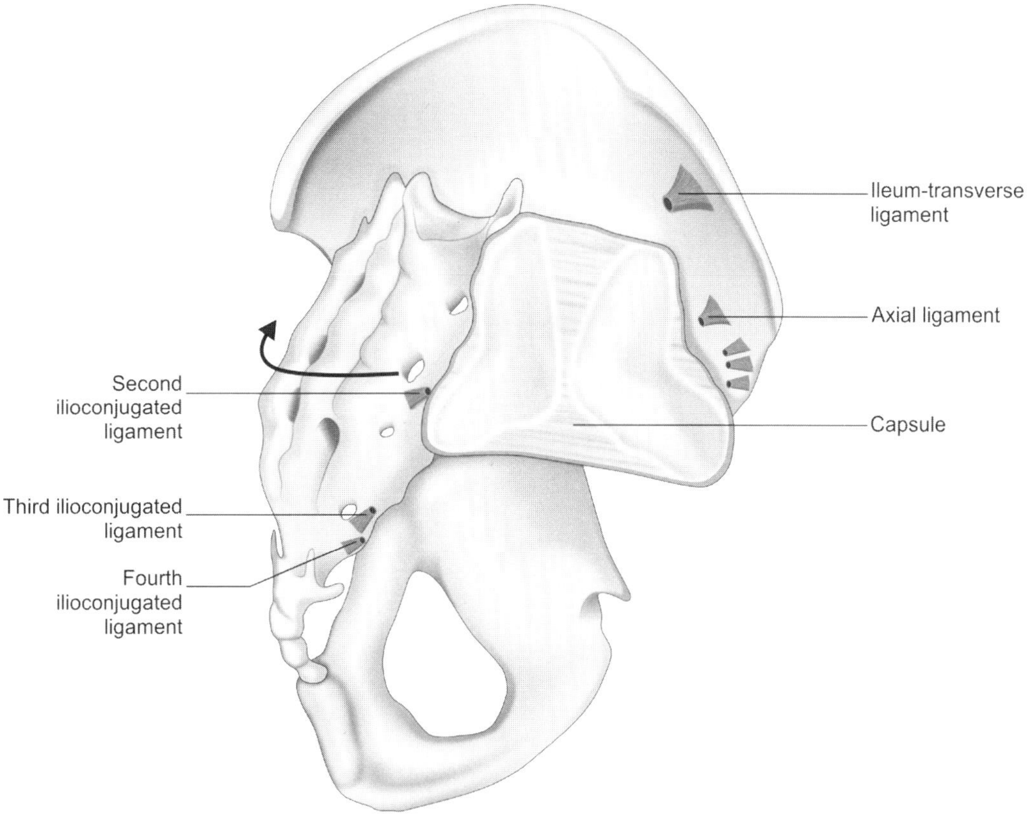

BIRTH CANAL (PASSAGEWAY)

Fig. 2.12: Right sacroiliac joint, (cut): Only the joint surface of the iliac bone has been left; the remaining portion has been removed (after Grégoire and Oberlin) (From P. Kamina, *Anatomia ginecologica ed ostetrica* DEMI, Rome)

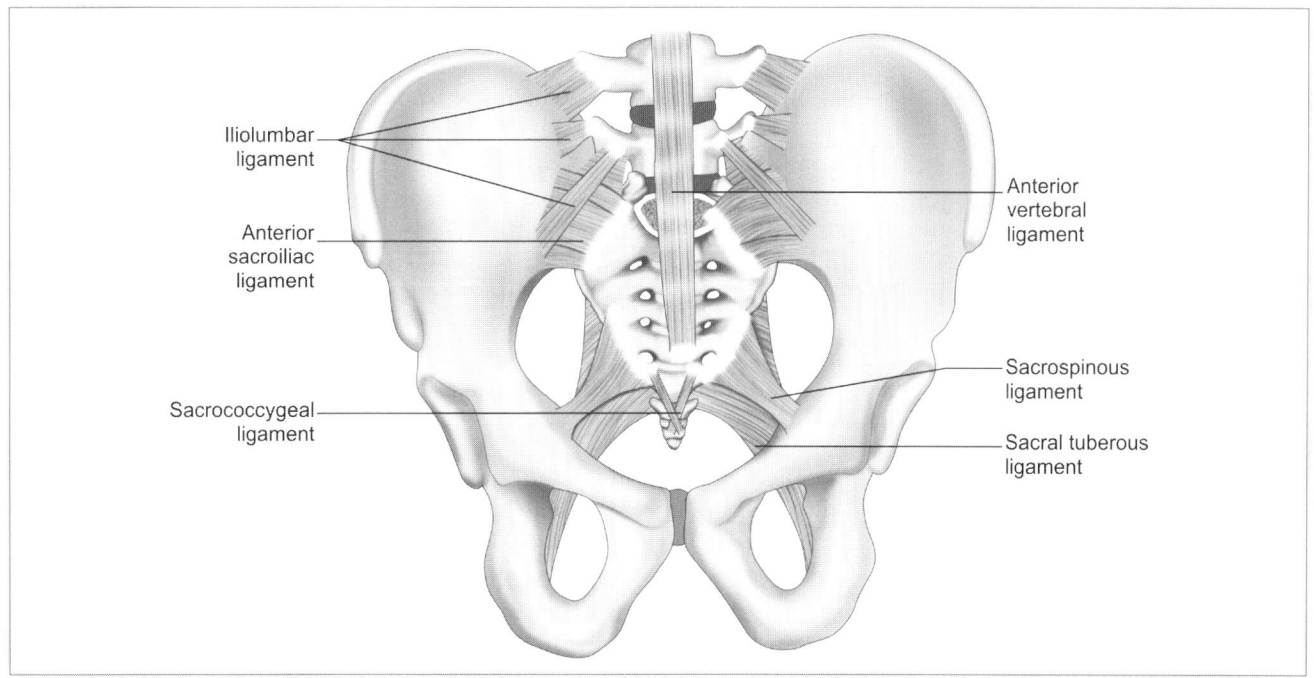

Fig. 2.13: Rigth sacroiliac joint

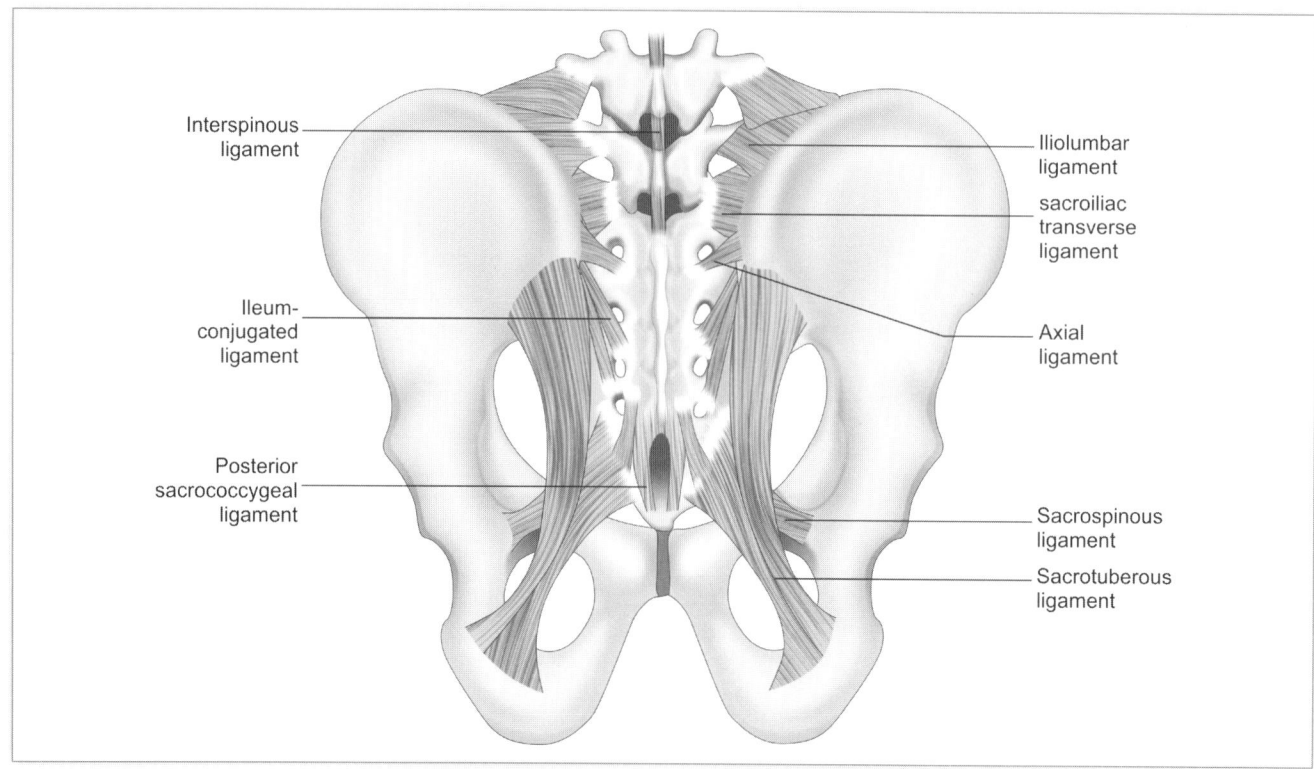

Fig. 2.14: Sacroiliac joint, posterior view
(From P Kamina *Gynecological and Obstetric Anatomy* DEMI, Rome)

- The *sacrospinous ligament* is triangular and thin, extending from the lateral border of the sacrum and coccyx to the spine of the ischium. It passes medially to the sacrotuberous ligament the iliopubic ligament.

During pregnancy the pelvic capacity is increased by:
- The *eccentric action* exerted on the pelvic walls by the uterine mass
- The *increased elasticity* of the pelvic ligaments, leading to greater mobility of the sacroiliac joint. This allows more expansive counternutation and nutation movements with a corresponding increase in the anteroposterior diameters of the superior and inferior pelvic straits (inlet and outlet).

It is worth noting that in Latin, *nutare* means to sway and so *nutation* and *counternutation* refer to the nodding movements made by the sacrum as it rocks on the axis of the sacroiliac joint.

Counternutation refers to the backward nodding of the base of the sacrum; this movement occurs in the upright position or in a person lying with their thighs in hyperextension, in what is known as Walcher's position.

The backward swaying of the base of the sacrum increases the anteroposterior diameter of the pelvic inlet, thereby promoting engagement. Forward displacement of the apex of the sacrum causes a reduction in the anteroposterior diameter of the pelvic outlet; the simultaneous wedge-like descent of the sacrum between the two pelvic bones drives them apart, which tends to bring the two ischial tuberosities closer together.

Nutation refers to a forward rocking (within the pelvis) of the base of the sacrum. This movement takes place during the passage from the horizontal to the vertical position, or in the *Detraine* and *Descombs position*, which consists in flexing and abducting the thighs strongly. The forward rocking of the base of the sacrum causes an increase in the anteroposterior diameter of the pelvic outlet and, at the same time draws the pelvic bones closer together, encouraging the ischial tuberosities to move apart. Additively, these two actions bring about an increase of the anteroposterior and transverse (bituberous) diameters of the outlet, facilitating disengagement of the presenting part.

Lumbosacral Joint (Fig. 2.15)

This is an amphiarthrosis (slightly mobile joint); the articular surfaces have a roughly elliptical shape with a transverse major axis (Fig. 2.8). The articular surface of the sacrum (Fig. 2.15) has a 45° anterior tilt; L5 has a tilt of 20°. Anterior slippage of L5 is prevented by the following mechanisms:

1. The protuberance of the sacral joint.
2. The interposition between L5 and S1 of the wedgeshaped lumbosacral disc, whose thickness is 15-20 mm anteriorly and 5 mm posteriorly (Fig. 2.15).
3. The lumbosacral diarthroses: The sacral superior articular process and the lumbar inferior articular process meet on a plane inclined at 45° to the mid-sagittal plane (Figs. 2.15 and 2.16).

True Pelvis

The bony pelvis has an *external or exopelvic surface* and an *internal or endopelvic one*; the latter (Fig. 2.1) divides into an upper portion, the *greater or false pelvis*, of no obstetric relevance, and a lower portion, the *lesser or true pelvis*, of fundamental obstetric relevance. The true pelvis is bounded anteriorly and caudally by the pubic symphysis and the superior rami of the pubis; superiorly and dorsally it is bordered by the sacrum and coccyx, and laterally by a broad, smooth, quadrangular area of bone, corresponding to the inner surfaces of the body and superior ramus of the ischium and that part of the ilium lying below the arcuate line. The relevant obstetrical structures of the true pelvis are the inlet, the midpelvis and the outlet.

Pelvic Inlet (Superior Pelvic Strait)

The superior pelvic strait, inlet, or brim is usually defined as "the plane passing through the promontory, the anterior margin of the sacral alae, the arcuate line of the ileum (linea terminalis), the iliopectineal eminence and the pubis". The promontory (Fig. 2.15), is generally referred to as "the angle formed by the fifth lumbar vertebra with the first sacral vertebra"; this definition is not always applicable, as sacralisation of the lumbar vertebrae (assimilation), and lumbarisation of the sacral vertebrae can occur; we will return later to the clinical significance of these phenomena. We therefore prefer to define the promontory as the *lumbosacral hinge*.

Under normal conditions, the above-listed structures—promontory, anterior margin of the sacral alae, the arcuate line of the ileum (linea terminalis) and pubis—lie at different levels: the promontory and anterior margin of the pubic symphysis is normally superior and the linea terminalis and the pubis inferior. For this reason the superior pelvic strait has a height of 3-4 mm, which can vary with lumbarisation or sacralisation. We therefore believe it more correct to define the inlet as "the bony ring, 3-4 mm thick, which connects the false to the true pelvis, having as its superior border the plane passing through the promontory, understood as the lumbosacral hinge, and as inferior border the plane passing through the linea terminalis and the pubis". The superior pelvic strait (Fig. 2.1) presents the following features:

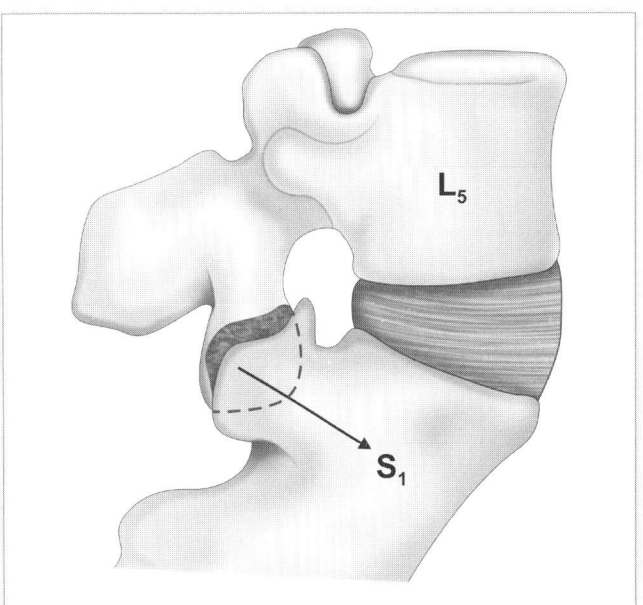

Fig. 2.15: Sacral promontory

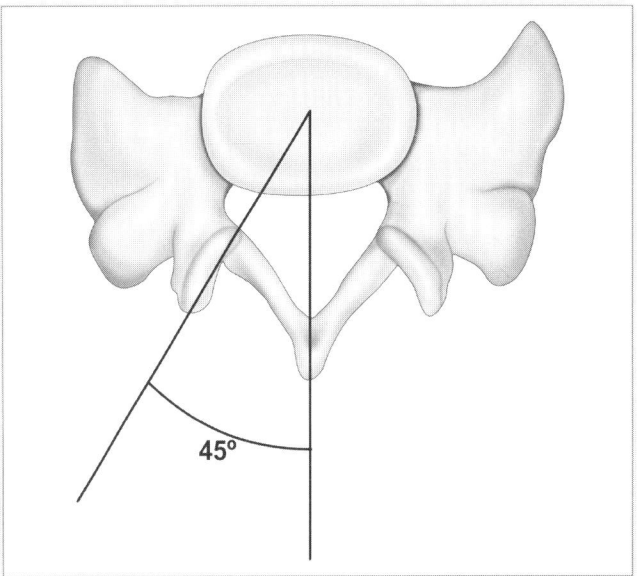

Fig. 2.16: Direction of the upper articular process which prevents the anterior slippage of L5 (from P. Kamina "Gynecological and Obstetric Anatomy" DEMI Turin)

Diameters

- *Anteroposterior diameters*: (Fig. 2.17) are the diameters between the pubis and promontory. As the posterior aspect of the pubic symphysis is convex, we distinguish between:
  - *Anteroposterior anatomic diameter* (Fig. 2.17, a), extending between the superior margin of the pubic

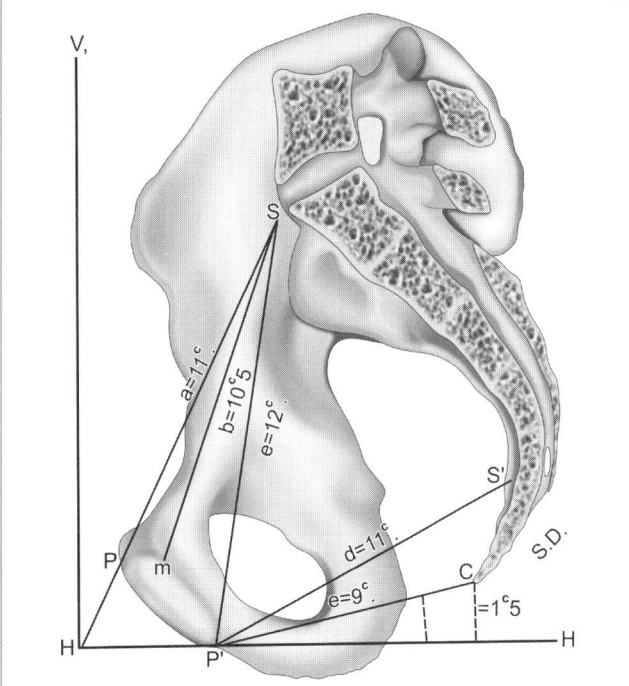

Fig. 2.17: Anteroposterior diameters of the inlet and outlet; proceeding caudally. The plane passing through the anatomical anteroposterior diameter of the pelvic inlet forms an angle of 60° with the horizon. (From Testut *Human Anatomy*, Utet, Turin; by kind permission)

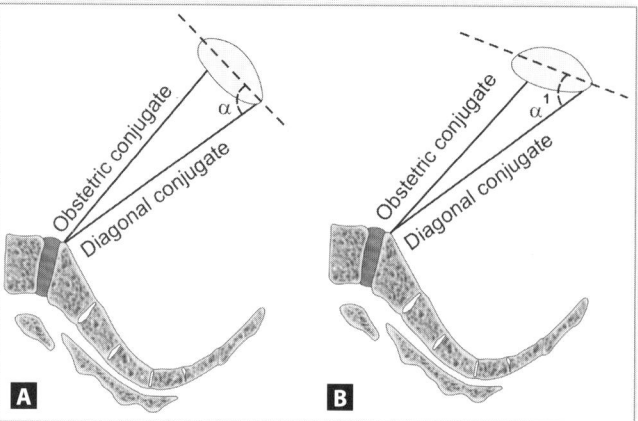

Fig. 2.18A and B: Diagrams illustrating how the angle formed between the major axis of the pubic symphysis and the diagonal conjugate (Jacobs' angle) is responsible for variations in length of the obstetric conjugate. In B, inclination of the pubic symphysis is very marked and results in a reduction of angle $\alpha 1$ and of the obstetric conjugate

symphysis and the promontory. Measuring 11 cm, it is of no obstetric interest
- *Anteroposterior obstetric diameter* or *obstetric conjugate* (Fig. 2.17, b), extending between the apex of the posterior convexity of the pubic symphysis and the promontory; typically measures 10.5 cm
- *Diagonal conjugate* (Fig. 2.17, c) this is the distance between the lower margin of the pubic symphysis and the promontory. It is believed that by subtracting 1.5-2 cm from the value of the diagonal conjugate, one obtains the value of the obstetric conjugate (see Chapter 6).

The angle formed by the major axis of the pubic symphysis with the diagonal conjugate is referred to as Jacobs' obstetric angle; its degree of obtuseness affects the value of the true conjugate (Fig. 2.18).

Oblique diameters: each oblique diameter extends from one iliopectineal eminence to the sacroiliac synchondrosis on the opposite side of the pelvis (Figs 2.1 and 2.19). They measure 12-12.5 cm. When the foetus is in cephalic presentation, engagement takes place along one of these diameters; the forehead and occiput (occipitofrontal diameter) are oriented along one of the oblique diameters and the parietal eminence (biparietal diameter) along the other one.

Transverse Diameters (Figs 2.19 and 2.20)

- These are projected at right angles to the *conjugate vera*. Two diameters are described: the *widest transverse diameter*, perpendicular to the anteroposterior diameter, which usually intersects it at a point about 5 cm anterior to the promontory. This represents the greatest distance between the linea terminalis on each side. It is too close to the promontory to be used by the foetal head for engagement

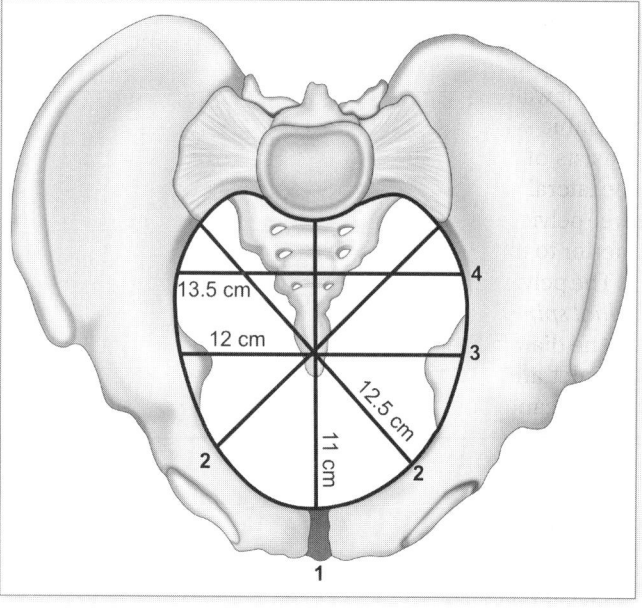

Fig. 2.19: Diameters of the pelvic inlet (superior pelvic strait): (1) Anteroposterior diameter; (2) Oblique diameters; (3) Transverse diameter; (4) Widest transverse diameter

BIRTH CANAL (PASSAGEWAY)

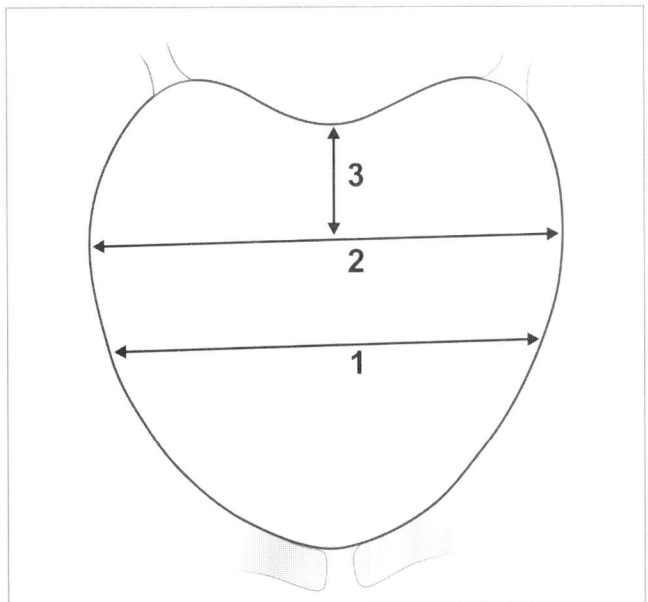

Fig. 2.20: Transverse diameters of the inlet (superior pelvic strait): (1) Available transverse diameter (used for the engagement of the presenting part); (2) Widest transverse diameter; (3) Thoms' posterior sagittal diameter

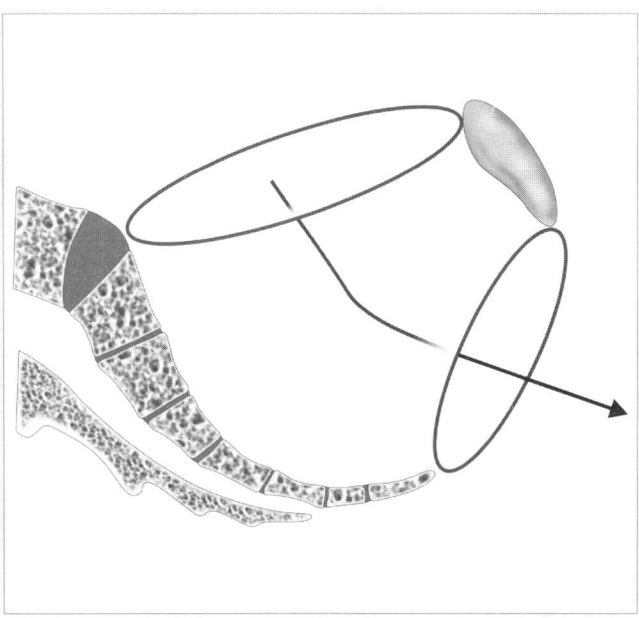

Fig. 2.21: Diagram of birth canal or pelvic axis

- *Median transverse or available diameter*: This is perpendicular to the anteroposterior diameter, intersecting it at its midpoint (Figs 2.19 and 2.20). Its average length is 12 cm. In 40% of cases (gynecoid pelvis) this is the diameter used by the foetal head for engagement.

Pelvic Cavity

Irregularly cylindrical in shape, the cavity begins to curve anteriorly in the region of the pelvic outlet (Fig. 2.21). The anterior wall, 4.5–5 cm long, consists of the posterior face of the pubic symphysis. The posterior wall, 12–12.5 cm long, consists of the pelvic face of the sacrum and the coccyx. The lateral walls correspond to the internal surfaces of the three pelvic bones (ilium, ischium, and pubis) in the section inferior to the linea terminalis.

The pelvic canal also has two pelvic bone eminences, the *ischial spines*, which mark the midpelvis.

The diameter of the pelvic canal narrows from 12 cm at the inlet and to 9–10 cm at midpelvis. An imaginary line passing caudally through the centre of the two pelvic straits and equidistant from the two lateral walls, passing through the pelvic cavity superoinferiorly, is known as the *birth canal* or *obstetric pelvic axis*.

There is disagreement among authors about the precise course of this line. Pajot leads the faction who believe that it is a curved line (Fig. 2.21). Others, led by Fabbri (1851), believe it to comprise two straight lines: the first, the *descending axis*, extends from the centre of the superior strait to the apex of the coccyx; the second, the *outlet axis*, is perpendicular to the first at the level of the 4th–5th sacral vertebrae, reaching the centre of the dilated vulva.

Pelvic Outlet (Inferior Pelvic Strait)

The pelvic outlet does not form one mathematical plane (Fig. 2.22), but consists of two triangular planes having a common base, formed by the intertuberous diameter. We distinguish an anterior (urogenital) triangle and a posterior (anal) triangle. The anterior plane (formed by the area below the pubic arch) has as its base the intertuberous diameter, the inferior pubic rami as its sides and the lower margin of the pubic symphysis as its apex.

The posterior and anterior triangles share the intertuberous diameter as their base. The sides of the posterior triangle are the sacrotuberous ligaments and its apex is the tip of the sacrum, not of the coccyx. The merger of the two triangles (anterior and posterior) forms, in the dry pelvis, a rhombus (lozenge) shape (Fig. 2.22); in the living, due to the presence of the sacro-iliac ligaments and levator ani muscles (Fig. 2.23), it takes on the shape of an anteroposterior ellipse; *disengagement*, therefore, must adapt to the anteroposterior diameter.

The pelvic outlet (Fig. 2.24) features:
- *Subpubic angle*, the three basic types are described in different ways by various authors:
  – *Android* and *anthropoid* pelvis; acute angle, pointed arch (height greater than radius), Gothic arch
  – *Gynecoid* pelvis: right angled, round arch (height equal to the radius), Roman arch

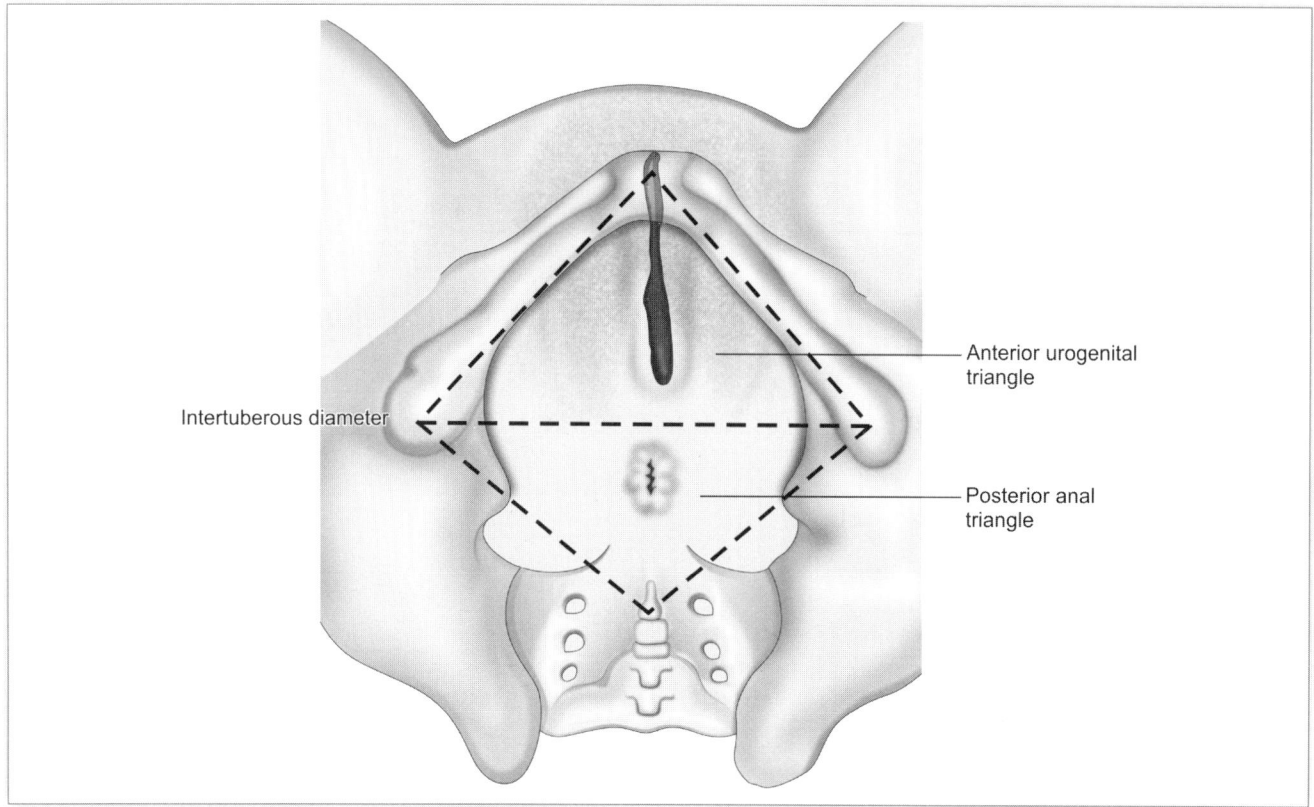

Fig. 2.22: Pelvic outlet (inferior pelvic strait): The outlet is divided into two triangles across the intertuberous diameter: an anterior or urogenital triangle and the posterior or anal triangle

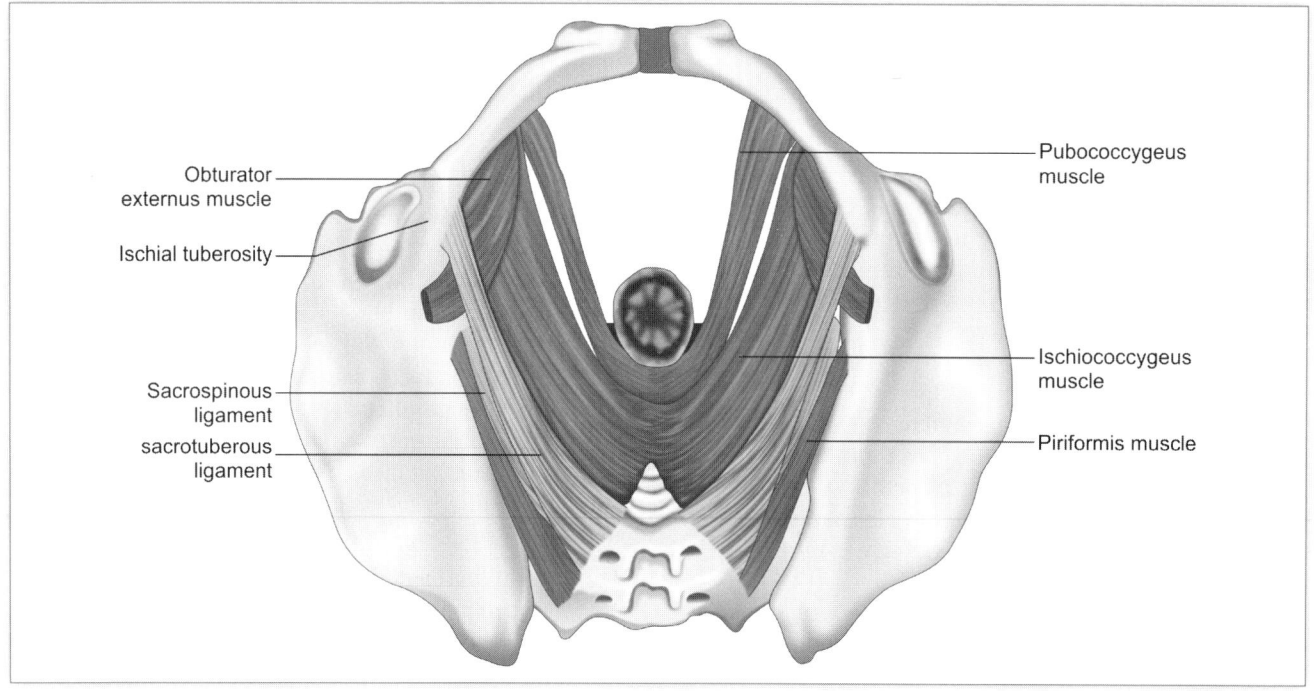

Fig. 2.23: Pelvic floor, viewed from below

- *Platypelloid* pelvis: obtuse angle, segmental arch (height lower than the radius), Norman arch, elliptical arch.
- The *anteroposterior or pubo-sacral diameter*, extends from the lower margin of the pubic symphysis to the tip of the sacrum (11.5 cm)
- The *anteroposterior or pubococcygeal diameter* has no clinical relevance; the anteroposterior diameter of the outlet should not be confused with the pubococcygeal diameter; the so-called *retropulsion of the coccyx* has no clinical significance, especially in the case of a hooked sacrum
- The *oblique diameter* is the distance between the midpoint of the inferior pubic ramus on one side, to the midpoint of the sacroiliac ligament of the opposite side; it measures 12 cm
- The *transverse or intertuberous diameter* is the distance between the internal edges of the two ischial tuberosities; it generally measures 11 cm.

We believe that other diameters, not taken into account in classic clinical obstetrics, are also of relevance: their clinical significance will be demonstrated in Chapter 6. These diameters are:
- The *anterior sagittal diameter* or McDermott conjugate (Fig. 2.24, a) is the height of the anterior triangle and generally measures 7.5 cm
- The *posterior sagittal diameter* (Fig. 2.24, b) is the height of the posterior triangle, measuring 6 cm

The *sacrococcygeal joint* can be located by introducing the index into the rectum up to the dorsal face of the coccyx, while the ventral face is grasped by the thumb inserted through the vagina; a manoeuvre of flex-extension will allow the joint to be identified.

Obstetric Pelvis

Of relevance for the purposes of engagement and progression of the presenting part are:
- Morphology and size of pelvis
- Length of pelvis
- Inclination of pelvis.

Morphology and Size of the Pelvis

The height of an adult woman and the morphology of her pelvis result from the following influences:
- Genetic
- Nutritional: Changes in the metabolism of calcium and phosphorus leading to excessive flattening of the pelvis are typical of the rachitic pelvis
- Action on the plastic bone structure of forces (Fig. 2.25) originating from: *above*, exerted by the head and trunk, which, via the spinal column, act on the last lumbar vertebra and on the base of the sacrum, pushing them ventrally and giving rise to the promontory (Fig. 2.15); this is shown by the absence of a sacral promontory in the foetal pelvis (Fig. 2.26).

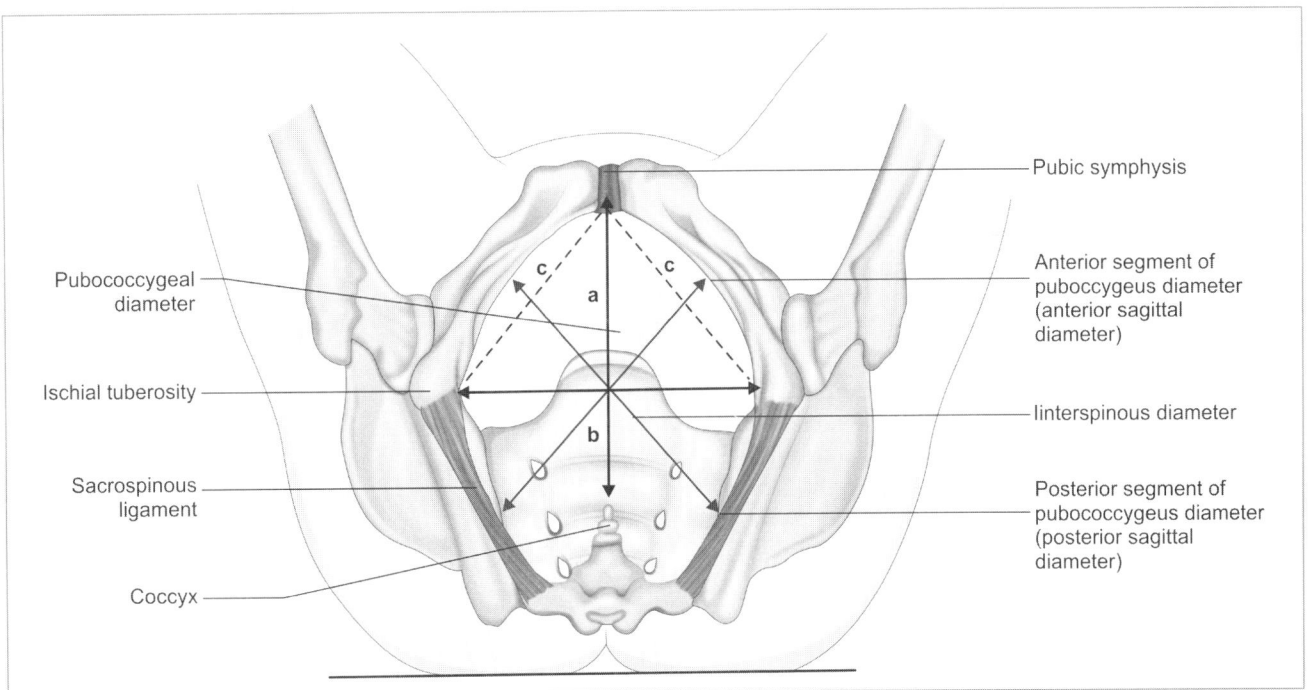

Fig. 2.24: Pelvic outlet (inferior pelvic strait). (a) Anterior segment of puboccygeus diameter (anterior sagittal diameter); (b) Posterior segment of pubococcygeus diameter (posterior sagittal diameter); (c) Cathetus of the anterior triangle, whose base is the intertuberous diameter (from P Kamina *Gynecological and Obstetric Anatomy* DEMI, Rome)

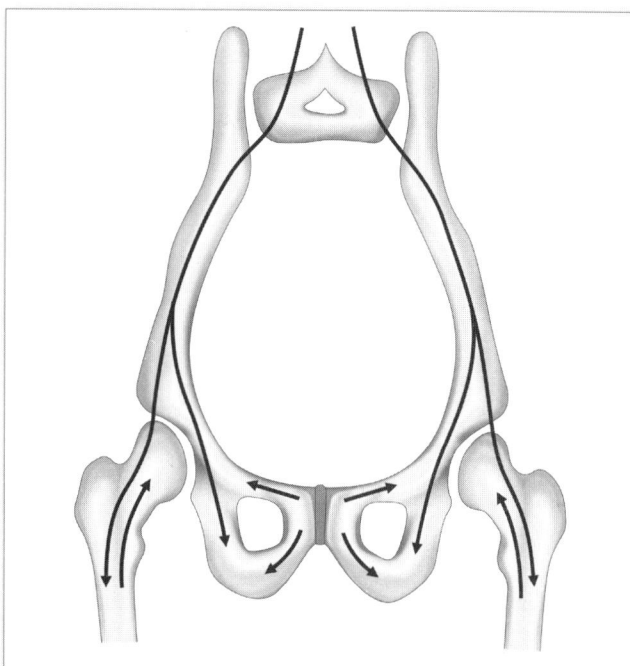

Fig. 2.25: Diagrammatic representation of forces acting on the pelvis

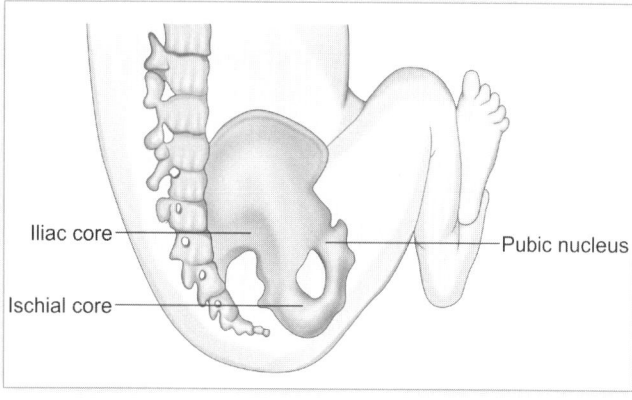

Fig. 2.26: Foetal pelvis: The sacral promontory is absent

The normal tendency for dorsal displacement of the sacral tip is prevented by the sacrotuberous ligaments (Figs 2.13, 4.5, 2.14, 7.8), thus forming the sacral concavity (Fig. 2.7). Subsequent loads bearing down from the head and trunk determine a wedge-like descent of the sacrum between the two pelvic bones, which would tend to separate if they were not blocked by the pubic joint. This joint tends instead to approach the sacrum, causing the process by which, in infant girls, the android pelvis becomes more gynecoid. If we add extra weight to the loads of the head and trunk, the symphysis approaches the promontory still further as a result. This phenomenon may be observed in farming populations of the Tropics and other populations where girls have to carry loads on their heads from childhood;

– *from below* exerted, in the erect position, by the femoral heads and, in the sitting position, by the ischial tuberosities (Fig. 2.25), whose counter-posed pressures tend to squash the pelvis transversely. This explains the frequency of *android* and *anthropoid pelvises in nomadic populations*.

In conclusion, **the morphology of the pelvis results from pressures exerted on it by the head and trunk and by the counter-pressure of the femoral heads, ischial tuberosities, ligaments and pelvic muscles.**

- Lifestyles, which may change the action of the forces that normally act on the pelvis, contribute to its morphology.

Classifications of the Small Pelvis

Over the centuries, one of the major concerns for obstetricians has been to find a method that would allow a patent pelvis to be distinguished from an impervious one; hence the *pelvimetric method*, with the study of one or more diameters consistent with pelvic patency (see Chapter 6 on obstetric diagnostics).

The first pelvic classification according to the shape of the inlet was made by Turner (1885) (Table 2.1), who classified three types on the basis of the ratio between the anteroposterior diameter, defined as the obstetric conjugate (OC) and the transverse diameter of the inlet:

Thoms (1923) (Table 2.2) added a fourth classification: *brachypellic*, in which the anterior-posterior diameter (OC) is less than the transverse by more (1–3 cm) than that observed in the *mesatipellic pelvis*.

Table 2.1

Turner classification

Dolicopellic	Anteroposterior diameter > transverse diameter
Mesatipellic	Anteroposterior diameter ≤ (max 1 cm<) widest transverse diameter
Platipellic	Anteroposterior diameter <3 cm widest transverse diameter

Table 2.2

Thoms classification

Dolicopellic	Anteroposterior diameter > transverse diameter
Mesatipellic	Anteroposterior diameter = Widest transverse diameter Anteroposterior diameter <1 cm widest transverse diameter
Brachipellic	Anteroposterior diameter <1–3 cm widest transverse diameter
Platipellic	Anteroposterior diameter <3 cm widest transverse diameter

Caldwell–Moloy Pelvic Classification

Caldwell and Moloy (1933, 1934, 1935) demonstrated that the shape of the pelvis is responsible for the type of engagement and progress of labour. They proposed a classifycation of the pelvis, still followed today. The criteria employed for classification are:

- Length of the anterior and posterior segments into which the anteroposterior diameter of the inlet is divided by its intersection with the widest transverse diameter
- Shape of the anterior and posterior pelves, into which the pelvis is divided by the widest transverse diameter; the anterior consists of an anterior or pubic arch, which corresponds to a circular arch with a radius slightly greater than 6 cm. The posterior pelvis, of greater importance in contributing to pelvic shape, consists of a posterior arch; this is made up in turn of two secondary arches, the so-called *sacroiliac sinuses*, corresponding to the wings of the sacrum and separated by the sacral promontory
- The geometric form of the inlet (triangular, anteroposterior elliptical, round, transverse elliptical).

According to this classification, we can distinguish four types of pelvis: *android*, *anthropoid*, *gynecoid* and *platypelloid* (Fig. 2.27, Table 2.3), with a relation between pelvis-type and type of physique. Recognising these different types of pelvis is not only of theoretical interest, but has a clearly defined practical relevance, as the mechanism of childbirth varies with the kind of pelvis (see Chapter 5).

Android (male: Fig. 2.27, Table 2.3): This is observed more frequently in white women (20–25% in Europeans, 16–18% in Africans), or when a woman has been subjected to strenuous physical activity during adolescence (Abitbol, 1996). It is typical of women with masculine build, or a short-set, square trunk and stocky lower limbs. The pelvic inlet has an irregular, wedge-like, triangular shape; the anteroposterior and transverse diameters are of the same length, with the latter very close to the promontory. The anterior pelvis is transversely flattened, while the posterior, being wide and flat quite often prevents (through not being rounded) the foetus from using the posterior pelvis for engagement.

The sacral angle (angle formed by the body of the first sacral vertebra with the anteroposterior diameter of the inlet) is ≤90° and the sacral line (line connecting the promontory with the apex of the sacrum) is not parallel to the pubic symphysis. Proceeding to the inferior pelvic strait, the lateral walls of the cavity side and posterior segment gradually reduce so that the pelvis assumes a funnel shape. The subpubic arch is narrow, with a very acute angle (<80°); the ischial spines are very prominent, the sacrum is long and narrow, and the sacral concavity is reduced. The foetal head engages occipitoposterior as the large occipital area fits better to the very wide posterior pelvis; the smaller frontal area uses the narrower wedge shaped anterior pelvis. As the head descends it meets increasing resistance caused by the funnelling of the walls of the lower pelvis. This may be sufficient to halt progress and prevent spontaneous rotation: deep transverse arrest is frequent if this occurs, the narrowing will make operative correction and delivery difficult.

Anthropoid (primates; Fig. 2.27, Table 2.3): This is more frequently observed in African women (41-45%) than in white women (20-25%) and when the child assumes the standing position after the normal developmental stage. It is typical of tall, slender women, with scapular circumference greater than that of the hips, or of short-limbed women with a sturdy trunk, slightly accentuated lumbar lordosis, short limbs and thin thighs that are closely positioned.

The anthropoid pelvis has an elliptical inlet; the anteroposterior diameter is greater than the transverse one, which is reduced; the anterosagittal diameter is longer than the posterior one; the anterior pelvis is narrow, the sacral angle is approximately 100°; the sacral line is parallel to the pubis; the lateral walls are parallel; the ischial spines are not prominent; the subpubic arch is narrow, but well formed (>80°); the depth of the pelvis is greater than in other pelves.

Prognosis is more favourable than in the android and platypelloid pelves: indeed, in about 2/3 of cases the head engages along the anteroposterior diameter. Engagement following the transverse diameter can take place only in a very broad pelvis. Occipitoposterior engagement is characterized by difficulty in rotation in the lower pelvis: "*persistent occiput posterior position*", but delivery can still take place. Engagement in occipitoanterior is the most favourable one, as it does not require rotation, and delivery is easier in occiput anterior.

Gynecoid (female: Fig. 2.27, Table 2.3): This is observed with slight predominance in Europeans (50%) and 42-47% in Africans. It is typical of women with a scapular circumference less than that of the hips, strong lumbar lordosis and abundant gluteal masses. The inlet is slightly ovoid with the anterior and posterior arches wide, rounded and equal in size. The widest transverse diameter and the medial transverse diameter (midway in the anteroposterior diameter) coincide. The subpubic arch is rounded: Roman arch. The sacral angle is approx. 100°; the sacral concavity is wide both vertically and transversely; the lateral cavity walls are parallel. Engagement takes place following all diameters.

Platypelloid (flat, Fig. 2.27, Table 2.3): This is the rarest of the four forms, with an incidence of 1–2%. It is observed when the child adopts the upright position before 14 months, or when girls carry loads on their heads from childhood. The platypelloid pelvis is transversely elliptical; the transverse diameter is slightly greater than the anteroposterior one,

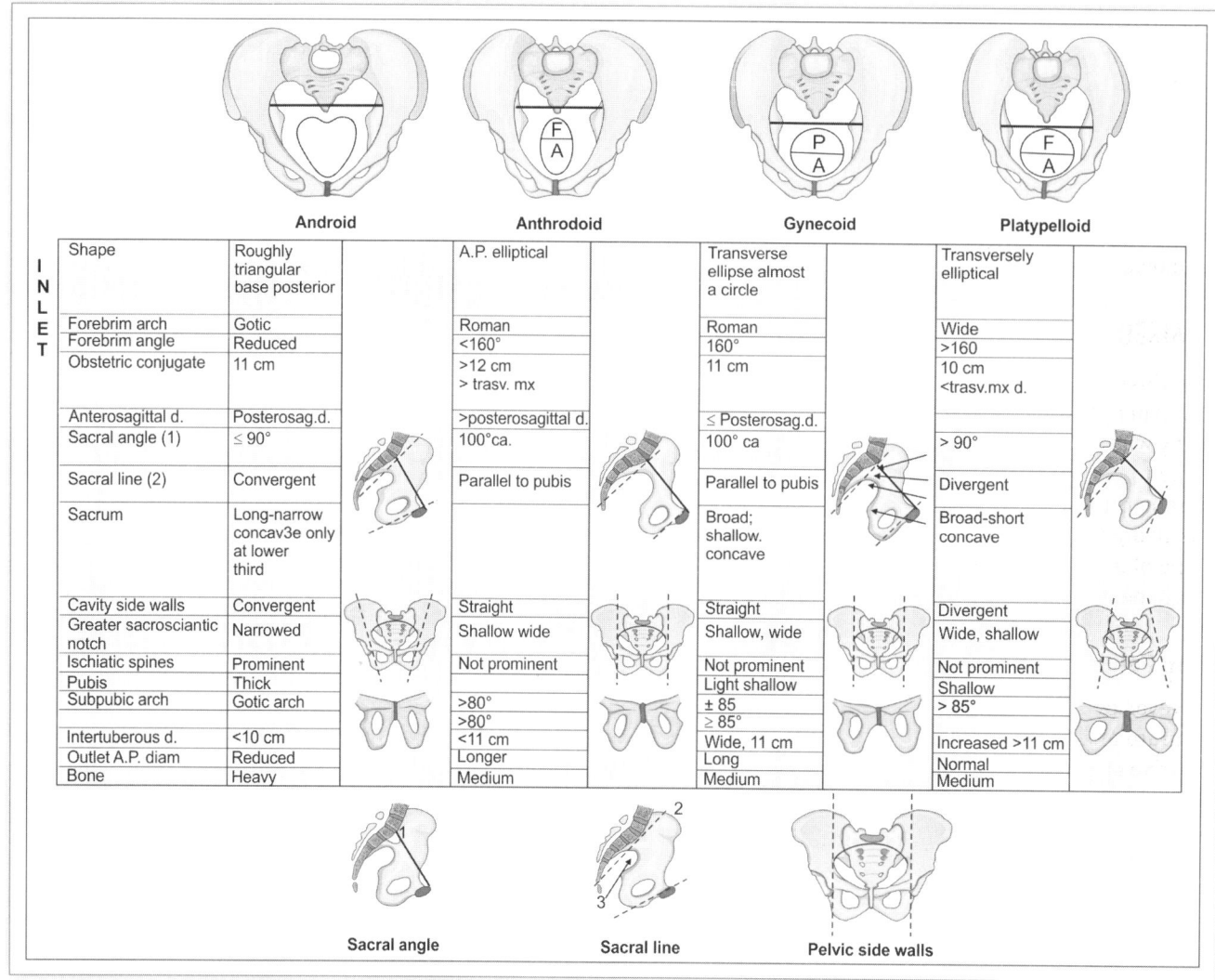

Fig. 2.27: Overview of the morphology of the pure pelvic types

Table 2.3

Synopsis of the four Pure Pelvic Types*

Android pelvis	d.s.a. > d.s.p d.a.p. > d.t.m. Frequently associated with a sixth sacral vertebra (assimilation pelvis according to Hirshoff). The two joined portions give rise to a triangular formation.
Anthropoid pelvis	d.s.a. = d.s.p d.a.p. > d.t.m. The two portions, joined, give rise to an elliptical formation, large anteroposterior axis
Gynecoid pelvis	d.a.p. = d.t.m. spinal ischial d. = 10 cm The two portions, joined, give rise to a round formation.
Platipelloid pelvis	d.a.p. < d.t.m. The two portions, joined, give rise to an elliptical formation large transversal axis.

*According to Caldwell & Moloy

Abbreviation: d.s.a = sagittal anterior diameter; d.s.p.= sagittal posterior diameter; d.a.p.= anteroposterior diameter; d.t.m.= transverse medial diameter which is reduced. Both the anterior and posterior arches are wide, flared and flat. The sacral angle is >90°. The cavity's lateral walls diverge caudally.

The head enters the pelvis in the transverse position; extreme moulding must occur before the biparietal diameter can be wedged in the superior strait. The head descends in transverse position until the occiput reaches the inferior pelvis; rotation does not usually occur until the head reaches the level of the perineum.

MIXED TYPES

After this classification was made, it was realized that about 35% of pelves (50% according to some authors) did not fall neatly within it, as the posterior segment may conform in shape to one standard type and the anterior to another, thereby producing *mixed types* (Fig. 2.28, Table 2.3). In classifying these mixed types, the first term indicates the shape of the dominant posterior segment and the second the shape of the anterior segment.

Long Pelvis According to Kirchhoff

However, even the classification now illustrated, although accurate and universally accepted, does not enable us to arrive at fully confident prognostic judgments. This is because it has often been observed that, even in a pelvis of normal size and morphology to which a normal-size head corresponds, engagement may not occur, and a clinical case of cephalopelvic disproportion follows.

In 1948 H. Kirchhoff introduced the concept of the "long pelvis", characterized by an abnormal extension of the birth canal, and identified two possible causes:

1. *Assimilation pelvis:* Assimilation (termed 'sacralisation' by some authors) is the anatomical and functional alignment of the fifth lumbar vertebra to the first sacral vertebra of a perfectly normal pelvis (Fig. 2.29); the alignment (assimilation) is defined as 1st or 2nd degree depending on whether the alignment is mobile or permanent. When it is permanent it results in:
   1. Double promontory: the lower promontory is formed by L5 with S1, while the upper one is the angle formed by L4 with L5 and which determines:
      - an almost vertical plane of the pelvic inlet; inclination dystocia may result (see Chapter 6)
      - elongation of the birth canal by 2-3 cm.
   2. *Pelvic arrest* (Fig. 2.30) this refers to the persistence in adults of a pelvis with neonatal features: raised promontory, vertical pelvic entrance and absence of sacral concavity. Under normal conditions these features are retained until puberty, when they then develop in a relatively short time into a final female pelvis through

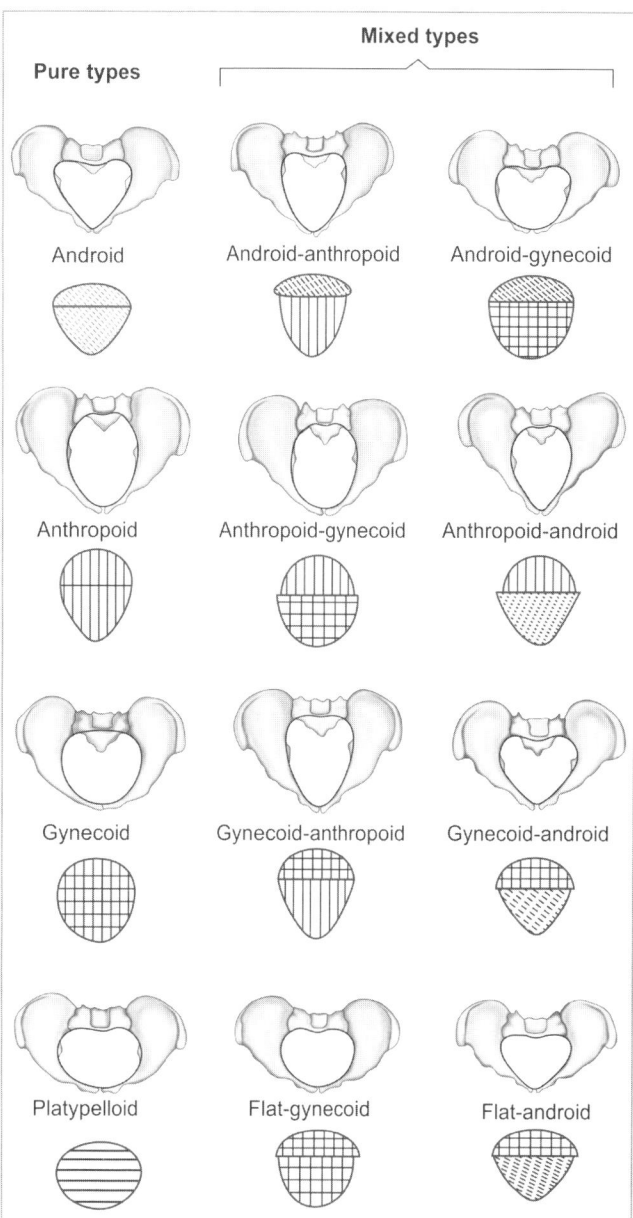

Fig. 2.28: Female pelvis: pure and mixed types of the Caldwell and Moloy classification; the first term indicates the shape of the posterior segment, which is dominant; the second, the shape of the anterior pelvis

lowering of the promontory and formation of a sacral concavity. An assimilation vertebra can be associated with "pelvic arrest".

Inclination of the Pelvis

In the standing position, the angle between the pelvic brim and the horizontal plane (Fig. 2.17) from top to bottom and from back to front, has an inclination of about 60° (Naegele),

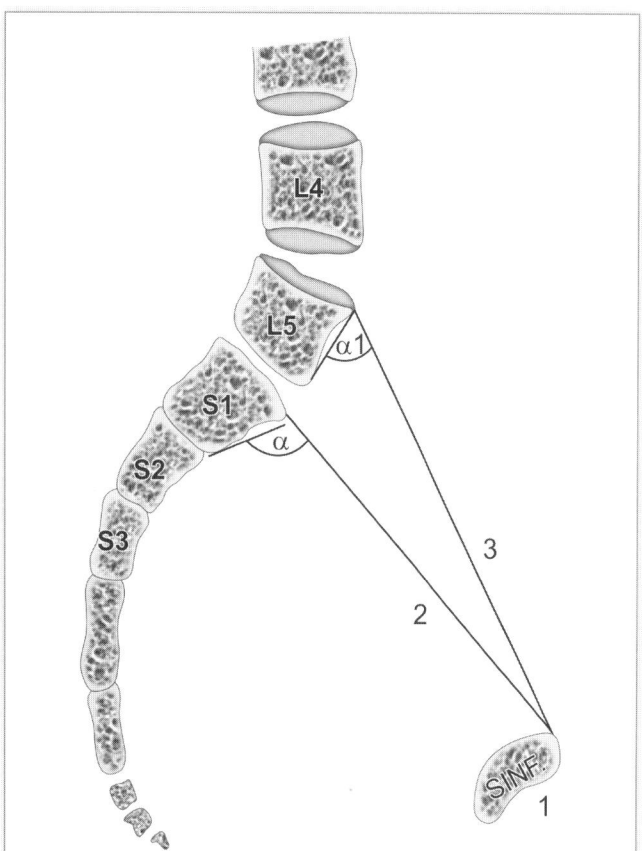 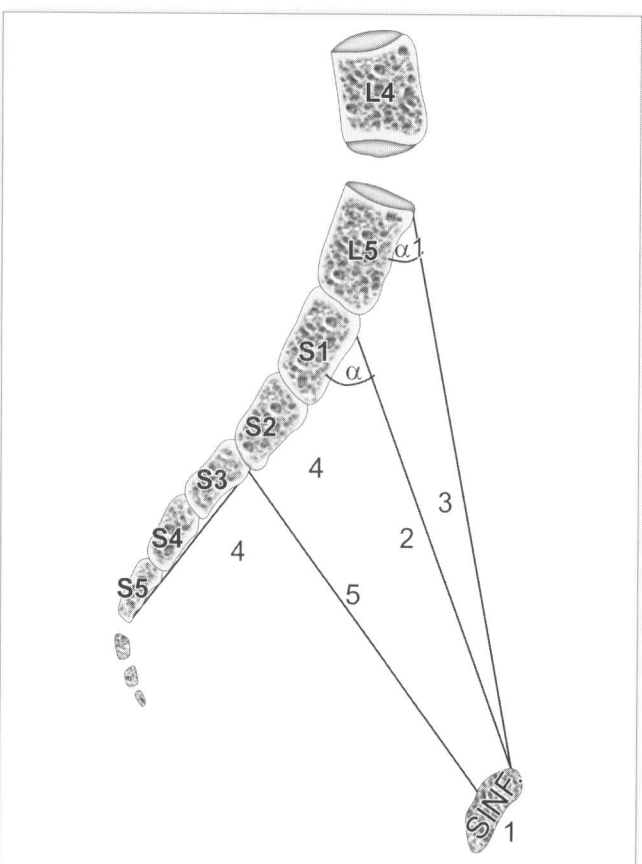

Fig. 2.29: Assimilation pelvis (Kirchhoff) with retention of the shape of the sacrum: sagittal section: L4 Fourth lumbar vertebra; L5 Fifth lumbar vertebra: assimilation vertebra; (alignment may be mobile or permanent. L4–L5 New promontory; 1. Symphysis, 2. Plane of normal pelvic inlet: Normal anteroposterior diameter of inlet; α Angle of inclination of pelvic inlet; (or sacral angle in normal pelves). Angle subtended by the body of the first sacral vertebra and the anteroposterior diameter of the inlet; 3. (L5-Symphysis) New plane of pelvic inlet; $\alpha1$ New angle of pelvic inlet, subtended between the body of the fifth lumbar vertebra (assimilation vertebra) and 3 (new anteroposterior diameter of inlet). $\alpha1$ is reduced compared to α; the inclination of the pelvis has increased and the plane of the pelvic inlet is almost horizontal

Fig. 2.30: Pelvic arrest (Kirchhoff); the morphology of the sacrum has been altered. Sacral concavity is reduced or absent. L5 assimilation vertebra, L4–L5, new promontory. 1. Symphysis, 2. Plane of normal pelvic inlet (symphysis–first sacral vertebra). 3 New plane of pelvic inlet (Symphysis–L4–L5),α, angle of pelvic inlet, $\alpha1$, new angle of pelvic inlet, subtended between the body of the fifth lumbar vertebra (assimilation vertebra) and 3 (new anteroposterior diameter of inlet). $\alpha1$ is reduced compared to α; the inclination of the pelvis has increased and the plane of the pelvic inlet is almost vertical. 4. The sacral line (projected between promontory and apex of the sacrum) is almost straight. 5. The narrowest point in the pelvis is not the obstetric conjugate, but is subtended between the apex of the posterior convexity of the symphysis and the junction of S2 with S3.

or of 35° and 75° according to Jacobs. In the woman in sacrodorsal position, it is approx. 42°. Abnormal inclinations lead to "inclination dystocia" (see Chapter 3).

BIBLIOGRAPHY

1. Abitbol MM. The shapes of the female pelvis. Contributing factors. J Reprod Med. 1996;41(4):242-50.
2. Caldwell WE, Moloy HC. Anatomical variations in the female pelvis and their effect in labour with a suggested classification. Am J Obstet Gynec. 1933;26:479.
3. Caldwell WE, Moloy HC, D'Esopo D. Further studies on the pelvic architecture. Am J Obstet Gynec. 1934;28:482.
4. Caldwell WE, Moloy HC, D'Esopo D. Further studies on the mechanism of labour. Am J Obstet Gynec. 1935;30:763.
5. Farabeuf M. Dystocie du détroit superieur, mécanisme, diagnostic, traitment, symphysèotomie. Gaz Hebdom de Mèd et de Chirurg. 1894.
6. Fabbri G. Alcune considerazioni ostetriche intorno alla pelvi. Mem. dell'Accademia delle Scienze di Bologna, 1856; vol VIII:113.
7. Kamina P. Anatomia ginecologica ed ostetrica. Marrapese Editore, DEMI, Roma; 1975.
8. Kirchhoff F. The assimilation pelvis as an obstetrical problem. Ztschr F Geburtsh U Gynaek. 1948;129:174.
9. Klima M. Anatomie des Menschen. W Frank'sche Verlagshandlung. W. Keller & Co. Stuttgart; 1984.
10. Testut L. Anatomia Umana. UTET, Torino; 1943.
11. Turner WM. The index of the pelvic brim as a basis of classification. J Anat Physiol. 1885;20(Pt 1):125-43.

CHAPTER 3

Uterus

MECHANICAL FUNCTIONS

The mechanical functions of the uterus are, at different times:
1. To prevent expulsion of the product of conception.
2. To deliver the uterine contents.

Preventing Expulsion of the Product of Conception

The retention of a product of conception as large as that of the human, if managed by a system based on muscle sphincters would require energy and be subject to fatigue; a viscous-elastic structure, such as a cervix made mainly of collagenous connective tissue overcomes these problems.

The shape and composition of the cervix render it ideal for retaining the product of conception: The cervix is tubular in shape and constituted mainly of fibrous tissue (connective tissue, collagen) with a smooth muscle component of just 15% (Danforth, 1954). The cervical connective tissue is not organised structurally, it has been hypothesized that there is a concentration of muscle tissue in the lateral and superior part, and a concentration of elastic and vascular tissue near the fibromuscular junction—the area in which muscle tissue transits into fibrous tissue at the internal cervical os. The cervical canal is between 3 and 5 cm in length, but in advanced pregnancy this reduces to 2–3 cm, and the structure disappears completely during labour.

Composition of Connective Tissue

Base substance: Glycoproteins, water and electrolytes. Glycoproteins are glycosaminoglycans formed by a long protein chain bound covalently to lateral unbranched polypolysaccharides, endowing them with a gel-like consistency. The entire protein–carbohydrate complex can be synthesized within the cells (fibroblasts, muscle cells) and secreted externally via cytoplasmic vesicles.

Collagen: Thanks to their small radius of curvature and close bonding with each other, collagen fibres are nonelastic and capable of withstanding dilatation with a minimum of circumferential tension (Laplace's law). Parturition occurs through an increase in compliance (adaptation to stress) by the fibrils and the basic substances, made possible by dynamic changes in their composition: fibrils become more dispersed and less stable, while the concentration of collagen reduces and there is an increase in the amount of structural proteins—water-retaining glycosaminoglycans.

Cellular components: The cellular components are muscle cells, fibroblasts and macrophages.

Delivering the Product of Conception

Smooth muscle fibre has the following properties:
- *It acts like normal muscle fibre*, so that it returns to its previous length following isotonic contraction (cf. the Braxton–Hicks contractions during gestation). This property is present for long periods during pregnancy and in the primigravida *one contraction per hour* is physiological. During labour, however, the *relaxation phase* is replaced by *fibre retraction*
- *It takes on the property of retraction*, that is, the tendency not to regain its original length at the end of a contraction and to start the next contraction from the length

previously attained. This means that each contraction is followed by a progressive shortening of the fibre, leading to a reduction in the overall volume of the uterus.

HISTOLOGY OF THE UTERUS

The uterus is constituted of peritoneal serous membrane, myometrium and mucosa (Fig. 3.1); only the myometrium is relevant for the purposes of this discussion.

Myometrium

The myometrium comprises a muscle and a connective tissue component.

Muscle Component

During pregnancy, a marked increase in the amount of muscle fibre can be observed. This occurs through two processes:

- Hyperplasia, or the multiplication of existing muscle cells
- Metaplasia, or the transformation of fibroblasts or of certain histiocytes into muscle fibres.

Muscle fibres increase in length from 40–60 μ to 250–500 μ and their width increases from 3–4 to 5–10 μ. 20–100 of these fibres combine to form one individual anatomical unit: the smooth muscle bundle. Muscle bundles or fascicles may be flat, ribbon-shaped, or rope-like. Separated from each other by the connective tissue, they organise into concentric coils in which each one lies in the same orientation, each being joined to the others by many terminal or lateral anastomoses.

At full term of pregnancy, the uterus consists of three muscle layers (Fig. 3.1).

Superficial Layer or Neomyometrium (Fig. 3.1A)

This comprises two arrangements of fibre: Longitudinal and transverse.

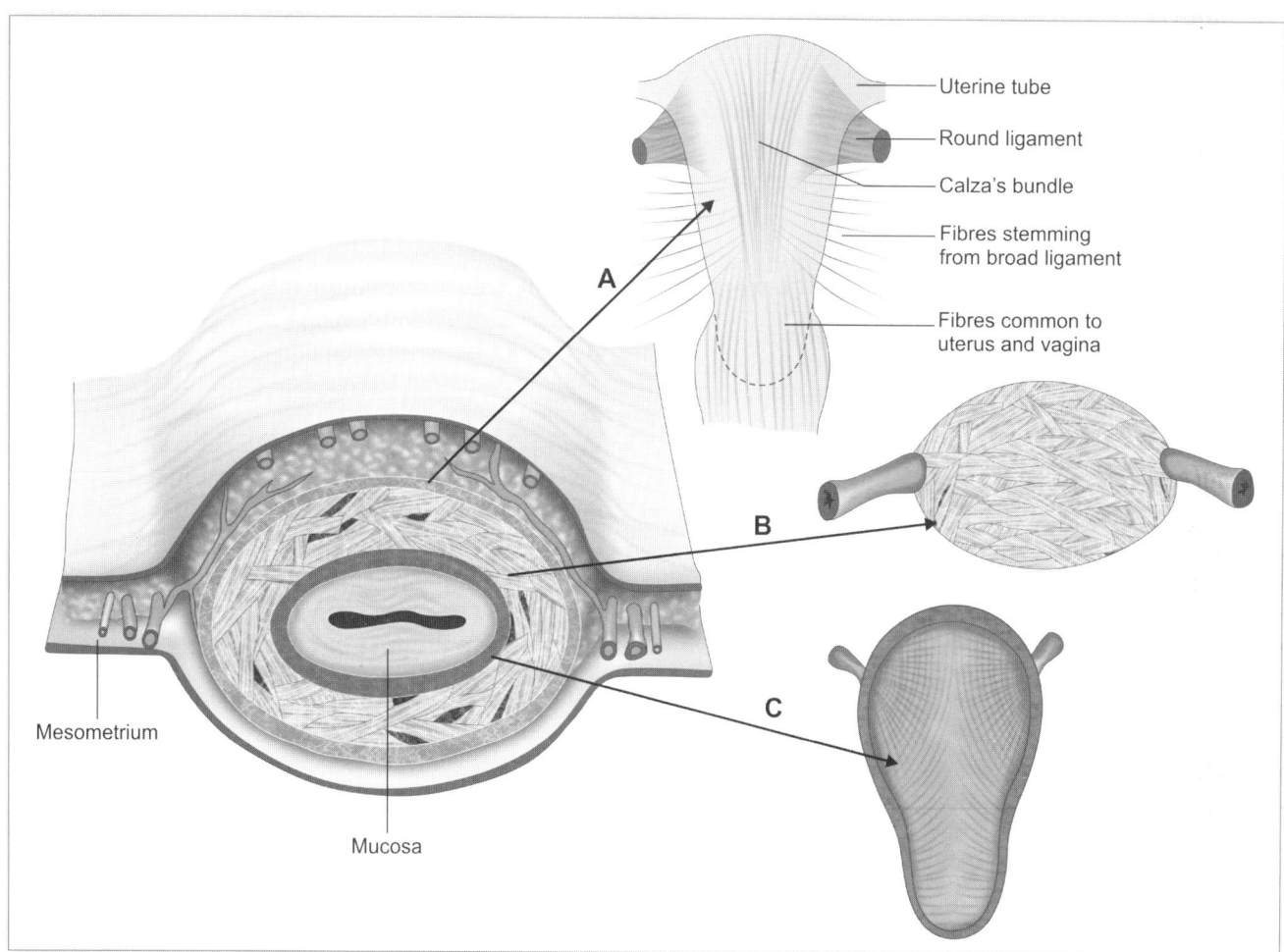

Fig. 3.1: Myometrium. (A) Superficial muscle layer or 'neomyometrium'; (B) Intermediate muscle layer or paleomyometrium (uterine fundus); (C) Internal muscle layer or subendometrial layer (From Kamina P *Anatomia ginecologica ed ostetrica*, DEMI Rome)

The longitudinal fibres form a flattened body: *Calza's bundle* (Fig. 3.1), which is 10-25 mm wide and clearly seen on the median face of the gravid uterus, covering its anterior, fundal and posterior aspects, taking on a horseshoe shape, whose median portion, which envelops the uterine fundus, is known as the *ansiform fascia of Helie*.

The transverse fibres form a continuous and regular plane, running bilaterally along the whole length of the uterine corpus. As these fibres reach the lateral borders:

- Some bend to form an arch, spanning from the anterior to posterior parts and vice versa, being crossed at this site by numerous vessels
- Others extend beyond the confines of the organ:
  - Into the body of the broad ligament (*ligamentum latum uteri* or broad ligament of the uterus), where they give rise to the muscle laminae that form the double-layered peritoneal sheet
  - Anteriorly to the round ligament (*lig. teres uteri*), these form the ligament of the ovary (*lig. ovarii proprium*), and, on the external layer of the ovarian tube's muscular coat, posteriorly in two distinct bundles directed toward the sacrum, they form the uterosacral ligaments.

Middle Layer, Plexiform or Paleomyometrium Layer (Fig. 3.1B)

This originates from the fusion of the Müller ducts; the muscle fascicles intertwine in every direction, including the venous vessels in their mesh. Such vessels are particularly abundant here, hence the name *Kreitzer's vascular stratum*. On contraction of the uterus, the lumina of vessels within this mesh are occluded, thereby considerably reducing any hemorrhaging.

Internal or Subendometrial Layer (Fig. 3.1C)

This originates from the muscle layer of Müller's ducts; it consists of circular muscle fibres disposed in a series of concentric rings around the uterine orifices. Cephalad, they circumscribe the outlets of the uterine tubes—the uterine ostium (*ostia uterina tubarum*), inferiorly, at the isthmus, they can clearly be seen, protruding beneath the mucosa of the internal uterine os.

Connective Tissue Component

An increase in collagen synthesis occurs during pregnancy, as is revealed by the high percentage of (newly formed) collagen III molecules on analytical ultracentrifugation. This leads to an increase in the amount of connective tissue in the myometrium. Distribution varies in different segments of the uterus: From 40 to 50% in the uterine corpus, rising to 90% at the uterine cervix. The collagen increase in the corpus performs a specific function: by interlacing itself between the muscle fibres, it promotes their sliding over each other and their displacement during uterine contractions.

Lower Uterine Segment

The lower uterine segment (LUS) is derived from the uterine isthmus, which, anatomically considered, is bordered by the *internal histological orifice* (the point of transition between the endometrium of the corpus and that of the cervix) and the *anatomical internal os*. The isthmus differentiates from the corpus during labour, when, the dispersal of muscle fascicles resulting from the increase in loose connective tissue during pregnancy, is augmented by disassociation of the collagenous and elastic fibres, leading to the so-called *demuscularisation* of the lower uterine segment.

Uterine Cervix

The contractile activity of the uterus and the reduction in compliance by cervical fibres are autonomous processes. It is in fact possible for flattening and dilatation (effacement) of the cervix to occur without any contractile activity, just as contractile activity can occur without any change in the cervix (cervical dystocia). During labour these two processes continue almost independently and become coordinated only at a certain point.

CONTRACTILE ACTIVITY

Contraction originates from the area of the uterine tubes and round ligaments, whence it spreads across the whole uterus. It has been thought that there are pace-makers located in the uterus, but a whole series of studies on the subject has so far identified no specific structures dedicated to this purpose.

In the course of a contraction, various segments of the uterus present different pressure gradients, high at the fundus and gradually decreasing caudad to a relatively inactive lower uterine segment. This relation indicates *normal uterine polarity*, which is promoted by a well flexed foetal head and a presenting part that is a good fit for the lower uterine pole.

If the myometrium were spherical in shape, retraction would mean that every contraction would be followed by a reduction in size of the cavity, but not by the expulsion of the product of conception. Expulsion is made possible by the uterus' *truncated conical shape*, with the (truncated) apex pointing distally.

Each contraction brings about two types of phenomena:
- Due to retraction, the uterine cavity progressively reduces in size
- Also due to the process of retraction, as the fundus is functionally dominant, the apex of the cone is stretched

upwards with each contraction (Fig. 3.2) and is forced to dilate. Concomitantly, flattening and dilatation of the cervix (cervical effacement) is taking place.

Two structures, therefore, two synchronised systems, connected together by the lower uterine segment, may be distinguished functionally: the corpus that contracts and shortens, and the cervix that flattens and dilates. Their harmonious interaction enables engagement and advancement of the presenting part.

Changes induced by a mechanical obstruction during labour, which can result in rupture of the uterus, are described in Chapter 23.

Physiology of Placental Circulation

At full term, uterine perfusion is commonly agreed to be between 500 and 700 mL/min. Of this, approx. 75% goes to the placenta (placental shunt), while the remainder permeates the myometrium (myometrial shunt). Flow volume depends on:
1. The maternal blood supply, in relation to the bore of the arteries and systemic arterial pressure.
2. Venous return.

Arterial blood, at a pressure of 70–80 mm Hg, enters the *intervillous space,* its pressure mirroring, at rest, that of the amniotic fluid, at 10 mm Hg, the blood is therefore projected upward toward the chorionic plate, passing through the villi with a vortex motion that promotes its mixing with the blood already present. Outflow is facilitated by the gradient between the intervillous space and the venous vessels, in which pressure is close to zero. The contractile activity of the myometrium interferes with blood flow to and from the intervillous space, and with foetal oxygenation.

Because of the squeezing action during the initial phase of contraction, blood escapes from the intervillous space and myometrium. This outflow, totalling approx. 200–300 mL, brings about a reduction in the volume of intervillous blood, which lasts until intramyometrial pressure is sufficient to cause the venous vessels to collapse.

Meanwhile, inflow of arterial blood (at a pressure of 80 mm Hg) continues until intramyometrial pressure and the pressure of the amniotic fluid become (at the acme of contraction) high enough to impede even this inflow.

Blood provision has nonetheless sufficed to replenish the initial volume with well-oxygenated blood and to enable effective gas exchange. It has in fact been shown that foetal oxygenation is at its highest at the peak of contraction. With the closure of the arterial vessels, intervillous blood is isolated from the external environment and gas exchanges between mother and foetus rapidly reach equilibrium.

During the relaxation phase, as soon as arterial pressure exceeds intramyometrial pressure, which has until now physiologically isolated the intervillous space, arterial flow resumes. As pressure finally ebbs, the collapsing of the venous vessels relents, allowing outflow of blood from the intervillous space.

It is well understood that the time of greatest danger for the foetus occurs during so-called *physiological isolation of the intervillous space*, characterised by very rapid transfer of O2 and the passage of CO_2 in the opposite direction.

It seems evident that if changes in the rate of blood flow, the properties of the placental membrane, or the timing

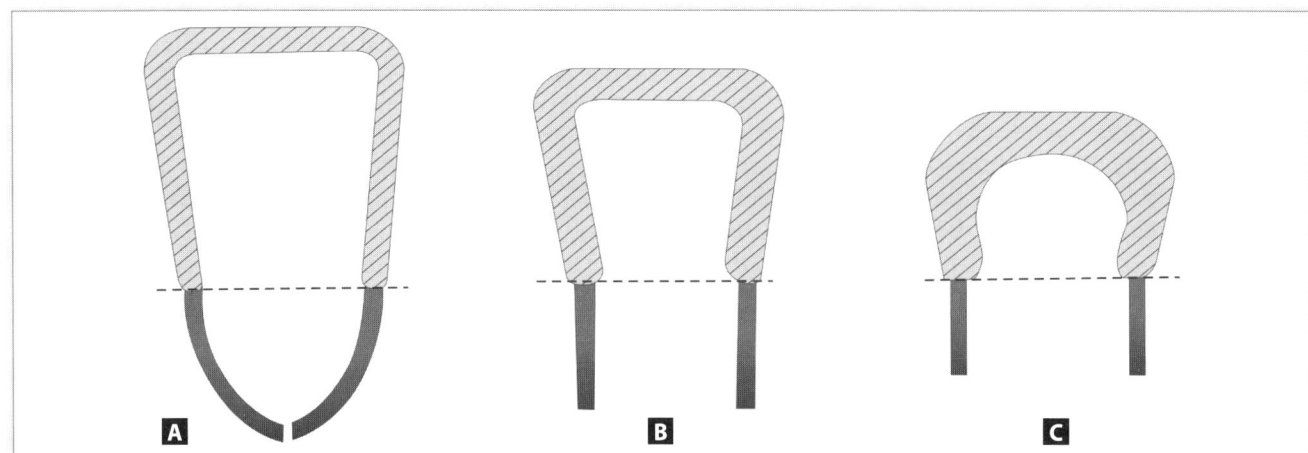

Figs 3.2A to C: Changes affecting the uterine corpus (hatched) and the LUS (in black) during normal labour: (A). At the start of labour, the corpus has the shape of a truncated cone; the LUS is hemispherical; (B). As the expulsive phase starts, the body reduces in height, concomitantly increasing its thickness, and the LUS takes on a cylindrical shape, due to an increase in its circumference and a simultaneous shortening and reduction in thickness; (C) During the expulsive phase, due to retraction, the height of the corpus is reduced still further. Simultaneously, the volume of the uterine cavity decreases. This is the mechanism by which the downwards progress and delivery of the product of conception takes place

and frequency of contractions occur, gas exchanges will be compromised and a rapid decrease in pO_2 and increase in pCO_2 will result.

A high frequency of contractions entails a shortening of the relaxation phase, compromising the inflow of arterial blood and prolonging the overall period of isolation of the intervillous space, with resulting foetal hypoxia and foetal hypercapnia.

Contractile Activity of the Myometrium

Uterine contraction is defined according to:
- *Polarity*: this indicates the direction of pressure gradients in a contraction. Polarity is normal when pressure gradients are high at the fundus and, proceeding towards the cervix, decrease progressively to a minimally active lower uterine segment. Uterine polarity may be:
1. *Preserved*, with functional domination by the fundus: Pressure gradients decrease as we proceed from the fundus to the cervix. Viewed functionally, this may be:
   a. Normal (Fig. 3.3(1)).
   b. Weak (Fig. 3.3(2)) Ineffective from the point of view of engagement or advancement of the presenting part.
   c. Hypertonic, caused by:
      » Obstruction to engagement or advancement of the presenting part (Fig. 3.3(3))
      » Cervical dystocia: The cervix is flattened, but an organic or functional cause is preventing its dilatation (Fig. 3.3(4)). Without rapid intervention, the upshot of both these conditions will be the formation of Bandl's ring, or pathological retraction ring (Fig. 3.3(5)).
2. *Inverted*, resulting from
   – Hypertonia of the lower uterine segment (Fig. 3.3(6))
   – Cervical stiffness, preventing the normal effacement of the cervix (Fig. 3.3(7)).
3. *Uncoordinated* due to colicky contractile activity that is:
   – Pure (Fig. 3.3(8))
   – Sustained by asymmetry between the two uterine hemispheres (Fig. 3.3(9)).

In the case of a prior hysterotomy, contraction polarity is a valuable indicator of the quality and extension of the uterine scar and its relation to the surrounding myometrium. Normal polarity indicates that the scar is not interfering with contractions. Incomplete transmission of the contraction wave associated with deviations or asymmetries of the uterus, having the scar as their epicentre, indicate impairment of myometrial structure or extensive adhesions between the uterine body and the abdominal wall. Confirmation will come through C-section.

Frequency: This expresses the number of contractions per unit of time, which in obstetrics is 10 minutes. Normal frequency is between 2 and 5; if below 2, contractile activity is ineffective, if above 5, it is aggressive (see section on the physiology of placental circulation).

Intensity: This expresses pressure variations in the amniotic fluid during a contraction compared to uterine basal tone. It is expressed in mm Hg.
- *Basal tone* refers to the minimum pressure achieved by the amniotic fluid during the interval between two consecutive contractions; it is approximately 10 mm Hg.

A close correlation exists between the intensity of uterine contractions and progress of labour:
- *Labour does not start or, if started, it arrests* if contraction intensity is below 15 mm Hg

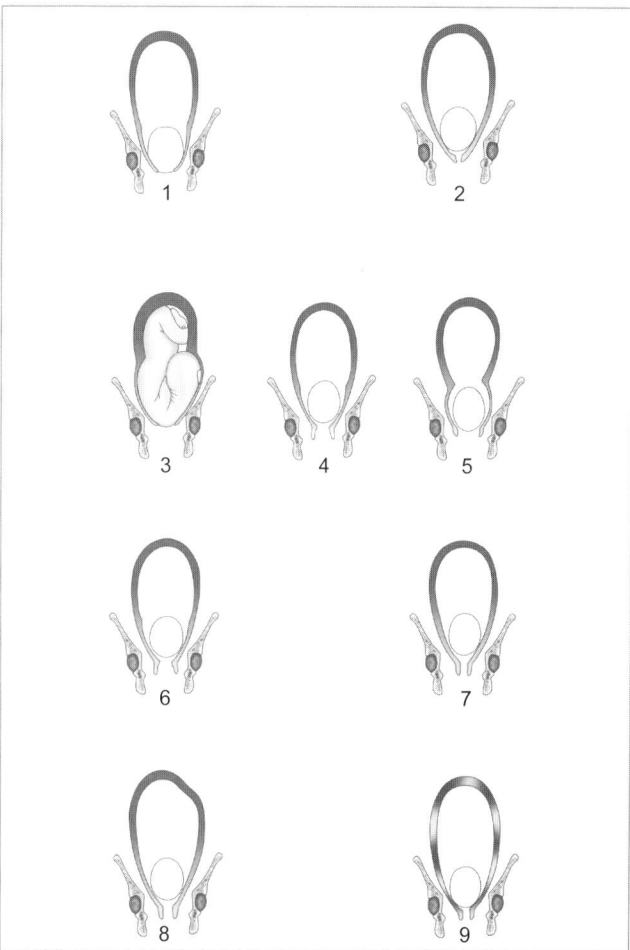

Fig. 3.3: Various forms of uterine polarity: Hatching indicates contractile activity and pressure gradients. (1) Normal polarity: Intensity of hatching, corresponding to pressure gradients, reduces proceeding caudad; (2) Hypotonic polarity; (3) Hypertonic polarity: obstruction represented by the passenger; (4) Hypertonic polarity: obstruction represented by cervical dystocia; (5) Hypertonic polarity: obstruction represented by Bandl's ring; (6) Inverted polarity due to hypertonia of lower uterine segment; (7) Inverted polarity due to cervical rigidity; (8) Uncoordinated contractile activity of colicky uterus; (9) Uncoordinated contractile activity due to asymmetry of the two uterine hemispheres

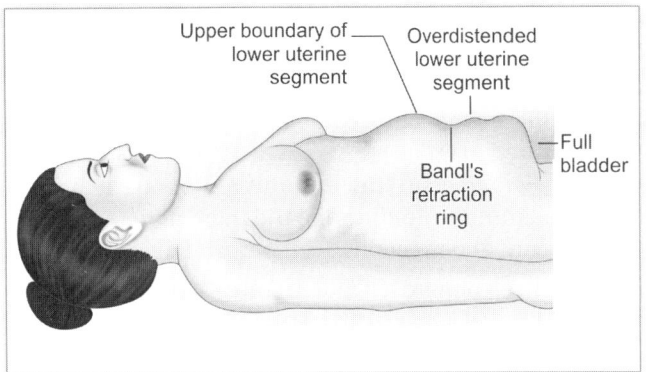

Fig. 3.4: Bandl's ring or retraction ring

- A minimum pressure of 15 mm Hg above basal tone (total pressure of 25 mm Hg) is necessary to dilate the cervix
- *Labour progresses*
- *Normally*, with pressure values between 25 and 50 mm Hg
- *Rapidly* and may result in a precipitate delivery, due to values between 50 and 60 mm Hg.

Duration: The uterine contraction curve can be divided into a rapid increment phase and a rapid decrement phase; both last 40–60 seconds, giving a total of 80–120 seconds, with a mean duration of 100 seconds.

Clearly, a cardiotocograph offers clear appreciation and definition of the features of uterine contraction referred to here. In resource-poor countries, however, this is not always available. Clinical science, however, offers evidential markers that enable a diagnosis of sufficient accuracy:

a. A contraction of the uterus becomes clinically salient only when it reaches 10 mm Hg above basal tone. Therefore, it actually lasts a little longer than can be identified by palpation.
b. The uterine wall can be indented by finger pressure as long as contraction intensity remains below 40 mm Hg. Above this value, it cannot be indented by the fingers.

When polarity is normal, anomalous uterine contractions can be divided into two main groups: hypoactivity and hyperactivity.

- *Hypoactivity* is diagnosed when there are fewer than two contractions every 10 minutes, or when contraction intensity is below 25 mm Hg (hypokinesia)
- *Hyperactivity* is diagnosed when there are more than 5 contractions every 10 minutes, when intensity is greater than 50 mm Hg (hyperkinesia), or when both are present
- *Hypertonia* is present when uterine basal tone is greater than 12 mm Hg. It may be caused by contractile incoordination, tachysystolia or overdistension of the myometrium due to polyhydramnios or multiple pregnancy.

Normal Uterine Polarity with Hyperkinesis (Overactive Contractile Activity)

Even in the presence of an obstruction to the engagement or progression of the presenting part, uterine contractile activity continues. The response of the myometrium to an obstruction consists in:

- Increased strength of contraction
- Increased frequency of contractions, which may reach the point of *uterine tetany*.

Due to the process of retraction, the height of the uterus will progressively reduce until it reaches a critical point, after which the truncated conical form is replaced by a spherical one. At this point propulsion gives way to compression.

The lower margin of the sphere thus formed at the junction with the overdistended lower uterine segment retracts away from the LUS, giving rise to *Bandl's ring or a retraction ring* (Figs 3.3(5), 3.4 and 3.5). This is to be distinguished from a *constriction or contraction ring* (Fig. 3.6).

The *constriction or contraction ring* (Smellie, 1743; White, 1916; Gilliat, 1933; Rudolph, 1937 Caldeyro-Barcia, 1958) is an isolated, persistent, annular contraction of circular fibres occurring in the absence of cephalopelvic disproportion or obstructed labour (Table 3.1).

A contraction ring may occur spontaneously in primigravidae, often preceded by contractile discoordination. It may also be seen in women who have given birth after an

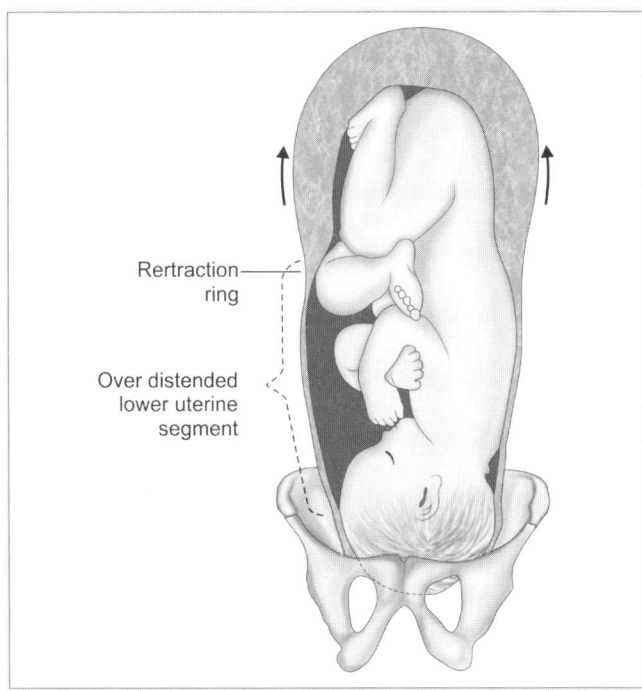

Fig. 3.5: Bandl's ring or pathological retraction ring: The lower uterine segment is overdistended

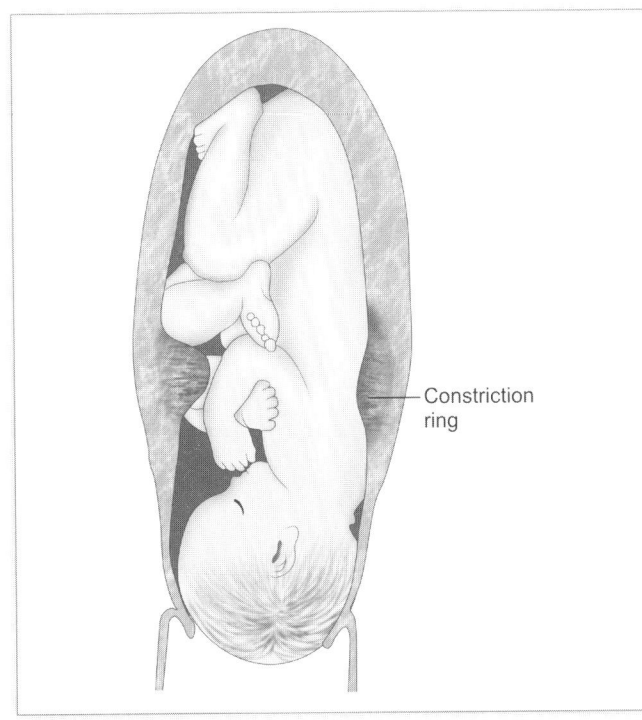

Fig. 3.6: Constriction or contraction ring: The contracted area follows the contours of a depression in the foetus; the lower uterine segment is not overdistended

Table 3.1
Distinguishing features of contraction ring and bandl's ring of retraction

Constriction ring	Bandl's or pathological retraction ring
During any period of labour	During dilatation
On the foetal body or an area of low resistance	At the junction between the lower uterine segment and uterine corpus
The uterine wall is thick in the ring area	
The uterine wall caudad of the ring is not thinned	The uterine wall is thinned
The uterine wall cephalad of the ring is not contracted	The uterine wall cephalad of the ring is contracted and hard
Once formed, the ring remains stable in that site	A retraction ring tends to rise
The round ligaments are not tensed	The round ligaments are tensed

insufficient administration of oxytocic agents (in hypertonic inertia or following I.M. administration of oxytocin), or may result from obstetrical handling.

The ring (Fig. 3.6) moulds onto a depression of the foetus: 45% are found at the neck; 21% around the foetal inferior pole; 15% on arms; 9% on the thorax, and 9% around the neck in breech presentation. At birth, signs left behind by a constriction ring on the foetal body can be clearly seen (Mills, 1949); it prevents foetal descent and, during contraction, the presenting part tends to recede.

Unlike the prognosis for Bandl's ring, with a constriction ring the lower uterine segment is not over dilated and there have been no reports of uterine rupture.

Uterine hypertonus, which is always present, compromises placental circulation and intrauterine asphyxia is common.

Complications vary depending on the stage of labour in which the ring appears:
- Prolonged dilatation stage, if it occurs at the uterine cervix
- Prolonged second stage, if around the neck or another part of the foetal body;
- Postpartum haemorrhage, responsible for the retention of the placenta.

THERAPY

- Pethidine during the dilatation stage
- General anaesthesia using volatile anaesthetic agents, in case of resolution of the ring, completion of the delivery by forceps or obstetric suction cap. If the ring fails to relax, C-section with vertical incision of the lower uterine segment is recommended.

BIBLIOGRAPHY

1. Brody S. Uterine distocia and constriction ring. Obstet Gynecol. 1961;18:502-6.
2. Caldeyro-Barcia R. Uterine contractility in Obstetrics. Main lecture. II World congress of International Federation of Obstetrics and Gynaecology. 1958.
3. El-Reyad M, Quinn M. Preterm uterine constriction rings and their consequences. J Obstet Gynaecol. 2008;28:440.
4. Gilliat W. The contraction ring in labour. J Obstet Gynecol Br Emp. 1933;40:1036.
5. Kaye Christopher H. Constriction ring dystocia. Can Med Assoc J. 1974;110:535-8.
6. Mills WG. Treatment of constriction ring dystocia. J Obstet Gynecol Br Commonw. 1949;56:838.
7. Rudolph L. Constriction ring dystocia. JAMA. 1937;108:532.
8. Smellie W. Treatise on the Theory and Practise of Midwifery. Edited with annotations by McClintock AH. London, New Sydenham Society, 1876; pp. 223.
9. White C. The contraction ring as a cause of dystocia, with the description of a specimen removed by hysterectomy during labour. Proc R Soc Med (Obst Gynaec). 1912;13:70.
10. White C. The contraction ring as a cause of dystocia, with the description of a specimen removed by hysterectomy during labour. Lancet. 1913;1:604.
11. White C. Five cases of labour obstructed by a contraction ring. Br Med J. 1916;2:752-3.

CHAPTER 4

Passenger (Foetus)

The spatial position of the foetus is defined according to:

The relation of the foetal longitudinal axis to the longitudinal axis of the uterus: *Lie*, which may be:
- *Longitudinal*: The two axes coincide
- *Oblique*: The major axis of the foetus describes an angle of less than 90° with that of the uterus
- *Transverse*: The major axis of the foetus is perpendicular to that of the uterus.

The relation that the major parts of the foetal body (head, lower extremities, shoulder) bear to the superior strait and felt through the cervix on vaginal examination is: *Foetal presentation and position*.
- *Presentation* refers to the major foetal part: Head, breech or shoulder, that first faces the upper strait. We therefore distinguish between cephalic, breech and shoulder presentation.

Cephalic presentations are classified according to the relation of the head to the body of the foetus (attitude); usually the head is sharply flexed, in this circumstance the vertex is the presenting part (*vertex presentation*) or partially flexed: When the large fontanel presents: *Sincipital presentation*, partially extended: *Brow presentation*, or the neck may be sharply extended so that the occiput and back come into contact and the face engages in the superior strait: *Face presentation*.

When the foetus *presents by the breech*: The thighs may be flexed and the legs extended over the anterior surface of the body: *Frank breech* or the thighs may be flexed on the abdomen and the legs upon the thighs: *Full breech presentation* or one of or both feet may be the lowest part: *Single or double foot or footling presentation*.
- *Position* refers to the relation that the point of direction (the landmark by which that foetal position is identified) has to the "relevant part" of the upper strait: The iliopubic, or iliopectineal eminence; the extremities of the transverse pelvic diameter and the sacroiliac synchondrosis.

CHAPTER 5

Mechanism and Physiopathology of Parturition

INTRODUCTION

Parturition is the transit of the product of conception (foetus, passenger) from the internal environment (the uterus) to the external one; the passageway is the birth canal (refer to Fig. 2.21), which we can subdivide into the *superior pelvic strait*—the *birth canal proper*—and the *inferior pelvic strait*.

According to classic obstetrics, there are two ways in which to divide the birth canal:

1. *The system of converging planes* (Fig. 5.1), in which we can distinguish:
   - The plane of the superior pelvic strait (pelvic inlet)
   - The *greater pelvic plane*, which passes anteriorly, between the point of greatest convexity of the pubic symphysis and posteriorly through the midpoint of the body of the third sacral vertebra. This is roughly circular in shape with a diameter of 12 cm
   - The plane of the middle strait is bordered by the inferior edge of the pubic symphysis anteriorly, by the ischial spines laterally and by a point situated on the 4th–5th sacral vertebra, whose height varies with the inclination of the sacrum
   - The plane of the inferior pelvic strait.
2. *Hodge's system of parallel planes* (Fig. 5.2)
   - The first plane coincides with the superior pelvic strait
   - The second plane is projected between the inferior border of the pubic symphysis and the centre of the body of the second sacral vertebra. It is the plane of greatest diameter of the pelvic canal
   - The third plane passes through the ischial spines
   - The fourth through the tip of the coccyx.

The space comprised between Hodge's first two parallel planes is the widest of the cavity, and forms Pigeaud's cylinder of descent. The space between Hodge's second plane and the plane of the inferior pelvic strait forms Fochier's disengagement triangle (Fig. 5.3).

In our opinion, we need distinguished only two planes in the pelvic cavity: one, superior and projected mainly horizontally, which forms, at the arcuate pubic ligament, a junction with a second, inferior, vertically projected plane (Fig. 5.3).

The birth canal has two features:

1. At the superior pelvic strait, the diameters favouring engagement are the *oblique and transverse diameters* (refer to Fig. 2.1). At the inferior pelvic strait, however, due to the presence of the ascending branches of the pubis and levator ani muscles (Fig. 2.23), the only favourable diameter lies anteroposteriorly. The angle subtended between the diameters (favourable to engagement) of the superior pelvic strait and the anteroposterior diameter of the inferior pelvic strait, with which they share a common centre, ranges between 45° and 90°. The differing orientations of these diameters requires of the presenting part that, in order to engage, it has to align its greatest diameter with one of the aforementioned diameters (oblique or transverse); for disengagement along the anteroposterior diameter of the inferior pelvic strait, this entails that the presenting part combine a rotational movement with its descent, resulting in a helical movement.

THE CAESAREAN SECTION

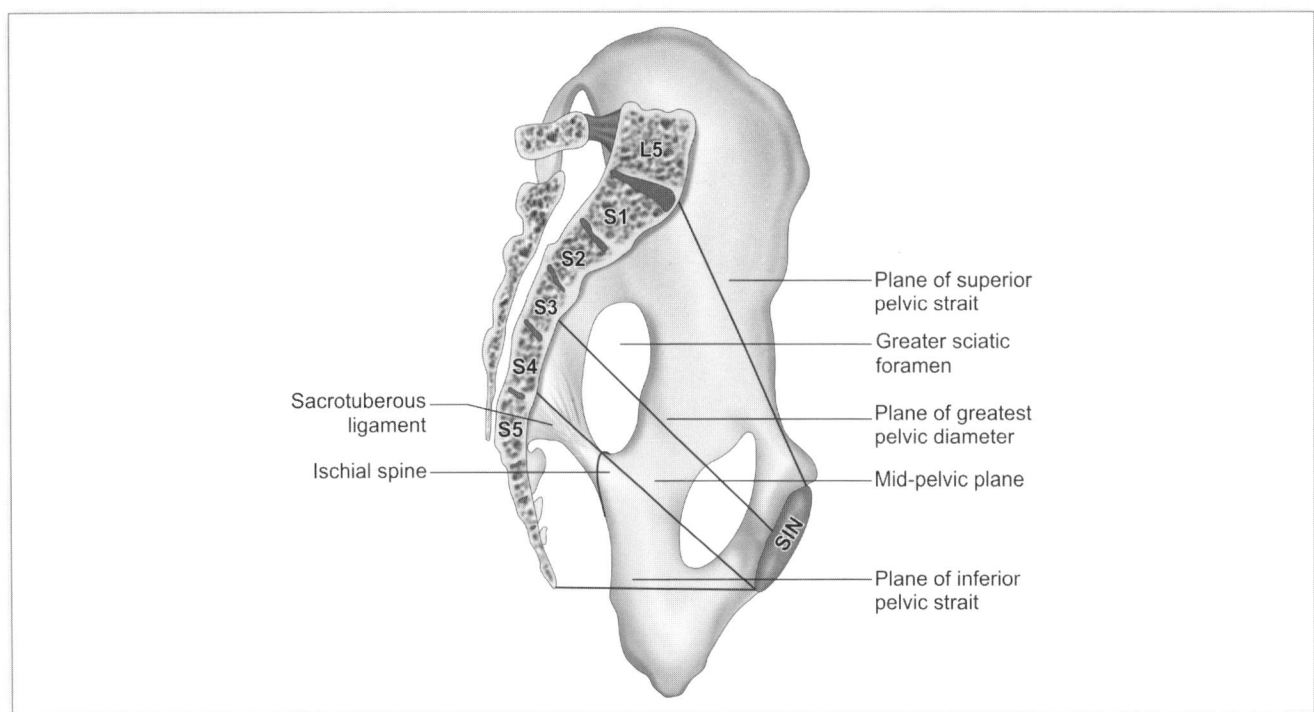

Fig. 5.1: Subdivision of pelvis into convergent planes

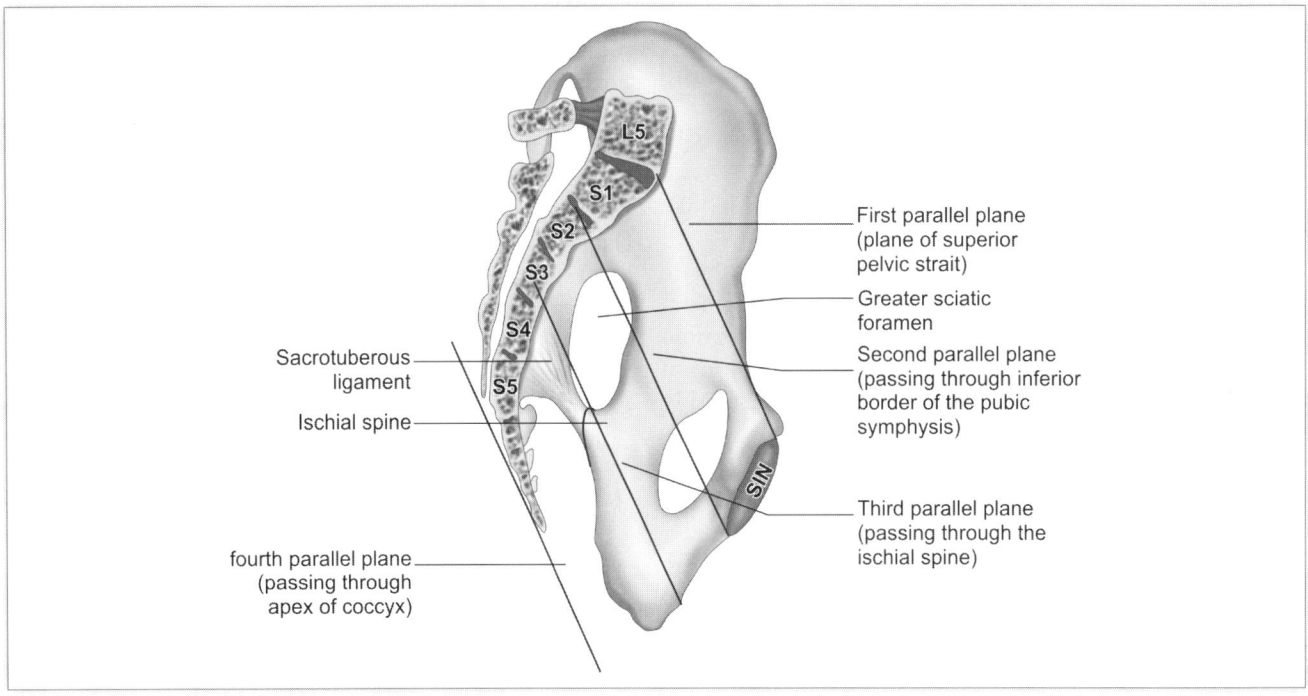

Fig. 5.2: Subdivision of pelvis into Hodge's parallel planes

MECHANISM AND PHYSIOPATHOLOGY OF PARTURITION

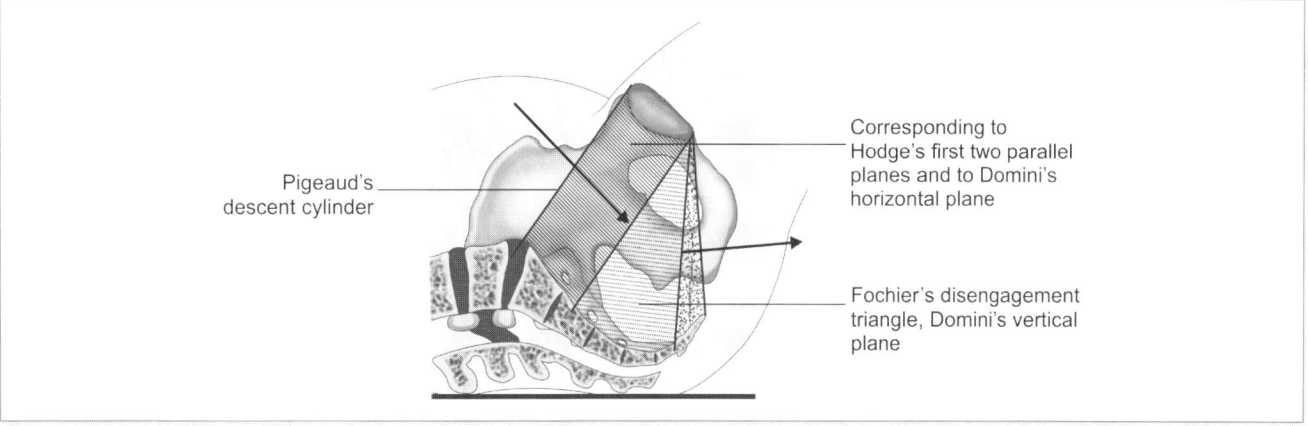

Fig. 5.3: 1. Pigeaud's descent cylinder (corresponding to Hodge's first two parallel planes and to Domini's horizontal plane)
2. Fochier's disengagement triangle; Domini's vertical plane

2. The birth canal does not describe a straight course, but a curvilinear, or *knee-shaped curvature* (refer to Fig. 2.21). The junction between the horizontally projected superior plane and the lower, vertical plane has as its landmark the arcuate pubic ligament with which the point of direction of the presenting part comes into contact, and around which it rotates as it passes along the sacral concavity in a "pendulum swing".

The *point of direction* refers to an arbitrary (usually the lowest) portion of the presenting part; in the usual cephalic presentation the point of direction is: *occiput* in well flexed head, *sinciput* (large fontanel presents) in partially flexed, *brow* in partially extended head, *chin* in extended head.

To summarise, within the mechanism of parturition, we distinguish two clearly distinct phases, unfolding at different times and in different planes:
1. The engagement, descent and rotation of the presenting part that unfold across a series of consecutive horizontal planes, during which a screw-like or helical manoeuvre is performed. These manoeuvres fall within Hodge's first two parallel planes, which coincide with Pigeaud's descent cylinder (Fig. 5.3).
2. Having completed these movements, the point of director of the presenting part makes contact with the arcuate pubic ligament, around which it rotates, entering Fochier's disengagement triangle and passing through the sacral concavity (vertical plane) until disengagement (Fig. 5.3).

MECHANISM OF PARTURITION

We may distinguish within the mechanism of parturition: presentation, engagement, descent with rotation, and progression.

PRESENTATION

The presenting part meets the superior pelvic strait and identifies, *during the course of a series of random movements*, an ovoid area: *area of engagement* whose spatial dimensions favour engagement. Areas of engagement vary with pelvic morphology:
- In the *gynecoid pelvis* (refer to Fig. 2.27), the major axes are the left or right oblique diameters and areas of engagement develop around these (Fig. 5.4). The transverse diameter is not used because, although larger in the dry pelvis, it is not *in vivo*, due to the psoas and iliacus muscles
- In the *android and anthropoid pelvis*, the major axis is the anteroposterior diameter
- In the *platypelloid pelvis*, the major axis is the transverse diameter.

Once this area has been individuated, engagement follows.

Table 5.1

Pelvic type and foetal position

Pelvic morphology	Favourable position	Unfavourable position
Android	OP - OT	OA
Anthropoid	OP - OA	OT
Gynecoid	OA - OT - OP	

ENGAGEMENT

Engagement refers to the achievement of overcoming the plane of the superior pelvic strait by the largest plane of progression for that particular presentation (Fig. 5.12A to C). This can be

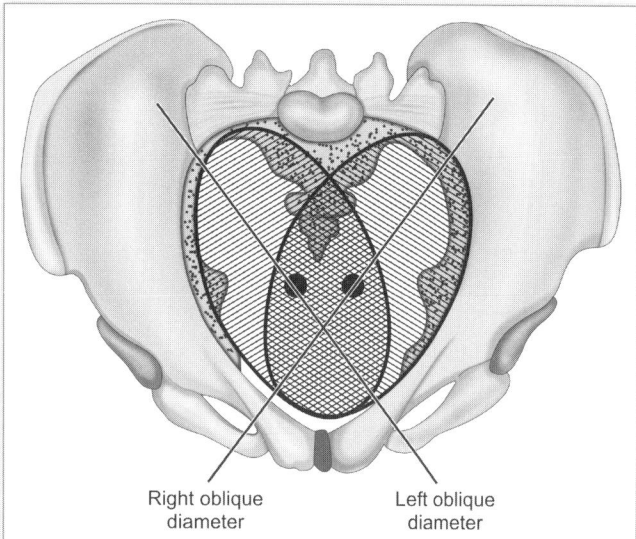

Fig. 5.4: Ellipsoids, or areas of engagement according to Renther: In the gynecoid pelvis, these are oval areas having an oblique diameter as their major axis. These have the most favourable ratio between capacity (containing aptitude) and the volume of the foetal head

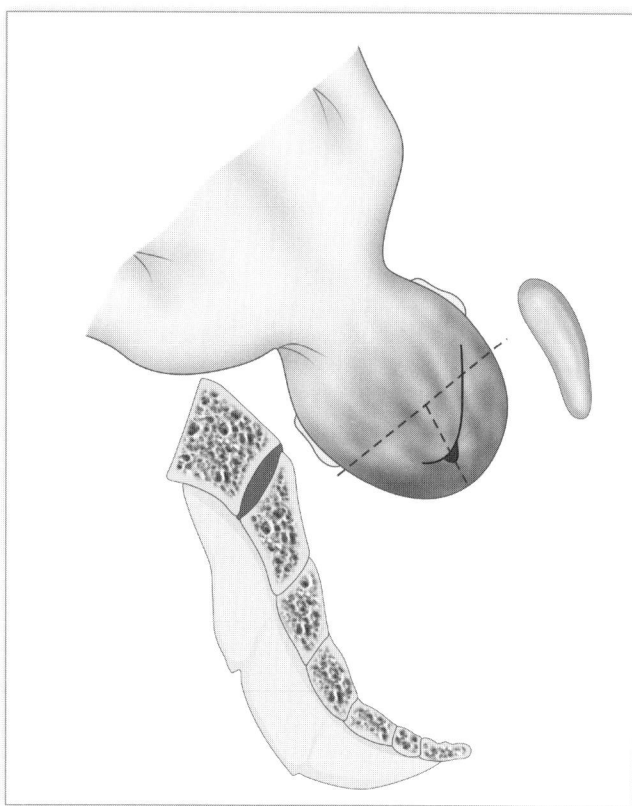

Fig. 5.5: Synclitism: Alignment of the cephalic plane with the superior pelvic strait occurs as a result of lateral flexion of the cervical vertebrae, with convexity in the direction of the abdominal wall

achieved only if there is a favourable relation between the dimensions of the presenting part and pelvic capacity. When this condition is met, the smaller the size of the *exposed or presenting surface*, the easier will the engagement be.

The minimum presented or exposed surface is therefore that feature which the presenting part makes ready for engagement. This occurs by means of two mechanisms: *alignment* and *diametral substitution, or flexion*, which take place in consecutive steps.

Alignment: The foetal head positions itself in a plane parallel (synclitism) to that of the superior pelvic strait (Fig. 5.5). The process by which, in a pelvis of normal morphology and inclination, the cephalic plane comes into alignment with that of the superior pelvic strait, is as follows: when a parietal bone bumps against the promontory, the head is held on that side and, due to the weight of the trunk bearing down from above, the cervical vertebrae undergo a slight lateral flexion, with a convexity directed towards the abdominal wall. This aligns the axis of the head perpendicularly to the plane of the pelvic inlet *synclitism*.

Failure to meet this condition is referred to as *asynclitism* and it leads to an increase in the area of sectional surface in direct proportion to the degree of obliquity, thereby impeding engagement.

With synclitism the major axis of the foetus, perpendicular to the plane of the superior pelvic strait, coincides with the axis of the birth canal (Fig. 5.6); engagement is thereby promoted by the weight of the foetal head.

We recall from Chapter 2 that in the standing position, the superior pelvic strait is inclined from top to bottom and from back to front, forming an angle of approx. 60° (Naegele) or of 35° and 75° (Jacobs) to the horizontal plane. In a woman in the sacrodorsal position, this angle equals approx. 42°.

The causes of asynclitism include as follows:

Normal Pelvis

- Inclination is normal, but due to a pendulous maternal belly, the major axis of the foetus adopts a nearly horizontal lie; engagement is not possible, leading to one of the causes of (posterior) uterine rupture, frequent among the multiparous
- The pelvis is either under- or over-inclined: *Inclination dystocia*. Under-inclination is typical among primigravidae, with the pelvic inlet lying almost vertically, and the maternal spine impeding correct alignment of the foetal spine and head. With over-inclination, the major foetal axis does not align with the axis of the birth canal.

Long Pelvis

Of which we distinguish two variants: the assimilation pelvis (refer to Fig. 2.29) and the arrest pelvis (refer to Fig. 2.30). Please refer to Chapter 2 for definitions.

MECHANISM AND PHYSIOPATHOLOGY OF PARTURITION

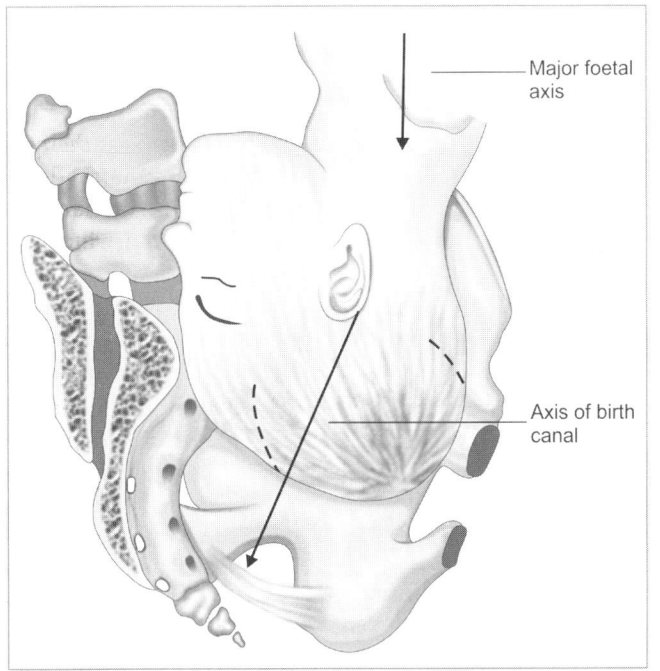

Fig. 5.6: 1. Major foetal axis 2. Axis of birth canal.

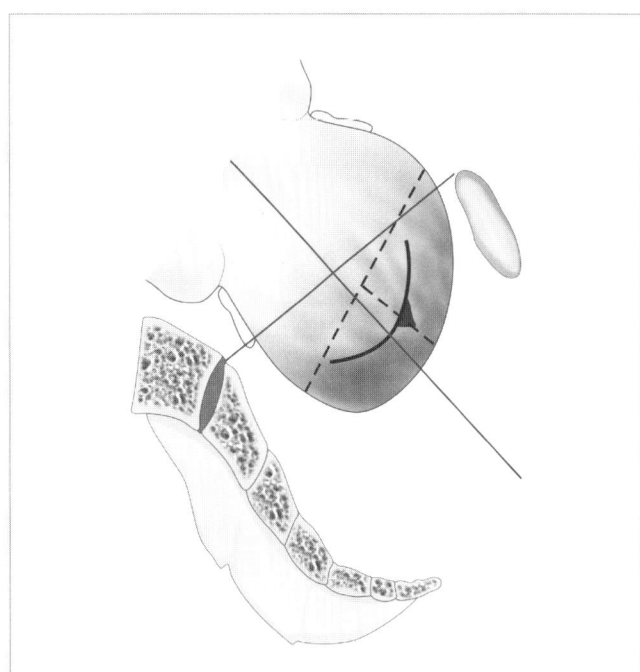

Fig. 5.7: Posterior parietal presentation at the brim (Litzman obliquity). The sagittal suture runs close to the symphysis

Here asynclitism may be posterior or anterior.

Posterior asynclitism, or posterior parietal obliquity, or *Litzman's obliquity* (Fig. 5.7): the posterior half of the head lowers into the pelvis, while the anterior half is held up on its descent. For this reason, the sagittal suture inclines toward the anterior pelvis and the foetal axis falls posteriorly to the axis of the superior pelvic strait. Aetiology may be traced to one or more of the following conditions:
- Platypelloid or mixed platypelloid pelvis (platypelloid android, or platypelloid-anthropoid)
- Pelvic inclination less than the norm <72°–40°
- Parous status (according to Deseigneux). This can be seen mainly in primigravidae, whose rigid abdominal wall compresses the uterus and the foetal body against the vertebral column, displacing the foetal axis posteriorly with respect to the pelvic axis.

Anterior asynclitism, or anterior parietal presentation, or *Naegele's obliquity* (Fig. 5.8): the anterior parietal bone presents inferior to the posterior; the sagittal suture inclines toward the posterior pelvic wall and the foetal axis lies posteriorly to the axis of the superior pelvic strait. Aetiology may be traced to one or more of the following conditions:
- Platypelloid or gynecoid platypelloid pelvis
- Pelvic inclination above the norm
- Parous status, in the multiparous with pendulous belly.

Once the cephalic plane has aligned with the plane of the superior pelvic strait, there follows the second mechanism, that of *diametral substitution* (reduction, flexion). When the

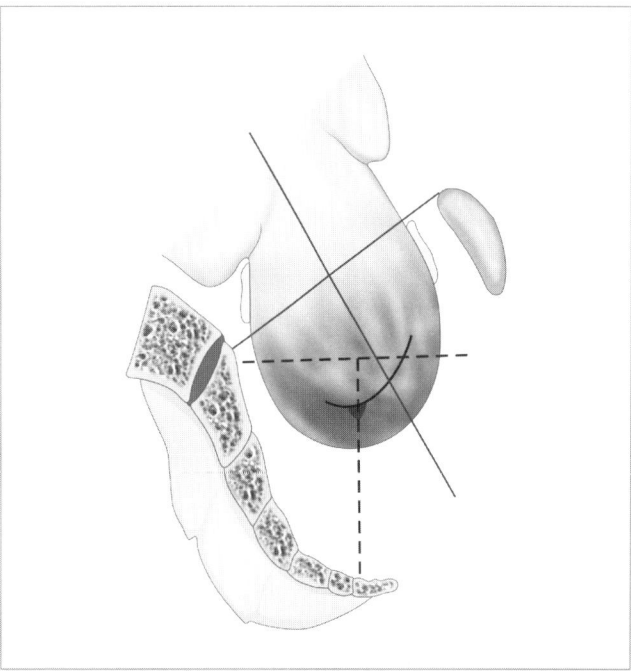

Fig. 5.8: Anterior parietal presentation at the brim (Naegele's obliquity). The sagittal suture runs close to the posterior pelvic wall

cephalic plane is parallel with that of the superior pelvic strait (Fig. 5.9), the presenting part faces the pelvic inlet in a bregma presentation (Figs 5.9 and 5.10B) in which

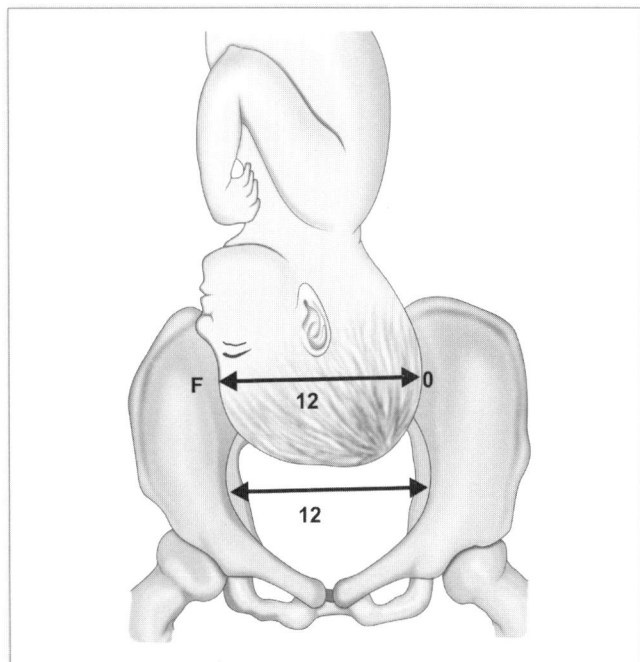

Fig. 5.9: The cephalic plane is parallel to the plane of the superior pelvic strait, the bregma presentation

the greatest diameter is the occipitofrontal diameter (Fig. 5.11) and the maximum advancig circumference is 34 cm (Fig. 5.12B).

This bregma presentation transforms into the vertex presentation (Figs 5.10 A and 5.14), replacing the occipitofrontal diameter (Fig. 5.11) with the suboccipitobregmatic or small oblique diameter, projected between the nape and the midpoint of the anterior fontanelle (9.5 cm). This decreases the maximum advancing circumference from 32 cm to 28 cm (Fig. 5.12A).

The *mechanism by which the head is flexed* can be described as follows (Fig. 5.13): The basis of the skull, from the frontal eminence (A) to the occipital protuberance (B), can be seen as a lever (occipitofrontal diameter) and its implantation on the spine (atlanto-occipital joint) as an (eccentric) fulcrum (F). Thereby a long arm (AF) is formed, from the frontal eminences to the atlanto-occipital joint, and a short arm (BF), from the atlanto-occipital joint to the occipital eminence. When the head meets a resistance from the superior pelvic strait, the point through which this force is transferred (the atlanto-occipital joint), becomes the fulcrum of the lever, and the resistance force applied to the longer arm predominates, for this reason the end of arm AF rises and the head flexes (Fig. 5.14).

Because engagement becomes easier as the amount of surface area facing the superior pelvic strait decreases, (as can be seen with the flexed head); it seems evident that in the opposite circumstances the increase of deflection of the head will lead to an increase of the presenting surface and of the cephalic advancing circumference, leading to greater difficulties with the engagement and progression of the presenting part.

The mechanism of flexion is influenced by the morphology of the head, which can be *dolichocephalic*, *mesocephalic* or *brachycephalic*. In dolichocephaly, the longitudinal axis prevail; in brachycephalic, the transverse one. The three cranial type of the skull are distinguished by the cephalic index (CI), which is obtained from the ratio between the biparietal and occiputofrontal diameters.

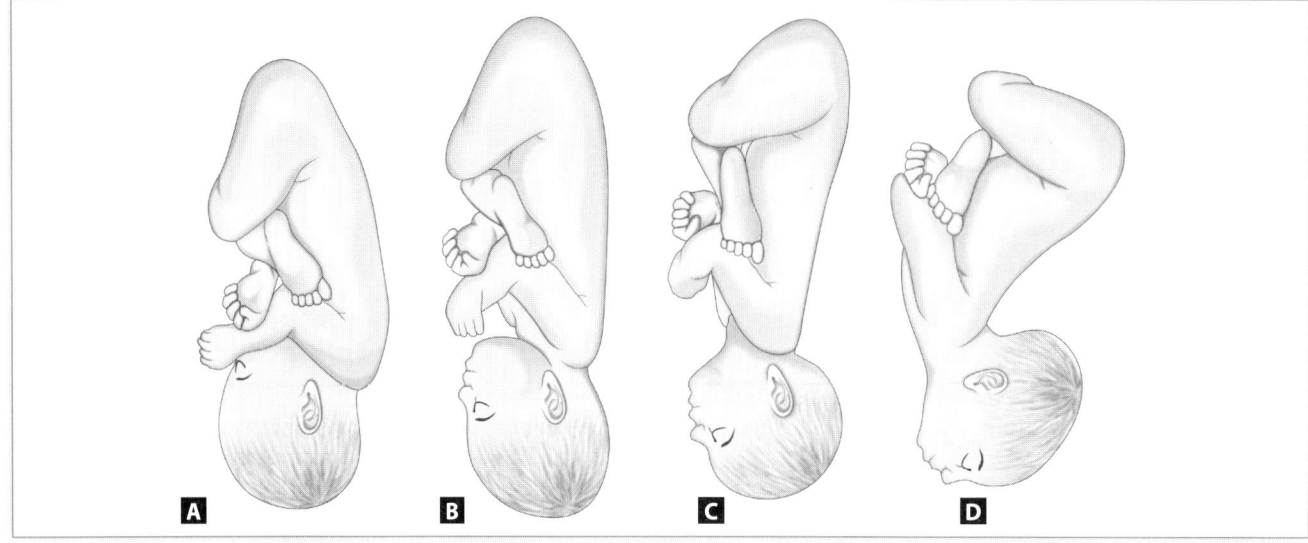

Fig. 5.10A to D: Various foetal head attitudes: (A) flexed (vertex presentation); (B) Partially flexed (bregma presentation); (C) Deflexed (brow presentation); (D) Extended (face presentation)

MECHANISM AND PHYSIOPATHOLOGY OF PARTURITION

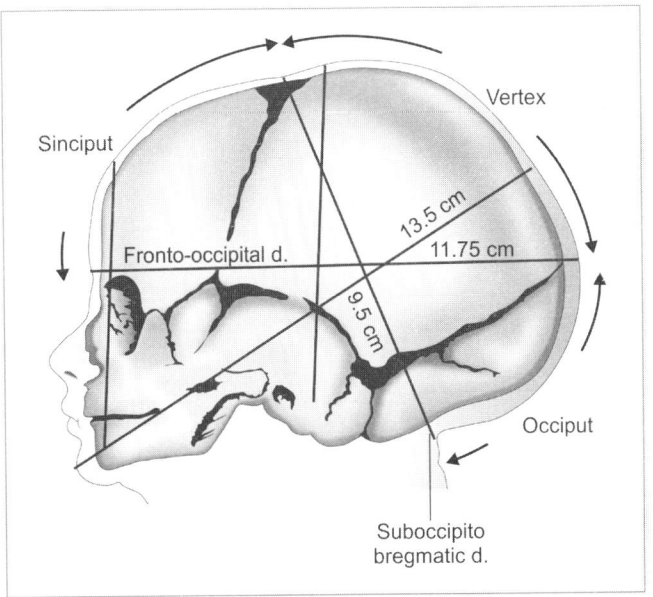

Fig. 5.11: Cranium of infant, major diameters, lateral veiws

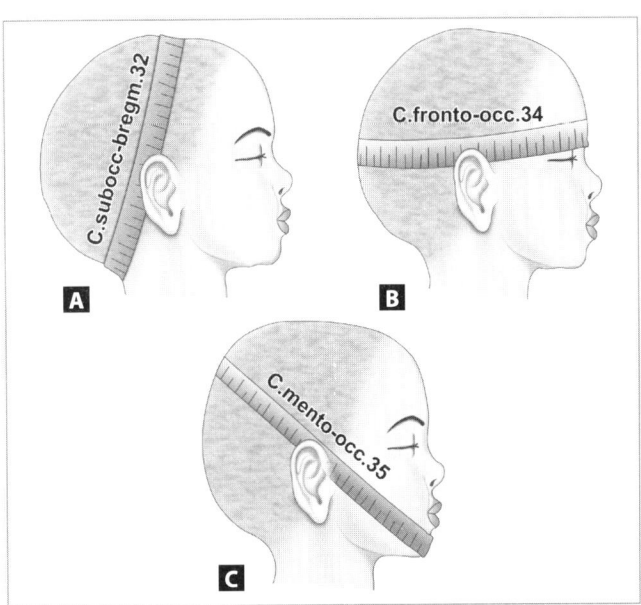

Fig. 5.12A to C: Maximum advancing circumference. (A). Vertex presentation; (B). Bregma presentation; (C) Brow and face presentation

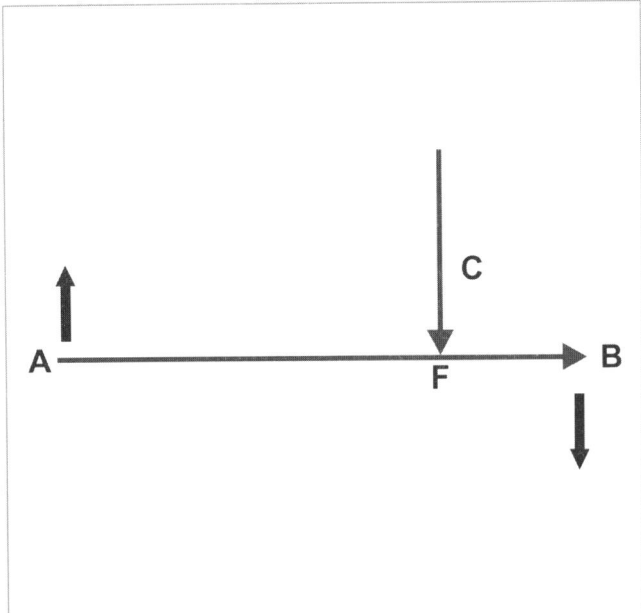

Fig. 5.13: Diagram showing lever action producing flexion of head. Conversion of occipitofrontal diameter into suboccipitobregmatic one

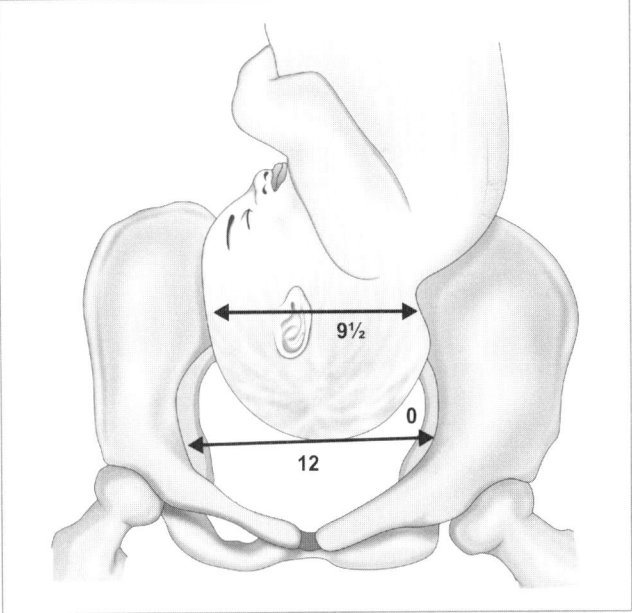

Fig. 5.14: Flexion has occurred: Engagement is along the suboccipitobregmatic diameter

Normal values range between 0.75 and 0.85; values above 0.85 indicate brachycephaly; values below 0.75, dolichocephaly.

When the cephalic index is close to an outlying value, the biparietal diameter cannot be used and is replaced by the cranial circumference.

The reason why the flexion mechanism is influenced by cranial morphology is intuitively clear: with dolichocephaly, the long arm (AF) of the lever is longer than in the mesocephalic case, and so flexion will be facilitated. The opposite holds in the brachycephalic condition, where flexion will be more difficult.

The *maximum advancing circumference*, which, as we have seen, is minimised with head flexed, increases with the degree of head deflexion (extension), and the theoretical obstacles to engagement increase proportionately. Engagement occurs:
- Along the occipitofrontal diameter (Fig. 5.11, projected from the brow to the most prominent point of the occiput, 12 cm) when the head is partially deflexed (bregma presentation, Fig. 5.10B). This corresponds to a maximum advancing circumference of 34 cm (Fig. 5.12B); Crichton's fifths are equal on each side (refer to Fig. 6.12).
- Along the occipitomental or major oblique diameter, 13.5 cm, projected from the chin to the most prominent point of the occiput, when the head is deflexed by a degree of deflexion just greater than in the bregma presentation. This corresponds to a maximum advancing circumference of 35–36 cm. Crichton's fifths on the occiput side now outnumber those on the sinciput side. Here we distinguish between:
  - Brow presentation
  - Face presentation: In the latter, the head is in maximum deflexion or extension. There are two variants of this:
    1. Dorsoposterior (chin in anterior position)—parturition possible.
    2. Dorsoanterior (chin in posterior position)—parturition impossible.

It seems clear that the greater the deflexion, the greater is the the circumference of the largest plane of progression and the more and the more the parturition mechanism is altered.

DESCENT, ROTATION AND PROGRESS

While engagement occurs exclusively through the power of contraction exerted by the uterus, descent and rotation are driven by two distinct and synergic mechanisms:
1. Force exerted from above.
2. The rotatory action of the levator ani muscles. These act in the following way: when the presenting part comes into contact with one muscle (right or left, depending on position), the muscle will compress and respond by contracting. Given the lateral position of the muscle, this translates into an impetus that completes the rotation. From this it is clear how cutting through or damaging one of the two levator ani muscles will slow down or compromise rotation in subsequent pregnancies.

After rotation is completed, there follows the second step, that of rotation of the presenting part around the arcuate pubic ligament, and its advancement. The point of direction (hypomoclion) comes into contact with and rotates around the pubic arcuate ligament, which represents the junction with the sagittal plane. This is to be traversed in a pendulum movement of the presenting part, until expulsion.

MECHANISM OF PARTURITION IN VARIOUS PELVIC TYPES

Gynecoid pelvis: As described above.

Android pelvis: Engagement of the head when possible is posterior occipital-iliac because the large occipital area fits better to the very wide posterior pelvic segment, while the smaller frontal area uses the narrower anterior pelvic segment. As the head descends, it meets increasing resistance caused by the funnelling of the walls at the android outlet. Labour progresses at a moderate pace and vaginal delivery, when it occurs, is difficult. Failure of rotation and deep transverse arrest are frequent. This constriction renders operative delivery problematic.

Anthropoid pelvis: The prognosis is more favourable than with android and platypelloid pelves: in about 2/3 of cases engagement is along the anteroposterior diameter. Engagement along the transverse diameter can take place only in a very broad pelvis. Occipitoposterior engagement is characterised by difficulty in rotation at the inferior pelvic strait: the '*persistent occiput posterior position*', but delivery can still take place in occipitoposterior engagement. Occipitoanterior engagement, which does not require rotation, is the most favourable and delivery is easier in this type of engagement.

Platypelloid pelvis: The greatest difficulties are encountered at engagement, which occurs along the transverse diameter, sometimes requiring a great deal of moulding. Having engaged, the head descends along the transverse diameter. As the platypelloid walls diverge, difficulty reduces as the foetus advances. Having reached the inferior pelvic strait, anterior rotation and delivery often occur at the perineum.

Assimilation pelvis: (refer to Figs 2.29 and 3.30) Difficulties associated with this condition are:
- The pelvic inlet has an almost vertical inclination: inclination dystocia
- Elongation of the pelvis.

CONCLUSION

An unfavourable relationship between presenting part and pelvis can present: (1) before engagement—in which case we are faced with *cephalopelvic disproportion*; (2) after engagement—here we are faced with *obstructed labour*, which may be traceable to:
- An anatomical obstruction (mechanical dystocia), present in various sections of the birth canal, which compromises advancement (descent and rotation) of the presenting part
- A functional obstruction: dynamic dystocia, contraction ring.

In either case, relevant *is not finding the causes, but swift detection of any signs of distress for the uterus, the foetus and the mother, whether of cephalopelvic disproportion or obstructed labour.*

SECTION 2

Diagnosis

- Diagnosis in Clinical Obstetrics
- Partograph

CHAPTER 6

Diagnosis in Clinical Obstetrics

INSTRUMENTS

a. Basic Equipment
   - Obstetric-gynaecological clinical record forms (Tables 6.1 and 6.2)
   - Midwifery ruler
   - Pen
   - Ruler
   - Weighing scale with built-in stadiometre. If the latter is not available, a normal builder's rule or a measuring tape fixed to a wall will suffice. Do not trust spring scales; they are unreliable in the tropics
   - Wall clock with clearly visible second hand
   - Sphygmomanometer with mercury column, preferably wall-mounted
   - Phonendoscope
   - Obstetrical stethoscope
   - Thermometer
   - Pelvimeter (Fig. 6.1)
   - Measuring tape
   - Reusable Cusco vaginal speculum (shun disposable materials; they take up space, are used up quickly and their procurement is difficult)
   - There is no need for sterile gloves; disposable polyethylene gloves are fine.
b. Advanced instruments
   - Haemoglobin test strips with colour scale
   - Microscope for fresh wet vaginal fluor examination
   - Microscopic slides and cover glass
   - Glass tray with lid, sulfochromic solution (for re-using slides)
   - Isotonic saline
   - Potassium hydroxide (KOH) solution at 10% for *Sniff test*; on contact with KOH, *Gardnerella vaginalis* releases aromatic amines; also for microscopic marking of fungal infection.

DIAGNOSIS IN CLINICAL OBSTETRICS

The cornerstones of clinical obstetric diagnostics are the following:
- Case history
- Physical examination.

These set out to detect the existence of risk factors (Table 6.3) on which to base prognostic clinical judgments, and to provide the basis for agreeing with the gravida which methodologies should be followed during pregnancy and labour.

Case History

A distinction is made between general medical history and obstetric anamnesis.

General Medical History

This includes the collection, for the purposes of diagnosis, of data concerning the gravida's individual and family physiological and pathological medical history, not related to the current obstetric case.

Previous Obstetric History

This is divided into past and recent obstetric history.

44 THE CAESAREAN SECTION

Past obstetric history

Parity represents a risk factor due to repeated uterine involutions and the resulting reduction in tone of the abdominal wall (see also Chapter 21: Uterine Rupture).

The patient's obstetric history may be summarised by the following formula: "gravida 0000 para". Reading from left to right: the first figure indicates the number of pregnancies carried to term; the second, premature parturitions; the

---

Antepartum risk assessment/Intervention form

Client's Name_____ Age_____ Parity _____
Planned Delivery site_____ Date booked_____
Blood group_____ Rh_____ Hemoglobin type_____
Height in cms._____ Partner supportive?_____ Family supportive?____
Expected date of delivery_____ Education level_____

Medical/surgical history

Anemia_____
Sickle cell disease (joint pains)_____
Diabetes_____
Chest disease (asthma, TB)_____
Cardiac disease_____
Hypertension_____
Seizures (epilepsy)_____
Laparotomy (specific reason)_____
Other surgeries (specify)_____
Previous accidents_____
Other medical problems (specify)_____

Previous obstetrical history

Number of term births_____
Number of pre-term births_____
Number of abortions (Induced)_____
Number of abortion (spontaneous)_____
Number of stillborn_____
Number of C/sections_____
Number of children currently alive_____
Age youngest child_____
History antepartum hemorrhage_____
History of postpartum hemorrhage_____
History of retained placenta_____
History of long or obstructed labour_____
History of abnormal presentation (transverse, breech, face)_____
History of hypertension/pre-eclampsia, eclampsia_____

Menstrual history

Age of menarche_____
Last menstrual period _____ Duration_____ Amount_____
Last normal menstrual period_____
Examined by_____ Today's date_____

[Weight in kg vs. weeks of gestation chart: y-axis 40–120 kg, x-axis 10, 20, 30, 40 weeks]

Table 6.1A: Antepartum risk assessment form (American College of Nurse Midwives): Front page

DIAGNOSIS IN CLINICAL OBSTETRICS

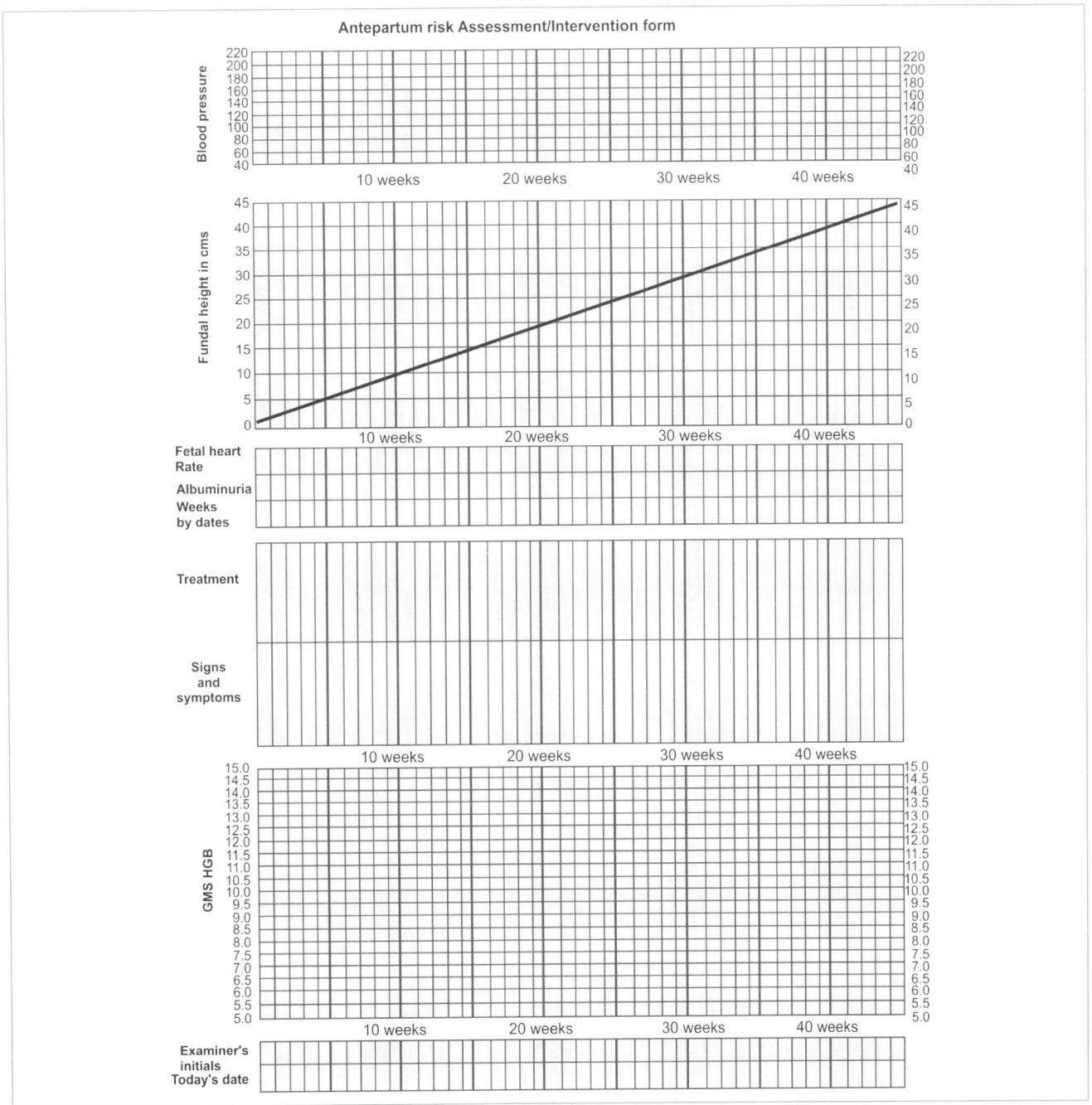

Table 6.1B: Antepartum risk assessment form (American College of Nurse Midwives): Back page

third, abortions or ectopic pregnancies; the fourth, the number of children now living. Therefore, a woman who has carried four pregnancies to term, three early childbirths and 1 abortion, all of whose children, both those born at term and those born prematurely are living, is *gravida 4 3 1 7 para* at x week (week of current pregnancy).

- *Uterine involution* is the process by which a postpartum uterus, weighing approx. 1 kg, returns to its prepregnant state, at a weight of approx. 100 grams.

The number of muscle-fibre cells remains unchanged: It is their volume that decreases through a process of autolysis, or enzymatic digestion of the cytoplasm, following activation of uterine collagenase and proteolytic enzymes. The proteins thereby released are conveyed to the capillary bed and hence eliminated with the urine.

The vascular component undergoes regressive processes, being replaced by fibrous tissue. Therefore, over the course of consecutive pregnancies, the uterine fibrous tissue/

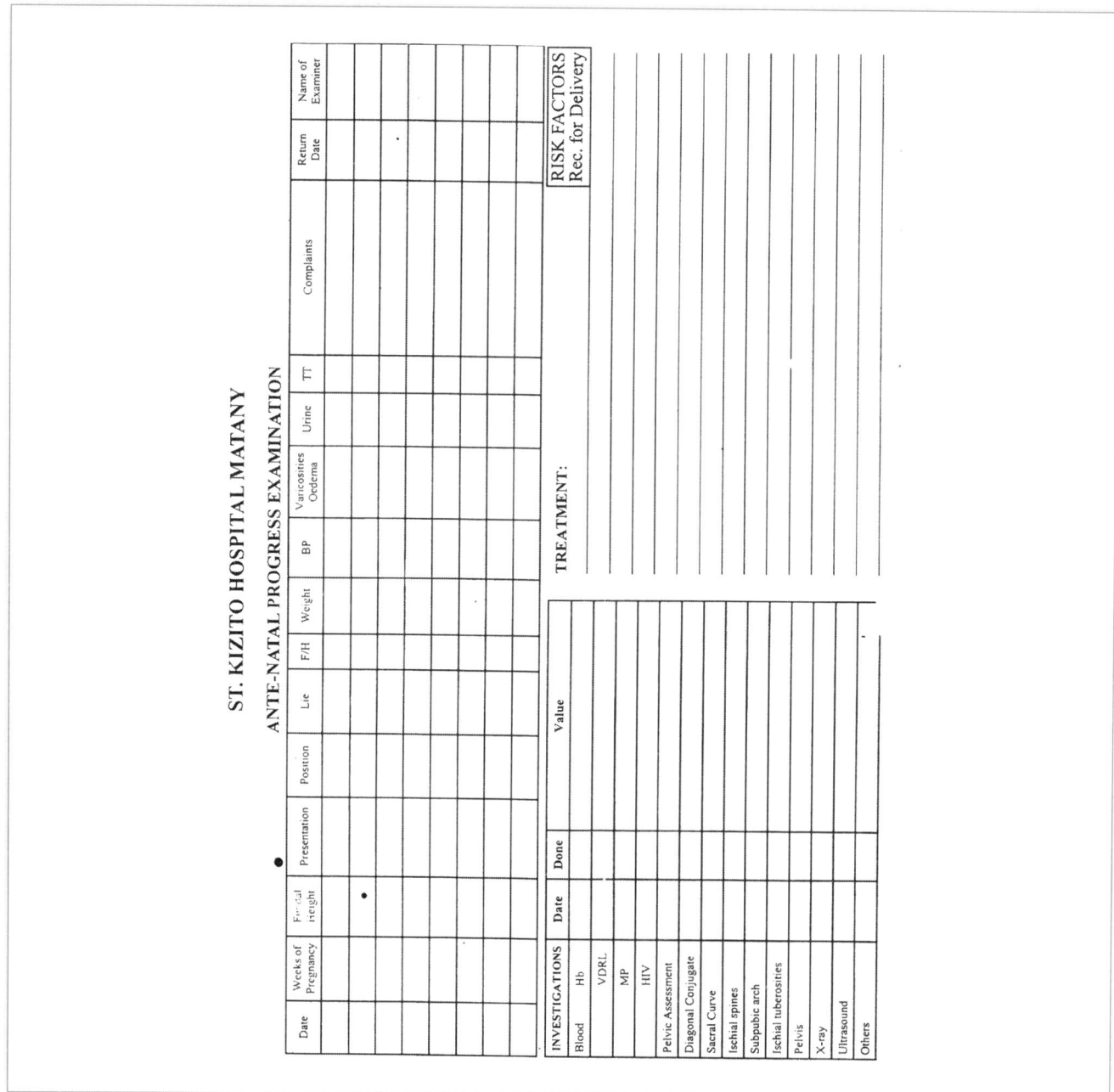

Table 6.2A: Antenatal monitoring form (Ugandan Ministry of Health): Front page

muscle tissue ratio alters in favour of the former. This gives rise to the following:

- Reduced tone of the myometrium, which is responsible for anomalies of foetal position, common among multiparae
- Hypokinesia during labour.

When associated with concomitant *deficit of the rectus abdominis muscles,* reduced myometrial tone will allow anterior displacement of the uterus: *Pendulous abdomen of the multipara.* As the major foetal axis is now no longer aligned along the axis of the birth canal, but towards the posterior LUS wall, posterior uterine ruptures are more common.

Table 6.2B: Antenatal monitoring form (Ugandan Ministry of Health): Back page

Obstetric history chart (Table 6.2B)

- *Urinary incontinence with postpartum onset:* Strain-related or continuous (vesicovaginal or ureterovaginal fistula)
- *Flatus or faecal incontinence*: Assess (see below) the condition of anal sphincters and rectum
- *Change in the quality of relationship with partner* following childbirth; assess the condition of the urogenital diaphragm.

Recent obstetric history

Active foetal movements: Period of appearance: From the 22nd week onwards in primigravidae, from 18th week onward in multiparae.

Pain

- *Affecting the LUS*, constant, where a hard, round structure is perceived; due to pressure exerted by the foetal head, *cephalic presentation*

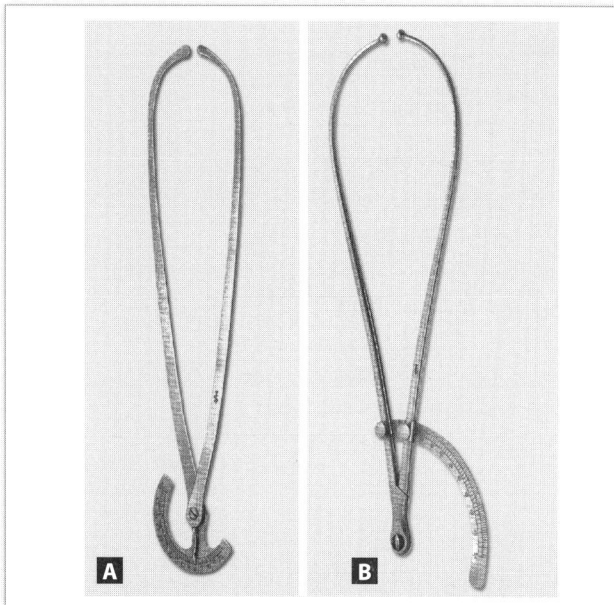

Fig. 6.1A and B: (A) Collin's pelvimeter; (B) Martin's pelvimeter

If the pain is located in the pubic area and is constant and intense, then, especially among primigravidae, a pelvic inclination incompatible with engagement should be ruled out. Where this possibility is excluded, we are most probably dealing with stress (distension) on the pubic symphysis joint; infiltrating the affected area with local anaesthetic will provide lasting relief.

- *On the lateral walls of the uterus*, from the inguinal canal to the uterine fundus, particularly during the final weeks of pregnancy and among primigravidae. This is due to stretching of the round ligaments and to dextrorotation of the uterus
- *At the LUS and round ligaments* concomitant with active foetal movements: A breech presentation is likely.

Physical Examination

A distinction is made between a general physical examination and an obstetric physical examination.

General Physical Examination

This takes the following factors into account (Tables 6.4 to 6.8):

Age: The female pelvis completes its development at around 18–20 years of age. In a gravida below this age, an incompletely developed pelvis should always be suspected

Height: A height below 152 cm is considered to be associated with pelvic anomaly in terms of capacity rather than morphology. Studies of a Congolese population (Liselele, 2000) have shown that the predictivity of this factor (21%) rises to 52% if it is associated with a transverse diameter of the lozenge of Michaelis of less than 9.5 cm.

Weight: Normal weight gain is 1 kg per month and it should not exceed 12 kg over the course of pregnancy, hence the advisability of faithfully recording weight gain at each obstetric examination.

In resource-poor countries, the two extremes of malnutrition and obesity are often observed. The latter is an expression of relative affluence and is becoming increasingly common. Both represent risk factors (Table 6.3).

Table 6.3
Risk factors

• Preexisting hypertension during pregnancy
• Immune system syndromes
• Nephropathy
• Diabetes
• Cardiopathy
• Epilepsy
• Prior systemic diseases
• Maternal age <17 or >35 years
• Hereditary, familial diseases
• Exposure to env. or teratogen risks
• Drug dependency
• Prepregnant weight < or >20% ideal BMI
• Smoker
• Alcohol
• Blood transfusion
• Allergies
	• Habitual abortion
	• Prior late abortion/pre-term delivery
	• Prior intrauterine death cause unknown
	• Prior foetal hypo-development or macrosomia
	• Prior foetal distress during labour
	• Prior gestational diabetes
	• Maternal–foetal isoimmunisation
	• Prior congenital anomalies
	• Prior surgery
	• Prior uterine surgery
	• Pregnancy following assisted fertilization
		• Abnormal ultrasound findings (retarded foetal growth, malformation, anomalous placenta insertion)
		• Gestational hypertension
		• Gemellarity
		• Oligo/polyhydramnios
		• Infections with risk of transmission to foetus
		• Cervical incontinence
		• Uterine myoma
		• Term breech presentation
		• Pathological laboratory data:
		  – Dysmetabolic syndrome
		  – Altered renal function
		  – Coagulopathies
		  – Altered hepatic function
		  – Maternal–foetal incompatibility

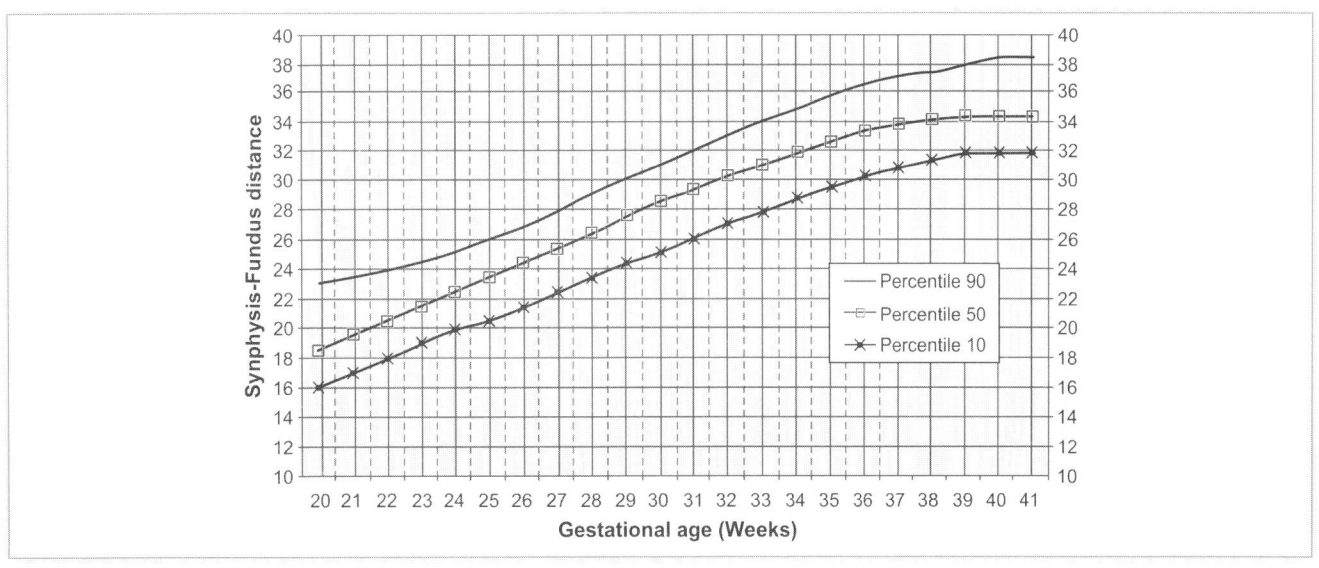

Table 6.4: Fundal height chart (SFD): On y-axis, fundal height expressed in centimetres; on x-axis, gestational age. Normal values lie within a range 2 cm above and below the mean (10th and 90th percentile)

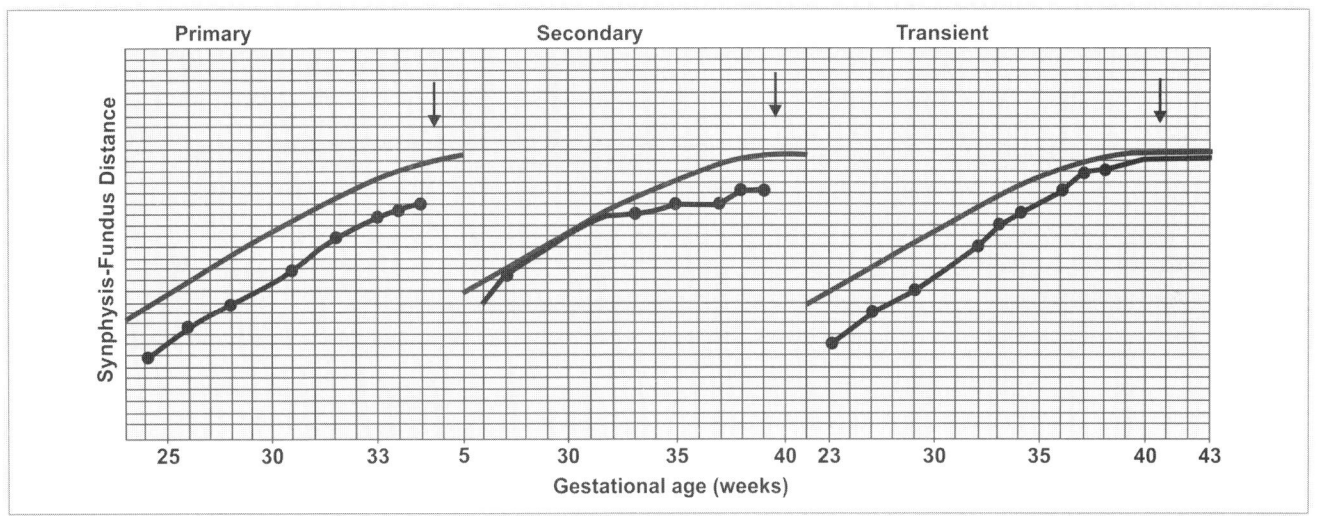

Table 6.5: Fundal height in different types of growth retardation: (from left to right) primary, secondary, transient

- *In malnutrition*: Foetus small for gestational stage
- *In obesity*: Cephalopelvic disproportion is a frequent observation. It is sustained by:
  - *Reduced pelvic diameters* resulting from the deposit of adipose tissue inside the pelvis (Sellheim's panniculus adiposus)
  - Foetus of a weight incompatible with the gravid patient's bone structure.

The nutritional condition of the gravid patient is found:
- *Within the first trimester* from:
  - The patient's body mass index (BMI): Weight divided by the square of height, or by using Table 6.7.

Risk conditions are represented by a BMI <18.5 or > 32.3;
Malnutrition Grade 1: BMI <18.5
Malnutrition Grade 2: BMI <17
Malnutrition Grade 3: BMI <16
Malnutrition Grade 4: BMI <14
Malnutrition Grade 5: BMI <13

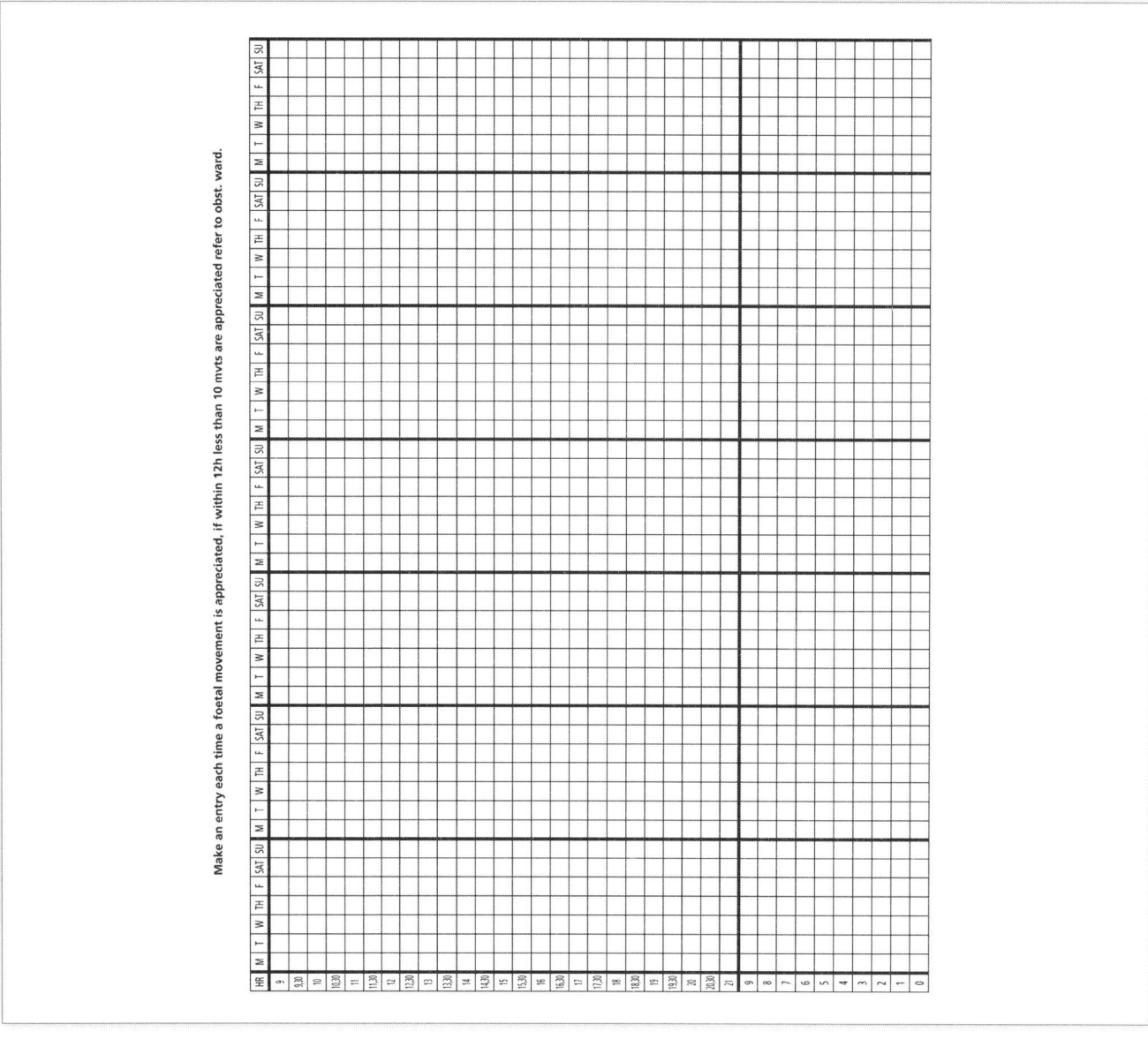

Table 6.6: Cardiff counting system for assessing foetal well-being. See text for explanation

- During the following trimesters, the middle upper arm circumference (MUAC) or brachial perimetry is used; the circumference of the median part of the arm measured using a simple tape.
  MUAC <190 mm: Moderate malnutrition (grade 3 malnutrition; needs food supplementation)
  MUAC <160 mm: Severe malnutrition (grade 5 malnutrition, extreme wasting), with recent weight loss and with bilateral lower leg oedema (other possible causes excluded)
  - *During the first three months of breastfeeding*:
  - Moderate malnutrition BMI = 16.0 to 16.9
  - Severe malnutrition: BMI <16.0 or MUAC <160 mm

Body surface area it is expressed in square meters and is obtained using the Dubois body surface nomograph (Table 6.8). Daily fluid requirement is 1,500 mL per square meter of body surface, which should be increased by 500 mL for every degree of temperature exceeding 37°C.

Skin: Normal, hydrated, dehydrated.

Mucosa: Anaemia, jaundice, cyanosis.

Organs and Systems

- *Respiratory system*: inspection, palpation, percussion and auscultation.
- *Cardiovascular system*: heart, cardiac silhouette, heart sounds

DIAGNOSIS IN CLINICAL OBSTETRICS

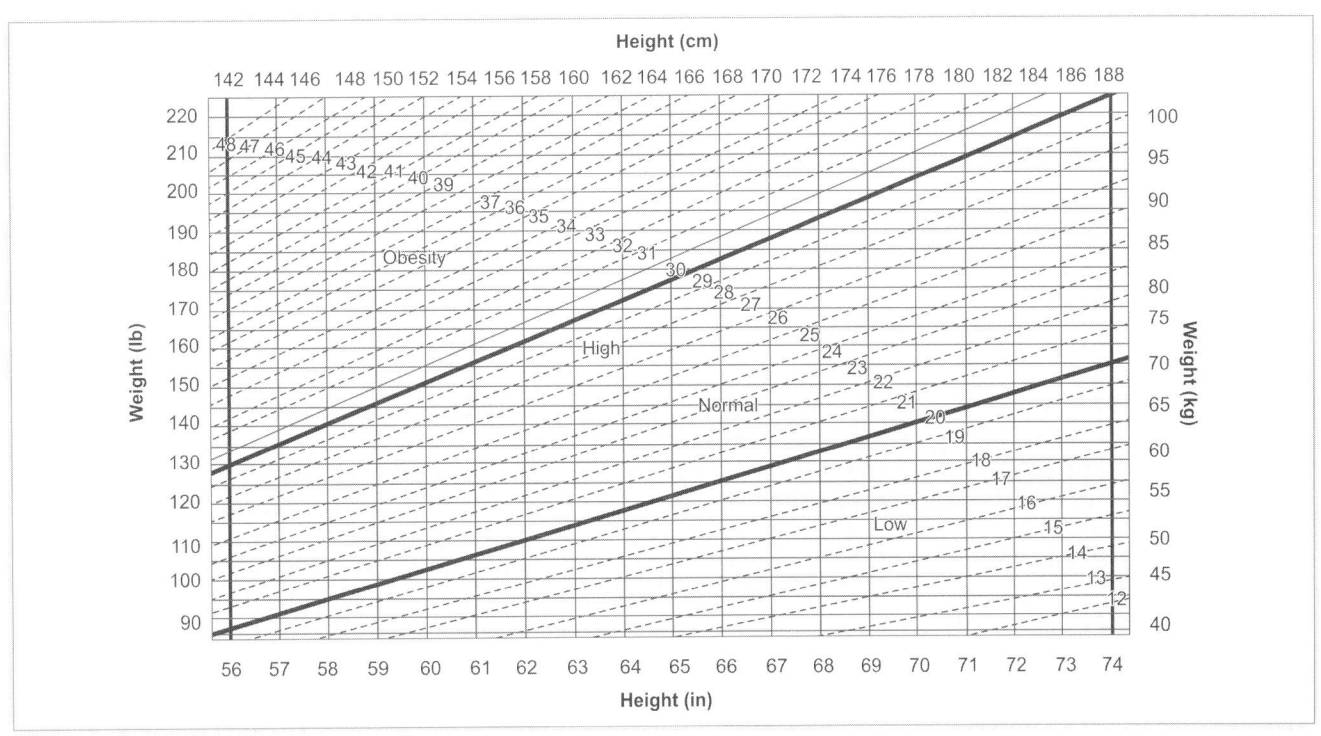

Table 6.7: Body mass index: The first column on the left shows height in centimetres; the top row shows weight in kilograms. Risk conditions are represented by a BMI of <18.5 or >32.3. See text for explanation.

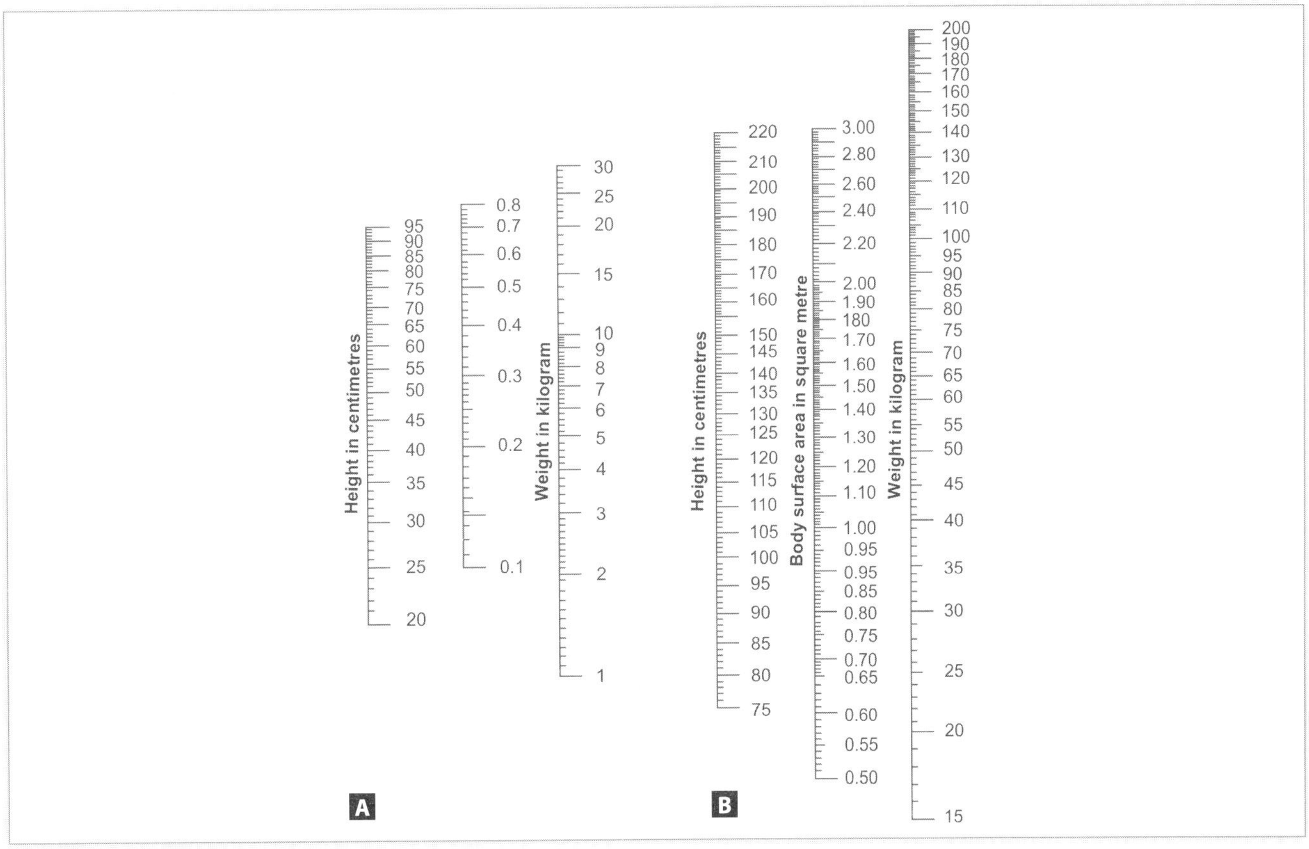

Table 6.8: Dubois body surface area nomograph: (A) Children; (B) Adults. A straight line joining the value for height with that for weight crosses the body surface area scale

Arterial pressure: This should be recorded faithfully at each obstetric examination, measured with the patient semi-seated at an inclination of 45°. The pressure cuff is placed at heart level. Confirmation of diagnosis requires numerous observations; the 5th Korotkoff sound indicates diastolic pressure.

We believe it also essential to determine *mean or integrated arterial pressure* corresponding to a diastolic pressure + 1/3 of the AP differential.

$$\text{Mean AP} = \text{Diast. P.} + \frac{\text{Syst. P} - \text{Diast. P}}{3}$$

For example: Left Humeral Arterial Pressure 170/110

$$\text{Mean AP} = 110. + \frac{170 - 110}{3} = \frac{60}{3} = 20; \quad 110 + 20 = 130$$

- *Capillaries* (capillary refill time in case of anaemia or dehydration) (Table 11.1):
- *Oedema* of the face, of the lower limbs: Measurement may be made of the ankle or foot circumference; more objective than just the fovea
- *Abdomen:* Morphology, scars, masses, effusions
- *Liver*
- *Spleen*: Palpation of the spleen is, in the Tropics, an essential step. Splenomegaly is measured as the number of transverse fingerbreadths distally to the costal arch that the inferior pole of the spleen can be palpated
- *Urinary system*
  - Palpation
  - Percussion
  - Ureteral points.

Often, in the tropics, it is not so easy to determine the exact location of pain. In our opinion, in diagnosing urinary and other pathologies, Jarricot's dermatome areas of cutaneous hyperaesthesia or 'areas of reflected dermatalgia' (Fig. 6.2) are of great assistance. The areas are identified by patient reaction, but especially through the operator's tactile perception.

The method is as follows: A fold of skin is grasped between the thumbs and forefingers of both hands, and it is rolled under the fingers; when you approach a painful area, an increase in the thickness of the skinfold can be appreciated, concomitantly with a pain reaction by the patient. Each area corresponds to a deep viscera.

- *Nervous system*
  Glasgow coma scale (Table 6.9)

The Glasgow coma scale provides a practical method for assessment of impairment of conscious level in response to defined stimuli; it is composed of three parameters: Best eye response, best verbal response, best motor response.

The GCS is scored between 3 and 15, 3 being the worst, and 15 the best; a coma score of 13 or higher correlates with

Table 6.9
Glasgow coma scale

Area assessed	Response	Points
Eye opening	Open spontaneously; open with blinking at baseline	4
	Open to verbal command; speech, or shout	3
	Open in response to pain applied to the limbs or sternum	2
	None	1
Verbal	Oriented	5
	Confused conversation, but able to answer questions	4
	Inappropriate responses: words discernible	3
	Incomprehensible speech	2
	None	1
Motor	Obeys commands for movement	6
	Responds to pain with purposeful movement	5
	Withdraws from pain stimuli	4
	Responds to pain with abnormal (spastic) flexion (decorticate posture)	3
	Responds to pain with abnormal (rigid) extension (decerebrate posture)	2
	None	1

a *mild brain injury*, 9-12 is a *moderate injury* and 8 or less a *severe brain injury*.

Note that the phrase "GCS of 11" is essentially meaningless, and it is important to break the figure down into its components, such as E3V3M5 = GCS11.

Reflexes

- *Corneal reflex*
- *Tendon reflexes*: These provide useful indications of whether seizure may be imminent, of the presence of hypertension or of a clinical picture compatible with preeclampsia. The *biceps* and *patellar reflexes* are tested
- The *biceps reflex* is provoked in a slightly flexed arm by tapping the tendon of the biceps brachii muscle inside the fold of the elbow: under normal conditions, the forearm will jerk. One proceeds as follows: if the patient is lying down, the arm is semi-flexed; if she is seated, the examiner supports the arm, rests his/ her thumb (Fig. 6.3A) or middle finger (Fig. 6.3B) onto the tendon (if it

DIAGNOSIS IN CLINICAL OBSTETRICS

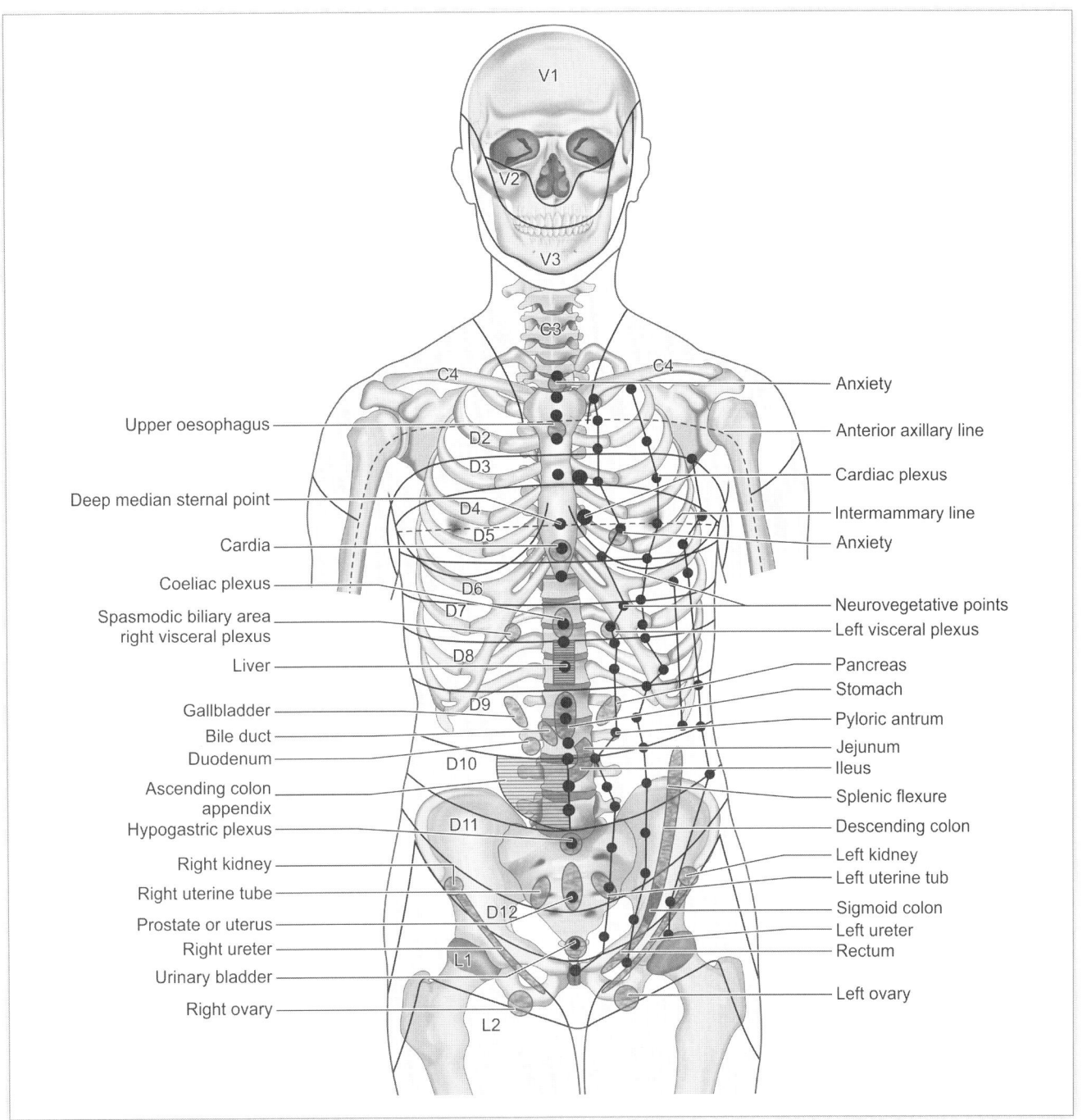

Fig. 6.2: Jarricot's reflex dermalgias and their metameric projections

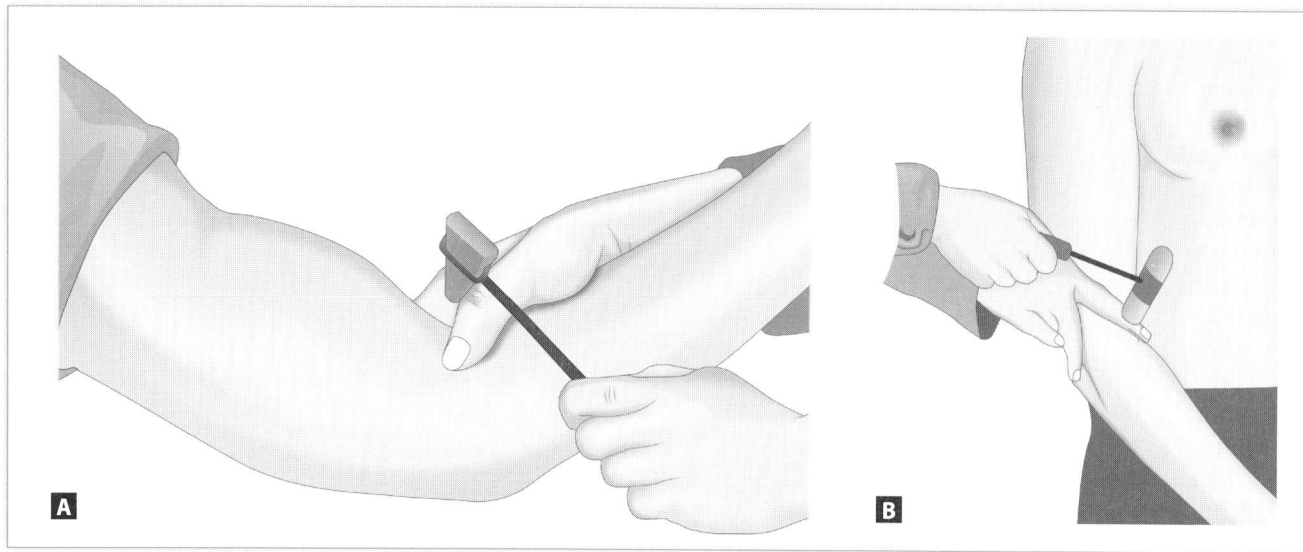

Fig. 6.3A and B: Testing the biceps reflex. (A) Thumb on tendon; (B) Index finger on tendon

is difficult to locate, flexing and extending the forearm will bring it out) and uses the tendon hammer to strike the nailbed of the thumb or middle finger, assessing the response.

- *Patellar reflex* (Fig. 6.4): this is obtained with the patient seated and leg overhanging the bed. Under normal conditions, tapping just below the patella one obtains an extension of the leg from the thigh due to contraction of the quadriceps muscle. In case of difficulty, move the leg until the tendon is detected, giving it a sharp blow. This reflex can also be tested for with the patient lying down; in this case, the leg is supported by the hand.

Point score
0 = no response
1 = reduced, but within norm
2 = normal response
3 = faster than normal
4 = accentuated, abnormal, may be accompanied by clonic contractions (rhythmic tremor).

If a preeclamptic patient presents hyperreflexia (+3 +4), there is a high probability of attacks developing. It is advisable to undertake appropriate treatment as soon as possible.

Obstetric Physical Examination

This comprises a clinical examination of the abdomen and of the pelvis.

Clinical Examination of the Abdomen

The essential steps are as follows:
- Observation
- Palpation
- Auscultation of foetal heartbeat
- Assessment of the dimensions, morphology and inclination of the pelvis
- Pelvic examination.

Correct observation and palpation of the abdomen can establish gestational age, lie, presentation and—in the case of cephalic presentation—engagement, position and flexion or deflection of the head. Our diagnostic pathway is as follows.

Observation

- *Abdominal morphology*:
  – Oval in longitudinal direction: longitudinal lie
  – Oval in transverse direction: transverse lie
  – Oval in oblique direction: oblique lie

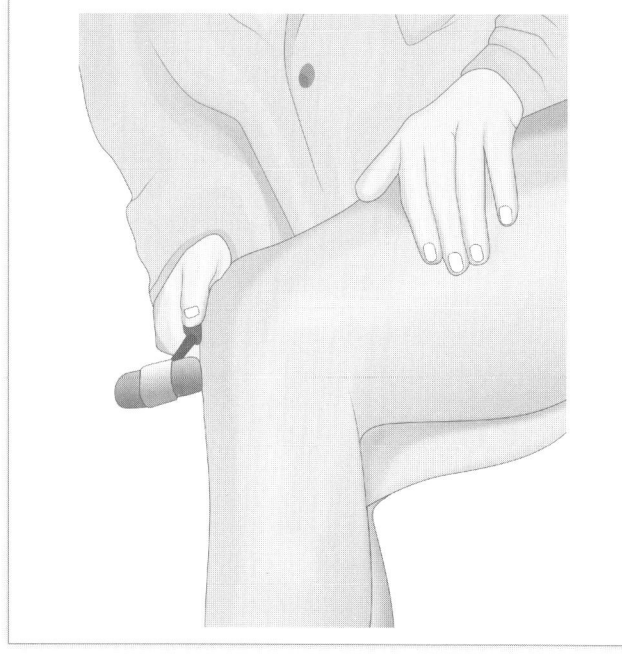

Fig. 6.4: Testing for patellar reflex

- Pointed, typical among primigravidae, with hypothesis of restricted pelvis
- Pendulous (see section above on medical history).
• *Examination of scars* and investigation of their significance: in the case of a prior C-section, an irregular scar with a keloid appearance, in which a high fibrous component is evident, (reducing relations with the underlying strata), is frequently associated with poor healing of a hysterotomy wound. A scar with these characteristics:
  - May interfere with contraction polarity during labour - the uterus takes on an asymmetric shape during contractions and a dystocia may follow
  - Can make it difficult to identify planes during surgery.

In the case of a prior C-section, pain at the scar site during pregnancy is due to distension of skin and inelastic scar tissue, not to the uterus; uterine rupture (dehiscence) during pregnancy is generally asymptomatic: *silent spontaneous rupture*.

• *Measurement of the abdominal circumference*, measurement passes over the umbilicus and it should be performed on each examination. There are no guiding tables; consistency between consecutive measurements or an anomaly between them should serve as guide to confirming a normal pregnancy or alerting to suspected retarded growth, oligohydramnios, macrosomia, multiple pregnancy or polyhydramnios. At term of pregnancy, in the case of a normally developed foetus with a normal amount of amniotic fluid and normal abdominal wall thickness, the measurement will be approx. 100–105 cm.

Palpation

Palpation starts with examination of the tone of the abdominal walls (see obstetric history) and aims at defining gestational age, lie, orientation of the back, presentation and, in case of cephalic presentation, attitude, position, engagement and flexion or deflection of the head.

Lie refers to the relation between the foetal longitudinal axis and the longitudinal axis of the uterus; lie may be *longitudinal, oblique or transverse*. An oblique lie in a primigravida generally correlates with a vitiated pelvis.

Presentation refers to the salient part of the foetal body (head, breech, shoulder) which is lies foremost towards the pelvic inlet; presentation may be cephalic, breech or transverse.

Foetal attitude here refers to the relationship between foetal head and trunk when passing through the birth canal. A normal attitude is that of a fully flexed head with the chin on the chest. Due to flexion, deflection or extension of the head, presentation will be vertex, bregma, brow or face (Fig. 5.10).

Position here refers to the relationship that the *point of direction*—the foremost descending part for that particular presentation (posterior fontanelle, bregma, brow, nose) adopts toto anatomical landmarks of the inlet, such as the iliopectineal eminence, the end point of the median transverse diameter and the sacroiliac synchondroses. Position will be right or left, and anterior, transverse or posterior.

With *engagement of the presenting part* we refer the transiting through the superior pelvic strait by the maximum advancing circumference typical for that particular presentation.

In the case of cephalic presentation, foetal position can be diagnosed either abdominally or vaginally.

In line with our Western obstetric traditions, we follow in this diagnostic pathway the five Leopold manoeuvres (the fifth was in fact first proposed by Zangenmeister). While abiding by their sequence, we will introduce some modifications that permit greater diagnostic accuracy

Approach by Examiner

The examiner stands facing the patient from the patient's right and level with the pelvis. The examiner first places their hands onto the fundus (first manoeuvre), then the hands slide along the abdominal walls (second manoeuvre); following this, the right hand grasps the presenting part (third manoeuvre). At this point the examiner turns side-on to the patient and places his/her hands flat on the area above the pubis (fourth manoeuvre), then one forefinger is placed over the symphysis and the other on the presenting part (fifth and final manoeuvre) and a comparison is made of the relation between the two forefingers.

First manoeuvre (Fig. 6.5): this aims to establish gestational age and to identify which salient foetal part lies at the uterine fundus. The examiner encompasses the uterine fundus with both hands: the ulnar side is in contact with the abdominal wall and opposite fingers are touching each other.
• Evaluating gestational age: the uterine fundus reaches:
  - the pubic symphysis at the 12th week
  - a point midway between the pubic symphysis and the transverse umbilical plane at the 16th week
  - the transverse umbilical plane at the 20th week
  - having crossed this line, we assume that each transverse fingerbreadth corresponds to two weeks.

For example: If the uterine fundus exceeds the umbilical line by two transverse fingerbreadths, gestational age corresponds to 24 weeks (2 supraumbilical transverse fingerbreadths × 2 = 4 + 20 weeks = 24/52).
• Which parts of the foetus are located in the fundus? In most cases, when a large portion of the foetal body is felt, it remains to be determined whether it is the breech or the head.

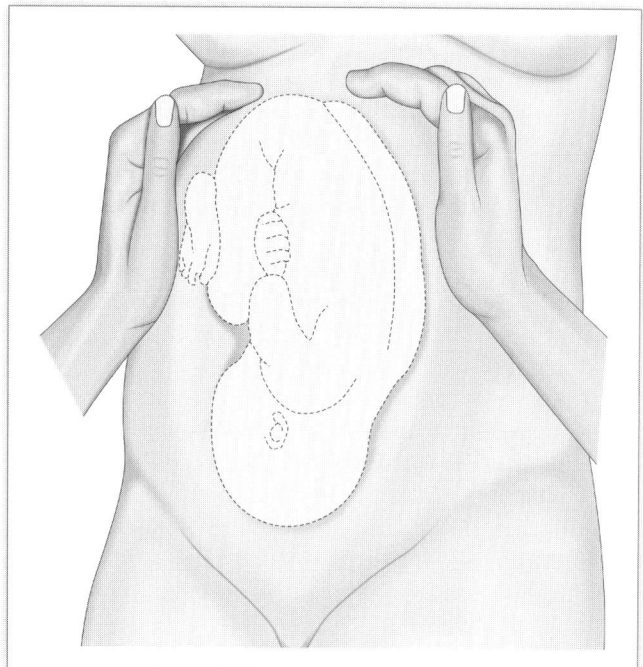

Fig. 6.5: First Leopold manoeuvre

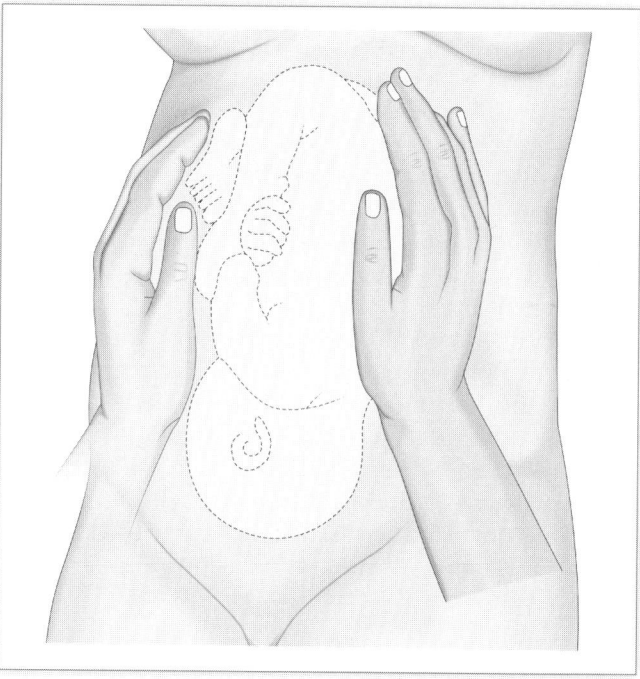

Fig. 6.6: Second Leopold manoeuvre

- The *breech* fills the uterine fundus more completely: it is smaller than the head; its surface is uneven, of heterogeneous consistency, not very mobile and ballottement is absent. Ballottement refers to the movement with which a large mass responds to pressure applied externally.
- The *head* is larger, regularly rounded with a hard, uniform consistency, smooth in outline, and ballottement is present.

Second manoeuvre (Fig. 6.6): This aims to identify foetal lie and which abdominal side corresponds to the foetal back. One proceeds as follows: both hands leave the fundus and slide, flat and parallel to each other, along the abdominal walls to stop at the level of the umbilicus. Where the lie is longitudinal, the back (Fig. 6.7) will be felt as a continuous, soft surface, while the abdominal surface of the foetus is characterised by the deep depression between breech and head: the *foetal triangle*, whose individual small parts can be traced (Fig. 6.10).

If identification of the back proves difficult, the following manoeuvres may be used:
- Using one hand, press with force on the uterine fundus; this will accentuate the curvature of the back, which is palpated more easily using the opposite hand (Budin manoeuvre).
- Alternating two-handed palpation of the lateral uterine surfaces, to identify which has more consistency, indicating the presence of the back.
- Auscultation of the foetal heartbeat (Fig. 6.8).

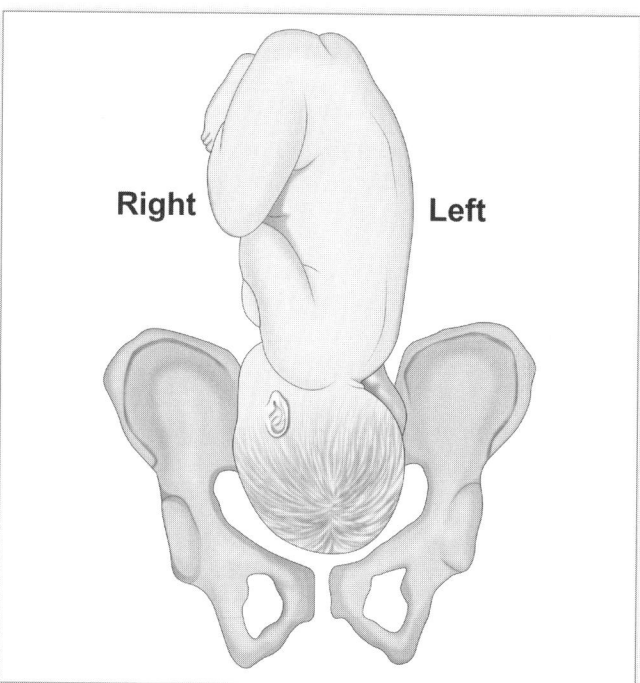

Fig. 6.7: Foetal back: A continuous surface of uniform consistency can be felt on the left

In the case of a transverse lie, one will be able to palpate a large foetal part, head and breech, on both sides (Fig. 6.9).

Third manoeuvre (Fig. 6.10): this may be performed only when the presenting part is still above the pubic symphysis.

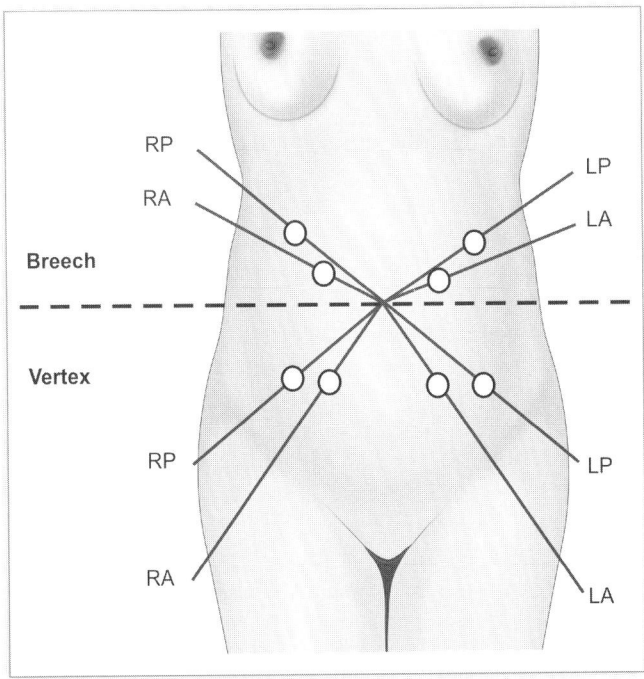

Fig. 6.8: Areas of auscultation of the foetal heartbeat

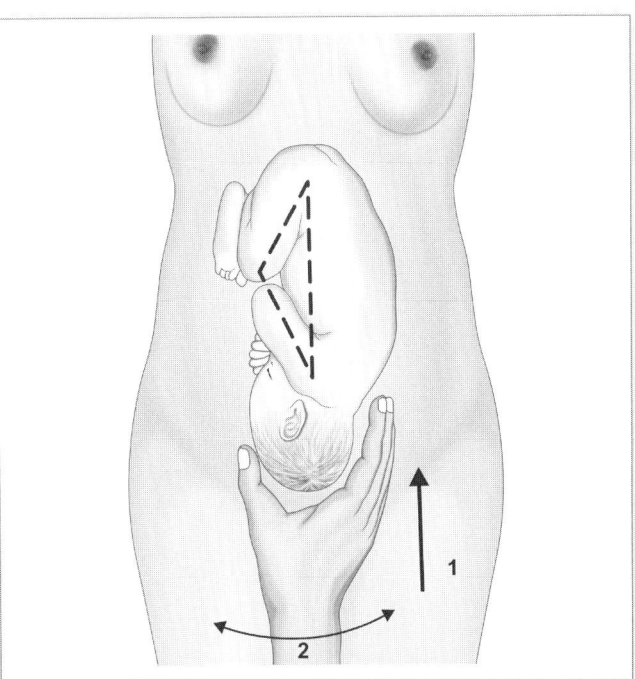

Fig. 6.10: Third Leopold manoeuvre: The back lies on the left, as indicated by the foetal triangle. 1. Cephalad push: the head has not engaged. 2. Direction of ballottement

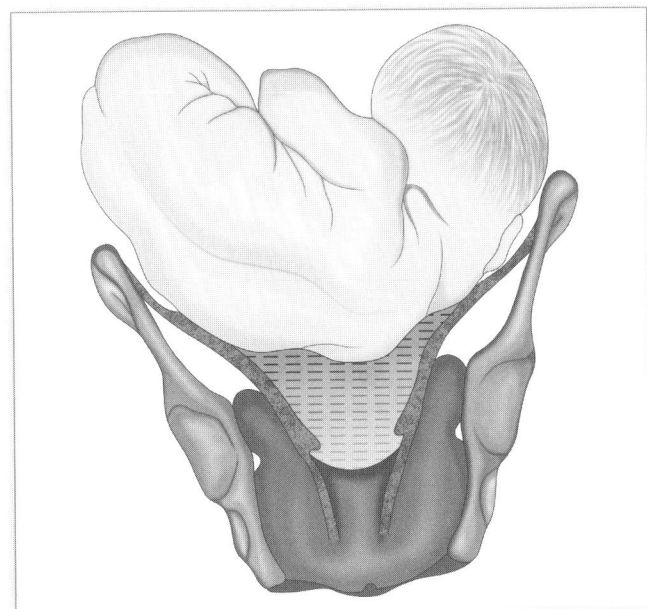

Fig. 6.9: Transverse lie: Two large foetal parts can be felt at the sides of the abdomen; the pelvic inlet is empty

The examiner moves back slightly, asks the patient to flex her knees and, using the thumb on one side and the index finger on the other, grasps the presenting part at the lower portion of the abdomen. The examiner first imparts a push in a cephalad direction (Fig. 6.10(1)); if the mass moves, the presenting part has not engaged. Secondly, the examiner imparts lateral movements (Fig. 6.10(2)) (ballottement test the rebounding movement of the foetus when displaced by the examiner). From the characteristics of the ballottement one can identify whether a head or a breech is presenting. In a cephalic presentation, there will be a degree of mobility and the push given to one part will be noticeable on the opposite side. The breech does not bounce, but gives a braking sensation.

With a transverse lie, *the pelvic inlet is empty* (Fig. 6.9).

Fourth manoeuvre (Fig. 6.11): the examiner turns side-on to the patient, whose knees are still flexed. The hands are placed on the lateroinferior areas of the abdomen, towards the pelvic floor; the fingertips are against each other. First they palpate, moving deeper to try and detect the presenting part, which will be felt with greater distinctness according to its degree of advancement.

Fifth manoeuvre: still side-on to the patient, the examiner places one forefinger over the symphysis and one on the presenting part, then compares the relation between the two forefingers. Where engagement has not taken place, the forefinger on the presenting part will be more cranial; if engagement has occurred, both fingers will be at the same level.

Zangenmeister's manoeuvre: the examiner sits on the edge of the bed, facing the patient, both hands placed close together, flat on the abdomen. Moving in a caudad direction, the hands palpate the lower uterine segment until they identify a depression lying in an oblique or

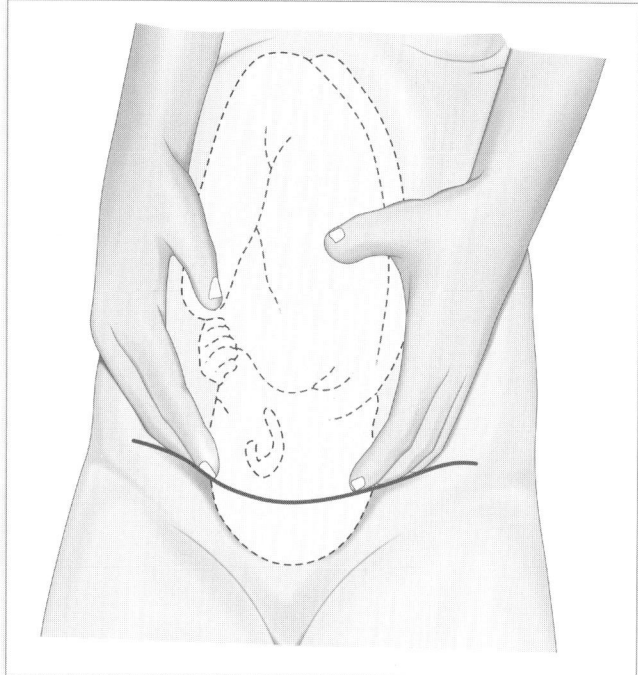

Fig. 6.11: Fourth Leopold manoeuvre

traverse position, corresponding to the fold of the foetal neck. When this lies transversely, the head is in the intermediate attitude (bregma) and the chin and occiput can be felt; if the fold lies obliquely, the head is in an attitude of flexion or deflection.

These manoeuvres have been outlined in due respect for the obstetric tradition and to establish points of contact with the reader. But, starting with the first manoeuvre, we follow a different diagnostic pathway, one that is perhaps more informative.

The first manoeuvre aims to identify gestational age, which can also be assessed by using the:

Graph of symphysis-fundal distance (Table 6.4): The y-axis shows the symphysis—fundus distance (in cm) and the x-axis shows gestational age (in weeks). Under normal conditions, each week will correspond to a different height.

The values shown on the graph will generate a curve which is bordered, above and below and at a distance of two cm, by two parallel curves, which correspond to the 90th and 10th percentiles respectively.

The symphysis-fundus distance chart can be used in two ways:
1. *If the date of the last menstruation is known*: measurement values are shown (distance in centimetres or manual determination) for each corresponding week. Manual determination of gestational age consists in calculating the number of transverse fingerbreadths cephalad between the uterine fundus and the umbilicus, where each transverse fingerbreadth corresponds to two weeks of pregnancy.
2. *If the date of the last menstruation is not known*, and no ultrasound dating is available: *gestational age* is established by noting the height of the uterine fundus, measured using a ruler or manually, at a given date; on the next examination, an assessment is made of whether the variation is to be expected from the time interval that has passed, or whether this variation is too great or too little.

If the symphysis-fundus distance a) coincides with gestational age, growth is normal; b) does not coincide, this could be due to:
- *Growth retardation*: values below 3 cm, if detected repeatedly, enable an early identification of growth retardation: primary, secondary, transient (Table 6.5). Among the recognised causes are: deferred conception (amenorrhoea in one month, followed by conception in the following month), growth retardation, oligohydramnios (the uterine walls cling to the foetus, whose parts may be noted clearly)
- *Excess growth*: errors in gestational calculation, multiple pregnancy, foetal macrosomia, polyhydramnios.

As the maximum fundal elevation occurs between weeks 38 and 39, followed by a moderate lowering over the following days, the height measured towards term of pregnancy does not have an absolute value. It may correspond either to the growth phase or to that of regression. Diagnosis should be guided by the following factors:
- The patient reports that the uterus has dropped and concomitantly:
  - *That breathing has become easier* (less elevation of the diaphragm due to the gravid uterus)
  - *That acid reflux*, from which she was suffering, has eased
  - *That she feels pressure on the bladder.*
- Abdominal palpation will reveal that the presenting part has moved to some extent into the pelvic inlet.
In general, lowering of the uterus usually precedes parturition by three week in primigravidae, and by two weeks in multiparae.

The second manoeuvre enables diagnosis of foetal lie and orientation of the back (right or left). Identifying the location of the back is a very important step for:
- *Diagnosing presentation*, as by following the contour of the back caudad, we will detect, in the case of cephalic presentation, a deep indentation—the fold of the neck—which is absent in the breech presentation. This depression is fairly large in the case of a vertex presentation, but very limited in face presentations (cf. Zangenmeister's manoeuvre)

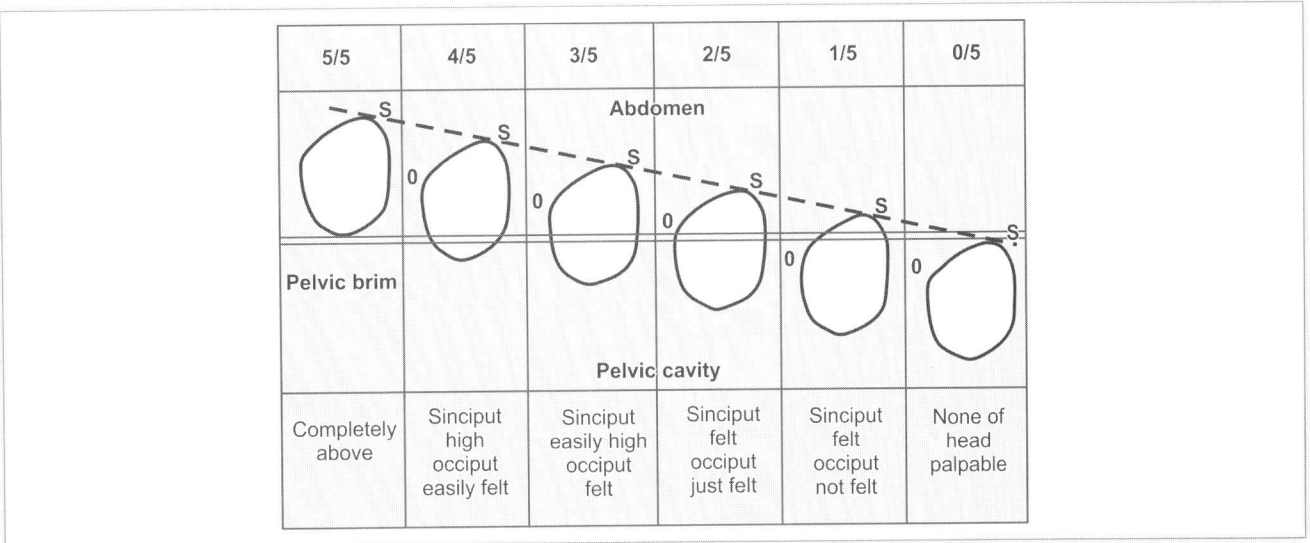

Fig. 6.12: Crichton's method for abdominal assessment of engagement and advancement of the head in the pelvic cavity: The head is divided into 5/5, with each fifth corresponding to a transverse fingerbreadth. Longitudinal foetal lie, cephalic presentation: the back is facing right. When only 2/5 of the head is detectable above the pubic symphysis, the head is engaged

- *Diagnosing position: the occiput faces the foetal back, forming an angle of 90° with the bisacromial diameter.* If we imagine a foetus in longitudinal lie, cephalic presentation and back to the right, when the back:
  - crosses to the left of the umbilical-pubic line, the occiput will be facing the iliopectineal eminence; therefore there will be a right occiput anterior (ROA) presentation
  - is located immediately within the umbilical-pubic line, the occiput will be facing the right extremity of the transverse diameter, and the presentation will be right occiput transverse (ROT)
  - is far behind the umbilical—pubic line, the occiput will be facing the sacroiliac synchondrosis and presentation with therefore be right occiput posterior (ROP).

  The *fourth manoeuvre* aims to establish the degree of engagement of the presenting part. In our opinion, the manoeuvres we illustrate offer better assessment of the degree of engagement, flexion or deflection of the presenting part.

- *Diagnosing engagement*: Crichton (1974) divides the distance between the base and vertex of the foetal head (10 cm in all) into five equal parts, with each fifth corresponding to 2 cm or approximately one transverse fingerbreadth. The method consists in determining the number of fingers (fifths) the head accommodates above the brim, which is the anatomical landmark used (Fig. 6.12).
  - Head accommodates (Fig. 6.13) full width of 5 fingers above the brim: the head is mobile above the brim.
  - The head accommodates 2 fingers above the brim: head is engaged.

This very simple and accurate method offers the following advantages:

- Assessment of the *flexion or deflection (extension) of the head*, as, if fewer head-fifths are detected on the occiput side (corresponding to the foetal back) than on the sinciput side (Fig. 6.14), the head will be flexed. If the reverse condition obtains, it will be deflected
- It may be used without limitation, avoiding vaginal exploration and therefore pollution of the birth canal or cervical dystocia
  - Unlike vaginal diagnosis (Fig. 6.31), assessment of engagement is not affected by the *caput succedaneum formation* (Fig. 6.15) which often leads the inexperienced to confuse *scalp descent* with *skull descent*.

If the head is mobile above the brim and shows no tendency of engaging when the examiner pushes while the patient is moving from a lying down to a sitting position, *cephalopelvic disproportion is probably* present. This manoeuvre is referred to as *fitting of the head* and should be performed from the 36th week onwards, the period during which engagement normally occurs in a primigravida. In a multigravida, engagement occurs at the time of labour.

The *round ligaments* play an important role during labour; their contraction causes forward displacement of the uterus and facilitates alignment of the foetal axis with that of the birth canal.

Locating them during pregnancy will help alert to possible uterine torsion. Particularly at term, these ligaments will be stretched more on the side opposite the twist; this may cause pain that is difficult to diagnose if this possibility has been overlooked.

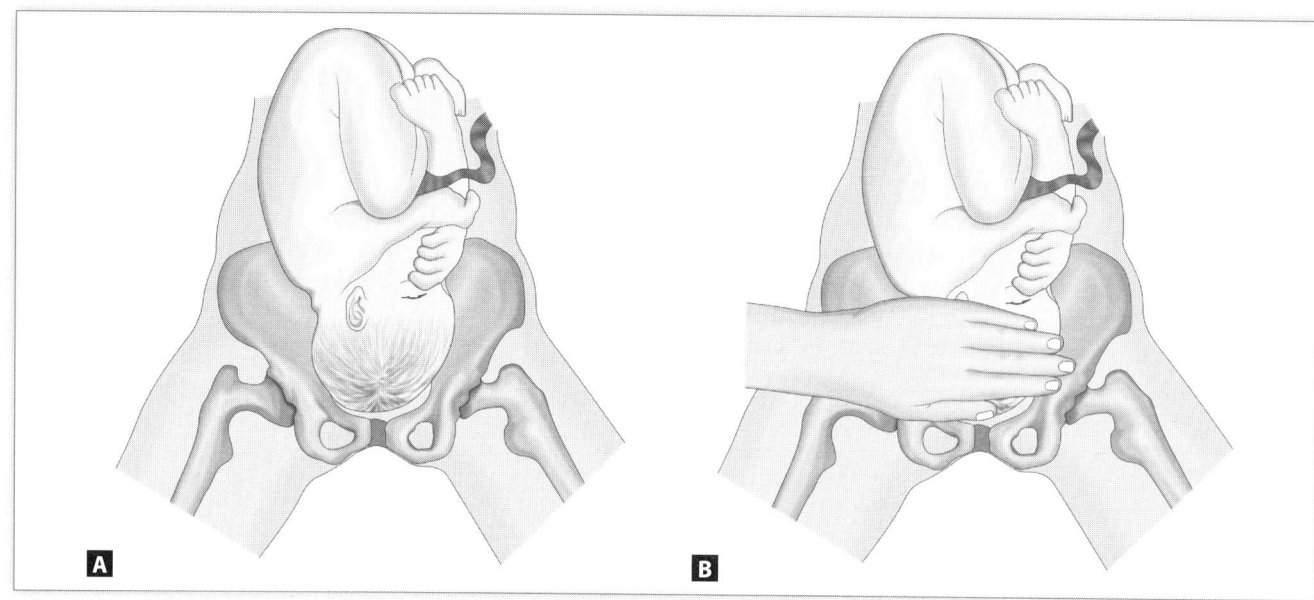

Fig. 6.13A and B: (A) Head is mobile above the brim = 5/5; (B) Head accommodates full width of 5 fingers above the brim

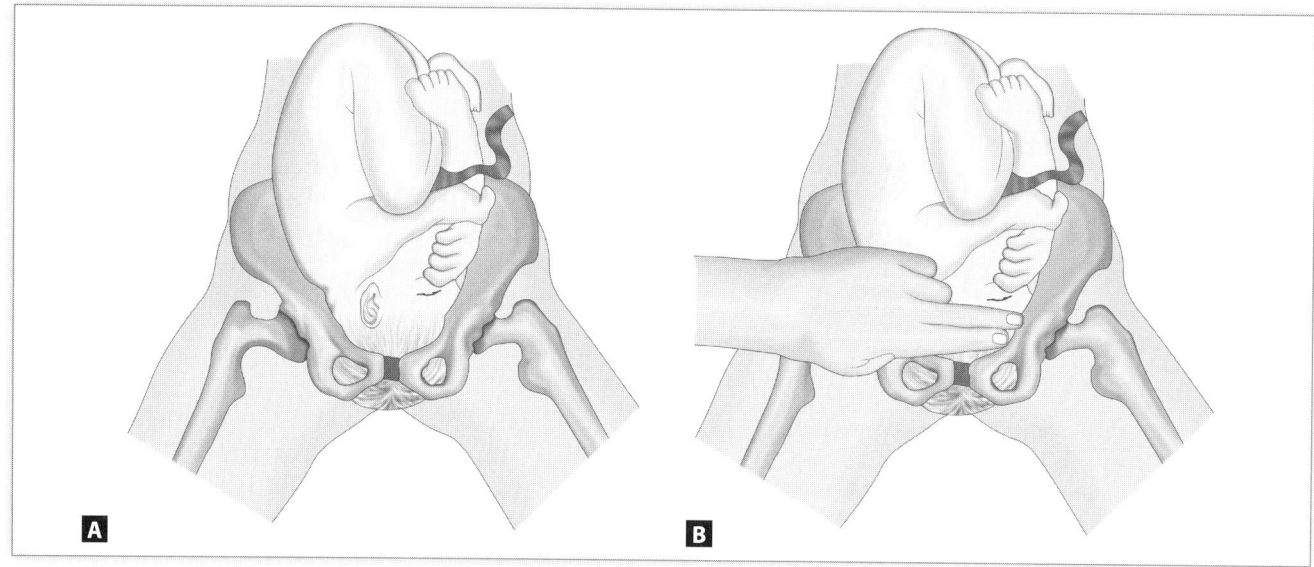

Fig. 6.14A and B: (A) Head is engaged; (B) Head accomodates 2 fingers above the brim

Round ligaments, stretched like strings, painful and prominent from the body of the uterus during labour, are among the signs associated with cephalopelvic disproportion or obstructed labour.

It is essential that the round ligaments are identified during a C-section, to ensure symmetry of hysterotomy.

Auscultation of Foetal Heartbeat

The focal point of maximum foetal heartbeat intensity varies with foetal presentation and position (Fig. 6.8). Umbilical cord murmur is a *muffled sound*, audible in synchronisation with the foetal heartbeat; it appears each time the cord is slightly compressed or stretched, when true knots or windings around the foetal neck or body are present.

Assessment of the True Pelvis

Engagement, descent, rotation and disengagement of the presenting part are possible only if there is a favourable (adequate) relation between the pelvic capacity and the volume of the presenting part.

DIAGNOSIS IN CLINICAL OBSTETRICS

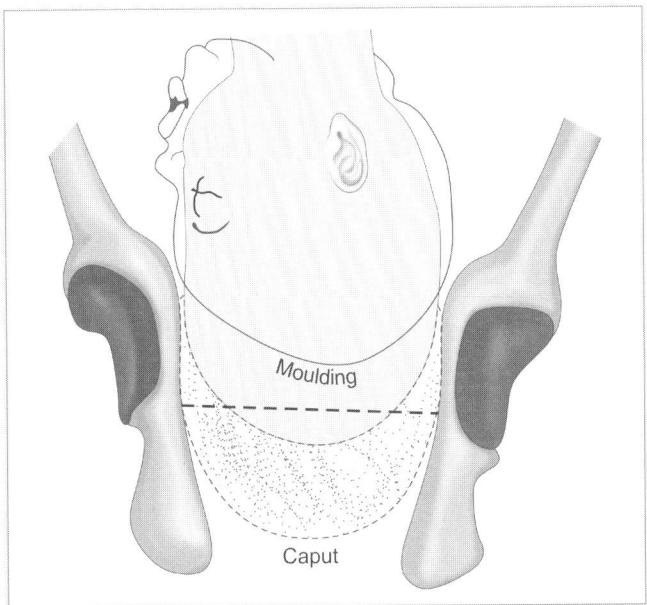

Fig. 6.15: How foetal skull moulding and caput formation prevent accurate diagnosis of engagement, when diagnosed vaginally

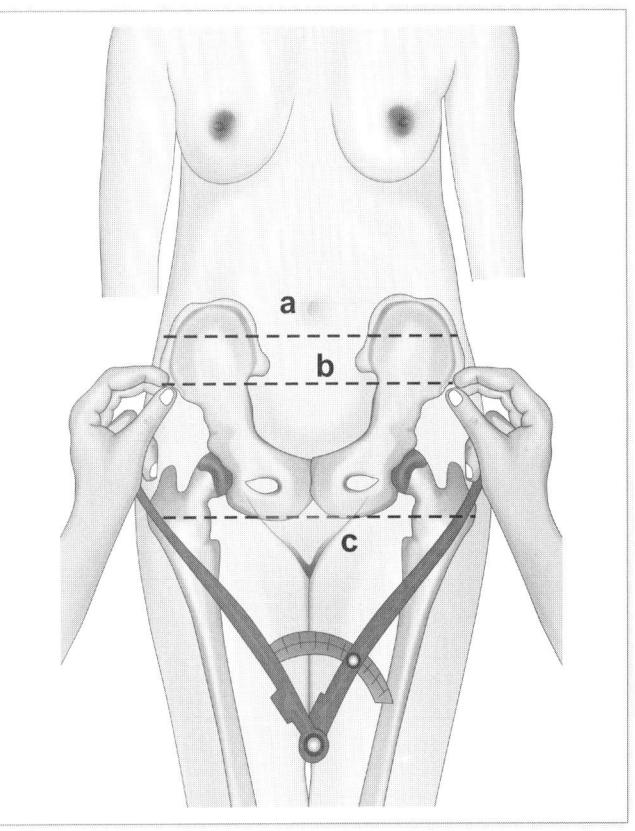

Fig. 6.16: External pelvimetry using a Martin pelvimeter Proceeding inferiorly: **a.** bicrestal diameter **b.** bispinous diameter **c.** bitrochanteric diameter. The tips of the pelvimeter are always within the anatomical landmarks. 1–2 cm is subtracted from the value obtained to allow for thickness of interposed skin

The capacity of the true pelvis (i.e. its containment ability) is determined by:
- Its size, morphology and inclination
- The volume of the presenting part.

The purpose of the examination is to determine whether there is a suitable relation between the pelvis and the presenting part.

Dimensions

The birth canal comprises a superior pelvic strait (inlet), an intermediate strait (midpelvis) and an inferior pelvic strait or outlet.

PELVIC INLET (SUPERIOR PELVIC STRAIT)

The evaluation of the pelvic inlet can be made only through indirect external and internal measurements, which are significant *only for values below normal.*

Indirect external measurements are made using specific instruments called pelvimeters (Fig. 6.1).
- The bispinous diameter (Fig. 6.16b) expresses the distance between the two anterior superior iliac spines; in a normal pelvis this is approx. 25-26 cm. The tips of the pelvimeter are held as one holds a pen and positioned at the *medial edge of each spine*
- The bicrestal diameter (Fig. 6.16a) expresses the distance between the two iliac crests; in a normal pelvis this measures 28-29 cm. It is found by using the pelvimeter to follow the iliac crests to their points of maximum divergence.

Of relevance in transverse measurements (bispinal and intercrestal) is not so much the individual value, but the relation between them. A difference of approx. 3 cm between them; is consistent with normal false and true pelvic; with differences of 1-1.5 cm, a flat pelvis should be suspected.
- The *bitrochanteric diameter* (Fig. 6.16c), expresses the distance between the most lateral points of the trochanters; in a normal pelvis this is approx. 31-32 cm. This measurement is less important than the above. Locating the trochanters can be facilitated by having the legs rotate externally
- The *external, or Boudeloque's conjugate* (Fig. 6.17) is greater than 20 cm in a normal pelvis. With values of 20-19 cm it is considered less than normal or verging on contraction and with values of 18 cm it is definitely contracted with certainty of a flat pelvis. Measurement is taken with the patient in a standing position or in lateral decubitus. The pelvimeter is placed between the thighs with one tip resting in the depression between the spinous processes of the 4th and 5th lumbar vertebrae; the other tip rests on the central portion of the superior border of the pubic symphysis

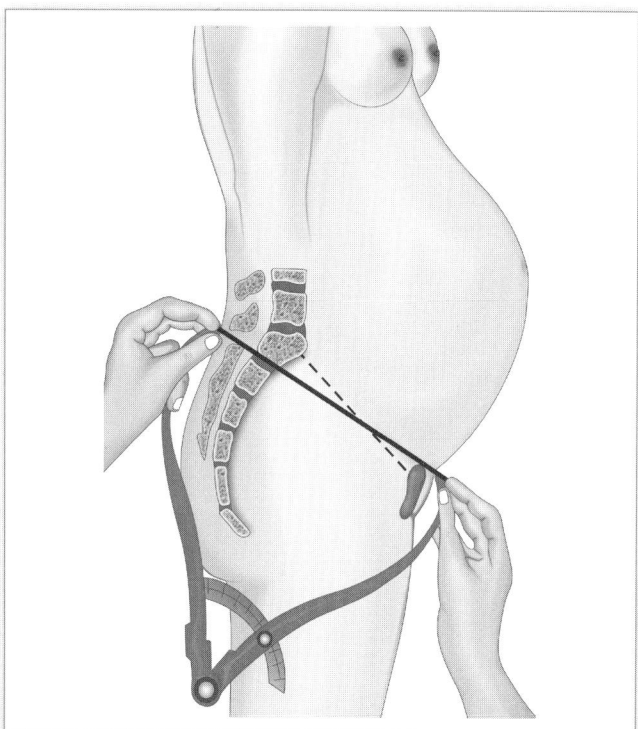

Fig. 6.17: External pelvimetry using a Martin pelvimeter: Measuring Boudeloque's external diagonal conjugate. The pelvimeter is placed between the patient's thighs

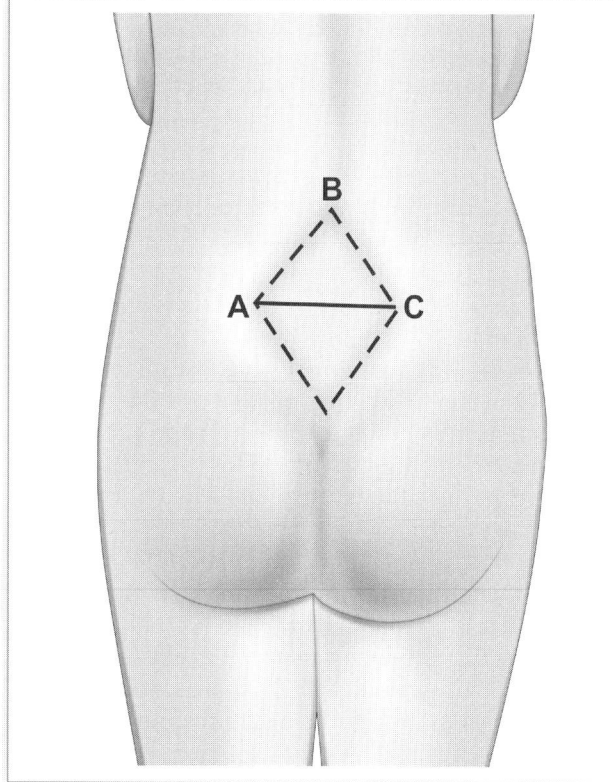

Fig. 6.18: Lozenge of Michaelis ABC—superior triangle

- The *superoposterior triangle* (Fig. 6.18 ABC), has as its base the distance between the posterior-superior iliac spines (approx. 10 cm). Its height is that of the lumbosacral hinge. A reduction in the size of the base expresses a reduction in the transverse diameter; the height of this triangle is important as it indicates the site of the lumbosacral hinge. In the normal pelvis, whose lumbosacral hinge corresponds to the fifth lumbar vertebra, the height is 4–5 cm and the triangle coincides with the upper triangle of the Lozenge of Michaelis (see below). Where sacralisation of the fifth lumbar vertebra occurs, as in Hirschhoff's assimilation pelvis (Figs 2.29 and 2.30), the height is greater and is accompanied by an increase in size of the diagonal conjugate. When inlumbarisation of the first sacral vertebra occurs (rare), height is reduced to less than 4 cm
- The *lozenge of Michaelis* (Fig. 6.18), located in the lumbosacral region, has the spinal process of the 5th lumbar vertebra (B) as its superior boundary and the top of the gluteal fold (D) as its inferior one. Laterally it is bounded by skin dimples corresponding to upper posterior iliac spines (A and C). Measurement must be taken from the patient in an upright position

Normal dimensions of the lozenge are 10 cm for the transverse diagonal and 11 cm for the vertical one. The transverse diagonal, correlated to the size of the transverse diameter of the pelvic inlet, divides the lozenge into two triangles: superior and inferior. It was once thought that the height of the superior triangle correlated with the anterior- posterior diameter of the pelvic inlet; currently this correlation is not believed to be so clear.

The lozenge of Michaelis (Fig. 6.19) has:
- A quadrangular shape in the normal pelvis
- An elongated, contracted shape, with acute superior and inferior angles, in the android or anthropoid pelvis
- A markedly obtuse superior angle in the flat pelvis
- An asymmetric quadrilateral form in the irregularly asymmetrical pelvis.

The *intertuberous diameter* (pelvic outlet) is the same as the transverse diameter of the pelvic inlet in anthropoid and gynecoid pelves, whose pelvic walls follow a parallel course (Fig. 6.28), while the walls of the android pelvis converge and those of the platypelloid pelvis diverge.

Indirect Internal Measurements

- The *obstetric conjugate* (Fig. 2.17b) is the shortest distance between the most prominent point of the symphysis and the promontory. It is obtained by subtracting 1.5 cm from the value of the diagonal conjugate, which is the distance between the inferior border of the pubic symphysis and the promontory. Therefore, an obstetric conjugate of 10 cm corresponds to a diagonal conjugate of 11.5

DIAGNOSIS IN CLINICAL OBSTETRICS

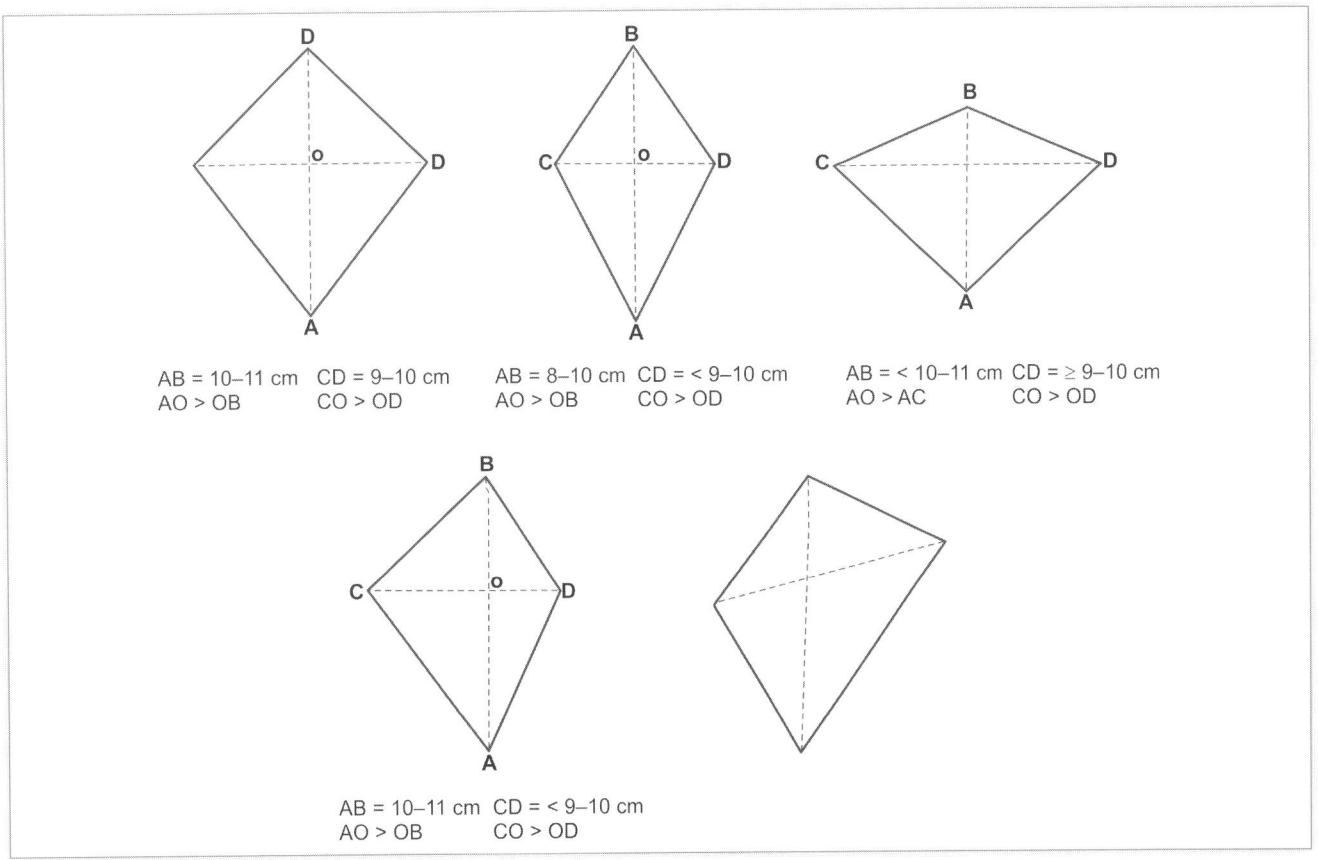

Fig. 6.19: Lozenge of Michaelis: From left to right, normal pelvis, fully and regularly contracted pelvis, flat pelvis, obliquely contracted pelvis, irregularly contracted pelvis

cm. Values below 11.5 cm (OC 10 cm) would indicate a constrained pelvic inlet.

The theoretical basis for this is as follows: by joining the upper and lower borders of the pubic symphysis to the promontory, one obtains a right triangle, whose hypotenuse is the diagonal conjugate and whose greater cathetus is the obstetric conjugate. It has been established empirically that for right triangles with these dimensions, by subtracting 1.5–2 cm from the hypotenuse (the diagonal conjugate), one obtains a reasonable approximation of the obstetric conjugate.

The reliability of this calculation is considerably limited (Fig. 2.18):
- The triangle is not always a right-angled one: often the angle subtended by the lesser cathetus (pubic symphysis) and the diagonal conjugate (Jacobs' angle) is less than 90° degrees, so: the superior border is closer to the promontory than assumed, and the obstetric conjugate is reduced even when a favourable diagonal conjugate is present
- The calculation does not take the thickness of the symphysis into account
- The calculation does not take into account the morphology of the pelvic inlet. Indeed, in the android and anthropoid pelves (Fig. 2.27), the anteroposterior diameter is long, but the accompanying difficulties in engagement, advancement and rotation are well known
- In the assimilation pelvis, as described by Hirshhoff (sacralisation of the fifth lumbar vertebra), the promontory is often not reached (Fig. 2.29)
- A recent study (Domini, Guidi, Guazzini, 2007) demonstrated the poor correlation between values for the obstetric conjugate obtained by vaginal examination and those found during caesarean section.

For these reasons, we recommend:
- the obstetric conjugate should always be determined
- its value should be taken as *predictive for values below normal*
- for normal values, it should always be correlated with the morphology of the pelvis
- the formula that *the promontory is not reached* is not a waiver, but constitutes a factor for suspicion.

Measuring the Diagonal Conjugate (Fig. 6.20)

A precondition is that every examiner should determine the distance that can be reached using the middle finger of the examining hand.

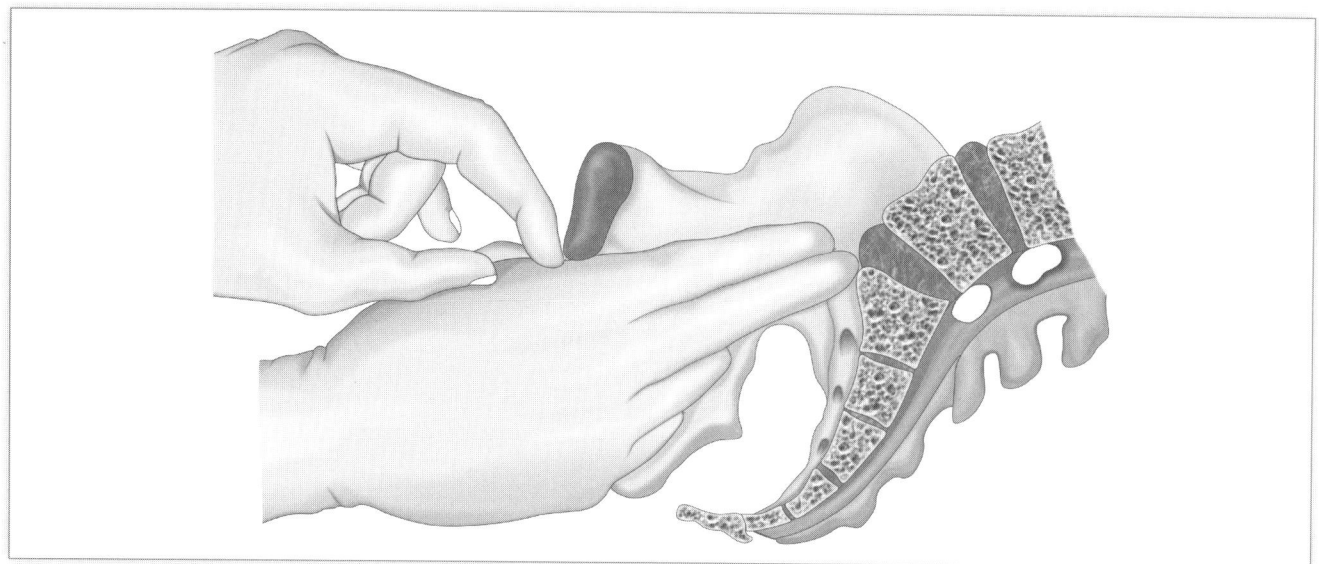

Fig. 6.20: Determining the diagonal conjugate

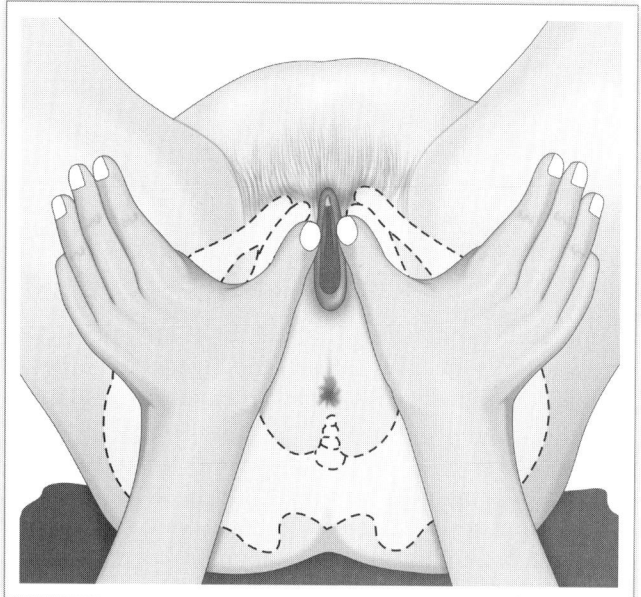

Fig. 6.21: Pelvic outlet; assessment of the morphology and breadth of the subpubic arch: modelling of the subpubic arch

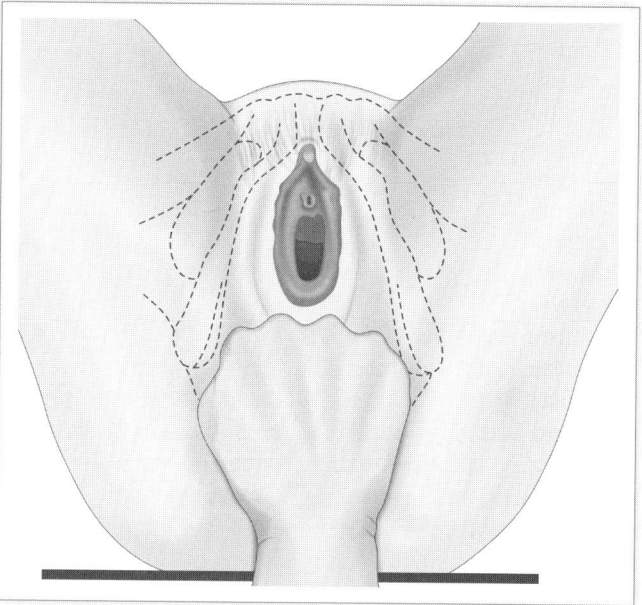

Fig. 6.22: Pelvic outlet; assessment of the intertuberous diameter according to Greenhill

Finger sensitivity increases as pressure on the fingertips decreases. Occasionally, when determining the diagonal conjugate, it will be necessary to overcome resistance; if it is the examining hand that does this, some sensitivity is lost. To obviate this problem, the foot corresponding to that hand is placed on a stool and the elbow is placed on the knee. Force is then exerted by moving the knee, and therefore the elbow, forward, so that the hand keeps all its sensitivity. On reaching the promontory with a fingertip, a mark is made, using a fingernail of the non-examining hand on the back of the exploring hand. The mark should be made with enough pressure so that one can make the measurement, with glove removed, without contaminating the instruments: ruler or pelvimeter.

Failure to reach the promontory may be due to the examiner (hand too small, incorrect technique), to poor patient compliance, or to pelvic morphology (android, anthropoid, assimilation pelvis). Therefore the formula *'promontory cannot be reached'* is not a 'get-out clause' in clinical diagnosis for two reasons: with the first two possible causes cited above, diagnosis has not yet been attained, and with the third, a very long anteroposterior diameter rules out a flat pelvis, but not an android or anthropoid pelvis whose pathologies of engagement and labour progress are certainly no less considerable than in the case of a flat pelvis.

Midpelvis

Bispinous diameter: In the past this was measured by placing one arm of the pelvimeter in the vagina and the other in the rectum. This practice has fallen into disuse and been replaced by a simple physical examination, during which it is assessed whether or not the ischial spines are prominent.

Pelvic Outlet (Inferior Pelvic Strait)

This is the dihedral angle (an angle formed by the intersection of two planes) formed by two triangles with a common base: the intertuberous diameter (Fig. 2.22). The anterior triangle has the ischial pubic rami as its sides, and the inferior margin of the pubic symphysis as its apex. The posterior triangle has the sacrotuberous ligaments as its sides and its apex is the apex of the sacrum, not the coccyx The pelvic outlet comprises (Fig. 2.24):
- *Angle of the pubic arch*: Its dimensions and morphology are assessed using:
- Pubic-arch modelling (Fig. 6.21)
- Digital evaluation: Using the forefinger and middle finger pronated, the amplitude and morphology of the pubic arch is assessed (Chapters 2 and 6, Section on pelvic exploration)
- *The intertuberous diameter* (Fig. 2.24) is projected between the borders of the two ischial tuberosities. It measures 10–11 cm and is determined either:
  - Manually: The Greenhill method (Fig. 6.22) consists in placing the clenched fist in contact with the perineum and counting the number of knuckles between the two ischial tuberosities. If there are four, or if the fi st advances between the two tuberosities, the intertuberous diameter is compatible.
  - Instrumentally: This may be carried out using:
  - Either a pelvimeter (Figs 6.1, 6.23A and B): The two nibs of the pelvimeter are rested on the medial margins of the ischial tuberosities. Two centimetres are added to the reading, corresponding to the thickness of the soft tissue (interposed between each tuberosity and nib).
  - Or a measuring tape: Tarnier's technique (Fig. 6.24) is the most widely used: With the patient in gynaecological position, the tape is held by the two thumbs placed against the medial faces of the ischial tuberositics. The intertuberous diameter is the distance between the two thumbs, plus two cm (thickness of soft tissue).
- *Anteroposterior or pubo-sacral diameter*: This is projected between the anterior border of the pubic symphysis and the apex of the sacrum. It measures 11.5 cm. Due to the

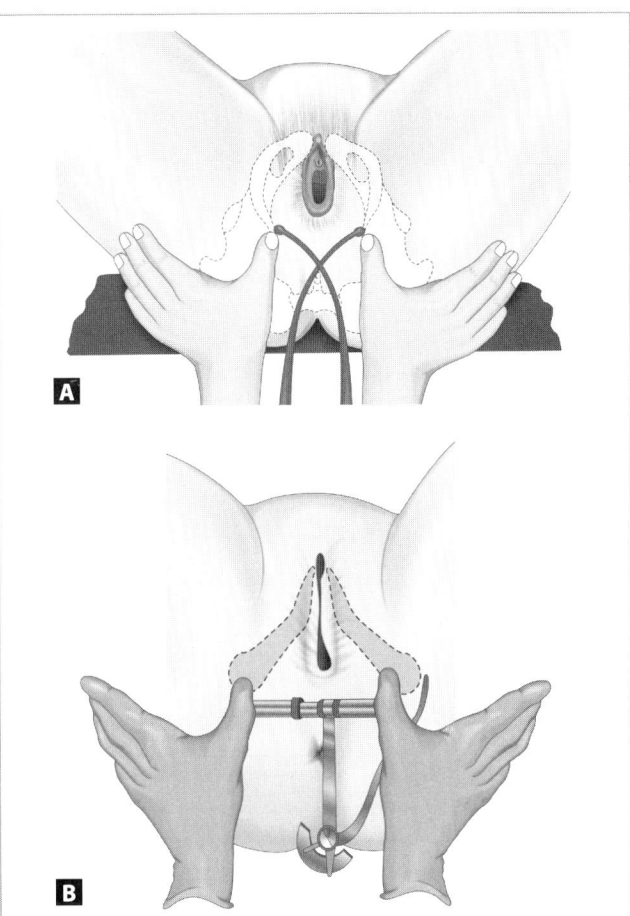

Fig. 6.23A and B: Pelvic outlet: measuring the intertuberous diameter using: (A) Collin's pelvimeter; (B) Thom's pelvimeter. 1–2 cm is subtracted from the reading, depending on the thickness of interposing skin

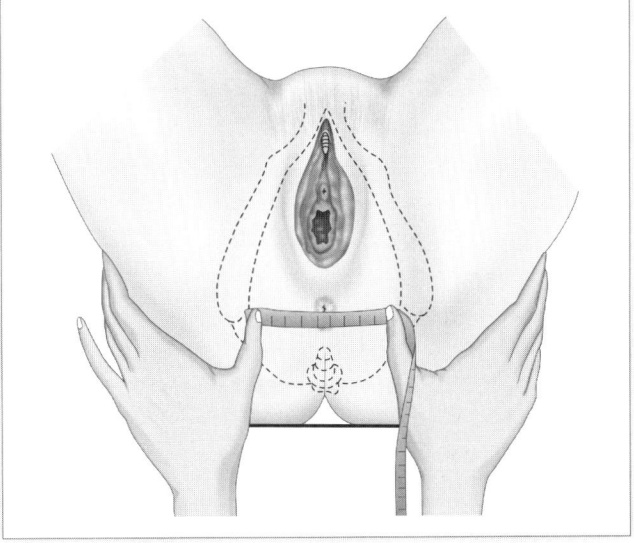

Fig. 6.24: Measuring the intertuberous diameter by Tarnier's method

presence of the sacrotuberous ligaments and levator ani muscles, disengagement is possible only as this diameter allows

- The *anteroposterior or coccyx-pubic diameter* has no clinical significance. So-called retropulsion of the coccyx does not always occur, especially in the case of a hooked coccyx.

The *sacrococcygeal joint* is identified by introducing the thumb into the rectum until it reaches the dorsal face of the coccyx; gripping the ventral face through the vagina using one's forefinger, the joint is identified through flex-extension. *This manoeuvre is especially useful for identifying the sacral hiatus when administering a sacral epidural.*

- *Oblique diameters* (Fig. 2.24): these are projected from the midpoint of the ischiopubic ramus on one side to the midpoint of the sacrotuberous ligament on the other. They measure 12 cm

- The *morphology of the sacral concavity* is evaluated by the number of sacral vertebrae detected on pelvic exploration. Where a good sacral concavity is present, only the fifth and fourth sacral vertebra should be detected. If the superior part or the entire third sacral vertebra is detectable, a reduced sacral concavity is suggested (Fig. 2.7).

Compass method: During a pelvic examination, using a tip of the middle finger, the portion of the sacrum closest to the promontory is identified. Contact is maintained and in the meantime the forefinger is placed on the pubic symphysis. Using the contact as a fulcrum, a compass-like movement

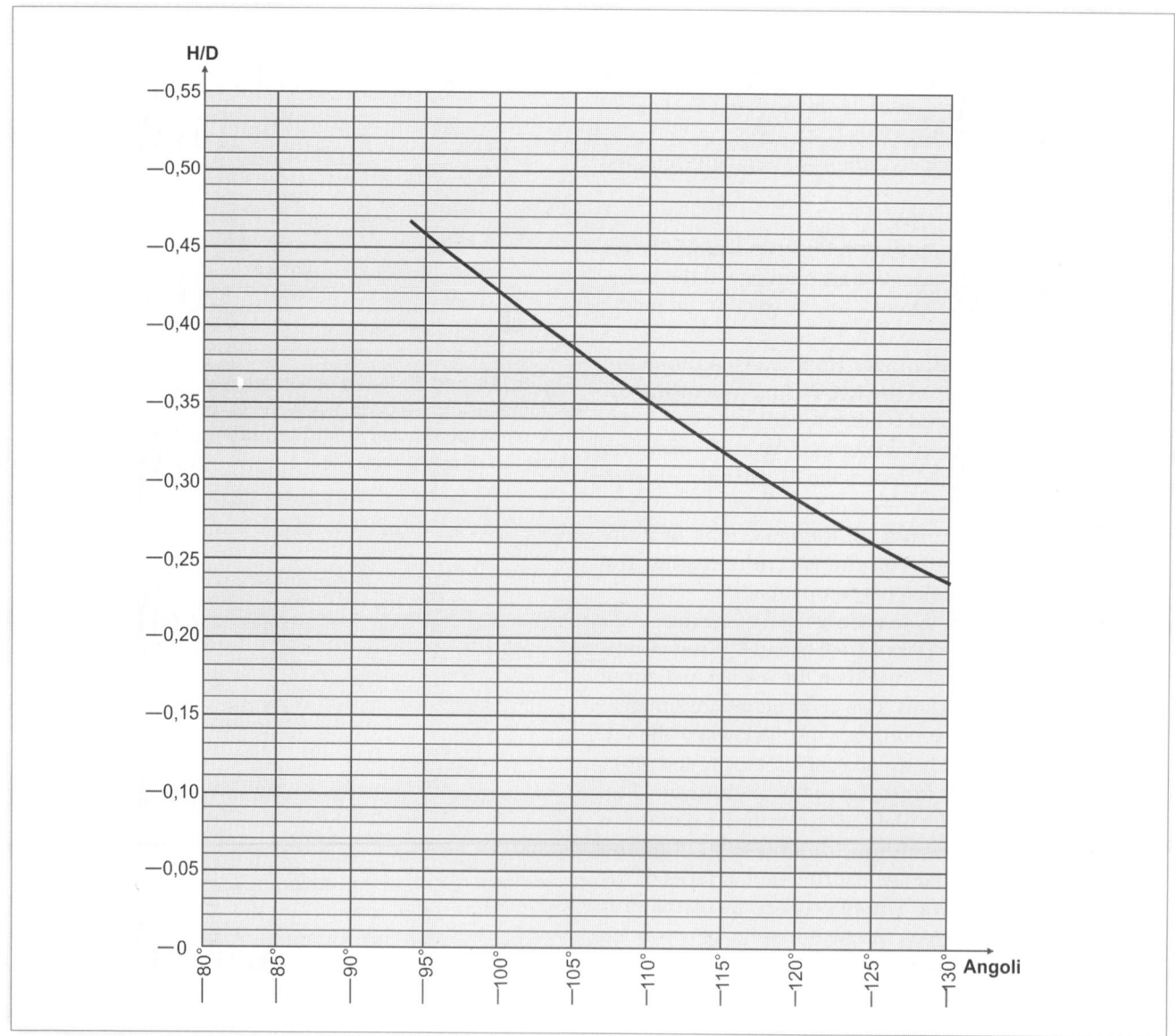

Table 10: Anthropometric index: On the y-axis, the anthropometric index; on the x-axis, the amplitude of the prepubic angle

is performed from back to front; under normal conditions, contact with the sacrum should rapidly be lost or reduced, to be regained near the coccyx.

Morphology

Returning to our remarks in Chapter 2, Caldwell and Moloy (1933, 1935, and 1935) should be credited with having pointed out how it is not the size as much as the morphology of the birth canal that affects progress of labour. Indeed, arrest of advancement by the presenting part is observed in 6% of gynecoid pelves, in 25% of an android pelvis and in 35% of parturients with a mixed type of android pelvis (see below).

Using radiographic images, the above-cited authors identified four pelvic types, codified the distinctive features of each and argued that from the morphology of the midpelvis and pelvic outlet, it was possible to deduce that of the pelvic inlet (Fig. 2.27). Having made their classification, it was realised that only in 35% (now 50%) of cases did the pelvis fall within the proposed classification. In the remaining cases it was found that the anterior and posterior pelvis, which comprises the inlet, could belong to different pure types. This problem was solved from a classificatory point of view by introducing the concept of mixed types (Fig. 2.28; Table 2.3). However it was not solved from a diagnostic point of view, in that the then prevalent clinical diagnostics (instrumental and digital pelvimetry) were not able to provide sufficient data to solve the problem.

This problem was further complicated by:
- Kirchhoff's (1948) introduction of the concept of the "long pelvis", which includes both the assimilation pelvis (sacralisation of the fifth lumbar vertebra) and the true long pelvis (see Chapter 2)
- Renewed recognition of the important role played in engagement by the inclination of the pelvic inlet (see Chapter 2).

The evaluation of pelvic morphology remains as topical a problem as ever, not only in resource-poor countries, but also in the West. Wischnik et al. (1992) demonstrated that, over the past 80 years, the anatomy of the pelvis has undergone profound changes. These are characterized at the level of the pelvic inlet through replacement of a transverse slightly elliptical shape with an elliptical shape whose major axis is anteroposterior, by contraction of the midpelvic area and by reduction of the sacral concavity. Generous use of Caesarean section has allowed and will continue to allow the transmission of these unfavourable characteristics. A further study conducted by Kraus et al. 1997, has shown that, with high frequency (61%), underlying an 'arrest of labour' was the presence of an "assimilation pelvis" (see Chapter 2).

Evaluation of Anterior Pelvis and Pelvic Inlet (Method Developed by the Authors)

It seems clear from the above sections that pelvimetry, understood as a series of measurements capable of defining pelvic patency, no longer has the relevance once ascribed to it, and that it is currently being replaced by manoeuvres designed to identify pelvic morphology—methods which may also make use of measurement. The problem now arises of which characteristics to take into account when defining the shape of the pelvis and, hence, its suitability for a normal vaginal delivery.

Width of the Forepelvis Angle (Prepubic Angle)

The width of the prepubic angle (Fig. 6.25A) varies with different pelvis types. In the android and anthropoid it is less than 90°; it is between 90° and 130° in the gynecoid pelvis and over 130° in the flat pelvis. It follows that we can deduce the morphology of the anterior pelvis from knowing the value of the forepelvis or prepubic angle.

By joining the extremities of the transverse diameter of the pelvic inlet to the pubic symphysis (Fig. 6.25B) we obtain an isosceles triangle (D1); by joining the two anterior-superior iliac spines to the pubic symphysis, we obtain a second isosceles triangle (D2).

If, using the pubic symphysis as fulcrum, we rotate D1 anteriorly until it is inscribed within D2, we find that the angle at its apex (αD1) is inscribed within αD2. The maximum deviation for αD1< αD2 = 5°. Therefore, from knowing αD2, we can deduce αD1.

If we divide the height of D2 by its base, we obtain (Table 6.10) an anthropometric index (Domini, Guidi, Guazzini, 2008) that corresponds to the apex angle αD2, in which it is included, with a maximum deviation of -5° αD1. From the width of D1 it is possible to deduce the morphology of the anterior pelvis.

Simply determining D1 is not sufficient for prognostic purposes. Indeed, if its height is 4 cm and its base 8 cm, the index will be 0.5; which is the same result as for a very different triangle with a height of 3 cm and base 6 cm. Therefore the important calculation is that of the area, which is obtained from base times height over 2. Under normal conditions, this should not be less than 70 cm squared.

So, now the final question arises: how representative is this area with regard to the area of the anterior pelvis? Its area should also be brought into relation with pelvic morphology, bearing in mind that the ratio between the maximum transverse diameter and the bicrestal diameter varies with the morphology of the pelvis.

In the android and anthropoid pelves, the transverse diameter is superior to the bicrestal diameter; in the gynecoid and platypelloid pelves, the transverse diameter

Table 6.11

Probable morphology of pelvic inlet obtained by combining the anthropometric index with measurement of the posterior bispinous diameter

Anterior pelvis	Bispinous dia.	Posterior pelvis
Android/Anthropoid	<9.5 cm	Android/Anthropoid
Android/Anthropoid	≥9.5 cm	Gynecoid
Gynecoid	<9.5 cm	Gynecoid/Android-anthropoid
Gynecoid	≥9.5 cm	Gynecoid
Platypelloid	=9.5 cm	Gynecoid
Platypelloid	>9.5 cm	Platypelloid

coincides (is aligned with) with the bicrestal diameter. "A very simple empirical method for assessing the morphology of the prepubic angle is to turn side-on to the patient and bring the ulnar side of one's hands into contact with the groin area in the space between the anterior-superior iliac spine and the pubis, holding the middle fingers in contact with each other. This forms a triangle, whose morphology and surface can be used to deduce the morphology and surface of the anterior triangle".

Evaluation of the Posterior Pelvis

Having defined the morphology of the anterior pelvis, it is possible to deduce that of the posterior pelvis by using the posterior bispinous diameter (projected between the two

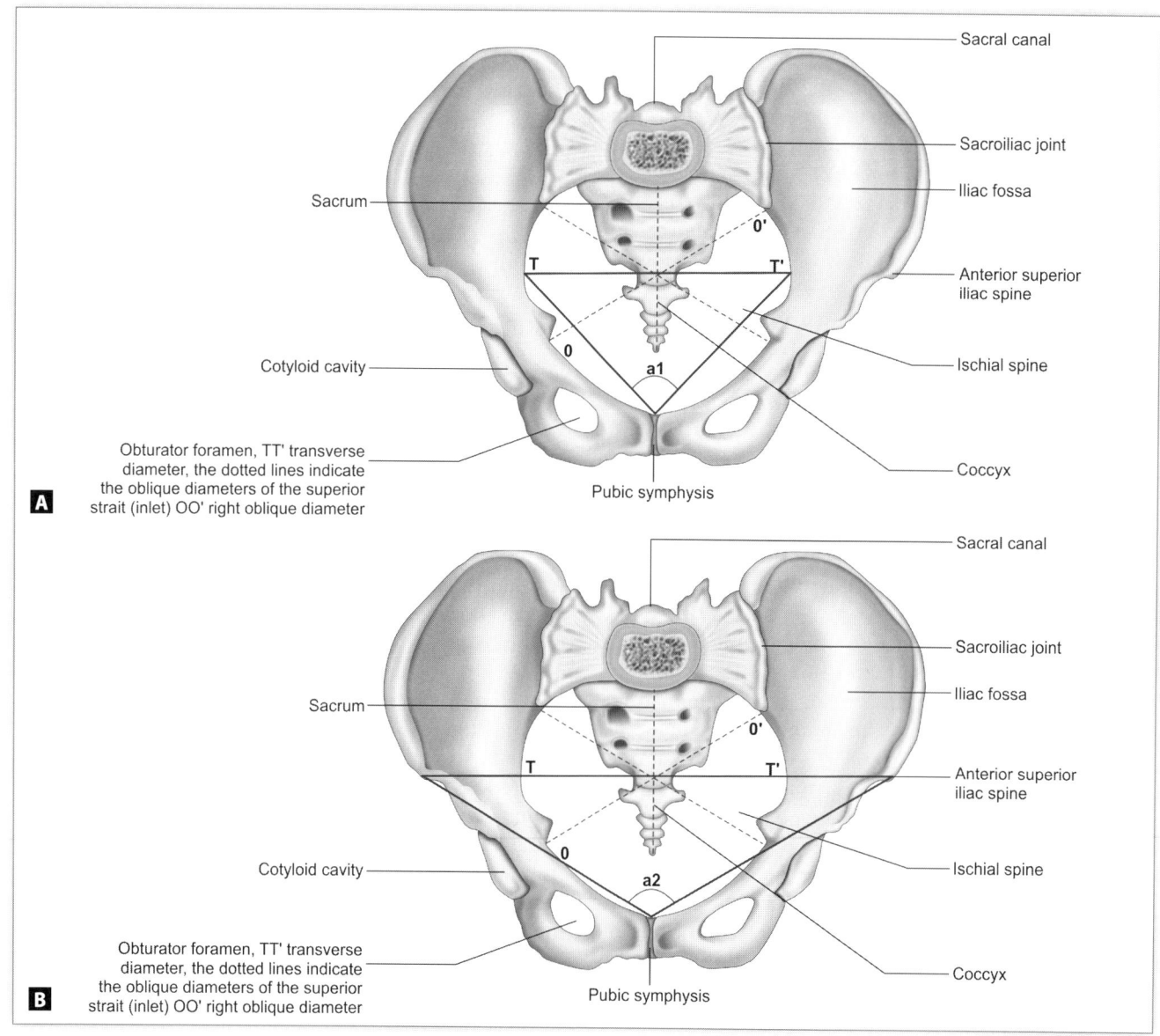

Fig. 6.25: From isosceles triangle (A) whose base is the bicrestal diameter and whose apex is the pubic symphysis, the anterior pelvis (B) can be derived

DIAGNOSIS IN CLINICAL OBSTETRICS

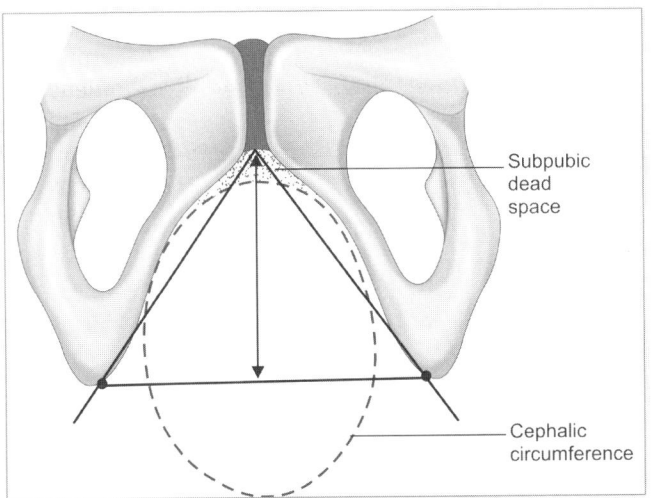

Fig. 6.26: Subpubic arch: 1. Subpubic dead space: The area of the subpubic arch not occupied by the presenting part is given the name 'dead space'. 2. Cephalic circumference

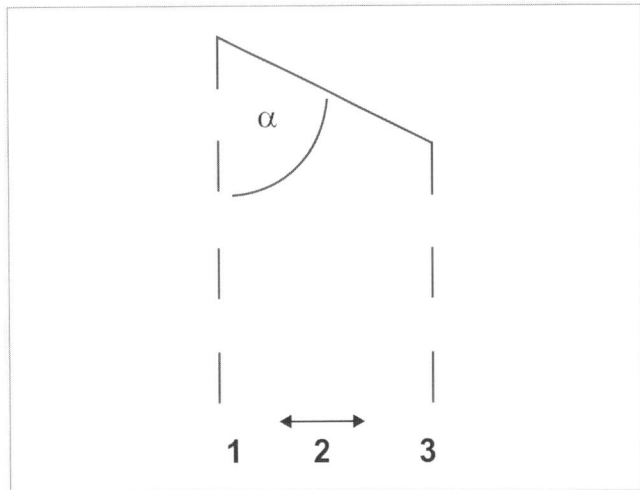

Table 6.12: 1. Distance from ground to posterior border of pelvic inlet 2. Space between the posterior and anterior borders of pelvic inlet 3. Distance from ground of anterior border α inclination of pelvic inlet

posterior iliac spines), which is representative of (correlates well with) the transverse diameter of the pelvic inlet (Table 6.11).

Site of Lumbosacral Hinge

This is obtained from the height of the posterior triangle (Table 6.11).

Inclination

Instruments Required
- A tape measure, (cut at the height of 180 cm), is attached to a wall (or to a door jamb)
- A second tape measure (200 cm) is divided into two equal portions (100 cm); the first is applied to a horizontal bar, which branches out at a right angle from the top end of the first measure; the second is set on the ground, branching from the foot of the wall measure.
  - a plumb bob
  - a goniometer

Method

The Patient stands below the horizontal bar with her feet on either side of the measure placed on the ground.

At a distance of 15 cm from the origin of the horizontal bar or door jamb a plumb bob is hung, whose end reaches half way up the base of the patient superior triangle (Fig. 6.18).

The length of the line is subtracted from 180 (or from the height of the architrave), thereby giving us the height of the posterior extremity of pelvic inlet. We note the datum, to scale, on a piece of graph paper.

Keeping patient's position unchanged, the plumb line is now held at the superior border of the pubic symphysis and allowed to slide down until it touches the measure set on the ground. This gives us:
- The distance from the origin; by subtracting 15 cm we obtain the interval between the posterior and anterior borders of the pelvic inlet. This value is noted on the graph paper
- The length, this value is noted (Table 6.12).
The angle is measured using a standard goniometer.

Pelvic Examination

Once completed the abdominal palpation and evaluation of the anterior pelvis: we proceed, with the patient in the standing position, to determine the posterior interspinous diameter (evaluation of the posterior pelvis) and the site of the lumbosacral hinge (height of the posterior triangle). The gravid patient is now placed in lithotomy position and pelvic exploration is continued.

As the birth canal consists of a bony part and soft tissues, a correctly conducted pelvic examination should assess both components: bone and soft tissues. The diagnostic pathway should proceed as follows:
a. Examination of soft tissues.
b. Determination of intertuberous diameter and its signifycance.
c. Assessment of subpubic arch.
d. Determination of retropubic angle.
e. Outline of pelvic inlet, characteristics of arcuate line of the ileum (linea terminalis).
f. Identification of promontory, its characteristics; diagonal conjugate.
g. Relationship between lateral walls of pelvis (parallel, convergent, divergent).
h. Characteristics of ischial spines.

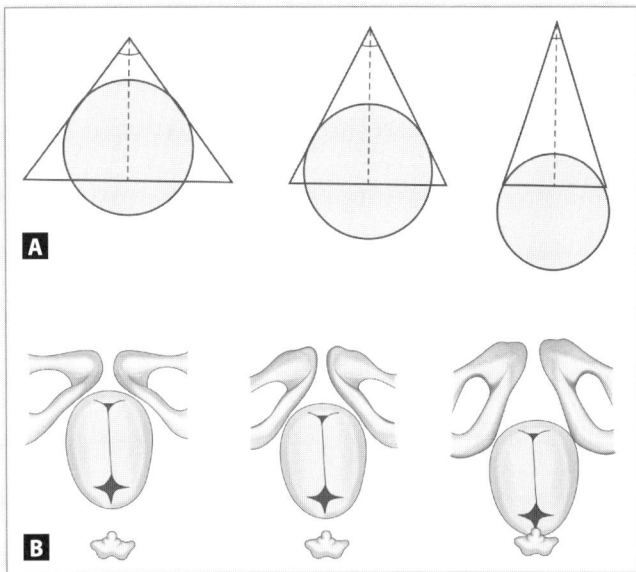

Fig. 6.27A and B. Illustration of how the area of inscription of a sphere within an isosceles triangle decreases (and dead space increases) as the angle of the apex is reduced. It shows: A. the direct relation between base and apex angle (the greater the base, the wider the angle); B. the inverse relationship between the triangle's height and the apex angle (as height increases, the angle narrows)

i. Characteristics of sacrum.
l. Evaluation of depth of fornices.
m. Assessment of characteristics of cervix - Bishop score.
n. Characteristics of membranes.
o. Diagnosis of presentation, engagement and position.
p. Abdominal pelvic score.

Examination of the Soft Parts

Simple observation of the external genitalia will establish whether the person is a primigravida or has already given birth, and, in the latter case, of the quality of obstetric assistance received.

A gaping vulvar fissure is a sign of a lesion of the urogenital diaphragm; if this is associated with protrusion of the anterior vaginal wall and verticalisation of the urethra, a concomitant lesion of the pubovesicocervical fascia has occurred.

A reduction in height of the perineal base (distance between the vaginal vestibule and the anus, usually 2.5 cm), is another sign of a lesion to the urogenital diaphragm.

The radiating contour of the anus, throughout its extension, indicates an intact sphincter; an interruption in the radiating folding reveals an injury to the sphincter at that point.

Height at which the intertuberous diameter crosses the external genitalia:
- Close to the vagina in the flat pelvis
- Midway between vagina and rectum in the gynecoid pelvis
- Posterior to this in the android and anthropoid pelves.

Determination of the Intertuberous Diameter and Significance

This diameter is projected between the borders of the two ischiatic tuberosities; it measures 10–11 cm and can be assessed using: the Greenhill method (Fig. 6.22), the Tarnier method (Fig. 6.24), or using a pelvimeter (Fig. 6.23A and B) —see section on evaluation of the pelvic outlet.

While the Greenhill method of measuring the intertuberous diameter is only of indicative clinical significance, a more accurate and, for our purposes, more useful measurement is that obtained using a pelvimeter or by the Turner method. A value obtained in these ways is of use because:

- A low value is itself an obstacle to advancement and disengagement of the presenting part
- When related to the height and morphology of the subpubic arch, the height of the pubic arch or anterior sagittal conjugate, or McDermott conjugate (Fig. 2.24, 7A), this is the perpendicular projected down from the apex to the intertuberous diameter (Fig. 6.26), or the height of the isosceles triangle that has the intertuberous diameter as its base and the ischiopubic rami as its sides. It measures 6.5–7.5 cm on average. A high arch is a poor prognostic indicator for disengagement in that disengagement becomes easier the easier it is for the head to fit into the subpubic space (Fig. 6.27).

The *dead space* below the symphysis should be as small as possible. It is easily assessed by comparing the subpubic arch (Fig. 6.26) with a disc of plastic material 9 cm in diameter. The lower the area of inscription, the greater will be the dead space and with it the difficulty of disengagement.

- When correlated with the relationship between the lateral pelvic walls, the intertuberous diameter allows us to deduce indirectly the median transverse diameter of the pelvic inlet (Fig. 2.27):
- If *the walls are parallel* (gynecoid and anthropoid pelves), the intertuberous diameter equals the median transverse diameter of the pelvic inlet (Fig. 6.28A).
- If *the walls are convergent* (android pelvis), the intertuberous diameter is less than that of median transverse diameter of the pelvic inlet (Fig. 6.28B).
- If *the walls are divergent* (platypelloid pelvis), the intertuberous diameter is greater than median transverse diameter.

At this point the examiner begins the pelvic examination. Access to the vagina and subsequent steps can take place using:
– A single finger (forefinger)

DIAGNOSIS IN CLINICAL OBSTETRICS

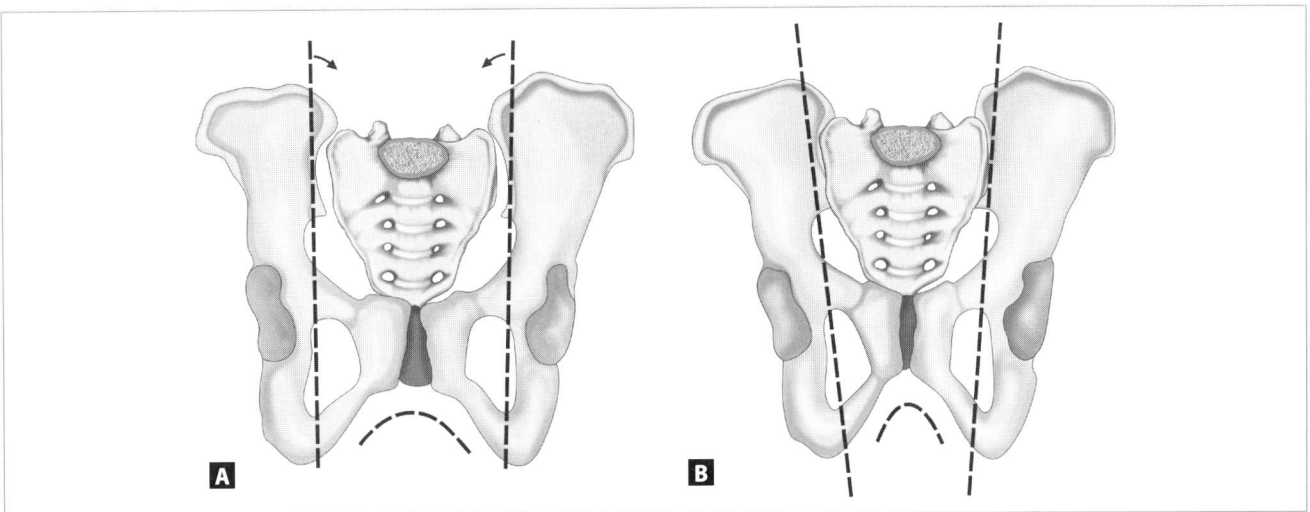

Fig. 6.28: (A) The pelvic walls are parallel (gynecoid and anthropoid pelves); the intertuberous diameter equals the median transverse diameter of the pelvic inlet, (B) The pelvic wall converge (android pelvis), the intertuberous diameter is less than the median transverse diameter of the pelvic inlet

- Two fingers (forefinger and middle finger), the volar side of the third phalanx of the middle finger of the not examining hand depresses the fourchette and the two fingers access the vagina, following the posterior vaginal wall, having accessed the vagina, the palm turns upwards (the hand in supination) and the two fingers evaluate now the subpubic arch.

Assessing the Subpubic Arch

The morphology may resemble:
- A Gothic arch in android and anthropoid pelves (Fig. 2.27, Table 6.2)
- A Roman arch (Fig. 2.27, Table 6.2) in the gynecoid pelvis, which easily receives the two fingers (forefinger and middle finger) of the hand in supination; the two fingers may separate
- A Norman arch, in the platypelloid pelvis.

At this point, with the hand still supinate, the two fingers go behind the pubis to assess the retropubic angle.

Determining the Retropubic Angle

The angle's amplitude and morphology (Fig. 6.26) are established; exploration continues of the pelvic inlet and characteristics of the *linea terminalis*.

Outline of Pelvic Inlet; Characteristics of the Linea Terminalis

In a cephalic presentation, the examining finger which follows the linea terminalis does not manage to follow the posterior third; assessment of the free spaces between head and pelvis provides futher useful information about pelvic morphology.

Identifying the Sacral Promontory, Its Characteristics, the Diagonal Conjugate

Interrelation between lateral pelvic walls

- Parallel (Fig. 6.28A), gynecoid and anthropoid pelves
- Convergent (Fig. 6.28B), android pelvis
- Divergent, platypelloid pelvis

Characteristics of the Ischial Spines

Locating them is relatively easy: having introduced two fingers into the vagina, one tries to locate the ischial tuberosity, then moving back and forth in a mediolateral direction, a small bony lump is detected: the ischial spine.

Locating the ischial spines is of crucial importance in obstetrics:
- In evaluating pelvic morphology—they are prominent in the android pelvis
- In diagnosing engagement by vaginal examination (see below, Fig. 6.31).

Assessment of the Sacral Cavity

Assessment of depth of fornices

This sign is not described in classic obstetrics, but in our opinion it should be thoroughly examined, as it is one of the earliest signs of a mechanical obstruction during labour.

The vagina enters the cervix at the level of the junction between the upper 1/3 with lower 2/3. At term of pregnancy and during labour, the LUS is formed: when it encounters an obstruction, the LUS distends and stretches cranially, and in doing so pulls with it the uterine cervix, which has by now (through effacement and dilation) lost its anatomical identity and consistency.

Table 6.13
Bishops's (1974) cervical scores

Points	0	1	2	3
Position of uterine cervix	Posterior	Middle	Anterior	
Effacement (lenght)	0–30%	40–50	60–70	80
Dilation of cervical os (cm)	0	1–2	3–4	> 4
Consistency	Normal	Medium	Soft	
Station of presenting part assessed in: cm above ischial spine fifths of head above symphysis	–3 5/5	–2	–1, 0 2/5	+1 +2

This cranial traction causes the vaginal fornices to be particularly deep, so the anterior fornix passes the superior border of the pubic symphysis and the lateral ones reach the linea terminalis. We will finally note how the cervix is adhering strongly to the presenting part.

Assessment of Characteristics of the Uterine Cervix; Bishop's Score

This is done by taking four parameters into account: position, effacement, dilation and consistency, which make up Bishop's cervical assessment score (Table 6.13). A fifth parameter is whether or not the head is engaged. Assessment of dilation can be done:
- *Using two fingers*—one finger accesses the cervix (2 cm), or two fingers (4 cm); if dilation is greater, the fingers are separated until they touch the margins
- *Using one finger only*—In our opinion, measurement is easier and more accurate using this method, also termed the *subtraction method*. We proceed as follows: the index finger moves along the cervix in a lateromedial direction; at 3 o'clock and at 9 o'clock the length of each side is evaluated in cm; the two results are added together and the result subtracted from 10 (full dilation): the difference is the degree of dilation.

A cervical score of between 0 and 13 is awarded. An at-risk condition is denoted by a score above:
- 2—in a primigravida before the 25th week or in a multipara before the 17th week
- 5—after these periods, both in primigravidae and in women who have already given birth previously

Induction may be conducted with certainty when the cervical score is ≥9.

Characteristics of the Membranes

Forebag (membranes) and amniotic fluid: The foetal head fits perfectly in a normal pelvis, thereby isolating the forewaters (forebag) from the amniotic fluid in the uterine cavity.

During labour, this quantity remains unchanged and the forebag takes on a hemispherical shape. In the contracted and in the flat pelvis, however, the forewaters are displaced, respectively, either laterally to the head or between the brow and posterior pelvis, and a free space opens up via which uterine waters can communicate with the forewaters. For this reason, at each new contraction, more amniotic fluid will pass forward and intrauterine pressure will be transmitted to the forewaters and membranes, which will at first protrude, remaining elastic and stretching into an elongated sausage, until they rupture prematurely.

Diagnosing Presentation, Engagement and Position
Recognition of foetal parts
- Distinguishing between head and breech: The head has uniform firmness; the sutures and fontanelles can be felt; the breech is not evenly firm, nor are any sutures or fontanelles detectable
- *Distinguishing between the posterior and anterior fontanelle* (Fig. 6.29): the posterior fontanelle is triangular and is located at the meeting point of three sutures: the sagittal and the two branches of the lambdoid suture. The anterior fontanelle is quadrangular in shape and located at the meeting point of four sutures: sagittal, frontal and the two branches of the coronal sutures
- *Distinguishing between the foot and the hand* (Fig. 6.30A): toes are roughly equal in length and are shorter than the fingers; fingers differ in their lengths; the thumb will extend, but the big toe does not (Fig. 6.30B).

When passing from the foot to the leg, one can feel (Fig. 6.30C) a change in direction, at right angles, which cannot be changed: this is the heel, which feels like a prominent and hard formation. When passing from the hand to the forearm, no change of direction is felt.
- *Distinguishing between elbow and knee:* The knee presents a cavity, in that the patella is not yet formed: the elbow has the prominence of the olecranon.

Diagnosing station by vaginal examination (Fig. 6.31): The distance between the pelvic inlet and ischial spines is 5 cm, while the distance between biparietal diameter of the foetal head and its vertex is between 2 and 5 cm. Therefore, when the vertex is 1 cm above or at the level of the ischial spines, the head will definitely be engaged. Using the ischial spines as an anatomical landmark, the number of centimetres that separate them from the foetal head provides the station of the vertex:

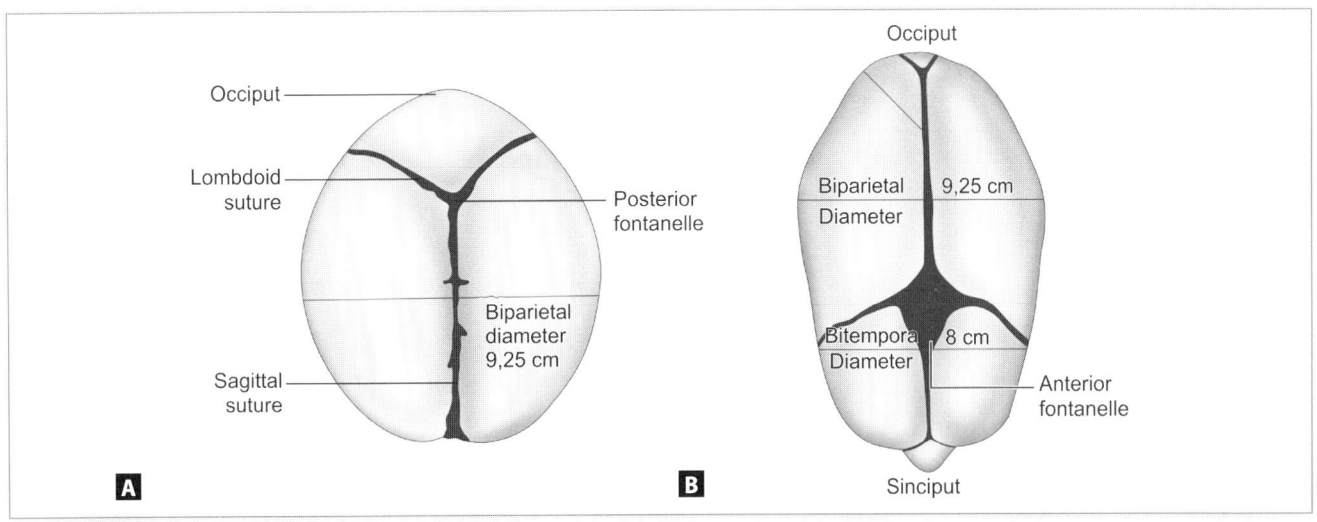

Fig. 6.29A and B: Sutures and fontanelles: (A) Posterior fontanelle, at the confluence of the lambdoid sutures with the sagittal suture; (B) Anterior fontanelle

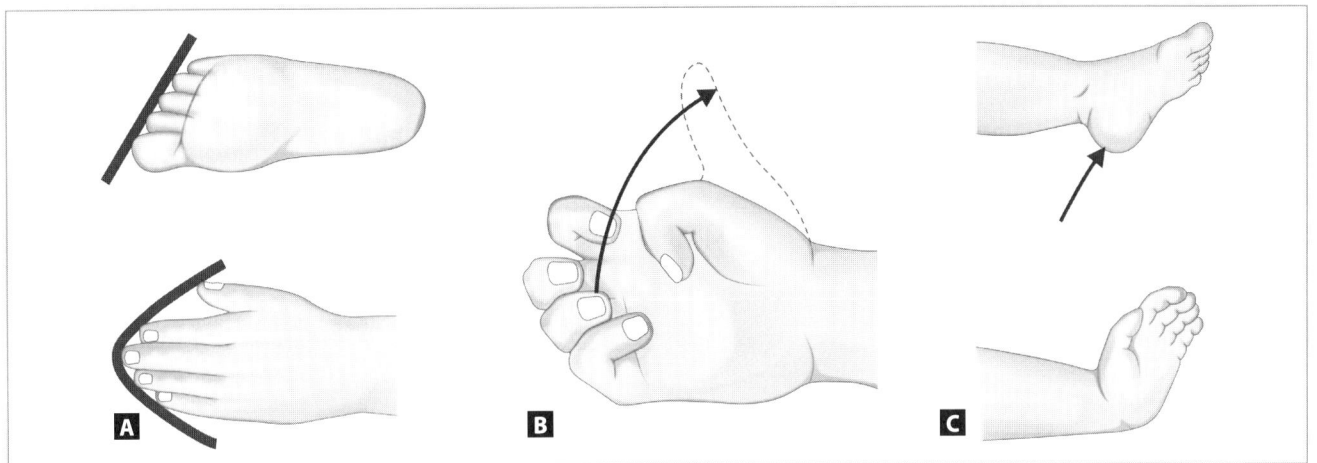

Fig. 6.30A to C: (A) Toes are shorter than fingers; (B) The thumb can extend; the big toe cannot; (C) When moving from foot to leg, the heel feels like a hard, prominent formation

- 3, 2, 1 centimetres above the ischial spines are indicated as -3, -2 and -1, respectively
- At the level of the ischial spines is indicated as zero = 0.
- Descent of the vertex from here onwards: 1, 2, 3 cm below the ischial spines is indicated as +1, +2 and +3, respectively.

Abdominal/Pelvic Scores (Knight, 1993)

When the sum of (Crichton's) head fifths and the moulding of skull bones is ≥3, there is cephalopelvic disproportion and vaginal delivery is not recommended.

Moulding of the foetal skull bones

This is an important indicator of the size ratio between foetal head and pelvis. It consists in assessing (Fig. 6.29) the relation between the parietal and occipital bones (lambdoid sutures) and the relation between the two parietal bones (sagittal suture). Points are scored as follows:

- O = Bones are separate and the sutures are detected easily.
- + = Bones are just touching each other.
- ++ = Bones are overlapping (imbricated), but easily separable by finger pressure.
- +++ = Bones overlapping (imbricated) and are not separable by finger pressure.
- Some authors (Stewart, KS, 1974) replace +, ++, +++ with 0, 1, 2, 3, respectively.

If imbrication of the lambdoid sutures is associated with imbrication of the sagittal suture, disproportion is more severe and the sagittal is given the same score as the lambdoid sutures. For example, separable overlapping of the lambdoid suture scores 2 points; if a separable

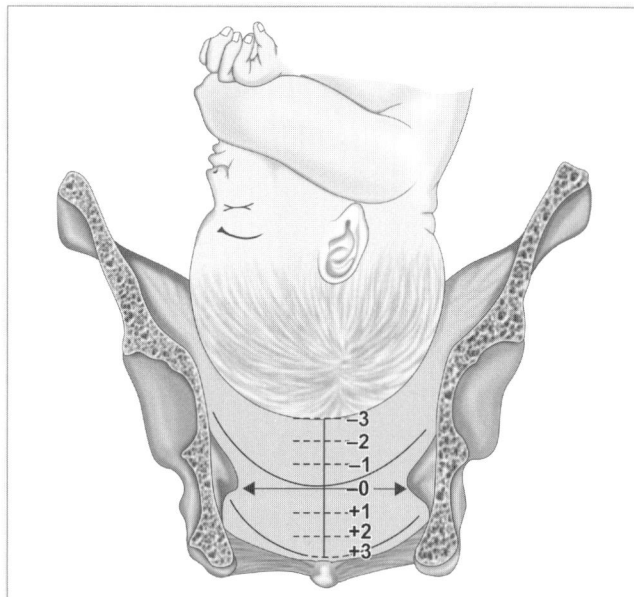

Fig. 6.31: Assessing engagement by vaginal examination: Engagement has occurred when the vertex reaches the level of the ischial spines

overlapping of the sagittal suture is concurrently present: 2 points, giving an overall score of 4.

Sharp overlapping (imbrication) of the cranial bones in a head that is still high in the pelvis, is an ominous sign of cephalopelvic disproportion (CPD).

A gradual increase in the moulding of the skull bones is an ominous sign of obstructel labour.

Soft-tissue Edema and Caput Succedaneum (Fig. 6.15)

After rupture of the membranes, the portion of the presenting part in contact with the cervix is subject only to the action of atmospheric pressure, while the remaining part of the foetal body is subject to the sum of pressures generated by the expulsive force and atmospheric pressure. This pressure gradient promotes the flow of fluid from the interstitial vessels of subcutaneous connective tissue. When the pressure exerted by the cervix on the foetal scalp is added to this, normal lymphatic and venous drainage is impeded and a limited area, a few millimetres in thickness, of infiltrated scalp and subcutaneous connective tissue is created. This is referred to as a caput succedneum, or soft tissue oedema. The volume of a caput is determined by the amount of time elapsed between membrane rupture and expulsion of the presenting part. When deformation is pronounced, it is referred to as a caput (protracted labour). With a pronounced caput, it may be difficult to assess the amount of moulding of the cranial bones, but a pronounced caput is itself already an expression of cephalopelvic disproportion or of obstructel labour. In concluding this Chapter, I would like to recall the often-repeated words of my teacher, (T Jeffeoate, Liverpool): "Dystocias of the pelvic inlet are difficult to diagnose during pregnancy, but easily recognized and easily managed during labour: Dystocias of the midpelvis and pelvic outlet are easily detected during pregnancy through pelvic exploration, but are difficult to treat during labour. Therefore, while one can tolerate failure to detect the former, one must be absolutely intolerant of failure to detect the latter."

BIBLIOGRAPHY

1. Bishop EH. A pelvic scoring for elective induction. Obstet Gyneecol, 1974;24:266.
2. Crichton D. Establishing the level of the foetal head. SAf Med J. 1974;48:784-7.
3. Domini E, Guidi M, Guazzini S, Vicentini S. Misurazione intraoperatoria della coniugata ostetrica. Giornale It Ostet Ginecol. 2007;29:283.
4. Knight D. A comparison of abdominal and vaginal examination for diagnosis of the engagement of the foetal head. NZ J Obst Gyn. 1993;33:155-7.
5. Kraus T, Osmers S, Westerfeld S, Metzger I, Puchta J, Kuhu W. Meaning of assimilation pelvis according to Kirchhoff in modern obstetrics. Z Geburtshilfe Neonatol. 1997;201:247-52.
6. Leopold GC, Pantzer MEC. Die Beschränkung der inneren und die grössmöglichste Verwertung der äusseren Untersuchung in der Geburtshilfe. Vierter Beitrag zur Verhutung des Kinderbettfie-bers mit einem Rückblick auf das Jahr 1889. Archiv für Gynäkologie, Ber- lin 1890; 38: 330.
7. Leopold GC. Die Leitung normaler Geburten nur durch äussere Untersuchung. Archiv für Gynäkologie, Berlin. 1894;42:394.
8. Leopold GC. Ueber die Leitung normaler Geburten nur durch äussere Untersuchung. Zbl für Gynäkologie. 1894; 21:498.
9. Stewart KS. The foetal response to cephalo-pelvic disproportion. J Obst Gyn Br Cmw. 1974;32:217.
10. Wischnik A, Lehmann KJ, Zahn K, Georgi M, Melchert F. Changes in pelvic anatomy in 8 decades-computerized tomography study of obstetrical relevant pelvic measurements. Z Geburshilfe Perinatol. 1992;196:49-54.

CHAPTER 7

Partograph

The partograph is a graphical representation of true labour and of maternal–foetal conditions. *It correlates cervical dilatation, descent of the presenting part and uterine contractions as functions over time* and its purpose is to alert to abnormal labour and anomalies in maternal and/or foetal well-being.

Partographs are applicable only to cephalic presentations with flexed head (vertex or bregma at most). Therefore, accurate and meticulous assessment of the gravid patient upon admission to the delivery room is an absolute requirement. This is the only way to ensure that presentation meets the above criteria and to exclude the presence of risk factors or emergency conditions.

A preliminary step consists of differentiating contractions of true and false labour (Braxton Hicks Contractions) (Table 7.1).

The partograph is *an indispensable obstetric instrument*, because, using very modest means:
a. It offers a simple means of monitoring true labour and of rapidly diagnosing an abnormal course of labour, thereby reducing maternal and foetal mortality and morbidity. The usefulness of keeping a partograph is so well established that *"not to introduce it might almost be considered criminal neglect".*
b. It indicates the point at which active intervention becomes necessary.
c. By requiring the recording of several clinic parameters, it develops the habit of observation, thus proving educational for medical personnel and obstetricians.

The only instrumentation required comprises: A chart, a pencil, an obstetric stethoscope, a wall clock with a second hand and a sphygmomanometer.

Table 7.1
The patterns of abnormal labour

False labour	*True labour*
Irregular intervals and duration	Regular intervals, gradually increasing
Painful uterine contractions	Painless uterine contractions
Intensity unchanged	Intensity increasing
Increased uterine tone	Notmal uterine tone
No cervical dilation	Cervical dilation occurs
Lower abdominal discomfort	Back and abdominal discomfort
Relief from sedation	No relief from sedation
Uterine contractions don't increase with physical activity	Uterine contractions increased with physical activity
It lasts fot 7–24–48 hours	It lasts fot 6–8 hours

It may happen that partograph charts are not available in a given environment. Supply can be ensured by the following contrivance: The partograph is placed under a white X-ray plate; observations are filled out on the plate itself, which is washable and reusable after each delivery.

INTRODUCTION

The first obstetrician to apply statistical analytical methods to the progress of labour was LA Calkin, who in 1955 published a book condensing results and findings from 16,000 deliveries recorded between 1933 and 1944.

We owe the theoretical basis of today's partograph to work by Friedman (1954) who, while acknowledging indebtedness to the pioneering work of Calkins, did not share Calkin's methodology, and was the first to portray cervical dilatation graphically in relation to time. The result was a sinusoid curve (Fig. 7.1) in which two phases were functionally distinguishable: Latent and active.

The *latent (or prodromal) phase* lasts from the onset of contractions until cervical dilatation of 2 cm; it has a duration of 8–10 hours as is characterised not only by dilatation but also by a progressive reduction in the length of the cervix (effacement).

- The *active phase* is characterised by rapid dilatation of the cervix from 2 to 10 cm. This phase may be subdivided into: *Acceleration phase* and *phase of maximum slope*, at the end of which dilatation of 9 cm is reached. These are followed by the reduced acceleration phase, or *deceleration phase*, leading to a complete dilatation (full cervical ripening) of 10 cm.

Finally, Friedman argued that the cervimetric curve for the primigravida differed from that for women who had already given birth, and therefore proposed two cervimetric curves: One for primigravidae (Fig. 7.1), and one for multiparae (Fig. 7.2).

Later Hendricks et al. (1970) showed that the active phase for primigravidae differed only slightly from that for multiparae; they also ruled out the existence of a deceleration phase.

The centimetric curve of cervical dilatation presents significant variations between different populations (Duignam et al., 1974; Lennox, 1981) and within one given population, due to obstetric clinical practice:

- In Texas, the use of epidural analgesia led to an extension of mean duration in the active phase from five to six hours (Alexander et al., 2002)
- In Ireland, following the introduction of a protocol for the active treatment of labour, duration of the active phase reduced to just 4.9 hours (Impey et al., 1997)
- In New Mexico, Rogers et al. (1997), using the Dublin protocol for active treatment of labour, reduced duration of labour and delivery among nulliparae from 11.4 to 9.7 hours.

All findings to date show that in every population and under all circumstances, *the rate of dilatation is consistently greater than 1 cm. per hour* and that *the lower limit will not be returned to again.*

We owe the present design of the partograph to Philpott (1972), who, while working in a Rhodesian hospital (in what is now Zimbabwe), sought an early warning system for prolonged labour.

A graphical system was developed, the partogram, in which the three essential components of the labour—foetal well-being, progress of labour, possible treatment—are represented. The original partogram included the two cervimetric curves as originally proposed by Friedman.

Another innovation was the representation of cervical dilatation and descent of the head on the same graph, correlating these in turn with the pattern of contractions. A final addition, providing a way of assessing engagement and descent of the presenting part, was Crichton's (1974) head-fifths method, as detected on the foetal dorsal side. As we have seen, 5/5 head corresponds to a nonengaged head; 2/5 to an engaged head (see Chapter 6).

Various changes have been made to Philpott's partogram over time; these can be seen in the WHO partograph (Fig. 7.3), which is the one in widest use in resource-poor countries. Its basic features are as follows:

- On Hendrick's (1970) recommendation, the two cervimetric curves have been replaced by a single one

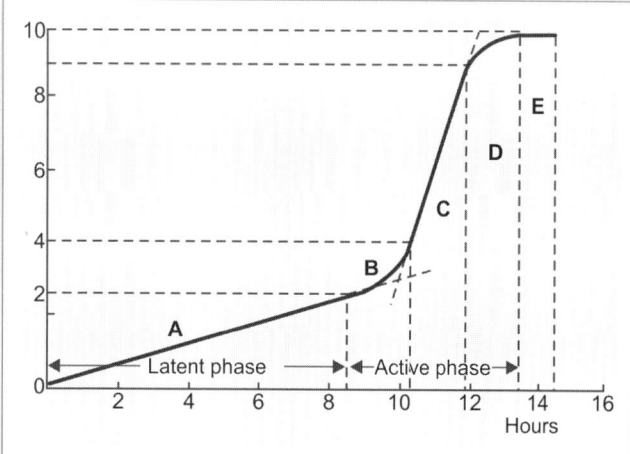

Fig. 7.1: Cervimetric graph for a primigravida—Friedman's curve: (A) Latent phase (note how the latent phase ends at 2 cm); (B) Acceleration phase; (C) Phase of maximum slope; (D) Deceleration phase; (E) Expulsive phase

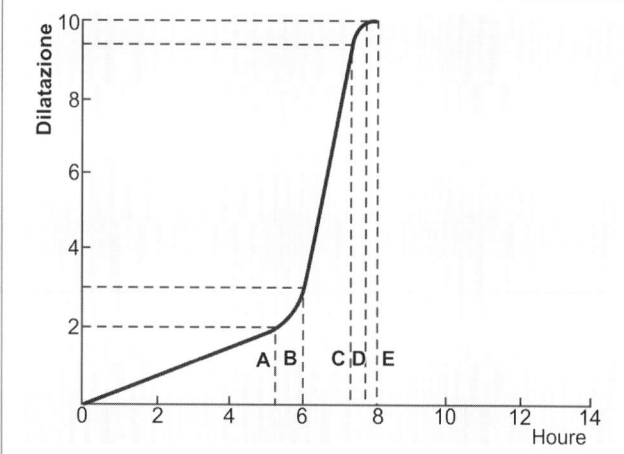

Fig. 7.2: Cervimetric graph of woman who has previously given birth: (A) Latent phase (note how the latent phase ends at 2 cm); (B) Acceleration phase; (C) Phase of maximum slope; (D) Deceleration phase; (E) Expulsive phase

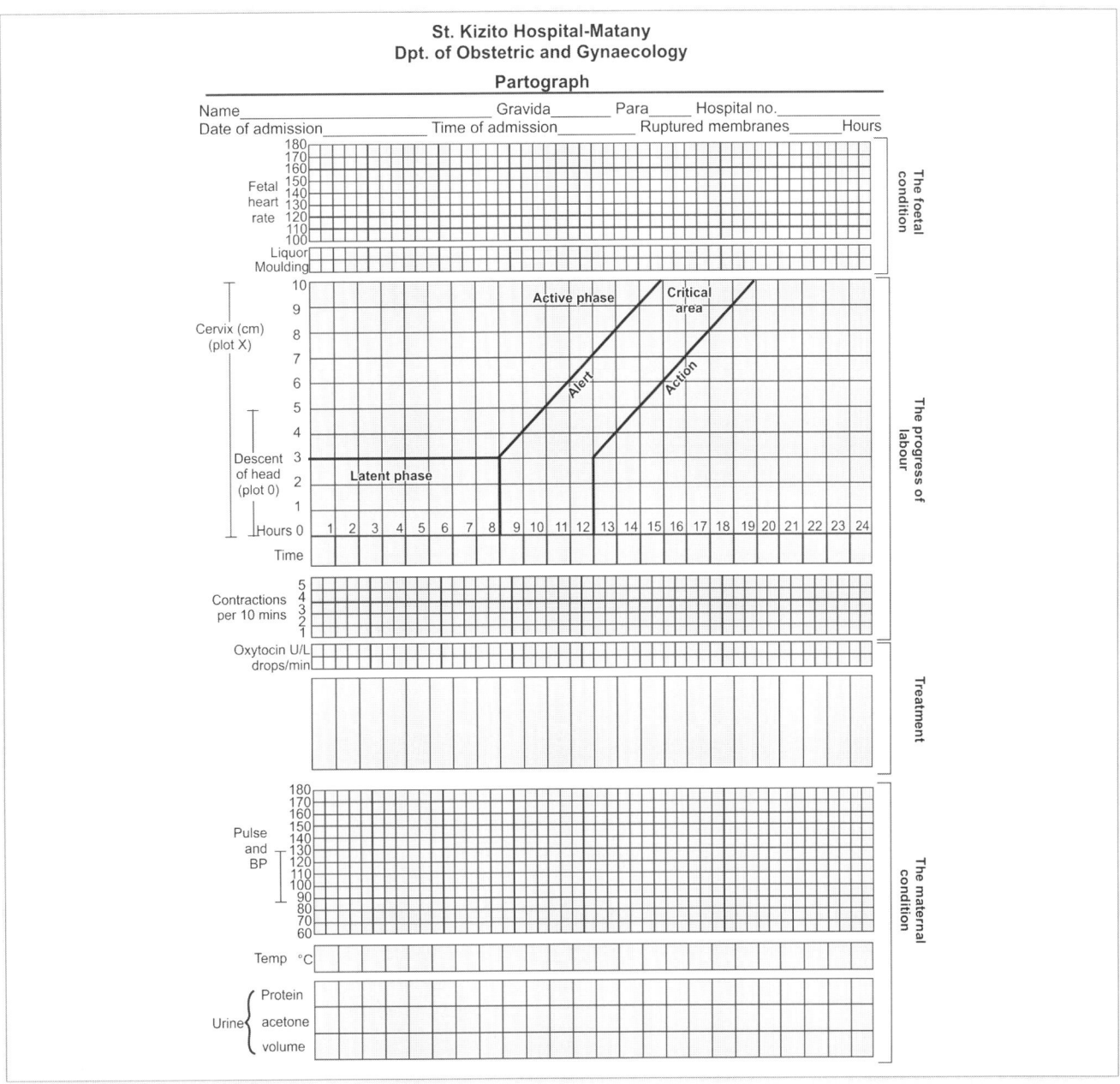

Fig. 7.3: WHO model partograph

- The latent phase ends at *3 cm* dilatation and must not exceed eight hours
- The active phase begins with 3 cm dilatation and has a minimum constant dilatation (constant inclination) of not less than 1 cm per hour
- A deceleration phase is no longer represented
- The cervimetric curve is flanked, on the right, (after a gap of 4 hours) by a second curve, called the *action line* (Philpot, 1972). Reaching this line is an indication that deceleration in the rate of dilatation and/or of descent by the presenting part is such that prolonging labour any further could prove harmful and that a decision has to be made. The area between the two curves is called the *critical area*. The consensus is that no repercussions on foetal well-being result from the four-hour interval between a deceleration in contraction rate and any intervention.

The original three sections—foetal well-being, progress of labour and any treatment given to the mother—have been augmented by a fourth section dedicated to maternal well-being.

THE CAESAREAN SECTION

STRUCTURE OF THE PARTOGRAPH

There are four sections. Proceeding from top to bottom:
a. The first concerns *foetal well-being* (foetal condition).
b. The second assesses *progress of labour* in its basic components of cervical dilatation, descent of the presenting part and contractions in relation to time.
c. The third describes *any medication given* (treatment).
d. The fourth covers *general maternal condition*.

This arrangement is not a random one, but follows specific graphical criteria. The central part of the chart, with greatest visual impact, is dedicated to the most significant section of the partograph: Progress of labour in its essential components of dilatation, descent and rate of contractions. Foetal well-being, treatment administered and maternal condition are positioned according to importance: Foetal well-being above with treatment and maternal well-being away from the centre. The intuitive place to begin, then, is with progress of labour.

PROGRESS OF LABOUR

The graph correlates contractile activity of the uterus (expulsive force) with cervical dilatation and descent of the presenting part (the passenger) as time functions.

The grid of the graph (Fig. 7.4) is a horizontal rectangle containing 11 horizontal and 25 vertical lines whose intersections provide 24 columns, each comprising 10 squares of equal size. The grid is bounded by orthogonal axis: A y-axis and an x-axis.

The y-axis features a numerical scale from 0 to 10, proceeding from the bottom upwards. Bracket alongside, the larger scale nearer the margin follows the entire height of the y-axis and traces cervical dilatation. To the right of this, a smaller square bracket follows the scale from 5 down to 0 and indicates the number of fifths of the foetal head detectable above the pubic symphysis.

The degree of cervical dilatation is marked by an X; descent of the presenting part is marked by a circle, 0.

The x-axis bears a scale of 24, each square corresponding to one hour; below each square is a space for noting the time of the clinical observation. The time of observation start is noted to the left of the word TIME.

Cervical dilatation: The cervical dilatation curve is shown on the grid where the horizontal course of the *latent phase*, lasting eight hours, is marked off from the *active phase*.

When marking out the curve of the active phase, it should be remembered that a normal rate of increase in diameter of external cervical os is *no less than 1 cm/hour*.

During normal labour the rate of dilatation is higher than 1 cm per hour; this means that the dilatation curve will always remain to the left of the alert line. If this theoretical line is reached, a deceleration has taken place. If the line is crossed, with the cervical curve now on its right, an alarm condition is indicated: Additional attention will now be required, as is indicated by the '*alert line*' label (Philpott et al., 1972).

It was also Philpott et al. (1972) who added a second line parallel to the alert line four hours on, calling it the 'action line'. Reaching this line signifies that a critical point has been reached, that further prolongation of labour could be harmful and that a decision must be made.

Within this range, the so-called *critical area*, any abnormality of labour is generally well tolerated and is unlikely to affect foetus or mother, thus avoiding

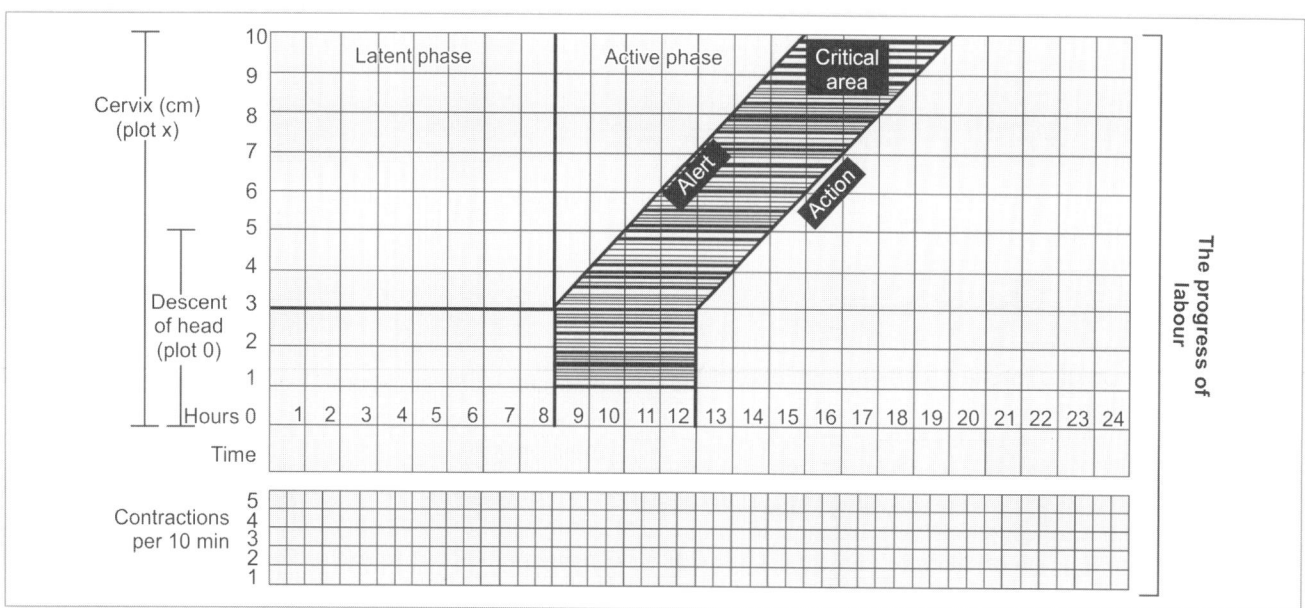

Fig. 7.4: Progress of labour; the critical phase is highlighted

unnecessary surgery. Some schools of thought question the arbitrary four-hour limit, arguing that decisions should be taken more promptly with multiparae. They therefore propose two action lines: One at 3 cm for multiparae and one at 4 cm (the present one) for primigravidae.

Descent and flexion of the head: Once the cervical os reaches a dilatation of 7 cm, the descent of the head, *indicated by a circle,* starts. Descent is expressed in terms of transverse finger breadth the head accommodates above the brim. Assessment by abdominal palpation (Chapter 6) has the following advantages:
- It is more accurate than vaginal examination (Figs 6.12 to 6.14), during which an inexperienced examiner may wrongly interpret what is in fact a caput as the leading part of the head (Fig. 6.15)
- It can be repeated several times
- It avoids the risk of vaginal contamination
- It allows the degree of flexion or extension of the head to be assessed. Figure 6.13 illustrates assessment of the head with the foetal back to the right and head flexed. It can be seen how fewer head-fifths are detectable on the dorsal side (occiput) than on the opposite (sinciput) side; when the head is deflected, the opposite occurs.

UTERINE CONTRACTILE ACTIVITY

Defined according to frequency and length (duration per contraction), contractions are shown on a grid bearing the title "Contractions per 10 minutes", positioned below the grid for progress of labour (Fig. 7.4).

This grid consists of a series of columns, each five squares high, extending along the whole length of the graph: Each (1-hour) square of the graph above corresponds to two 30-minute columns in the contractions grid.
- *Frequency* indicates the number of contractions in 10 minutes, with the 10-minute count starting as a contraction begins. This contraction rate is noted in the column corresponding to the time of observation (Fig. 7.4).

The uterine contraction rate is measured hourly during the latent phase and every half hour during the active phase; observation lasts 10 minutes and takes place during the last 10 minutes of every hour or half hour.

The reader is reminded that:
- During the latent phase, labour is under way when there are two or more contractions every 10 minutes, each lasting 20 seconds or more
- During the active phase, labour is under way when one or more contraction occurs, lasting 20 seconds or more, every ten minutes. As labour progresses, contractions become more frequent and each one lasts longer. We strongly recommend that the direction of contraction wave, i.e. its polarity, also be noted.
- *Duration* indicates how long an individual contraction lasts. Contractions are therefore defined as *mild* (lasting less than 20 seconds), *moderate* (20–40 seconds) and *strong* (more than 40 seconds), and are recorded using conventional graphic symbols: For *mild*, the square is filled with dots; for *moderate* it is filled with diagonal hatching, and for *strong* it is shaded in completely (Fig. 7.5).

FOETAL WELL-BEING

This is noted in the upper part of the partograph (Fig. 7.3), which records: Heart rate, condition of membranes and amniotic fluid, moulding of foetal skull.
- *Heart rate*: The graph features two horizontal lines in bold at 120 and 160 bpm, indicating the upper and lower extremes of physiological fluctuation.

Heart rate is taken every half hour, with the mother in left lateral decubitus. Initially, heart rate outside a contraction is established to determine the basal heart rate. Then, starting straight after the phase of greatest contractive intensity, auscultation is conducted for 1 minute. A frequency higher than 160 bpm is referred to as *tachycardia*: A rate of less than 120 bpm is *bradycardia*; either may be an indicator of foetal distress. When a nonreassuring rate is detected, the observation is repeated every 15 minutes, at the end of a contraction, during the dilatation period, and every 5 minutes during the expulsive phase. If the abnormality persists over more than three consecutive observations, surgical intervention is required, provided that delivery is not imminent.

A heart rate below 100 signifies that severe acute foetal distress is under way, requiring intervention without delay.

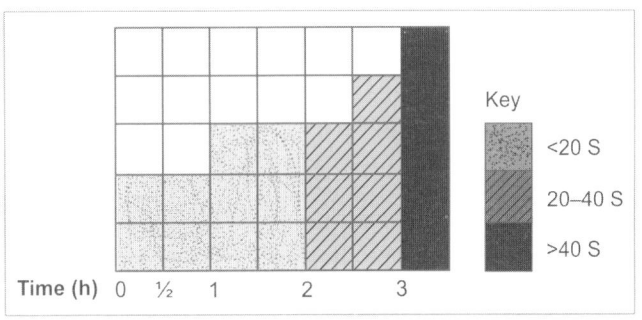

Fig. 7.5: Contractile activity: Graphic indication of duration. Key: Dotted infill: Duration less than 20 seconds; Diagonal hatching: Duration between 20 and 40 seconds; Fully shaded in: More than 40 seconds. From left to right: First hour: Two contractions observed every half hour, each lasting less than 20 seconds. Second hour: Three contractions observed every half hour, each lasting less than 20 seconds. Third hour: Three contractions observed during the first half hour, each lasting between 20 and 40 seconds; in the following half hour the number of contractions rise to 4, each lasting between 20 and 40 seconds. First half of fourth hour: Five contractions are observed, each lasting more than 40 seconds. Number of contractions exceeding five in 10 minutes is defined as "hyperkinesia"

The following methods of auscultation may be used:
- The standard method of auscultation, which begins immediately after a contraction and is continued for 30 seconds
- The Whitfield method of auscultation, in which marked abnormalities in the foetal heart rate (FHR) are noted. By this method, FHR is monitored at 5-second intervals both during and after contraction, and for periods of 5 seconds. The lowest value obtained, multiplied by 12, indicates the most marked bradycardia, which is indicated on the partograph by an arrow.

The number of 5-second periods that elapse between the end of a contraction and the first FHR value which, when multiplied by 12, gives a frequency higher than 120 provides a *reliable indicator of delay in recovery*.

Bradycardia should be related to different phases of contraction. Bradycardia needs be related to different phases of contraction (↑) or relaxation (↓) using the following symbols: ↑-, +, ++, +++, ↓++.+, -.

This will help distinguish deceleration bradycardia, which coincides with the peak of the contraction (type 1 dip), from late deceleration, occurring after 30 seconds (type 2 dip).
- *Early deceleration* (type 1 dip) coincides with contraction peak; its cause is stimulation of the dorsal vagus nucleus through increased intracranial pressure, which is induced by the contraction.

This type of deceleration appears in every labour once 5 cm dilatation has been reached, and is eight times more frequent among parturients whose membranes have ruptured than among those with intact membranes. Return to normal FHR follows swiftly.
- *Late deceleration* (type 2 dip) appears at the end of the contraction and is due to disturbed uterine-placental gas exchange. The prognosis will be poorer as
  - Deceleration increases in magnitude
  - The time interval increases between deceleration and return to normal frequency (recovery delay, see above).

Where malaria is endemic in the tropics, severe decelerations are commonly observed during apparently normal and unexceptional progress of labour, with nothing of relevance (neither cord compression nor placental abruption) detected postpartum. These apparently 'causeless' severe decelerations result from reduced placental perfusion, caused by:
- *Infarction of the intervillous space* by erythrocytes that have been sequestrated by *Plasmodium falciparum*. It has been shown that the parasite is particularly attracted to chondroitin sulphate A receptors (Lekana Douki et al., 2002) and to hyaluronic acids within the cells of the intervillous space
- *Fibrin deposits* by macrophages (Imamura, T. et al., 2002) within the placenta.

The mechanism of action appears to be as follows: A contraction is followed by hypoxia and acidosis; myocardial hypoxia causes bradycardia, while hypoxia and acidosis stimulate chemoreceptors, which in turn apparently stimulate the dorsal nucleus of the vagus, hence bradycardia.

The body's response to hypoxia and acidosis is by so called centralisation of circulation: A protective phenomenon which prioritises circulation to certain areas (brain, kidneys, heart) at the expense of others (skin, visceral plexus).
- *Forebag (membranes) and amniotic fluid*: Intactness of the forebag and characteristics of the amniotic fluid are checked every 4 hours, during pelvic examination. The condition of the membranes is recorded as follows:

  I = intact membranes; membrane integrity (forebag and hindwater) is not the only parameter to consider; morphology is also relevant.
- The foetal head fits perfectly in a *normal pelvis*, acting as a ball-valve and thereby isolating the forewaters (forebag) from the hindwaters. This is why the amount of forewater remains unchanged and the forebag takes on a hemispherical shape
- In the contracted and in the flat pelvis, however, the forewaters are displaced, respectively, either laterally to the head or between the brow and posterior pelvis, and a free space opens up via which the hindwaters can communicate with the forewaters. For this reason, at each new contraction, more amniotic fluid will pass forward and intrauterine pressure will be transmitted to the forewaters and to the membranes, which will at first protrude, remaining elastic and stretching into an elongated sausage, until they rupture prematurely. This does not occur in the normal pelvis.

  C = ruptured membranes, clear fluid

  M = ruptured membranes, fluid stained with meconium (see Chapter 26 for more on the significance of meconium in the amniotic fluid).

Recent experimental research and clinical studies (Arbay et al., 1998) have suggested that the mere presence of meconium in the amniotic fluid is not itself an indicator of acute foetal distress, but rather indicates an impairment of the fluid clearance system, linked to problems of circulation.

It is argued that during the 3rd trimester, amniotic fluid is completely replaced every 24–48 hours through foetal urine, ingestion, respiratory expiration and via the transamniotic pathway.

Amniotic fluid ingestion helps stabilise its volume and plays an important role in the mechanism of clearance; swallowing breaks down in conditions of foetal distress. It is thought, therefore, that the staining of amniotic fluid with meconium is not due to the passing of amniotic fluid following distress, but rather to the break-down of clearance mechanisms for the amniotic fluid, which now holds meconium from in-utero defecation.

The presence of meconium in the amniotic fluid damages the amnion epithelium and compromises the transamniotic clearance mechanism; it also exerts vasoconstrictive action on the umbilical veins (Altshuler et al., 1989) causing foetal hypotension. De-epithelialisation of the amnion and constriction of the umbilical veins are two further mechanisms by which the clearance of amniotic fluid is compromised, thus initiating a vicious cycle.

A = ruptured membranes, absence of fluid. In resource-poor countries, because of the danger of bacterial ascent, amniotomy should be performed only on carefully evaluated obstetric grounds and preferably not performed to induce labour. An untimely amniotomy can necessitate a C-section.

- *Moulding of the foetal skull* (Fig. 6.15) is assessed every four hours along with vaginal examination. This is an important indicator of the size ratio between foetal head and pelvis. It consists of assessing the relation between the parietal and occipital bones (lambdoid sutures) and the relation between the two parietal bones (sagittal suture). See Chapter 6 for more. Points are scored as follows:

O = Bones are separate and the sutures are detected easily.

+ = Bones are just touching each other.

++ = Bones are overlapping (imbricated), but easily separable by finger pressure.

+++ = Bones overlapping (imbricated) and are not separable by finger pressure.

Some authors (Stewart, K. S., 1974) replace +, ++, +++ with 0, 1, 2, 3, respectively.

If imbrication of the lambdoid sutures is associated with imbrication of the sagittal suture, disproportion is more severe and the sagittal suture is given the same score as the lambdoid one. For example: Separable overlapping of the lambdoid suture scores 2 points; if a separable overlapping of the sagittal suture is concurrently present, 2 points, giving an overall score of 4.

Sharp overlapping (imbrication) of the cranial bones in a head that is still high in the pelvis; this is an ominous sign of cephalopelvic disproportion (CPD).

A gradual increase in the foetal skull bones in an engaged head is an ominous sign of obstructed labour.

With a pronounced caput, it may be difficult to assess the amount of moulding of the cranial bones, but a pronounced caput is itself already an expression of cephalopelvic disproportion.

TREATMENT

In the area of the partograph below that dedicated to *progress of labour,* any administered drugs (fluids or oxytocins) are registered. This position was chosen to facilitate correlation between the administration of oxytocin and uterine contractile activity.

MATERNAL CONDITION

This is assessed by recording:
- *Temperature*: Every two hours or more frequently, if required
- *Heart rate*: Every half hour
- *Blood pressure*: Every 4 hours
- *Volume and characteristics of urine*: Low amounts of concentrated urine indicate a faulty fluid household. Dehydration, with all its consequences, can easily arise, particularly in obese women. 1 kg of adipose tissue contains only 100 mL of water, while 1 kg of muscle contains 720 mL: Dehydration should be corrected promptly, preferably using 10% glucose solution. If you suspect the patient is diabetic (polydipsia, polyuria) and no test strips are available, one trick is to pour her urine near an anthill; if the ants are attracted to it, glucose is present in a significant concentration
- On admission, dilatation is 1 cm, with two contractions every 10 minutes; after 4 hours dilatation has risen to 2 cm, and after another 4 hours to 3 cm; dilatation then proceeds rapidly and is complete after 4 hours
- On admission, head admits 5/5 above the brim; after 4 hours (2 cm dilatation), 4/5, and after a further 4 hours, 2/5
- *Urine ketones test*: The presence of ketone bodies in urine indicates that normal energy radicals of the myometrium (glycogen) have been exhausted and that body fat has been used in their instead. The presence of ketonic bodies can be detected by using test strips, but if these are unavailable, the patient's breath may be a guide.

FILLING IN THE PARTOGRAPH

Preconditions to begin recording the partograph are as follows:
a. *Labour has started.*
b. *Careful assessment of the parturient.*

a. *Onset of labour*

Labour has started when one or more contractions occur every 10 minutes; if this condition is present, we proceed as follows:
- Record the characteristics of the contractions: *Frequency* (the count of 10 minutes starts from the beginning of a contraction) and *duration*, but do not record them on the graph just yet.

Thorough pelvic examination, with two objectives
- Evaluate the pelvis, particularly the pelvic outlet and midpelvis (if this has not already been done), to exclude bone or soft-tissues abnormalities of the birth canal

- Determine the characteristics of the cervix (effacement, dilatation and the characteristics of its margins), foetal station (head height) and characteristics of the membranes.

It is dilatation that indicates whether labour is in the latent or active stage.

Assessment of dilatation: When the cervical os will admit one finger, dilatation has reached 2 cm; if slightly more, then it is 3 cm. If it admits two fingers (forefinger and middle finger), dilatation is 4 cm. Any greater degree of dilatation is detected using either:

- On admission dilatation is 1 cm; after 4 hours, it is 5 cm, at which point it is transferred to the alert line (dotted curve). After another 3 hours, dilatation is complete
- On admission foetal station is 5/5; after 4 hours, 4/5, and station is transferred to the alert line (dotted curve). After another 3 hours, it is at the perineal level
- The *two-finger method*: Forefinger and middle finger are introduced into the cervix and spread apart until they touch the cervical edges. Dilatation corresponds to the amount of divarication of the fingers. There is considerable intra- and inter-personal variation of measurement; in addition, one often unconsciously exaggerates divarication with the fingers (Fig. 7.6)
- Or the *one finger method*: Introducing just one forefinger into the vagina, on both sides assessment is made of the distance between the fornix and the cervical margin. These distances in centimetres are added and then subtracted from 10 (full cervical ripening) to give the degree of dilatation. For example: If we measure 3 cm on each side, we have: 3 + 3 = 6; 10 cm (full cervical ripening) – 6 = 4. Dilatation is 4 cm. This method is more accurate and less traumatic, and so better tolerated by the patient.

Vaginal exploration should be performed as seldom as possible; an interval of four hours between two consecutive examinations is generally sufficient.

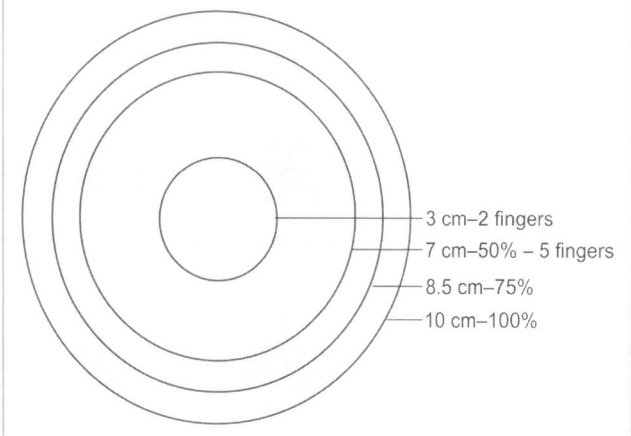

Fig. 7.6: Correspondence between examining fingers and centimetres while assessing the dilatation of the cervix.

Occasionally, cervical dilatation may be observed outside labour either in multiparae or in primigravidae affected by cervico-isthmic insufficiency. Hence, when monitoring parturition, the problem arises of how to distinguish whether dilatation is due to the ongoing labour or to these conditions.

Here medical history is useful; also, in a primigravida with cervico-isthmic insufficiency, there is a certain looseness of the cervical margins; the edges are irregular, sometimes scarred, and in a multipara the cervix may be partially preserved. In normal effacement, the cervical margins display a degree of tone, are regular and as labour progresses they thin out almost to a cutting edge.

At this point, having established whether we are dealing with the latent or active phase of labour, we note our observations on the graph (Fig. 7.7). The first thing to enter is the *dilatation* (symbol **X**),

- This we enter on the y-axis (the first vertical line), if labour is in the latent stage (Fig. 7.7)
- If in the active phase, our first entry is on the active phase line (Fig. 7.8)

Next we fill in, from top down in the appropriate squares:

- *Time of first observation*, recorded to the left of the word TIME. The times of subsequent observations are written in the square corresponding to the degree of dilatation, making it easier to determine the duration of labour
- *Station of foetal head* (symbol **O**), defined in terms of the number of head-fifths detectable above the pubic symphysis. When the measure of dilatation and the number of head-fifths coincide, the X is written inside O
- *Number of contractions*, as described above and bearing in mind that during a *normal latent phase*, two or more contractions are to be observed every 10 minutes, with contraction duration of no less than 20 seconds. During a *normal active phase* one or more contractions are observed every 10 minutes, with contraction duration of no less than 20 seconds
- On admission dilatation is 3 cm and is therefore recorded on the alert line. After 4 hours it is 6 cm and the alert line has been crossed; we are therefore in the critical area. After a further 4 hours, dilatation is 7 cm, the action line has been crossed and the decision is made for surgical intervention
- On admission, foetal station is 5/5; after 4 hours, 4/5, and after a further 4 hours it is still 4/5.

b. *Careful assessment of the parturient* (See Chapter 6).

Subsequent Recording

- *Dilatation* (**X** symbol): The first measurement is made on registering the partograph; subsequent recordings are made at four-hour intervals. With multiparae this frequency may be increased, particularly in advanced labour. During normal labour, dilatation should never cross over to the right side of the alert line (Fig. 7.6).

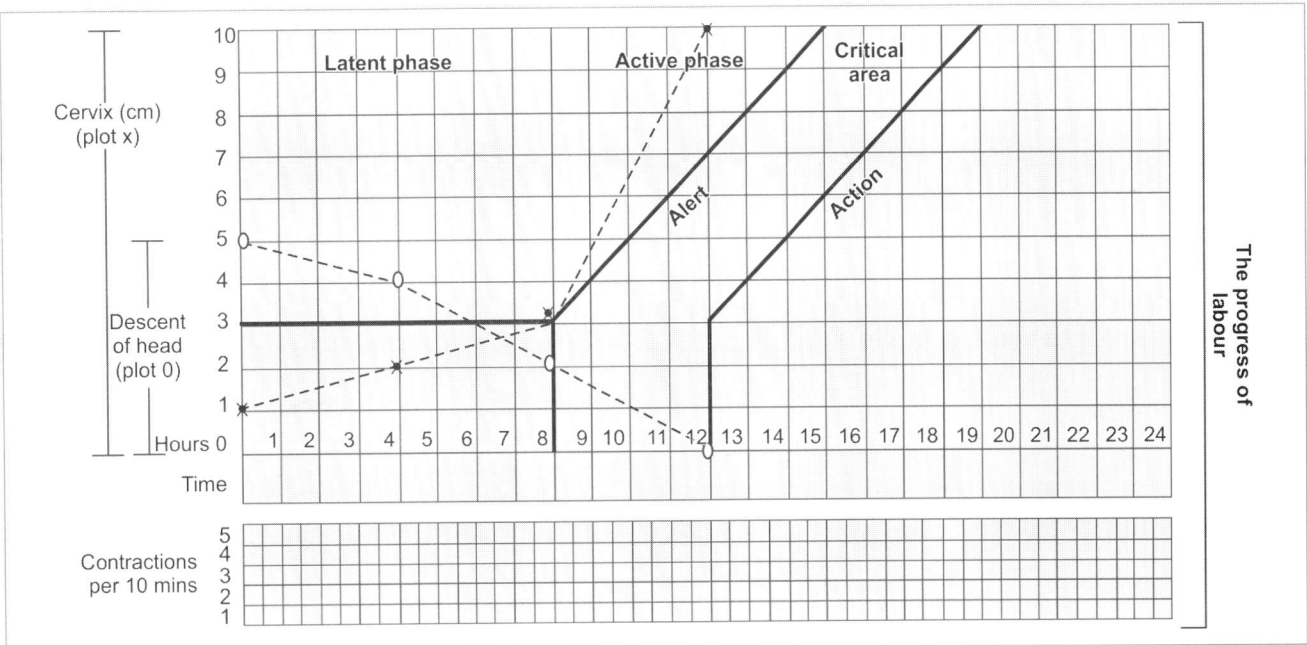

Fig. 7.7: Cervicograph and graph of head descent:
- On admission, dilatation is 1 cm, with two contractions every 10 minutes; after 4 hours dilatation has risen to 2 cm, and after another 4 hours to 3 cm; dilatation then proceeds rapidly and is complete after 4 hours.
- On admission, head admits 5/5 above the brim; after 4 hours (2 cm dilatation), 4/5, and after a further 4 hours, 2/5.

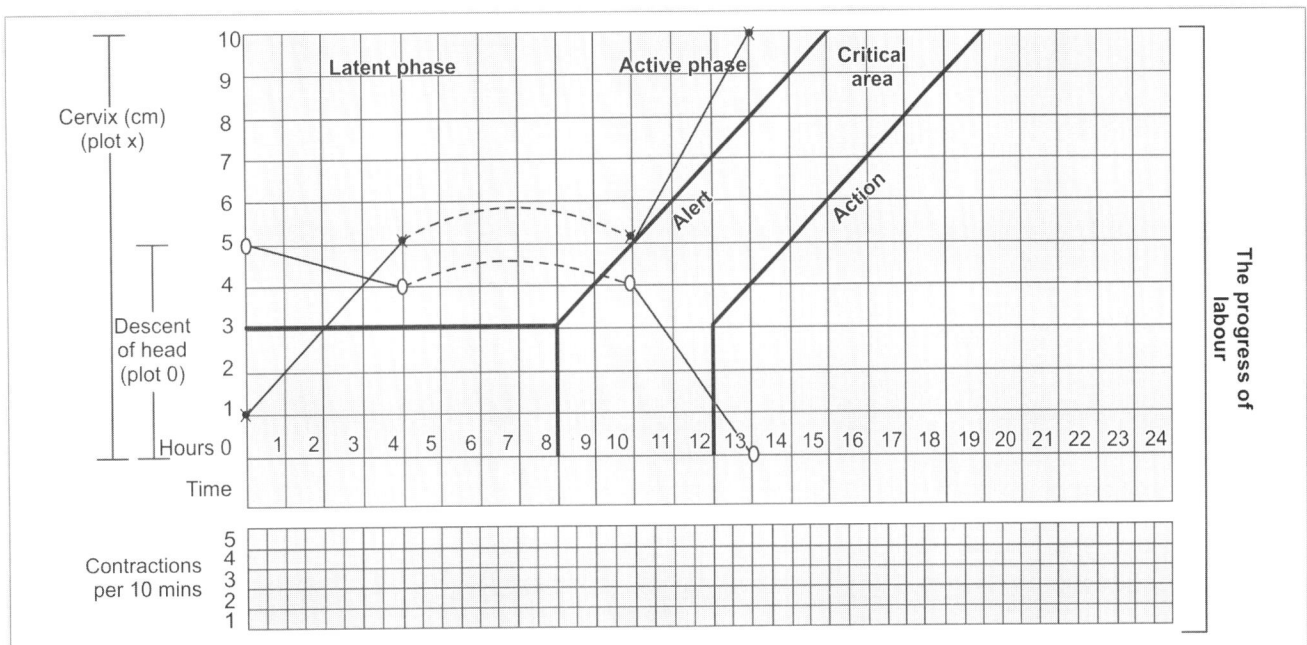

Fig. 7.8: Cervicograph and graph of head descent:
- On admission dilatation is 1 cm; after 4 hours, it is 5 cm, at which point it is transferred to the Alert Line (dotted curve). After another 3 hours, dilatation is complete.
- On admission foetal station is 5/5; after 4 hours, 4/5, and station is transferred to the Alert Line (dotted curve). After another 3 hours, it is at the perineal level.

When labour passes from the latent to the active phase (3 cm dilatation), measurement is recorded on the alert line of the cervimetric curve (Fig. 7.8).

- *Descent of the head*, indicated by **0**; Assessment is made with bladder empty, should *always* precede vaginal examination, and may be made independently of vaginal examination
- *Uterine contraction rate* is measured hourly during the latent phase and every half hour during the active phase of labour. Contractions are counted during the final ten minutes of each hour or half hour (Fig. 7.5).

Suggested Protocols

The protocols suggested here are to be adapted to working conditions; every obstetrician will obviously make the changes they consider necessary.

A. Latent Stage

(Primigravidae and multiparae)

a. *Normal*:

- Rupture of membranes (amniotomy) is not performed
- There is no need to enhance labour with oxytocin infusions, unless complications arise.

b. *Protracted*: If this phase is prolonged for more than 8 hours with at least two contractions every 10 minutes, this is a signal for alarm. Diagnosis is made on the basis of cervical characteristics and condition of the membranes:

- *The woman is not in labour*, membranes are intact; in a primipara the cervix is preserved and closed and, in a multipara, the cervix is preserved, even when a two-cm dilatation is present
- *Contractions are irregular, with uterine hypertonicity*, placental abruption can be excluded: Look for the areas of uterine contraction; infectious process with fever (malaria, infection of urinary tract).

If none of the above is detected, if foetal heart rate is normal and if amnioscopy (where possible) shows no staining of fluid, the partograph may be discarded and 100 mg of pethidine administered IM.

In cases of false onset of labour, contractions will very often disappear, but if it is true labour, contractions will resume after a period of repose:

- *The woman is in labour,* the membranes are still intact, cervical effacement is complete, but dilatation sticks at 2 cm; or both effacement and dilatation of the cervix progress very slowly.

It is important that *cephalopelvic disproportion* is ruled out; once we have ruled out cephalopelvic disproportion,

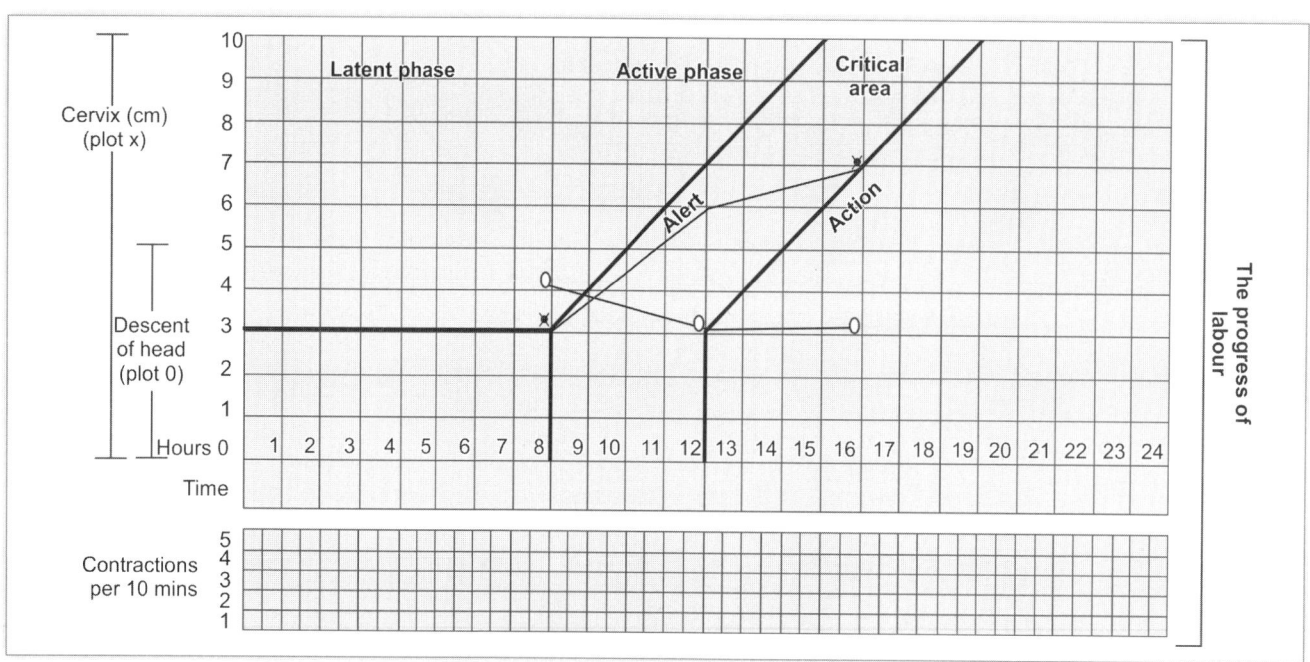

Fig. 7.9: Cervicograph and graph of head descent (obstructed labour):
- On admission dilatation is 3 cm and is therefore recorded on the Alert Line. After 4 hours it is 6 cm and the Alert Line has been crossed; we are therefore in the Critical Area. After a further 4 hours, dilatation is 7 cm, the Action Line has been crossed and the decision is made for surgical intervention.
- On admission, foetal station is 5/5; after 4 hours, 4/5, and after a further 4 hours it is still 4/5.

foetal distress or medical complications that indicate operative delivery by caesarean section, three pathways are open:
1. Administration of pethidine (100 mg IM), repeated if necessary.
2. Invite the patient to try walking.
3. Perform amniotomy and, after a period of time (1–2 hours), start infusing oxytocin, which should be administered until a rate of 3-4 contractions every 10 minutes is attained, each contraction lasting 30–40 seconds. This frequency can be maintained throughout the second or third stages of labour. However, the authors are in two minds about this approach.
4. Oxytocin infusion is indicated when the cervix is normal but contractions are of short duration, are ineffective, and with a frequency of less than 2 every 10 minutes. It should be preceded by re-establishing the parturient's energy reserves and correcting her fluid household.
The administration of oxytocin is strongly contraindicated in gravidae with previous hysterotomies or whose parity is greater than five.
5. Method of administration for oxytocin:
   - *Dosage*: The drug oxytocin is measured in milliunits (mU); 1 UI = 1,000 mU
   - *Dosage regimen* is patient-specific; two protocols are proposed:
     a. *Stepwise increase*: Starting with 1 mU/min, moving on to 2 mU/min after 15 minutes, increasing by 2 mU/min every 15 minutes (but not exceeding 20–25 mU/min), until a rate of 3-4 contractions every 10 minutes, with contraction duration of 20–30 seconds, is reached. At this point we scale back the quantity by 1 mU/min every 10 minutes until reaching a minimum concentration at which the desired effect is maintained.
     b. *Doubling every 15 minutes*: Starting with 1 mU/min (two drops), doubling every 15 minutes and stopping at 32 mU/minute.
   - *Infusion*: Saline solutions should be avoided, especially in patients with gestosis (PIH, pregnancy-induced hypertension) to reduce Na+ intake. Glucose solutions at 10% should be preferred
   - *Dilution*: We find a 500 mL intravenous drip infusion ideal, to which we introduce one.
The calculation runs as follows:
   500 mL contain 5000 mU.

Therefore

1 mL contains 10 mU; and as
1 mL = 20 drops,
20 drops will contain 10 mU therefore
2 drops will contain 1 mU.
6. Injection site: A needle of a gauge sufficiently large to prevent blood clotting should be applied preferably on the forearm, not at the fold of the arm, to allow mobility, allowing the arm to contribute its strength when pushing.

Stimulation should not be extended beyond six hours, as a retrospective study has shown this to be the maximum time limit within which a change can be induced. There is no point in persisting beyond this.

Amniotomy is not recommended under these circumstances, because if ineffective and entails a series of additional risks to the mother.

Continue with vaginal observation every four hours for a maximum of 12 hours. Caesarean section is indicated if:
- Active phase is not reached within eight hours of infusion
- Active phase is reached within eight hours, but dilatation is less than 1 cm/hour, calculated from start of infusion.

During infusion with oxytocin, *maternal* heart rate should be checked every 30 minutes.

If the membranes have been ruptured for more than 12 hours, administer antibiotics (see Chapter 11, section on the administration of antibiotics).

B. Active Phase

a. *Normal*
   - Amniotomy may be performed at any time during the active phase.

b. *Abnormal*

Abnormal active phase in primigravidae

The active phase is abnormal once the alert line has been crossed and the curve enters the so-called critical area between alert line and action line.

An active phase may approach the action line because of:

a. *Uterine inertia*:

   One proceeds as follows:
   - *Correct dehydration and ketosis*, using a 5% dextrose infusion. This has the advantage of spreading rapidly through the interstitial compartment, correcting intravascular hypertonia
   - Bladder catheterization
   - Analgesia using pethidine 100 mg, and promethazine 25 mg, both intramuscular, not in the same syringe.

   If we are sure that the patient is in true labour and dilatation has reached 3 cm.
   - Perform amniotomy, if the membranes have not ruptured already. In resource-poor countries, because of the danger of bacterial ascent, an amniotomy should be performed only on carefully evaluated obstetric grounds and preferably not performed to induce labour. An untimely amniotomy may necessitate a C-section
   - *Oxytocin infusion*: Monitor progress of labour and foetal well-being; decisive here is foetal heart rate; fluid stained with meconium is of relative importance. If dilatation progresses at a rate slower than 1 cm/h

or if the head does not descend (see below) within six hours of the start of infusion, then perform a C-section.

Frequently, contributory factors to uterine inertia are cephalopelvic disproportion or obstructed labour; recourse to oxytocin should always be considered very carefully.

b. *Mechanical obstruction*: The most common obstructions are cephalopelvic disproportion or obstructed labour.

Cephalopelvic disproportion is a sign of an altered relation between the volume of the pelvic inlet and that of the foetal head. This may be incurred through a contracted or vitiated pelvis in the mother or by foetal head abnormalities (hydrocephalus), by anomalies of presentation (deflected, bregma, brow, face) or by primary or secondary asynclitism. On abdominal palpation, 4/5 of head can be detected above the pubic symphysis and there is a large amount of foetal skull moulding on pelvic examination. This condition accounts for approximately 18% of indications for C-section.

Deflected and extended presentations are responsible for cephalopelvic disproportion, as the condition of *minimum plane of passage* is not observed (see Chapter 2). The maximum circumference of passage is greater than that in vertex presentation.

Occiput posterior position:

Maximum plane of progression circumference of passage: 32 cm

Bregma presentation: Maximum plane of progression circumference of passage: 34 cm

Brow presentation:

Maximum plane of progression circumference of passage: 35–36

Face presentation:

Maximum plane of progression circumference of passage: 34 cm.

Asynclitism is primitive when it is due to an altered inclination—over-inclination or under-inclination—of the pelvis (see Chapters 2 and 6) or to pelvic morphology (platypelloid pelvis or mixed platypelloid android forms); it is secondary when it is due to a pendulous uterus, typical of multiparae.

Obstructed labour (Fig. 7.9): A contributory factor is a particular pelvic morphology which, on engagement and with effective contractions, prevents descent and/ or rotation of the presenting part. Labour may also be obstructed by anomalies of foetal lie: Oblique, breech or transverse. This condition accounts for 33% of C-section indications.

To differentiate obstructed labour from a simple delay in progress of labour, we look at the ensuing secondary signs and complications, i.e. marked moulding of the presenting part, caput succedeum, foetal distress, overdistension of the lower uterine segment, bloody urine, uterine rupture, bladder lesions and fistulas.

Do not use just head-fifths to diagnose obstructed labour: Other accessory criteria may be subdivided into abdominal and vaginal signs:
- Contractions are preceded by pain
- Overdistension and tenderness of the lower uterine segment
- The round ligaments are tense, painful, contracted, almost standing out from the edges of the uterus
- Rising of vaginal fornices (see Chapter 6)
- Obstructed labour score.

Mechanical impediment (cephalopelvic disproportion and obstructed labour) is an *absolute indication* for caesarean section.

Abnormal Active Phase in a Multipara

This situation is graver than the above, and requires careful assessment of the patient. When cephalopelvic disproportion or obstructed labour cannot be excluded with certainty, the use of oxytocic agents is contraindicated: These are absolutely prohibited in gravidae with a parity greater than 5. Some authors suggest that oxytocic agents should never be administered during labour to women who have given birth previously.

In diagnosing mechanical obstruction, anamnestic criteria are of little value: Cephalopelvic disproportion and obstructed labour can present even in mothers with histories of 6 or 8 normal deliveries. Cephalopelvic disproportion is frequently associated with secondary asynclitism, due to a pendulous uterus.

MATANY PARTOGRAPH

The partograph opposite (Fig. 7.10), now in use at Matany, has two interesting features:
- *The three areas* (normal labour, critical and action areas) of the progress of labour graph (dilatation and descent of foetal head) are shown in different colours: Green, yellow and red, respectively. This arrangement enhances, we think, its visual impact and attracts the attention of birth attendants to the gravity of the transition from normal to critical to action zones
- *Diagnostic indicator of mechanical obstruction score* (cephalopelvic disproportion—CPD and obstructed labour): During normal labour, when distension of the LUS reaches a certain value, it remains stable, while the head-fifths score tends to decrease. Where there is mechanical obstruction, (cephalopelvic disproportion, obstructed labour or cervical dystocia), the height of the LUS tends to grow and to form, in extreme conditions, a retraction (or Bandl's) ring, while descent of the head remains unchanged.

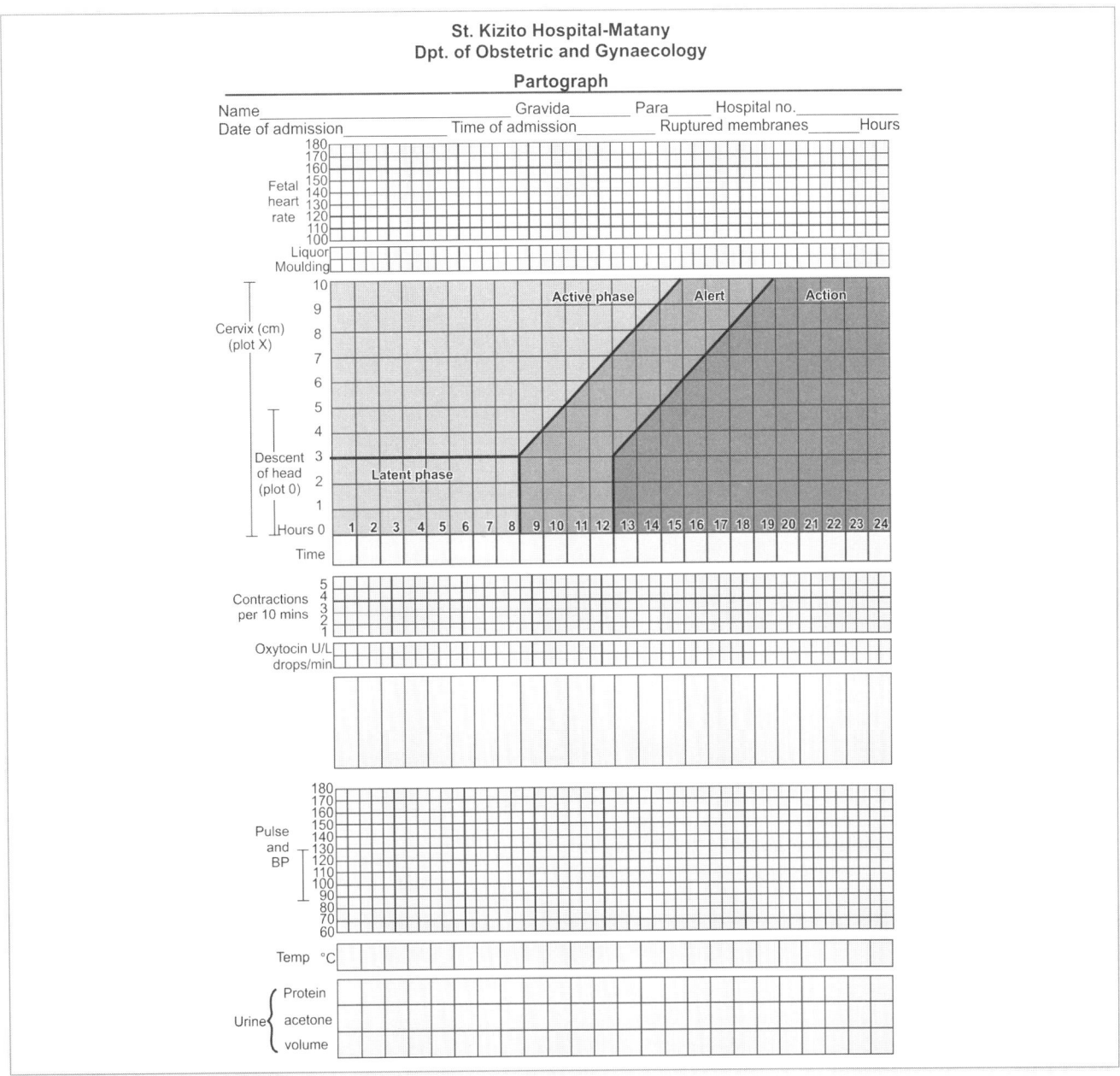

Fig. 7.10: Partograph according to Matany—Differs from the WHO model partograph in: 1) The three areas for normal labour, critical and action areas are in different colours, giving greater visual impact and drawing the attention of the person following the labour. 2) Includes a diagnostic indicator for obstructed labour (LUS score)

As distension of the lower uterine segment and descent of the head are closely related, by comparing these two indicators with each other, we obtain a reliable indicator of progress of labour.

Acting on this principle, we have developed a diagnostic index (Domini, Guidi and Guazzini, 2006), which consists of multiplying head fifths by height of LUS, expressed in transverse fingerbreadths above the pubic symphysis.

Example 1: Normal labour—head 4/5, LUS 6 fingerbreadths = diagnostic index of 24

Example 2: Cephalopelvic disproportion—head 5/5, fingerbreadths 5 = diagnostic index = 25. After 2 hours, head 5/5, transverse fingers 7 = 35.

This index is recorded in a box placed between those for time and contractions.

In our opinion, clinical observation of progress of labour and promptness in reaching a decision may be improved by the following observations, not shown in a normal partograph:

- Obstetric examination at the time of admission to delivery: This should include, in addition to the

determination of stature and careful examination of the size and morphology of the pelvis, also the relationship between the major longitudinal axis of the foetus and the inclination of the pelvic inlet; a factor often not taken into account
- Distention and tenderness of the lower uterine segment
- Morphology of the uterus at rest and under contraction
- Relationship between pain and contraction: In a normal delivery, pain is synchronous with or follows the contraction; with cephalopelvic disproportion or obstructed labour, it precedes the contraction
- Characteristics of the round ligaments (stretched, prominent, painful due to the presence of a mechanical impediment)
- Changes in polarity of contractions.

BIBLIOGRAPHY

1. Alexander JM, Sharma SK, Mcintire DO, Leveno KJ. Epidural analgesia lengthens the Friedman active phase of labour. Obstet Gynecol. 2002;100:40-50.
2. Altshuler G, Hyde S. Meconium induced vasoconstriction: A potential cause of cerebral and other fetal organs hypoperfusion and of poor pregnancy outcome. J Child Neurol. 1989;7:137-42.
3. Arbay O, Ciftci AO, Tanyel FC, Bingol-Kologlu M, Sahin S, Buyukpa-mokcu N. Foetal distress does not affect in utero defecation, but does impair the clearance of amniotic fluid. J Ped Surg, 1999;34(2):246-50.
4. Beazley JM, Kurjak A. Influence of a partogram on the active management of labour. Lancet. 1972;348-51.
5. Bird GC. Cervicographic managemen to flabour in primigravidae and multigravidae with vertex presentation. Tropical Doctor. 1978;4:163-5.
6. Calkins LA. Normal labour. Springfield, IL:Charles C. Thomas;1955.
7. Crichton D. A reliable method for establishing the level of the fetal head in obstetrics. S Afr Med J. 1974;48:784-7.
8. Domini E, Guazzini S, Vicentini S, Urso M. "Obstructed labour score" Giorn. It. Ost. Gin. Vol XXVIII, 5,209.
9. Duignan NM, Studd JW, Hughes A. The characteristics of normal labour in different racial groups. Br Med J. 1974; 34:223-5.
10. Friedman EA, Kroll BH. Computer analysis of labour progression. I. Distribution of data and limits of normal. J Reprod Med. 1971;6:20-5.
11. Glick E, Trussel R. The curve of labour used as a teaching device in Uganda. J Obst Gyn Brit Commw. 1970; 77: 1003-6.
12. Friedman EA, Kroll BH. Computer analysis of labour progression. J Ob Gynaecol Br Commonw. 1969;76: 1075-9.
13. Friedman EA. Graphic analysis of labour. Am J Obstet Gynecol. 1954;68:1568-75.
14. Friedman EA. Labour clinical evaluation and management 2nd ed. New York: Appleton Century-Crofts; 1978.
15. Friedman EA. Prinigravid labour-a graphico statistical analysis. Obst Gynaecol. 1955;68:567-8.
16. Hendricks CH, Brenner WE, Kraus G. Normal cervical dilatation pattern in late pregnancy and labour. Am J Obstet Gynecol. 1970;106:1065-82.
17. Imamura T, Sugiyama T, Cuevas LE, Makunde R, Nakamura S. Expression of Tissue Factor, the Clotting Initiator, on Macrophages in *Plasmodium falciparum*-Infected Placenta. J Infect Dis. 2002;186(3):436-40.
18. Impey L, Hobson J, O'Hierlihy C. Graphic analysis of actively managed labour; perspective computation of labour progress in 500 consecutive nulliparous women in spontaneous labour at term. Am J Obstet Gyne. 2000;183: 438-43.
19. Knight D. A comparison of abdominal and vaginal examination for diagnosis of the engagement of the fetal head. NZ J Obst Gyn. 1993;33:155-7.
20. Lekana Douki JB, Traore B, Costa FT, Fusai T, Pouvelle B, Sterker Scherf A, Gysin J. Sequestration of Plasmodium falciparum infected erythroci chondroitin sulphate A, a receptor for maternal (malaria: monoclonal antibodies against the native parasite ligand rei panreactive epitopes in placenta) isolates. Blood. 2002;15;100(4):1478-83.
21. Lennox CE. The cervicograph in labour management in the Highlands of Papua New Guinea. Papua New Guinea Medical Journal. 1981;24(4):286-93.
22. Philpott Rh, Castle WM. Cervicographs in the management of labour in primigravidae. I. The alert line for detecting abnormal labour. J Obst Gyn Br Commwel. 1972;79:592-8.
23. Philpott Rh, Castle WM. Cervicographs in the management of labour in primigravidae. II. The action line and treatment of abnormal labour. J Obst Gyn Br Commwel. 1972;79: 599-602.
24. Philpott Rh, Sapire KE, Axton JHM. Normal labour and its management. In: Obstetrics, family planning and paediatrics. Natal Witness (Pty) Ltd; 1976. 61L.
25. Philpott RH. Foetal quality preserved in cephalopelvic disproportion in the primigravida. S Afr Med J 1973;47: 2021.
26. Rogers R, Gilson GJ, Miller AC, Izquierdo LE, Curet LB, Qualis CR. Active management of labour, does it make a difference? Am J Obstet Gynecol. 1997;177:599-605.
27. Stewart KS. The foetal response to cephalo-pelvic disproportion. J Obst Gyn Br Cmw. 1974;32:217.
28. Studd J. Partograms and nomograms of cervical dilatation in management of primigravide labour. Br Med J. 1973;4: 451-5.
29. Webber RH. Simplified cervicograph for rural maternity practice. Trop Doctor. 1987;17:81-4.
30. World Health Organization, The partograph: A managerial tool for the prevention of prolonged labour. WHO documents MCH/88.3.
31. Ye Yinyun. Clinical application of the partogram Shangai First Maternity and Infant Health Institute. WHO Collaborating Centre for Research and Training on Maternal and Infant Care. Shangai. 1986.
32. Zang J, Troendle JF, Yancey MK. Reassessing the Labour curve in nulli-parous woman. Am J Obstet Gynecol. 2002: 187(4):824-8.

SECTION 3

Caesarean Section and Management

- Indications for Caesarean Section Outside Labour
- Indications for Caesarean Section During Labour
- Trial of Labour
- Preparing for the Operation
- Anaesthesia
- Laparotomies
- The Various Types of Hysterotomy—Criteria of Choice
- Transverse Hysterotomies
- Vertical Hysterotomies
- Management of Intraoperative Complications
- Tubal Sterilization
- Abdominal Wall Closure
- Perimortem and Postmortem Caesarean Delivery
- Uterine Rupture
- Monitoring Caesarean Section: Postoperative Recovery
- Complications of the Laparotomic Wound Suture
- Postcaesarean Wound Dehiscence
- Obstructed Labour Injury Complex
- The Newborn

CHAPTER 8

Indications for Caesarean Section Outside Labour

We take caesarean section (C-section) to refer to the delivery of foetus, placenta and membranes following the 28th week of gestation by means of an incision of the abdominal and uterine wall; before this gestational stage, the operation is referred to as a *transabdominal hysterotomy*.

Indications for C-section are all conditions in which vaginal delivery either cannot be effected or is associated with high risks for the mother and/or foetus.

Indications are classified as *maternal* or *foetal* and may arise (Fig. 8.1):
- Outside labour, and have an elective or urgent character;
- During labour.

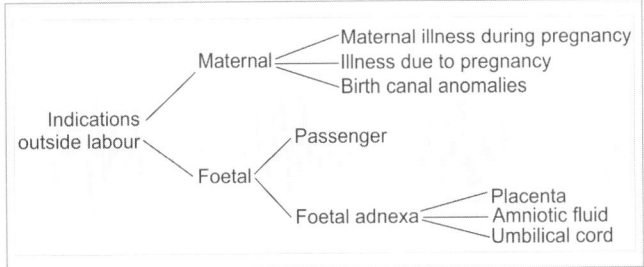

Fig. 8.1: Indication of caesarean section outside labour

MATERNAL INDICATIONS

- Maternal illness during pregnancy
- Maternal illness due to pregnancy
- Birth canal pathologies.

Maternal Illness During Pregnancy

Cardiopathy

The NYHA defines cardiopathies under four functional classes:

- Class 1: No limitation
- Class 2: Ordinary physical activity results in fatigue, dyspnoea, palpitation, angina, slight limitation of physical activity (can walk for a distance of 7 km on even ground; can do gardening work)
- Class 3: Comfortable at rest. Less than ordinary activity causes fatigue, palpitation, or dyspnoea. Can wash, change the bed, walk up to 4 km on even ground
- Class 4: Above symptoms even at rest.

In functional classes 1 and 2, if there is no obstetric contraindication, vaginal delivery is possible, using the following stratagems:
- During labour, the patient is placed in orthopneic position (semi-seated or Fowler's position) with oxygen mask (Fig. 8.2);

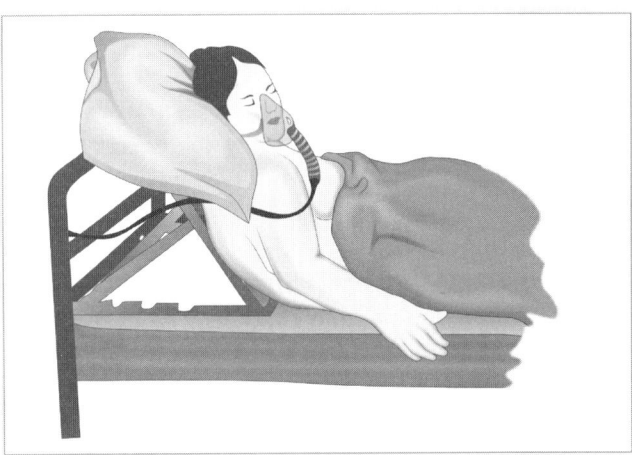

Fig. 8.2: The cardiopathic (class I, II) gravida should preferably be placed in orthopneic position during labour (also known as Fowler's or half-sitting position)

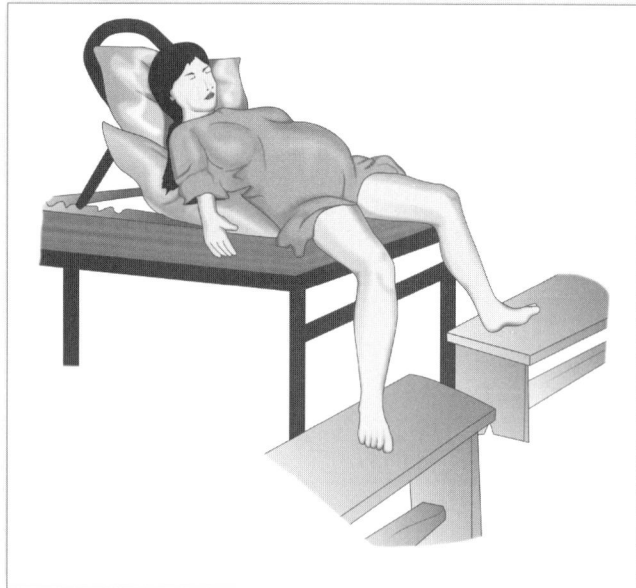

Fig. 8.3: The patient sits on the edge of the bed with her feet resting on footstools. The lithotomy position should be avoided during the expulsive phase. Duration of the expulsive phase should be reduced by use of vacuum extractor or forceps

- Reducing duration of the expulsive stage by using vacuum extraction or forceps
- Postpartum, the legs should be kept low (Fig. 8.3) to avoid cardiac overload due to the abrupt removal of the ileocaval obstacle to venous blood flow from the uterus and lower limbs. The veins of the lower limbs increase in caliber during pregnancy.

Some schools take a more restrictive view and allow classes 1 and 2 to perform a trial of labour lasting 4 and 2 hours respectively. Class 1 and 2 patients are allowed to breastfeed. C-section is indicated for functional classes 3 and 4 to avoid major strain on the heart during labour. The increased postpartum blood flow from the uterus and lower limbs is relieved by sloping downwards the lower limbs and in severe cases and in severe cases the patient should be ventilated with continuous positive pressure (something hard to implement in resource-poor countries).

Lung disease: the second stage of labour should be reduced by use of vacuum extractor or forceps. Should C-section be decided on, it is advisable to use spinal anaesthesia, not anaesthesia by inhalation.

Maternal Illness Due to Pregnancy (3rd Trimester Gestosis)

Gestational Oedema Proteinuria Hypertension (GEPH)

Classification:

- *Gestational (transient) oedema:* G E+ P0 H0 (oedema at the ankles and above)
- *Gestational (transient) proteinuria* G E0 P+ H0 (proteinuria above 300 mg/l over 24 hours, or more than 1g/l (1-2+) in two separate samples (six hours apart) collected via catheter or mid-stream
- *Gestational (transient) hypertension* (G E0 P0 H+).

Gestational Hypertension (G E0 P0 H+)

Pressure should be measured with the patient semiseated at an inclination of 45°. The pressure cuff is placed at heart level. It is the 5th Korotkoff sound that indicates diastolic pressure. Confirmation of diagnosis requires numerous observations.

Gestational hypertension refers to a finding of diastolic blood pressure (DBP) values ≥90 mmHg and systolic (SBP) pressure of ≥140 mmHg in a previously normotensive woman after the 20th week of pregnancy, confirmed in two consecutive measurements separated in time (6 hours).

Gestational hypertension resolves within three months postpartum, is not accompanied by significant proteinuria, organ damage or clinical and laboratory signs typical of preeclampsia and/or of HELLP syndrome;

Development of gestational hypertension into preeclampsia is observed in 15–25% of cases overall; this rises to 45–50% when it appears within the 34th week of pregnancy; no certain factors or data are available that allow us to predict the risk of developing preeclampsia.

Hypertension is defined as severe in the presence of DBP ≥110 mmHg and/or SBP ≥160 mmHg (National Institute of Health Blood Pressure Education Program. Am J Obstet Gynecol 2000).

Therapy

Four therapeutic goals are set:
1. Controlling arterial pressure.
2. Prophylaxis of the preeclampsia, that is, impeding development of gestational hypertension into preeclampsia.
3. Collateral measures.
4. Timing of parturition.

a. Control of arterial pressure

The therapeutic approach will differ according to whether we are facing mild to moderate or severe hypertension.

- *Mild to moderate hypertension*: A Cochrane review of the advisability of antihypertensive therapy came up with no definitive answer.

Twenty-four trials demonstrated that while the use of antihypertensive agents in mild-to-moderate hypertension reduced the risk of developing severe hypertension by 50%, their use did not lead to major differences in the final outcome in terms of the risks of proteinuria, pre-eclampsia or reduction in the percentages of preterm births or caesarean deliveries.

Furthermore, no significant differences were found in the efficacy of various antihypertensive drugs. On subgroup analysis, calcium blockers appeared to have increased the risk of preeclampsia, while beta blockers appeared to have reduced it, but their use appeared to be associated with a greater risk of foetuses too small for their gestational age. The advisability of setting up pharmacological therapy remains very controversial in the West, where it is by now accepted that a diastolic arterial pressure of up to 100 mmHg does not entail an increased risk for mother or foetus.

A recent critical review (Paruk, Modley 2006) suggested that, ahead of definitive clarification on the subject, antihypertensive therapy is indicated especially in resource-poor countries where gravidae may not be able to have their blood pressure monitored frequently, or to receive prompt assistance in the presence of danger signs, such as persistent headache.

Hypertension should also be assessed in view of age and parity; particularly at risk are primigravidae under 18 years of age. For this reason, primigravidae aged 16 with 140/90 should be treated as moderate hypertension and a 15-year-old primigravida with pressure of 150/100 should be treated as having severe hypertension. With the above-mentioned limitations, drugs that may be used in controlling hypertension in pregnancy are enlisted in Table 8.1 and discussed below:

- Centrally acting antihypertensive drugs
  Methyldopa: 250 mg 2-3 times per day up to a maximum of 4 g per day
  Clonidine (Hartikainen et al., 1987) may also be administered transdermally

- Calcium antagonists
  Nifedipine: 10 mg 3-4 times in fast-release formulation or 20-30 mg 1-2 times per day in slow-release formulation up to a maximum of 120 mg per day (*Gruppo di Studio Ipertensione in gravidanza* [Hypertension in Pregnancy Research Group], 1998; Bortolus et al., 2000). Severe hypotension may arise in the presence of hypovolaemia

- Beta blockers are the medication of choice only in the event of severe maternal tachycardia or as second-line medication in the event of severe hypertension
  Labetalol: 100 mg 2-3 times per day up to maximum of 2400 mg per day

- ACE inhibitors (inhibitors of the angiotensin-converting enzyme) should be avoided in the second and third trimesters of pregnancy. Their use is associated with oligohydramnios, IUGR, bone malformations, neonatal renal failure, anuria, renal dysgenesis, persistent ductus Botalli (ductus arteriosus), pulmonary hypoplasia, RDS, foetalneonatal deaths; these adverse outcomes are not observed if ACE inhibitors taken early on in pregnancy and are suspended as soon as possible. Similar effects are caused by angiotensin receptor blockers

- Arterial dilators
  Hydralazine HCL is the preferred medication in severe hypertension: (SBP ≥160 mmHg and/or DBP ≥110 mmHg); it increases cardiac output, improves placental perfusion, particularly of the kidney, as often demonstrated by the increase in diuresis.

Administration is IV, IV/IM or by infusion. When the direct IV route or infusion are used, a cannula that has been used for magnesium sulphate should preferably not be reused, nor, ideally, should the same arm.

Maternal tachycardia is a limiting side effect of hydralazine.

- *Intravenous route:* 5 mg slowly, directly into a vein, repeated every 20 minutes, up to a maximum of 20 mg; maintenance dose 5 mg IV every hour or 12.5 mg IM every 2 hours, or by infusion
- *Infusion*: 80 mg (four ampules) are diluted in 500 ml of saline or Hartman's solution (not glucose solution), obtaining a concentration of 1 mg/6 ml; infusion rate is 1-20 mg/h.

Blood pressure is measured every 30 minutes, if diastolic BP is still above 100 mmHg one hour after starting the infusion, the infusion rate is increased to 5 mg/h. The action of hydralazine lasts 4-6 hours; a dosage of 200 mg per day should not be exceeded.

In approx. 10% of severely hypertensive patients, hydralazine may produce no effect or act only partially. If this occurs in the presence of hypervolemia or congestive heart failure, use of a diuretic such as Furosemide is indicated.

In the absence of a volume overload, the addition of a beta-blocker such as Propranolol at a dose of 5-15 mg IV may increase the action of hydralazine.

Table 8.1

Antihypertensive drugs used during pregnancy

Medicinal product	Intravenous	Oral
Centrally acting	250 mg 4 times per day	250 mg-1 g x 4
a. Methyldopa		0.1-0.3 mg x 2
b. Clonidine		
Calcium antagonist		
Nifedipine		
(fast-release formulation)		10 mg x 3-4
(slow release formulation)		20-30 mg x 1-2
Beta-blockers		100 mg x 2 (MX 2.4 g/per day)
a. Labetalol		
b. Atenolol		
ACE inhibitors		
Arterial dilators		
Hydralazine HCL		

b. Prophylaxis against preeclampsia (using acetylsalicylic acid)

The use of aspirin in prophylaxis against preeclampsia (Beaufils et al. 1985; Wallenburg et al., 1986; Benigni et al., 1989; It. "Study of Aspirin in pregnancy", 1993; CLASP, 1994) was the subject of a Cochrane review in 2000 (Knight, M., Duley, L. 2000). Its findings may be summarised as follows:

- Aspirin is probably capable of preventing the early and severe forms of preeclampsia (15% reduction in the risk of preeclampsia in patients at both high and medium risk), or at least of improving pregnancy outcomes by slowing the onset of the syndrome
- The efficacy of aspirin is probably dose-related, with variation between individuals: the minimum dose should be 100 mg per day, but this should be modulated on the basis of partial thromboplastin time
- There is a slight decrease (8%) in preterm deliveries
- Perinatal mortality is reduced by 14% overall, although the studies examined showed very wide confidence intervals (between 25% and no reduction)
- There is no significant effect on the incidence of placental abruption.

c. Collateral measures

- Administer crystalloid solution at a rate not exceeding 85–100 ml/hour. In patients with elevated blood pressure and low central pressure, volume expansion, can sometimes dramatically improve severe hypertension
- In case of oliguria, do not exceed the urine output of the previous hour by 30 ml
- Do not administer diuretics except where there is risk of pulmonary oedema
- Maternal monitoring: Daily evaluation of:
  - blood pressure
  - Weight.
- Proteinuria
- Diuresis.

d. Timing of labour

- A gravid patient with non-complicated gestational hypertension can give birth vaginally at term
- There are no indications in the literature on the advisability of expediting delivery early, except in cases where the following conditions are present:
  - Aggravation of the clinical picture of hypertension and/or failure to respond to pharmaceutical therapy
  - IUGR and/or foetal distress
  - it is not advisable to postpone delivery beyond the 40th week of gestation.

Preeclampsia

Preeclampsia refers to a finding of blood pressure values ≥ 140/90 mmHg associated with proteinuria values greater than or equal to 300 mg in 24-hour urine, or a proteinuria/creatinine ratio equal to or greater than 30 mg/ mmol, in previously normotensive and non-proteinuric women after the 20th week of pregnancy.

Preeclampsia is considered severe where:
- BP ≥160/110 mmHg;
- BP <160/110 mmHg, but is associated with one or more of the following signs:
  - proteinuria [3] ≥ 5 g in 24-hour urine
  - oliguria, diuresis < 500 ml/24 h or < 80 ml/4 hours
  - neurological signs: frontal and/or occipital headache; dizziness, restlessness, confusion, sensory obfuscation
  - visual disturbances, scintillating scotoma, visual uncertainty (the patient cannot count fingers held in front of her eyes), double images, papilledema
  - hyperreflexia (see Chapter 6)
  - convulsions
  - irespiratory rate: pulmonary oedema
  - appearance of epigastric pain and/or pain in right hypochondrium (liver tenderness)
  - ascites
  - arenal failure (ARF)
  - disseminated intravascular coagulation (DIC)
  - rapid weight gain (*oedema*): This sometimes precedes the clinical onset of preeclampsia and is a common sign of preeclampsia in process or of imminent eclampsia. Weight gain is rapid, as it is driven mainly by water retention. A gain of over 1 kg in a week or 3 kg in one month is considered significant. As the disease progresses, weight gain can reach 5 kg in a month. Weight gain during normal pregnancy is 250 g per week and does not exceed 500 g. Oedema is first detected in the lower limbs, then as water retention increases, particularly during the latter stages of preeclampsia, it becomes clinically evident periorbitally or in the fingers, particularly in the morning.
- Retarded foetal growth
- Changes in laboratory test values (ALT or ASP above 70 U/l)
  - Platelet count <100,000/mm[3]
  - Elevated creatinine
  - HELLP syndrome: H (haemolysis), EL (elevated liver enzymes), LP (low platelet count)
  - Proteinuria.

The classifications of moderate and severe preeclampsia are purely heuristic; all forms of preeclampsia are considered serious. Preeclampsia is associated with prematurity, perinatal morbidity and mortality and with maternal death.

The development from simple gestational hypertension to eclampsia is often all the more rapid and dramatic in geographical areas where the pathology is less frequently diagnosed.

Epidemiology

Preeclampsia is observed more frequently among primigravidae (65%); frequency increases when the primigravida is under 17 or over 35-year-old, and with multiple pregnancies. In resource-poor countries it has an incidence of 2.3% (Villar and Voll, 2003).

Gravidae with severe preeclampsia are at increased risk of developing eclampsia and of dying from it; it is estimated that 1–2% of women with severe preeclampsia will develop eclampsia.

Monitoring for Preeclampsia

Respiratory system: An increased respiratory rate may be an early sign of pulmonary oedema: auscultate the lung.

Circulatory system: Measure pressure, heart rate and, if possible, oxygen saturation.

Diuresis: An accurate fluid household should be set up to monitor the fine balance between renal insufficiency exacerbated by restriction hypovolemia and pulmonary or cerebral oedema. Fluids to administer: 1000 ml/12h normal saline or Hartmann's solution;

If oliguria is present (diuresis <30 ml/h over 4 hours), stimulation using 250 ml normal saline is indicated.

The definitive treatment for preeclampsia and eclampsia is delivery of the foetus.

Treatment of Mild Preeclampsia

See treatment for hypertension during pregnancy.

Treatment of Severe Preeclampsia

- Bed rest
- *Hydration: crystalloid solution* 85 ml/hour (2000 ml/24 hours)
- *Antihypertensive therapy:* This should be initiated if diastolic BP exceeds 100 mmHg. Currently, there is no evidence to recommend the use of one antihypertensive rather than another. The most commonly used drugs are:

a. Treatment of attacks:

- Nifedipine 10 mg/os (20 drops or 1 tablet) repeatable every 15–30 minutes up to a maximum of 30 mg.
- Labetalol 10–20 mg bolus; subsequently infusing 40 mg/hour, doubling the dosage every 10 minutes up to a maximum of 160 mg/hour (cardiac monitoring required) until reaching diastolic arterial pressure (DAP) <100 mmHg. If DAP remains <100 mmHg, commence maintenance therapy, possibly using the same medication as for treatment of attack.

b. Maintenance therapy

Nifedipine retard (20 mg capsule) up to a maximum of 120 mg per day, or Labetalol (100 and 200 mg capsules) up to a maximum of 800 mg per day.

- *Monitoring diuresis*:
    - If *diuresis* is above 0.5 ml/kg/hour, continue the maintenance hydration. If *diuresis* is less than 0.5 ml/kg/hour, assess the need for application of CVP, review input and composition of fluids and consider the need to prescribe diuretics or dopamine.
- *Anticonvulsant prophylaxis*: The MAGPIE Trial (2002) justified the use of magnesium sulphate in severe preeclampsia, in eclampsia prophylaxis and in the treatment of convulsions.

This historic study concluded that:
- Prophylaxis reduces the risk of eclampsia and should be implemented in women with preeclampsia, who are at risk of an eclamptic attack
- It is probable that magnesium sulphate also contributes to reducing the risk of maternal deaths correlated with preeclamptic disorders.

At the dosage and mode of administration used in the MAGPIE TRIAL, magnesium sulphate does not cause any harm to mother or foetus; a quarter of the women treated presented irritating side effects.
- Duration of treatment should not exceed 24 hours; nothing is known about the safety for the mother and child at longer exposure times to the drug.
- Blood monitoring is not necessary with this medication.
- Clinical monitoring of the drug may be performed by suitably trained medical or paramedical personnel.

Magnesium sulphate is a very economical medication.

Among patients with severe preeclampsia, BP ≥160/110 and/or CNS symptoms compatible with progression to eclampsia, administration of magnesium sulphate reduced the risk of eclampsia by 58% and the risk of placental abruption to 27%. The mortality rate was also reduced compared to the placebo group.

No significant differences in foetal mortality were found between the two groups.

During labour, patients with severe preeclampsia present a high risk of convulsions: anticonvulsant prophylaxis is indicated. The recommended regimen is:

- Loading dose: Ringer's solution or normal saline 400 ml to which 10 ampules of magnesium sulphate are added (1 ampule = 2 g in 10 ml); we thus obtain 20 g in 500 ml = 2 g per 50 ml
- Dosage for attacks: 4 g IV (100 ml) in 20 minutes (infusion pump at 300 ml/hour for 20 minutes)
- Maintenance: infusion of 1 g/hour (25 ml) for 24 hours
- Hourly monitoring of: tendon reflexes, respiratory rate (> 16/m'), diuresis

- Ask about scotoma, headache, convulsions; evaluate reflexes.

Mortality increases with every fresh attack; it is the obstetrician's task to prevent the occurrence of new attacks.

Timing of Delivery

A. Expedite delivery immediately in the case of:
   a. Foetal indications:
      » Gestational age ≥34 weeks
      » Foetal distress
      » Oligohydramnios
      » Severe foetal growth retardation
      » Reverse umbilical artery flow and diastolic flow absent
      » Intrauterine foetal death.
   b. Maternal indications:
      » Hypertension not controlled by antihypertensive therapy
      » Pulmonary oedema
      » Acute renal failure
      » Persistence of neurological disorders
      » Thrombocytopenia (<100,000/nl)
      » Pathological transaminase levels (AST, ALT) with epigastric pain and/or radiating upper-quadrant pain
      » Eclampsia.
B. In the absence of maternal and/or foetal indications for immediate expedition of delivery, clinical management depends on the response to therapy. Where there is improvement, expectant management should be pursued until foetal maturation; otherwise delivery is expedited following induction of foetal lung maturation by administering Betametasone 12 mg IM x 2 days.
C. **Mode of expediting delivery:** vaginally, either spontaneous or induced, possible if:
   b. the foetus is in cephalic presentation
   c. gestational age is ≥34 weeks
   d. true labour has begun
   e. cervical conditions are favourable
D. Type of anaesthesia: local-regional anaesthesia is not contraindicated either in labour or during C-section in the event of severe preeclampsia (Hogg et al., 1999), unless a coagulopathy is present, due to the potential risk of haemorrhagic complications.

Postpartum Clinical Management

The puerpera is monitored intensively for 48–72 hours, repeating biohumoral tests at short time intervals, partly to permit prompt detection of possible serious complications such as: DIC, pulmonary oedema, IRA, cerebral oedema, retinal detachment, hepatic haematoma, etc.

Eclampsia

Eclampsia is one of the major health problems in resource-poor countries. Its incidence is not well defined, varying from 1:100-1,400 or 1:100-1,700 deliveries, (Bianchi et al, 1998; Castro M, 2003), against 1:2,000 in Western countries (Douglas & Redman, 1994; Saftlas et al., 1990). It is estimated that approx. 50,000 women die from eclampsia every year, most of them in resource-poor countries (Maharaj B., Moodley, J. 1994).

Eclampsia affects not only maternal but also foetal morbidity and mortality; a survey conducted in South Africa (Saving Babies 2003. Fourth perinatal care survey of South Africa) found a greater than 50% correlation between perinatal mortality and maternal hypertension; weights ranged between 1,000 and 2,000 grams. Death was intrauterine in most cases, 29% of mortality being linked to respiratory distress.

Aetiopathogenesis

There is a broad consensus that eclampsia is the natural conclusion of a progressive and gradual process, a "continuum" that begins with the accumulation of fluid (oedema) signalled by weight gain, followed by hypertension and proteinuria, and which terminates in the appearance of convulsions. This view is validated by the effectiveness of magnesium sulphate therapy in both preventing and combatting convulsions.

But there is also a form of eclampsia, defined in the past as *"eclampsia sine eclampsia"* which is not necessarily related to the degree of proteinuria or hypertension, as shown by the following:

- Only 1–2% of gravidae affected by severe preeclampsia go on to develop eclampsia
- A study of 399 eclampsia cases (Mattar 2000) found no hypertension in 16%, no proteinuria in 14% and oedema was absent in 26% of cases
- In 60% of cases, convulsions were the first sign of eclampsia; these were not preceded by preeclampsia (Katz et al., 2000).

For this reason, the view presented above should be augmented by the hypothesis that eclampsia is a probably primitive, cerebrovascular disease and not simply the deterioration of preeclampsia. Eclampsia may therefore appear before other manifestations.

This view appears to receive indirect confirmation by the greater effectiveness of magnesium sulphate, which acts on the muscles and on the endothelium of vessels, in comparison to anticonvulsant drugs whose action is neuronal.

Onset

The 50% percent of eclampsia cases are antepartum 20% are intrapartum and the remaining 30% occur postpartum. Of postpartum cases, 50% are observed within the first 48 hours and the others never beyond the 4th postpartum week ('late eclampsia').

In a study by Douglas and Redman (1994), 2/3 of antepartum forms occurred pre-term, while 2/3 of the intraor postpartum forms occurred at term.

Sequence of Symptoms

The sequence of symptoms is as follows:
- *Prodromal period* characterised by exacerbation of the cardinal signs of preeclampsia (headache, epigastric pain, visual disturbances and hyperreflexia), with the following incidence: headache 63%; visual disturbances 32%, other signs at lower percentages (epigastric pain, nausea and vomiting, behavioural disturbances, irritability)
- *Invasive period*: Fibrillar contractions of the facial muscles, tremors of the hands and arms, hands and feet, dilatation of the pupils
- *Tonic contractions*, hands clench into fists, teeth grind, breathing stops, face turns blue, and later, other effects appear:
- *Clonic contractions*, affecting the whole body; contractions of the nuchal muscles push the head back, contractions of the dorsal muscles arch the vertebral column; the patient hits herself with hands and legs, during an attack, reflexes are inactive and blood pressure increases. After one minute, the convulsive state recedes with a deep, snoring breath; the patient remains still and unconscious for some time.

Diagnosis

An eclampsia diagnosis generally comes out of a prior preeclampsia. However, in countries where malaria is endemic, when faced with a normothermic gravida in coma, in whom hypertension and proteinuria are absent, the possibility of eclampsia should always be suspected nonetheless. Where it is not possible to determine the presence of a parasite in the peripheral blood, dual therapy is always justified (quinine and magnesium sulphate IV). Perhaps, in this way, the number of maternal deaths from "therapy-resistant cerebral malaria" will be reduced. Different criteria which might be able to direct diagnosis are shows the Table 8.2.

Therapy

Therapy should consider both the well-being of the mother and of the foetus.

Table 8.2
Criteria to diagnose eclampsia and malaria

Criteria	Eclampsia	Malaria
Locally resident	Resident	Non-resident
Parity	Primigravida	Primigravida
Coma, preceded by convulsions	constantly	rarely
Reawakens	after attack	persistent coma
Hypertension	present, but not always	occasional
Hyperthermia (*)	rarely present	present
Oedema	present and marked	present, not very marked
Proteinuria	not always present	sometimes (see below)
Contraction diuresis	present	rare (renal insufficiency)
Convulsions	during attacks	not present
Placenta affected	present	Blockage of space intervillous
Foetus	distress	
Maternal lesions	Present	Absent
Ex adjuvantibus (*)	Magnesium sulphate	Antimalaris
Fundal examination (oedema)	present	Present
Fundal examination crossings	Present	absent

Well-being of the Mother

Control of convulsions: As a preliminary consideration, it is pointed out that the less common eclampsia is in that particular geographical area, the more likely it is that its progress will be dramatic. Often, hospitals in resourcepoor countries do not have the organisation or the facilities to treat severe cases adequately. As gestosis is a "diseases due to pregnancy" and delivery of the foetus is the definitive treatment, we suggest control of hypertension and convulsions, stabilisation of the mother and expedition of delivery, bearing in mind that in these countries the mother's survival, not that of the foetus, *has priority*. Magnesium sulphate stops the convulsions through its curariform action on neuromuscular junctions. It should be used only where calcium gluconate is available (magnesium antagonist).

Elimination of the drug takes place mainly via the kidneys. The stated doses are sufficient to maintain serum potassium values within safe limits where there is normal renal function. Where urine output is less than 120 ml/4h, overdose reactions are to be expected: These include hypotension and arrhythmia, reduced tendon reflexes presaging respiratory depression, respiratory depression and neurological disorders (drowsiness, limited speech function, diplopia, nausea and vomiting).

Administration regimens for magnesium sulphate: Administration may be intravenous, intramuscular and intravenous, or intramuscular.

Intravenous administration:

- Magpie Trial Regimen
  a. Dosage for attacks, 4 g IV, at intervals of 20–30 minutes.
  b. Maintenance dosage.

One proceeds, essentially, as follows: the $MgSO_4$ is available in 50% solution in 50 ml vials; 100 ml is drawn from a 500 ml bottle of saline solution or 5% glucose solution; the contents of two 50 ml vials are injected. This will yield 100 g of $MgSO_4$ in 500 ml of solution, i.e. 1 g per 5 ml of solution.

An attack dose is 4 g: As 5 ml contain 1 g; 4 g = 5 ml x 4 = 20 ml, to be administered over a period of 20 minutes.

Since intravenous lines are calibrated so that 20 drops correspond to 1 ml, the rate of infusion will be 20 drops per minute for 20–30 minutes.

Maintenance Dose: 1 g/h; i.e. 5 ml per hour, followed by 1 drop every 40 seconds

If contractions persist or if there is a new eclamptic attack, administer the dosage for an attack dose; when faced with continuous attacks, administration of $MgSO_4$ increases from 1 g/h to 1.2–2 g/h.

The total dose of $MgSO_4$ administered intravenously over the first hour should not exceed eight (8) grams.

Intravenous administration
- Witlin Sibai regimen (1998)
  a. Attack dose (IV): 6 g in 20–30 minutes
  b. Maintenance (IV): 2–3 grams/hour

Intravenous and intramuscular administration
- Pritchard regimen
  a. 4 g (IV) within 3–5 minutes, to which is added: 2.5 g IM in each buttock, giving thereby a total loading dose of $MgSO_4$ of: 4 g IV + (2.5 × 2 IM) 5 g IM = 9 g If convulsions do not stop, administer 2 g slowly intravenously over 2 minutes; if convulsions persist, consider administration of 5 mg diazepam IV or 1 mg of lorazepam (bear in mind the possibility of respiratory depression).
  b. Maintenance dose: 5 mg IM every 4 hours

Intramuscular administration:

a. Dosage for attacks: 5 grams magnesium sulphate in each buttock; as an IM injection of MgSO4 is very painful, combine 1 ml 2% lignocaine in the same syringe. The intramuscular route should be used as an emergency measure in locations where healthcare assistance is limited; where there is a minimum level of assistance, the combined IV and IM route should be preferred;

b. Maintenance dose: This is administered every 4 hours, alternating in each buttock; 2.5 g IM, after ascertaining that there are no signs of overdose (see next Section).

Monitoring

Excessive dosage is shown by:
- Hypotension and arrhythmia
- Reduced tendon reflexes, followed by respiratory depression
- Respiratory depression
- Neurological disorders: Drowsiness, impaired speech function, diplopia, nausea, vomiting.

Therefore, monitoring consists in continuous monitoring of:
- *Blood pressure and heart rate*
- *Patellar reflex*, every two hours. In case of:
  - *reduced or absent patellar reflex:* If respiratory function is normal, discontinue infusion until reflexes return;
  - *reduced or absent patellar or bicipital reflex with concomitant respiratory depression*: Reduce or discontinue infusion; administer calcium gluconate IV at a dosage of 1–2 g; slowly (over three minutes). Repeat administration at 30-minute intervals until respiratory activity resumes with normal frequency. If necessary resuscitate
- *Respiratory rate*: It is useful to establish the basal frequency before starting the infusion, in case of:
  - *respiratory depression:* Administer oxygen by mask, 1 g calcium gluconate IV over three minutes; discontinue therapy with magnesium.
- *Respiratory arrest*: Intubate and ventilate the patient; administer 1 g calcium gluconate
- *Diuresis*: In case of
  - *oliguria* (urine output less than 30 ml/h, 120 ml over past 4 hours, or, according to other authors, less than 25 ml/h over past 4 hours) or *reduction in respiration* where oxygenation remains optimal: *Halve the maintenance dose*
  - *oliguria* associated with: *Respiratory rate <16 breaths/minute, reduced or absent bicipital or patellar reflexes*: see above.
- Cognitive function.

Alternative Regimens to Magnesium Sulphate

If magnesium sulphate is not available, it is possible to use the following alternative regimens:

- *Diazepam* may be used at the beginning of any anticonvulsant therapy, or in the absence of magnesium sulphate, to counter contractions that are under way or to maintain constant sedation. Administration is intravenous or by infusion (which would require an infusion pump), rectal, intramuscular or oral.

Intravenous Administration

Dosage for attacks: 10 mg IV slowly, over the course of two minutes; if contractions do not stop, repeat the attack dose.

Maintenance dose: 40 mg of diazepam in 500 ml of saline or Ringer's lactate solution, rate of infusion 30 drops/minute; adapt dosage to keep patient sedated, but not asleep. Do not exceed a dosage of 100 mg over 24 hours.

Rectal administration: fill a 10 ml syringe with 20 mg of diazepam; remove the needle and insert half of the length of the syringe into the rectum, and inject. Leave the syringe in situ for 10 minutes to avoid the expulsion of the medication. The drug can also be administered by urinary catheter into the rectum. If convulsions are not under control within 10 minutes, introduce a supplementary dose of 10 mg per hour, adjusting the dose to the patient's body weight.

Intramuscular administration: Not recommended; absorption is less than per os and efficacy is not predictable.

Diazepam has the property of placental transition; a single dose, to control an eclamptic attack, may be given freely and is unlikely to cause neonatal respiratory depression, which is, however, possible with prolonged use (more than 36 hours before labour). In case of prolonged use, the neonate, especially if preterm or exposed to placental ischaemia, will be flaccid and subject to attacks of cyanosis.

- *Clomethiazole* 'Heminevrin' is a sedative and anticonvulsant, administered by intravenous infusion at a concentration of 0.8% clomethiazole edisylate; initially 5–15 ml (40–120 mg/min) up to a maximum of 40–60 ml.
- Pethidine-based (50 mg) *lytic cocktail,* Promethazine (50 mg), chlorpromazine (50 mg), the first dose may be administered intravenously, the subsequent ones IM after 4–6 hours. With chlorpromazine, do not exceed 300 mg over 24 hours.
- *Phenytoin* can be administered orally: 150–200 mg, 1 or 2 times a day, or intravenously at the same dosage.

Foetal Well-being

In addition to monitoring foetal heart rate, it is important to count foetal active movements (Cardiff system or foetal kick count chart; see Chapter 6).

Delivery should be expedited within 12 hours of start of convulsions. If the Bishop pelvic score is not favourable for induction, cervical ripening may be assisted using a Foley catheter or using Prostaglandins. If this is not possible, expedite delivery by C-section; locoregional (spinal) anaesthesia is the method of choice.

Birth Canal Anomalies

- Pelvic dystocia: Abnormalities in the size and morphology of the pelvis
- Soft tissue dystocia, which may affect:
  - Uterine corpus: Prior hysterotomies for: C-section, metroplasty, myomectomy, prior tumours
  - Cervix: Scar tissue from prior cervical lesions; cervical lesions, particularly lateral ones, generally indicate elective C-section due to possible cranial extension of scar with involvement of the uterine arteries
  - Vagina: Prior repair of vesicovaginal fistula, prior repair of anterior vaginal profile
  - Bladder: Grafts, fistulas
  - Rectum: Prior repair of rectovaginal fistulas, prior colpoperineorrhaphy surgery
  - Female genital mutilation
  - Inflammatory pathology of distal genital tract: Genital herpes, Chlamydia, condylomatosis.

FOETAL INDICATIONS

A. *Dystocias of the passenger*
   - Abnormal lie: Transverse, oblique, that has not proven possible to correct by external version
   - Longitudinal lie, complication of presentation: breech presentation incompatible with parity, foetal size, morphology and size of the pelvis, previous uterine surgery
   - Abnormal cephalic presentation: Asynclitism, brow and face presentation
   - Labour dystocia due to foetal macrosomia
   - Growth defect
   - Abnormal duration of pregnancy
   - Late-age primigravida
   - Monoamniotic twins with first twin in breech presentation and second in cephalic presentation, risk of interlocked twins
   - Crossed factors: The concomitant presence of factors that, in isolation, do not indicate C-section, but become an indication when associated
   - Maternal-foetal isoimmunisation.

B. *Pathology of the foetal adnexa*
   a. Placenta:
      » *Third trimester haemorrhage* (APH – antepartum haemorrhage); in resource-poor countries these often occur on anaemic terrain. They include:

» Abruption of normally inserted placenta
» Anomalies of pregnancy site: Placenta praevia.

The indication for C-section is made only after assessing the percentage of placenta praevia (Fig. 8.4). If this is less than 30%, delivery may be expedited vaginally. Profuse bleeding during the C-section: This sometimes requires uterine artery ligation. Where we can clamp only the ascending branches, not the descending ones, and as the latter permeate part of the area of placental insertion, this continues to bleed profusely. Here we suggest either figure of- eight haemostatic sutures in the area of haemorrhage or transvaginal clamping of the cervical branches.

This simple and effective measure is described in Chapter 17.

a. *Placental insufficiency*: Intrauterine growth retardation (IUGR, small for dates), which may be:
   - *Primary*
   - *Secondary*: Following infarction of the intervillous spaces by erythrocytes recruited by the malarial Plasmodium.
   - *PROM* (premature rupture of membranes) with chorioamnionitis.

b. *Amniotic fluid pathology*:
   - *Deficit*: Oligohydramnios and anhydramnios
   - *Excess*: Polyhydramnios, where abnormal presentation is also present.

c. *Umbilical cord pathology*:
   - Variation in length: *Excessive length* (loops or encirclement) or unusually short
   - Knots, true knots occur in about one per 200 deliveries, if tight will cvause fetal asphyxia and death. False knots are with no clinical relevance
   - Procidentia and prolapse.

The term *procidentia* refers to an umbilical cord that precedes the leading part, *with membranes intact*. *Prolapse* refers to an umbilical cord that precedes the leading part, *with membranes ruptured*. In the case of prolapse, emergency manoeuvres consist in quickly filling the bladder with 500 ml of normal saline (to prevent engagement of the presenting part), placing the gravid patient in a genupectoral position and assessing whether it is possible to extract the foetus immediately by breech extraction, or, with cephalic presentation, using vacuum extraction. A condition for this is cervical dilatation of at least eight centimetres.

BIBLIOGRAPHY

1. American College of Obstetricians and Gynecologists. Chronic Hypertension in pregnancy. ACOG practice bulletin no 29. Obstet Gynecol. 2001;98:177-85.
2. Barton JR, O'Brien JM, Bergauer NK, Jacques DL, Sibai BM. Mild gestational hypertension remote from term, progression and outcome. A J O G. 2001;184:979-83.
3. Beaufils M, Uzan S, Donsimoni R. Prevention of preeclampsia by early antiplatelets therapy. Lancet. 1985;1:840.
4. Benigni A, Gregorini G, Frusca T. Effect of low-dose aspirin on fetal and maternal generation of tromboxane by platelets in women at risk for pregnancy-induced hypertension. N Engl J Med. 1989;321:357.
5. Bianchi LR, Navarrete AI, Ortega I, Eckolt E, Caroca A, Sandoval L, Vargas E, Palavecino L. Estudio Clinico de la eclampsia. Revista Chilena de Obstetricia y Ginecologia. 1998;53:128-33.
6. Bortolus R, Ricci E, Chatenoud L, Parazzini F. Nifedipine administration in pregnancy: Effect on the development of children at 18 months. Br J Obstet Gynaecol. 2000;107: 792-4.
7. CLASP. Collaborative Low-dose Aspirin Study in Pregnancy Collaborative Group: A randomized trial of low-dose aspirin for prevention and tretment of preeclampsia among 9364 pregnant women. Lancet. 1994;343:619.
8. Douglas e Redman. Br Med J. 1994;309:1395.
9. Gruppo di Studio Ipertensione in Gravidanza. Nifedipine versus expectant management in mild to moderate hypertension in pregnancy. Br J Obstet Gynaecol. 1998; 105:718-22 (Level I).
10. Hartikainen-Sorri AL, Heikkinen JE, Koivisto M. Pharmacokinetics of clonidine during pregnancy and nursing. Obstet Gynecol. 1987;69:598-600.
11. Hogg B, Hauth JC, Caritis SN, Sibai BM, Lindheimer M, Van Dorsten JP. Safety of labor epidural anaesthesia for women

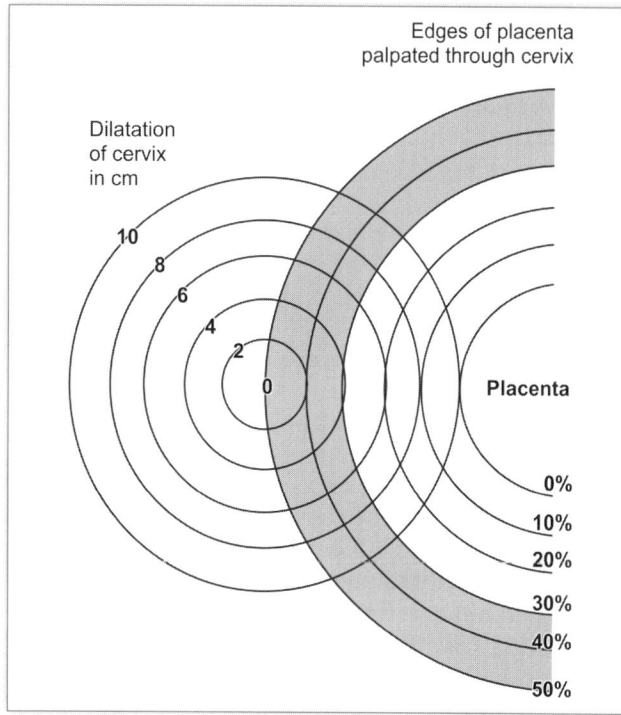

Fig. 8.4: Relation of percentage placenta praevia to cervix

with severe hypertensive disease. National Institute of Child Health and Human Development. Maternal-Fetal Medicine Units Network. Am J Obstet Gynecol. 1999;181:1096-101.
12. Italian Study of Aspirin in pregnancy. Low-dose aspirin in prevention and treatment of intrauterine growth retardation and pregnancy-induced hypertension. Lancet. 1993;8842: 396-9.
13. Knight M, Duley L, et al. Antiplatelet agents for preventing and treating preeclampsia. The Cochrane Database of systematic reviews; 2000.
14. Magee LA, Elran E, Bull SB, Logan A, Koren G. Risks and benefits of beta-receptor blockers for pregnancy hypertension: Overview of the randomized trials. Eur J Obstet Gynecol Reprod Biol. 2000;88(1):15-26.
15. The Magpie Trial Collaborative Group. Do women with pre-eclampsia, and their babies, benefit from magnesium sulphate? The Magpie Trial: a randomised placebo-controlled trial. Lancet. 2002;359:1877-90.
16. Maharaj B, Moodley J. Management of hypertension in pregnancy. Continued Medical Education. 1994;12:1581-9.
17. Mattar F, Sibai BM. Eclampsia. VIII. Risk factors for maternal morbidity. Am J Obstet Gynecol. 2000;182(2):307-12.
18. Paruk F, Moodley J. Management of mild to moderate hypertension during pregnancy: RHL practical aspects (last revised: 19 Septmber 2001).
19. The WHO Reproductive Health Library, No 9, Update Software Ltd, Oxford, 2006.
20. Report of the National High Blood Pressure Education Program Working Group on High Blood Pressure in Pregnancy. Am J Obstet Gynecol. 2000;183:S1-S22.
21. Saftlas AF, Olson DR, Franks AL, et al. Epidemiology of preeclampsia and eclampsia in the United States, 1979-1986. Am J Obstet Gynecol. 1990;163(2):460-5.
22. Saving mothers. Report on confidential enquiries into maternal deaths in South Africa, 1998. Pretoria (South Africa): Department of Health 1999.
23. Sibai BM, Mabie WC, Shamsa F, Villar MA, Anderson GD. A comparison of no medication versus methyldopa or labetalol in chronic hypertension during pregnancy. Am J Obstet Gynecol. 1990;162:960-6; discussion 966-7.
24. Sibai BM. Hypertension in pregnancy. Obstet Gynecol Clin North Am. 1992;19:615-33.
25. Sibai BM. Chronic Hypertension in Pregnancy. Obstet Gynecol. 2002;100:369-77.
26. Villar J, Say L, Gulmezoglu AM, Merialdi M. Eclampsia and preeclampsia: a worldwide health problem for 2000 years. Preeclampsia, London: 2003.
27. Wallenburg HCS, Dekker GA, Makovitz JW. Low-dose aspirin prevents pregnancy-induced hypertension and preeclampsia in angiotensine-sensitive primigravidae. Lancet. 1986;1:1.
28. Witlin AG, Sibai BM. Magnesium sulphate therapy in preeclampsia and eclampsia. Obstet Gynecol. 1998;92: 883-9.

CHAPTER 9

Indications for Caesarean Section During Labour

PRELIMINARY CONSIDERATIONS

In setting indications for C-section, we should concentrate not on the aetiology of the condition—which may become apparent on surgery—but rather on rapid detection of its consequences. These may be summarised as follows:

a. *Compromise of maternal–foetal gas exchanges,* that are made clinically manifest by changes in foetal heart rate.
b. *Failure of engagement and descent by the presenting part* in the case of mechanical obstruction, accompanied by so-called *secondary signs*, which occur much earlier and are more significant than simple failure of descent. These signs include: Alterations in uterine morphology, overdistension of the (LUS) to the point of forming a retraction ring, stretching of the round ligaments, marked tenderness of the LUS, pain that precedes uterine contractions rather than, as in normal labour, coming after them.

The *secondary signs* are associated with the complex of symptoms known as *"maternal distress"*, characterised by anxiety, restlessness and ketoacidosis.

These considerations also apply in abnormal foetal lie (transverse and oblique) and to noncephalic longitudinal lies (breech).

Indication for caesarean section should be preceded by pelvic examination to detect whether conditions allow vaginal delivery (Table 9.1). Often full cervical ripening is associated with an intact forebag, whereby an amniotomy may enable rapid expedition of delivery.

Table 9.1

Methods of expediting delivery

Level of head above pelvic inlet	Foetal distress	Moulding of foetal skull	Method of expediting delivery
3/5	Absent	Present	C-section
3/5	Absent	Absent	attempt vacuum extraction
2/5	Present	Present	C-section or symphysiotomy
2/5	Absent	Present	Attempt forceps or vacuum extraction, but generally C-section or symphysiotomy
1/5	Present	Present	Symphysiotomy then forceps, Malmström extractor or C-section
1/5	Absent	Present	Malmström extractor or forceps
0/5	Absent	Present	Malmström extractor or forceps

Indications for C-section may be summarised as follows:
1. Compromise of maternal–foetal gas exchange.
2. Obstruction to engagement and descent of the passenger.

3. The above two indications in varying relations to each other.
4. Maternal indications (hyperthermia, gestosis, haemorrhage).

COMPROMISE OF MATERNAL–FOETAL GAS EXCHANGE

Contributory factors:
- *Uterine hyperkinesia* (number of contractions greater than five), see Chapter 7, Fig. 7.5 for more details
- *Placental insufficiency, reduction of surface for placental exchanges*
- *Infarction of the intervillous spaces* by *Plasmodium falciparum* infected erythrocytes which adhere both in the intervillous spaces and on the villous surface of the placenta due to binding to two receptors: Hyaluronic acid (Beeson et al. 2000) and chondroitin sulphate A (Lekana Douki et al, 2002), present in the placental tissue. Infarction is responsible for abortion, IUGR (Jelliffe, 1991, Menendez et al., 2000) and for intrauterine death (Guyatt et al., 1995)
- Due to *placental abruption or placenta praevia:* Where the latter is present, C-section is indicated only after assessing the percentage of placenta praevia; when this is less than 30%, expedition of delivery can take the vaginal route, if more than 40%, C-section will be indicated (Fig. 8.3).

Umbilical Cord Pathology

- *Loops* around the neck, trunk or limbs
- *Shortness*
- *Procidentia*, which refers to the presence of umbilical cord in front of or near the presenting part, where the umbilical cord is not subjected to compression and where the membranes are intact. The hazard presented by this condition is that it usually precedes cord prolapse.

Classical obstetrics offers a series of measures aimed at bringing the cord back in a cranial direction. As noted, the cord floats in amniotic fluid and thus, will always tend to move upwards. Among these measures are: Genupectoral position, decubitus with the pelvis raised by two pillows, and lateral decubitus with the pelvis raised on the side opposite that of the cord. These measures are followed, on full cervical ripening, by amniotomy and a concomitant push to the foetal head from outside to facilitate its engagement and descent. These manoeuvres are difficult to execute and attain modest results even when performed by experienced hands. We therefore strongly recommend *expedition of delivery* by caesarean section.

Cord prolapse: Presence of the cord anteriorly or near the presenting part after rupture of membranes: C-section is here indicated if conditions are not present for immediate extraction of the foetus by vacuum extraction, with cephalic presentation, head engaged and dilatation of at least 8 cm, or by breech extraction where full cervical ripening is present.

While awaiting C-section, *emergency manoeuvres* aimed at preventing engagement of the head and compression of the cord, consist in quickly filling the bladder with 500 ml saline solution and placing the patient in the genupectoral position.

When indicating C-section, consideration should be given to the gestational age of the foetus, and whether this is compatible with its survival. When these conditions are absent, and in view of the limited resources often available, it is preferable to allow delivery to go ahead by the vaginal route, thereby sparing the mother a pointless and potentially harmful hysterotomy. Not infrequently, cord prolapse is the consequence of an incorrectly executed amniotomy, a correct procedure requires:

- The patient in semi-seated position, (also called Fowler's position)
- During the pelvic examination preceding amniotomy, no space is found between head and pelvis which would allow for passage of the cord
- After performing the amniotomy, the head should never be pushed back to allow the fluid to flow more rapidly.

Uterine Rupture

The concept of compromised maternal–foetal gas exchange, generically referred to as "foetal distress", it encompasses two distinct conditions: *Foetal asphyxia* and *foetal anoxia*.

- *Foetal asphyxia* refers to a condition in which gas exchange, even though reduced, is still present; here the time conditions are present for performing a C-section under regional anaesthesia
- *Foetal anoxia* refers to the complete interruption of maternal–foetal gas exchange due to: Complete compression of the cord, maternal bradycardia, tetanus uteri or uterine rupture; this can be lethal within less than 10 minutes. The anaesthetic of choice is ketamine.

All the conditions described above are clinically manifested by variations in foetal heart rate.

OBSTACLES TO THE ENGAGEMENT AND PROGRESS OF LABOUR

The following factors may contribute to obstructing engagement and descent of the presenting part:

Unfavourable Foetal Lie or Presentation

Due to multiple pregnancies or retained second twin.

Unfavourable Foetal Lie

Oblique or transverse.

Unfavourable Presentation: Breech

- In primigravidae
- In contracted pelvis
- Foetal macrosomia.

Unfavourable Presentation: Cephalic

Obstacle to engagement by:

Presenting Part

This may relate to:
- *Flexion or deflection of the head:* We recall from Chapter 5 that engagement occurs
- *With the head flexed:* (vertex presentation), along the suboccipitobregmatic diameter or minor oblique diameter (projected from the nape to the midpoint of the anterior fontanelle, 9.5 cm). This corresponds to the *smallest possible plane of passage* (suboccipitobregmatic circumference) of 32 cm; Crichton's fifths on the occiput side outnumber those on the sinciput side
- *With the head partially deflected* (bregma presentation) along the occipitofrontal diameter (projected from the brow and most prominent point of the occiput, 12 cm) corresponding to a largest plane of passage of 34 cm; Crichton's fifths are equal on each side
- *With the head deflected* (a degree of deflexion just above that of bregma presentation) along the occipitomental or major oblique diameter, 13.5 cm, (projected from the chin to the most prominent point of the occiput), corresponding to a largest plane of passage of 35–36 cm.

The number of Crichton's fifths detectable on the occiput side outnumber those on the sinciput side; here we distinguish between:
- Brow presentation
- And face presentation: In the latter, the head is in maximum deflexion
- *Dimensions of the head*: Hydrocephalus.

Pelvis

- *Dimensions*: Diameters of pelvic inlet, midpelvis or pelvic outlet incompatible with a normal head. Please refer to Chapter 2, Section 5 and to the section on intraoperative measurement of the obstetric conjugate (Chapter 12)
- *Morphology*: Please refer to Chapter 6 "Diagnosis in Clinical Obstetrics", which deals in some detail with the pure types of pelvis (android, anthropoid, gynecoid and platypelloid), as well as with mixed ones
- *Lack of alignment between major axis of foetus and that of the birth canal or 'inclination dystocia',* which can be traced to

- *Altered inclination of the pelvis:* Pelvic inclination refers to the angle that the plane of the pelvic inlet subtends with the horizon. In the standing position, this varies between 35 and 75°; under normal conditions, inclination is 60° to the horizon. In obstetrics, position is the orientation of the fetus in the womb, identified by the location of the presenting part of the fetus relative to the pelvis of the mother.

Variations from this in excess or deficit: Beyond given values, this angle will impede alignment of the major foetal axis with the axis of the birth canal, so the principle of the *smallest possible plane of passage* (synclitism and flexion) breaks down. This principle is indispensable for engagement of the presenting part (see Chapter 5); for this reason, we observe cephalopelvic disproportion.

Variations in this angle may be:

- *In excess*: The plane of the pelvic inlet has a tendency to assume an almost horizontal position. This is observed particularly among primigravidae, whose lumbosacral hinge is only slightly accentuated and who have good muscle tone in the abdomen. The presenting part tends to bear down against the pubic symphysis, which explains how uterine ruptures are mainly anterior among primigravidae
- *In deficit,* found most often among multiparae. Accentuation of lordosis leads to an inclination of the pelvic inlet of less than 60°, so that it tends to assume an almost vertical position.

In most cases, this variation of inclination is accompanied by a similar variation in the major foetal axis, caused by the anterior inclination of the uterus—the pendulous abdomen due to decreased tone of the abdominal wall, observed among multiparae. For this reason we observe abnormal engagement (anterior asynclitism), where inclination of the major foetal axis exceeds that of the pelvis. If this is not detected and treated early, it can lead to uterine rupture, particularly to posterior ruptures.

- *Engagement* refers to "the passage through the pelvic inlet of the largest circumference for that particular presentation". Engagement occurs as a result of random movements during which the foetal presenting part identifies the area compatible with engagement, the *area of inclusion.* In order for this to happen, it is essential that there is a favourable ratio between the capacity (ability to contain) of the true pelvis and the volume of the presenting part. A size ratio incompatible with the engagement may be caused by:
  - The *passenger*: Because of its lie (shoulder presentation), oblique lie
  - Or in the case of cephalic presentation, to abnormality of the head: Hydrocephalus
  - *Asynclitism,* under normal conditions the head enters the plane of the pelvic inlet perpendicularly (synclitism); when this condition breaks down, we

have *asynclitism*, which is in turn divided into *anterior* and *posterior* (See Chapters 5 and 6).

The above factors (presenting part/pelvis) in varying relations with each other.

A leading limb

Changes in Uterine Morphology

Due to:
- Congenital causes: Uterus didelfus, arcuate uterus
- Acquired causes: Scars, parietal adhesions, prior myoma, pathology of contraction and/or of cervical dilatation (cervical dystocia), change in contractile polarity, uterine inertia unresponsive to oxytocics.

Changes to the Soft Tissue of the Birth Canal

- Anomalies of dilatation—dynamic dystocia
- Outcomes of repairs to bladder or vaginal rectal fistulas
- Outcomes of anterior or posterior vaginal repair
- Female genital mutilation
- Inflammatory processes, sexually transmitted infectious diseases.

Hyperthermia

Unless dehydration is a contributory factor.

Expulsive Phase Anomalies

If, after 30 minutes of pushing, 2/5 of the head is still above the pelvic inlet, we are faced with obstructed labour, which is to be treated appropriately.

Finally, it should be noted that there is a "point of no return" during labour, represented by a head at the inferior part of the pelvic cavity, or at the pelvic floor, accompanied by effective uterine contractions. Dystocia of the pelvic outlet may be:
- Osseous: If the abdominal pelvic score (calculated as the sum of fifths of head detectable above the pubic symphysis and the degree of moulding of the foetal skull at full uterine dilatation) is equal to or greater than three, we strongly discourage vaginal expedition of delivery, unless preceded by a symphysiotomy
- Of the soft tissue, a bilateral mediolateral episiotomy is preferable to a unilateral mediolateral episiotomy, which is often a Schukhardt incision with section of the anus levator muscle, this is rarely recognised and repaired.

THE TWO INDICATIONS PRESENTED ABOVE IN VARYING RELATIONS TO EACH OTHER

Maternal Indications

- Hyperthermia
- Gestosis.

BIBLIOGRAPHY

1. Beeson JG. Adhaesion of *Plasmodium falciparum* infected erythrocytes to hyaluronic acid in placental malaria. Nature Medicine, 2000;6:86-90.
2. Guyatt Hl, Snow RW. Malaria in pregnancy as an indirect cause of infant mortality in sub-Saharian Africa. Trans R Soc Trop Med Hyg. 2001;95(6):569-76.
3. Lekana Douki JB, Traore B, Costa FT, Fusai T, Pouvelle B, Sterker Scherf A, Gysin J. Sequestration of *Plasmodium falciparum* infected erythrocytes: chondroitin sulfate A, a receptor for maternal malaria: monoclonal antibodies against the native parasite ligand panreactive epitopes in placenta isolates. Blood. 2002;100(4):1478-83.
4. Menendez C, Ordi J, Ismail MR, Ventura PJ, Aponte JJ, Kahigwa E, Pont F. Alonso PL. The impact of placental malaria on gestational age and birth weight. J Infect Dis. 2000;181(5):1740-5.
5. Ordi J, Ismail MR, Ventura PJ, Kahigwa Fr, Hirt R, Cardesa A, Alonso PL. Massive chronic intervillositis of the placenta associated with malaria infection. Am J Pathol. 1998;22(8):1006-11.

CHAPTER 10

Trial of Labour

By trial of labour here is meant the conducting, in the absence of contraindications and within well-defined clinical and time constraints, of a spontaneous or induced labour for the purpose of assessing the compatibility of the birth canal or of the force of uterine contractions with a normal delivery. A precondition for conducting a trial of labour is access to an operating theatre *within 30 minutes of indicating a C-section operation*.

Two phases can be clearly differentiated in a trial of labour:
- Preliminary assessment of suitability for labour
- The actual labour, within well-defined clinical and temporal constraints.

PRELIMINARY ASSESSMENT OF THE GRAVID PATIENT
(presence of the criteria for admissibility to labour)

The diagnostic approach will vary according to whether or not patients have undergone a hysterotomy, as these will present differing complications:
a. For patients who have not undergone a hysterotomy, possible complications will be cephalopelvic disproportion or an obstructed labour.
b. For patients with previous C-section (VBAC-TOL or vaginal birth after caesarean trial of labour), we must add to the above complications that of uterine rupture. More common than among patients who have not undergone a hysterotomy, the frequency of rupture of the uterus is approximately 1%, but this can vary with other risk factors present (McMahon, 1996; Rageth, 1999; Mozurkewich, 2000; Lydon-Rochelle et al., 2001).

Suitability for Trial of Labour for a Patient Who has not Undergone C-section

This is normally a primigravida in whom an incompatibility between foetus and pelvis is suspected: Borderline pelvis or foetal macrosomia in a woman who has already given birth to foetuses of normal size with difficulty in engagement or in expulsion of the presenting part. Careful clinical assessment is here decisive (see Chapter 6).

Suitability for Trial of Labour for a Patient who has Undergone C-section

To be excluded are multiple pregnancies, breech presentation and foetal macrosomia.

In addition to precise assessment of the pelvis, diagnosis is complicated by the need to classify the previous C-section according to the following considerations:

Anamnestic Criteria

Maternal age: According to McMahon (1996) and Gregory et al, (1999) a maternal age of 35 years or more presents a greater risk of uterine rupture. After weighting for variables, such as foetal weight, time period since previous caesarean section and present pregnancy, induction of labour and increase in uterine contraction activity, Shipp et al. (2002) found that a maternal age above 30 years presented a risk of uterine rupture 3.2 times higher than a maternal age below 30.

Number of previous C-sections: Women with two or more previous c-sections are at greater risk of uterine rupture than women with one previous C-section only; percentages vary across age groups. In the largest survey of cases conducted to date (12,707 women with uterine scars from a previous C-section admitted to trial of labour), Miller (1994) reports a percentage of 1.7% for uterine rupture among women with two or more scars compared to 0.6% for women with one only.

According to Asakura et al, (1995), these percentages were 1% and 0.5%, respectively. Subsequently a multifactorial analysis by Caughey et al. (1999) found that during a trial of labour, the percentage of uterine rupture among women with two or more previous C-sections was 4.8 times higher than for those with one previous C-section.

Previous vaginal deliveries: Vaginal deliveries, whether preceding or subsequent to a C-section, reduce the risk of uterine rupture during a trial of labour. According to Zelop et al. (2000), the percentage of uterine ruptures is in this case 0.2%, against 1.1% for women with no previous vaginal delivery.

Time interval between previous C-section and current pregnancy: According to Shipp (2001), at an interval of less than 18 months the incidence of uterine rupture is 2.3%, but is 1.1% for longer periods. However, these findings are not confirmed by Huang et al. (2002).

In a recent survey of 1,527 cases, Bujold et al. (2002) found that, while 1.1% of ruptures occurred after longer intervals, 2.3% of uterine ruptures occurred after interdelivery intervals of less than 24 months; furthermore, uterine closures using single-layer technique increased this latter percentage to 5.6%.

Type of hysterotomy: With vertical hysterotomy, the incidence of uterine rupture varies according to whether or not the hysterotomy reaches the fundus. Where it does, the percentage is 12%, (Rosen et al., 1991; ACOG, 1999) and trial of labour is not attempted; where it does not, incidence falls to 1.1% (Naef et al., 1995).

Further confirmation of the safety of a vertical but low hysterotomy is provided by Shipp et al. (1999), who compared percentages of uterine rupture between low vertical (1.6%) and transverse low-segment (1.3%) hysterotomies. Data provided by Flamm (1990, 1994) and Martin vary only slightly from the above: Uterine rupture for transverse hysterotomies is less than 1%.

Single or double layer closure: Two factors should be weighed in considering whether to perform closure in a single or double layer:
- *Operating time and postoperative recovery:* A series of studies (Hauth JC et al., 1992; Jelsema RD et al., 1993; Ohel G et al., 1996; Ferrari AG et al., 2001) have demonstrated that single-layer uterine suturing reduces operating time and postoperative morbidity. What these studies did not consider were possible long-term outcomes of this technique, particularly outcomes for a trial of labour
- *Long-term outcomes:* Tucker et al. (1993) found no significant differences between the two techniques (single and double layer). These results were confirmed by Chapman (1997), whose sample size was, however, too small to be significant. In a wide-ranging critical review of the issue, Bujold et al. (2002) showed that for women whose uterine wound was closed using a single-layer of sutures, incidence of uterine rupture was *four times higher* than for those with double-layer closures.

Postoperative recovery complicated by fever: Defining fever as "the presence of a temperature above 38°C", Shipp et al. (2003) found among uterine ruptures during trials of labour that fever complicated previous CS postoperative recovery in 15% of cases.

Obstetric Physical Examination

- Assessment of the pelvis, situation, foetal presentation and position: See Chapter 6
- *Characteristics of the laparotomy scar:* There is a moderate correlation between the morphologies of the laparotomic and uterine scars. We assess the morphology, the thickness, the relation with deeper layers of the laparotomy scar and any asymmetries of the uterus due to adherences between the anterior wall of the uterus and the abdominal wall.

  During labour, we assess the diffusion (polarity of contraction) and asymmetries of the uterus
- *LUS thickness:* Measurement of the thickness of the LUS, where possible, helps identify scars at risk of dehiscence/rupture. According to Asakura et al. (2000), there is very low risk of dehiscence/rupture when LUS thickness is greater than 1.6 mm.

ACTUAL LABOUR

The concept of a trial of labour has evolved over time. In the past, before deciding whether or not delivery could be carried out vaginally, labour was allowed to continue for a period of two hours after full dilatation of the cervix. This approach is no longer current as, for example, where there is cephalopelvic disproportion, full dilatation will never be reached.

The current orientation is to conclude, before full dilatation occurs, whether vaginal delivery may be safely carried out either, according to some authors, within the first two hours of the period of dilatation or, according to others, within 4–6 hours of active-phase labour.

Onset of labour for a patient who has undergone a previous CS may take place: *spontaneously* or be *induced*.

Spontaneous Onset of Labour

- Every effort should be made to obtain the previous Caesarean section operative report to determine the type of uterine incision used
- Provided there are no contraindications, a woman with one previous transverse low-segment Caesarean section should be offered a trial of labour (TOL) with appropriate discussion of perinatal risks and benefits
- Women delivering within 18–24 months of a Caesarean section should be counselled about an increased risk of *uterine rupture* in labour
- Although the rate of uterine rupture was not statistically increased during oxytocin augmentation, use of oxytocin in such cases should proceed with caution (ACOG, 2003)
- The available data suggest that a trial of labour in women with more than 1 previous Caesarean section is likely to be successful but is associated with a higher risk of *uterine rupture*
- Diabetes mellitus, suspected foetal macrosomia, postdatism, multiple gestation are not a contraindication to TOL
- Continuous electronic monitoring of women attempting a TOL after Caesarean section is recommended
- Suspected *uterine rupture*—signs are persistent suprapubic pain, repetitive foetal heart rate and variable decelerations followed by bradycardia require urgent attention and expedited laparotomy to attempt to decrease maternal and perinatal morbidity and mortality
- An approximate time frame of 30 minutes should be considered adequate in the set-up of an urgent laparotomy
- Uterine rupture is rare; it occurs in between 0.3% and 0.7% of labours; the terms *"rupture"* and *"dehiscence"* are not used consistently.

Elective Induction of Labour

Conditions may arise in term pregnancies that make the accomplishment of the delivery, necessary; but "choosing the route of delivery after caesarean birth" is not an easy task as the risk of failed induction and the possibility of uterine rupture are major concerns of clinicians caring for women undergoing a trial of labour after a previous caesarean delivery (TOLAC).

The best method, efficacy, and safety of cervical ripening and/or labour induction in this population has not been established (Alfirevic Z., 2006). Available evidence is inconclusive, the data are insufficient for many reasons, including inconsistent definitions of uterine rupture and dehiscence, wide variation in induction protocols (eg, timing and dosage of prostaglandins and/or oxytocin administration), heterogeneity in patient populations, and inconsistency in primary outcome measures (Kayani SI, Alfirevic Z, 2006).

At least 50 percent of inductions in women with a prior caesarean delivery are successful, with the highest chance of success in women with a prior vaginal delivery and favourable cervix (Bishop score ≥7); compared with spontaneous onset of labour in previous CS, induction results in a lower vaginal delivery rate than spontaneous labour (mean vaginal delivery rate 68 versus 80 percent (McDonagh MS, 2006).

The *latent phase* (Stout MJ, 2015), in women who are induced after a previous caesarean delivery, is longer, while the *active phase*, compared with women who experience spontaneous labour after a caesarean delivery, is similar. When making the diagnosis of a protraction or arrest disorder in women who undergo induction of labour after caesarean delivery, it is reasonable for clinicians to apply the same criteria as in women without a previous caesarean delivery (Sondgeroth KE et al., 2015).

Induction (artificial stimulation of uterine contraction) may be performed by medical (oxytocin or prostaglandins, which have different indications) or by surgical means.

Induction by Medical Means

The drug of choice is related to the degree of cervical readiness for induction.

- *Favourable cervix (Bishop score ≥7),* under this score the myometrial oxytocin receptors are globally well espressed and small amounts of oxytocin are reguired to induce labour.

Induction of labour with oxytocin has been the subject of two large-scale studies; in the first, Rageth et al. (1999) found that out of 17,613 admissions to a trial of labour following C-section, among the uterine rupture group, labour had been induced in 63% of cases. In a subsequent study, (Lydon-Rochelle et al., 2001) uterine rupture among women whose labour had been induced stood at 0.77%, against 0.52% where labour developed spontaneously.

We recommend the following therapeutic regimen: 5 IU oxytocin in 500 ml isotonic solution; initial infusion rate is 8 drops/minute (0.4 ml/min = 4 mU/min). The rate of infusion may be gradually increased until the desired outcome is attained (maximum infusion rate 20 drops/minute.

Under these favourable conditions, amniorrhexis is optional, unless urgent expedition of labour within the shortest timespan possible is indicated, as in cases, such as gestational hypertension, pre-eclampsia, etc.

Conclusion: Medical induction of labour with oxytocin is associated with an increased rate of uterine rupture in gravid women with one prior uterine scar, in comparison with the rate among women in spontaneous labour, and should therefore be used carefully and after appropriate counselling.

- *Bishop score of 5–6*: In intermediate conditions, assess contractile activity, and where the condition of the cervix is compatible with rapid ripening, and there are signs of contractile activity, proceed with the above regimen, repeating if need be on the following day.
  If the condition of the cervix is not consistent in a fast ripening cervix, its ripening, and induction of labour, may be obtained through prostaglandins
- *Unfavourable cervix: Bishop score <5–6*, in a woman with an unfavourable cervix, no previous vaginal delivery and a single previous CS the increased risk of UR must be balanced against the lower chances of a successful delivery Dodd et al., 2006.
  The use of vaginal prostaglandin to induce labour in women with one previous CS is controversial (Scott, 2011); while early reports were reassuring, there is now an emerging consensus that caution should be exercised especially with the sequential use of prostaglandin and oxytocin
- *Misoprostol* (Prostaglandin E1), labour induction with misoprostol, use of which is indicated for labour induction when the cervix is not yet ripened; some preliminary studies (Bennet, 1997; Scissione et al., 1998; Wing et al., 1998; Cunhas et al., 1999; Plaut et al., 1999; Gherman et al., 2000; Hill et al., 2000) highlighted how the use of misoprostol for cervical ripening in the induction of labour represents a significant risk for women who have undergone a caesarean section.
  A Cochrane review of the matter (Hofmeyr et al., 2000) found that the smallness of the data set does not support definitive conclusions. While it allows trial of labour after a previous C-section, ACOG (2002) discourages the use of misoprostol. A study by NICE (National Institute for Clinical Excellence, 2004) found that out of 10,000 induced labours with previous C-section, 80 uterine ruptures were observed among those induced with oxytocin, against 240 among those induced with misoprostol.
  Compared with prostaglandin E2, misoprostol is more effective in cervical ripening and induction of labor, is as safe for patients who do not have a history of caesarean birth, *may carry a higher incidence of uterine rupture, and should not be used for patients attempting vaginal birth after previous cesarean delivery*" (Blanchette HA et al., 1999).
  This is reflected in the more recent ACOG and RCOG guidelines. Particular caution should be exercised with misoprostol (prostaglandin E1), which is associated with a high risk of *uterine rupture*. According to Ravasia et al., "The relative risk of uterine rupture with PGE2 use versus spontaneous trial of labour was 6.41"

- *Dinoprostone* (prostaglandin E2) is associated with an increased risk of uterine rupture and should not be used except in rare circumstances and after appropriate counselling; the currently used protocol consist of 2 mg in gel applied to the cervix for three times with an interval of 6 hours.

Complications are as follows:

- *Uterine hyperstimulation* (more than 5 contractions in 10 minutes, or contractions lasting more than 2 minutes). This complication appears in between 1% and 5% for all indications, and in 31% of cases associated with FHR anomalies. Recommended treatment is tocolysis induced by means of IV infusion (bolus) di *Atosiban* (oxytocin receptor antagonist). In 98% of cases, this allows the foetal heart rate to be normalised within five minutes. Caesarean section is recommended for the remaining cases
- *Failed induction*: Failed induction refers to cases in which three administrations have not been followed by active-phase labour, or where latent-phase labour has lasted more than 12–18 hours. Failure of induction occurs in approximately 15% of cases, and should be distinguished from cases in which progress of labour fails through dystocia
- *Mifepristone* (Lelaidier, C., et al. 1994): Current dosage is 200 mg of mifepristone on days one and two of a four-day observation period
- *Oil-based purgative* for the induction of labour by reflex uterine hyperactivity may be harmful, are often unsuccessful and are not recommended; to our experience a single dose of castor plant proved, at term, being quite often successful.

Induction by Surgical Means

According to Al-Zirqi (2010) "induction should be discouraged in mothers with previous caesarean section, as it carried the highest risk, and most catastrophic consequences, of uterine rupture for both mother and neonate. If needed, mechanical induction should be used instead of medical induction by prostaglandins".

Michael Marsh, BJOG deputy editor-in-chief, said: "women should be aware that although trial of labour was associated with greater risk of uterine rupture, as compared to arranged repeat caesarean section, the *absolute risk of uterine rupture is low*; the study does, however, caution against the use of medical induction of labour for women with previous caesarean section.

Possible alternatives to medical induction are as follows:

- *Foley balloon in the cervical canal*: The procedure is as follows: A N° 16 Foley balloon catheter is introduced into the uterine cavity, not into the cervical canal, and filled with 30 ml of saline. The end of the catheter is attached to

the thigh with tape and the gravid patient is encouraged to walk. Downward traction is exerted with each step on the internal os of the uterus and thereby a stimulation (Ben- Aroya et al., 2002; Jozwiak M. et al., 2014)
- *Sweeping or stripping of the lower pole of the membranes*: Not recommended
- *Amniotomy or disruption of the membraners*: With great circumspection; not recommended.

Progress of Labour is to be Monitored Carefully

Anomalies and arrests of labour occur frequently during both spontaneous and induced labour.
- *Augmentation of labour with oxytocin*: According to Zelop (2000), the percentage of uterine ruptures in gravid patients with previous C-section is 2% compared to 0.7% observed among patients without uterine scars; Blanchette et al. (2001) found similar results (1.4% against 0.34%)
- *Monitoring foetal well-being during labour*: Variations in foetal heart rate accompany and precede clinical manifestations of uterine rupture. Early identification of such variations therefore allows the necessary provisions to be put in place for accomplishment of the delivery. Decelerations of any kind and bradycardia should be treated as suspicious; tachycardia has never been observed.

According to Meniham (1998), decelerations: Variable (73%), late (36%) and early (27%) preceded bradycardia (82%), which presages and accompanies impending rupture and rupture of the uterus.

According to Ayres et al. (2001) late decelerations, present in 88% of cases, precede terminal bradycardia (50%).

According to Leung et al. (1993), prolonged decelerations following on from late decelerations characterize the contractions that precede uterine rupture; here by prolonged deceleration is meant foetal heart rates below 90 beats/minute extending over a minute without returning to baseline rate.

Prolonged decelerations are a constant observation with expulsion of foetus into the abdominal cavity.
- *Foetal outcomes following uterine rupture*: Compromise of a foetus involves a constant timeline; prompt resuscitation does not manage to prevent severe acidosis and foetal death; even when this does not occur, long-term outcomes are not favourable.

Bujold (2000) compared foetal outcomes in relation to the time elapsed between rupture of the uterus, umbilical cord prolapse and completion of the delivery (laparotomy); mean time for uterine rupture was 18 minutes compared to 17 for cord prolapse. At the moment of birth, pH values of <7.1 were present in 47% of uterine ruptures against 3% of cord prolapses; at 5 minutes an Apgar score of <6 was present in 33% of the first group against 3% in the second; at six months hypoxic-ischemic encephalopathy was present in 20% of the first group against 0% (zero) of the second. Data from Leung (1993) highlight how foetal asphyxia is already present in a foetus extracted within 10 minutes of uterine rupture when late decelerations precede the prolonged decelerations during those very contractions that result in rupture of the uterus.

BIBLIOGRAPHY

1. Alfirevic Z. Induction of labour with previous caesarean delivery: where do we stand? Curr Opin Obstet Gynecol. 2006;18:636.
2. Al-Zirqi I, Stray-Pedersen B, Forsén L, Vangen S. Uterine rupture after previous caesarean section. BJOG. 2010;CD 0528.
3. American College of Obstetricians and Gynaecologists. Vaginal birth after previous caesarean delivery. Practice Bulletin No. Washington (DC): ACOG, 1999.
4. American College of Obstetricians and Gynaecologists. Induction of labour for vaginal birth after caesarean delivery. ACOG Committee Opinion 271. Obstet Gynecol. 2002;99:679-80.
5. American College of Obstetrics and Gynecology Committee on Practice Bulletins-Obstetrics. ACOG Practice Bulletin Number 49, December 2003: Dystocia and augmentation of labor. Obstet Gynecol. 2003;102:1445.
6. Asakura H, Myers SA. More than one previous caesarean delivery: A 5-year experience with 435 patients. Obstet Gynecol. 1995;85:924-9.
7. Ayres AW, Johnson TRB, Hayashi R. Characteristics of foetal heart rate tracings prior to uterine rupture. Int J Gynaecol Obstet. 2001;74:235-40.
8. Ben-Aroya Z, Hallak M, Segal D, et al. Ripening of the uterine cervix in a post-cesarean parturient: prostaglandin E2 versus Foley catheter. J Matern Fetal Neonatal Med. 2002;12:42.
9. Bennett BB. Uterine rupture during induction of labour at term with intravaginal misoprostol. Obstet Gynecol. 1997;89:832-3.
10. Blanchette H, Blanchette M, McCabe J, Vincent S. Is vaginal birth after caesarean safe? Experience at a community hospital. Am J Obstet Gynecol. 2001;184(7):1478-84; discussion 1484-7.
11. Blanchette HA, Nayak S, Erasmus S. Comparison of the safety and efficacy of intravaginal misoprostol (prostaglandin E1) with those of dinoprostone for cervical ripening and induction of labor in a community hospital. Am J Ob Gyn. 1999;180:1551-9.
12. Bujold E, Gauthier RJ. Comparative study of neonatal morbidity associated with uterine rupture during VBAC versus cord prolapse. Am J Obstet Gynecol. 2000;182:S160.
13. Bujold E, Bujold C, Hamilton EF, Harel F, Gauthier RJ. The impact of a single-layer or double-layer closure on uterine rupture. Am J Obstet Gynecol. 2002;186:1326-30.
14. Bujold E, Mehta SH, Bujold C, Gauthier RJ. Interdelivery interval and uterine rupture. Am J Obstet Gynecol. 2002;187:1199-202.

15. Caughey AB, Shipp TD, Repke JT, Zelop CM, Cohen A, Lieberman E. Rate of uterine rupture during a trial of labour in women with one or two prior caesarean deliveries. Am J Obstet Gynecol. 1999;181:872-6.
16. Chapman SJ, Owen J, Hauth JC. One-versus two-layer closure of a low transverse caesarean: The next pregnancy. Obstet Gynecol. 1997;89:16-8.
17. Cunha M, Bugalho A, Bique C, Bergstrom S. Induction of labour by vaginal misoprostol in patients with previous caesarean delivery. Acta Obstet Gynecol Scand. 1999;78:653-4.
18. Dodd JM, 2004; Crowther CA, Huertas E, Guise JM, Horey D. Planned elective repeat caesarean section versus planned vaginal birth for women with a previous caesarean birth. The Cochrane Database of Systematic Reviews 2004, Issue 4. Art. No. CD004224.
19. Dodd JM, Crowther CA, Huertas E, Guise JM, Horey D. Planned elective repeat caesarean section versus planned vaginal birth for women with a previous caesarean birth. The Cochrane Database of Systematic Reviews 2004, Issue 4. Art. No. CD004224.
20. Ferrari AG, Frigerio LG, Candotti G, Buscaglia M, Petrone M, Taglioretti A, et al. Can Joel-Cohen incision and single layer reconstruction reduce caesarean section morbidity? Int J Gynaecol Obstet. 2001;72:135-43.
21. Flamm BL, Newman LA, Thomas ST, Fallon D, Yoshida MM. Vaginal birth after cesarean delivery: Results of a 5-year multicenter collaborative study. Obstet Gynecol. 1990;76:750-4.
22. Flamm BL, Goings JR, Liu Y, Wolde-Tsadik G. Elective repeat cesarean delivery versus trial of labor: A prospective multicenter study. Obstet Gynecol. 1994;83:927-32.
23. Gherman RB, McBrayer S, Browning J. Uterine rupture associated with vaginal birth after cesarean section: A complication of intravaginal misoprostol? Gynecol Obstet Invest. 2000;50:212-3.
24. Hauth JC, Owen J, Davis RO. Transverse uterine closure: One versus two layers. Am J Obstet Gynecol. 1992;167(4 Pt 1):1108-11.
25. Hill DA, Chez RA, Quinlan J, Fuentes A, LaCombe J. Uterine rupture and dehiscence associated with intravaginal misoprostol cervical ripening. J Reprod Med. 2000;45:823-6.
26. Hofmeyr GJ, Gulmezoglu AM. Vaginal misoprostol for cervical ripening and induction of labour (Cochrane Review). Cochrane Database Syst Rev. 2003;1:CD000941.
27. Huang WH, Nakashima DK, Rumney PJ, Keegan KA, Chan K. Interdelivery interval and the success of vaginal birth after caesarean delivery. Obstet Gynecol. 2002;99:41-4.
28. Jelsema RD, Wittingen JA, Vander Kolk KJ. Continuous, non-locking, single-layer repair of the low transverse uterine incision. J Reprod Med. 1993;38:393-6.
29. Jozwiak M, Dodd JM. Methods of term labour induction for women with a previous caesarean section. Cochrane Database Syst Rev. 2013;3:CD009792.
30. Jozwiak M, van de Lest HA, Burger NB, et al. Cervical ripening with Foley catheter for induction of labor after cesarean section: a cohort study. Acta Obstet Gynecol Scand. 2014;93:296.
31. Kayani SI, Alfirevic Z. Induction of labour with previous caesarean delivery: where do we stand? Curr Opin Obstet Gynecol. 2006;18:636.
32. Lelaidier C, Baton C, Nifla JL, Fernandez H, Bourget Ph, Frydman R. Mifepristone for labour induction after previous caesarean section. BJOG. 1994;101(6):501-3.
33. Leung AS, Leung EK, Paul RH. Uterine rupture after previous cesarean delivery: Maternal and fetal consequences. Am J Obstet Gynecol. 1993;169:945-50.
34. Lydon-Rochelle M, Holt VL, Easterling TR, Martin DP. Risk of uterine rupture during labour among women with prior cesarean delivery. N Engl J Med. 2001;345:3-8.
35. Martin JA, Hamilton BE, Ventura SJ, Menacker F, Park MM, Sutton PD. Births: Final data for 2001. National Vital Statistics Reports 2002;51(2):1-103.
36. McDonagh MS, Osterweil P, Guise JM. The benefits and risks of inducing labour in patients with prior caesarean delivery: a systematic review. BJOG. 2005;112:1007.
37. McMahon MJ, Luther ER, Bowes WA, Olshan AF. Comparison of a trial of labour with an elective second caesarean section. N Engl J Med. 1996;335:689-95.
38. Menihan CA. Uterine rupture in women attempting a vaginal birth following prior cesarean birth. J Perinatol. 1998;18:440-3.
39. Miller DA, Diaz FG, Paul RH. Vaginal birth after caesarean: A 10- year experience. Obstet Gynecol. 1994;84:255-8.
40. Mozurkewich EL, Hutton EK. Elective repeat cesarean delivery versus trial of labour: A meta-analysis of the literature from 1989-1999. Am J Obstet Gynecol. 2000;183:1187-97.
41. Naef RW, Ray MA, Chauhan SP, Roach H, Blake PG, Martin JN. Trial of labour after caesarean delivery with a lower-segment, vertical uterine incision: Is it safe? Am J Obstet Gynecol. 1995;172:1666-74.
42. Ohel G, Younis JS, Lang N, Levit A. Double-layer closure of uterine incision with visceral and parietal peritoneal closure: Are they obligatory steps of routine caesarean sections? J Matern Fetal Med. 1996;5:366-9.
43. Plaut MM, Schwartz ML, Lubarsky SL. Uterine rupture associated with the use of misoprostol in the gravid patient with a previous cesarean section. Am J Obstet Gynecol. 1999;180:1535-42.
44. Rageth JC, Juzi C, Grossenbacher H. Delivery after previous caesarean: A risk evaluation. Obstet Gynecol. 1999;93:332-7.
45. Ravasia DJ, Wood SL, Pollard JK. Uterine rupture during induced trial of labor among women with previous cesarean delivery. Am J Obstet Gynecol. 2000;183:1176.
46. Rosen MG, Dickinson JC, Westhoff CL. Vaginal birth after cesarean: A meta-analysis of morbidity and mortality. Obstet Gynecol. 1991;77:465-70.
47. Sciscione AC, Nguyen L, Manley JS, Shlossman PA, Colmorgen GHC. Uterine rupture during preinduction cervical ripening with misoprostol in a patient with a previous caesarean delivery. Aust NZ J Obstet Gynaecol. 1998;38:96-7.
48. Shipp TD, Zelop CM, Repke JT, Cohen A, Caughey AB, Lieberman E. Intrapartum uterine rupture and dehiscence in patients with prior lower uterine segment vertical and transverse incisions. Obstet Gynecol. 1999;94:735-40.

49. Shipp TD, Zelop CM, Repke JT, Cohen A, Lieberman E. Interdelivery interval and risk of symptomatic uterine rupture. Obstet Gynecol. 2001;97:175-7.
50. Shipp TD, Zelop C, Repke JT, Cohen A, Caughey AB, Lieberman E. The association of maternal age and symptomatic uterine rupture during a trial of labour after prior caesarean delivery. Obstet Gynecol 2002; 99: 585-8.
51. Shipp TD, Zelop C, Cohen A, Repke JT, Lieberman E. Post-cesarean delivery fever and uterine rupture in a subsequent trial of labor. Ob Gynecol. 2003;101:136-9.
52. SOGC (Canada) clinical practice guidelines. Guidelines for vaginal birth after previous caesarean birth. Int J Gynaecol Obstet. 2005;89(3):319-31.
53. Tucker JM, Hauth JC, Hodgkins P, Owen J, Winkler CL. Trial of labor after a one – or two – layer closure of a low transverse uterine incision. Am J Obstet Gynecol. 1993;168:545-6.
54. Zelop CM, Shipp TD, Repke JT, Cohen A, Caughey AB, Lieberman E. Uterine rupture during induced or augmented labor in gravid women with one prior cesarean delivery. Am J Obstet Gynecol. 1999;181:882-6.
55. Zelop CM, Shipp TD, Repke JT, Cohen A, Lieberman E. Effect of previous vaginal delivery on the risk of uterine rupture during subsequent trial of labor. Am J Obstet Gynecol. 2000;183:1184-6.
56. Wing DA, Lovett K, Paul RH. Disruption of prior uterine incision following misoprostol for labour induction in women with previous caesarean delivery. Obstet Gynecol. 1998; 91:828-30.

CHAPTER 11

Preparing for the Operation

Adequate preparation is just as important as—if not more important than—the operation itself.

PREOPERATIVE FASTING

For elective caesarean section the following preoperative fasting is considered necessary:
6 hours for solid food.
4 hours for milk, breastfeeding.
2 hours for liquids without added carbon dioxide or containing any solids.

INTRAVENOUS ACCESS

Obtaining venous access may sometimes be difficult, particularly in dehydrated patients; never allow anyone to undertake it who is not expert in venepuncture. If veins are hard to detect, allow the arm to hang over the side of the bed—this already impedes the return flow of venous blood and the veins will swell; after a minute, apply a tourniquet above the elbow (Fig. 11.1A), tightened to the point at which the peripheral pulse can be noted (Fig. 11.1B), alternatively, apply a pressure band and inflate it to a pressure of 30 mmHg. The function of the tourniquet or pressure band is to allow the inflow of arterial blood but to impede the outflow of venous blood.

Always begin venepuncture from the hand (Fig. 11.2), rising as required to the forearm (Fig. 11.3). Do not work in the opposite direction as this would render the lower veins unusable. Stabilise the needle or cannula with an adhesive plaster.

Access to two veins is useful and prudent. When it is difficult to access peripheral veins, consider access to the femoral vein, which is easier and safer than the jugular or subclavian veins.

Access to the femoral vein: An assistant carries out a light traction and abduction of the leg and, by exerting pressure on the knee, prevents it from flexing.

Having prepared the infusion and with the intravenous line, the operator takes up a position on the patient's right (the procedure is described for a right-handed operator) and, using the index, middle and ring fingers

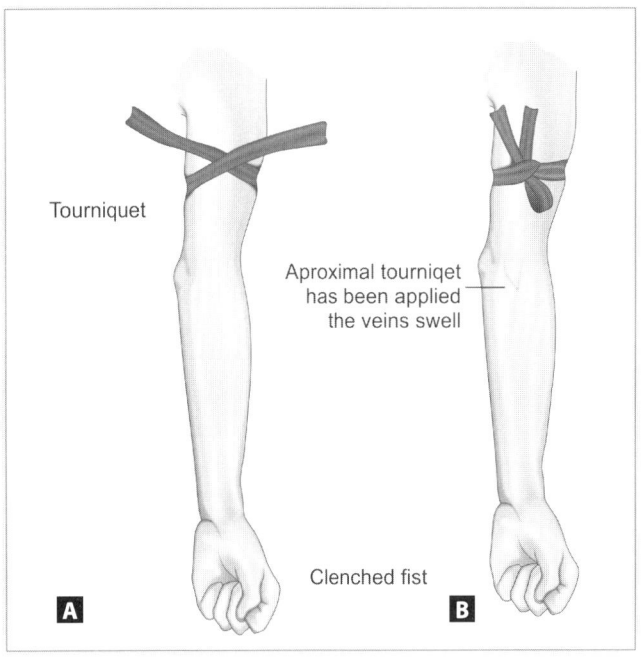

Fig. 11.1A and B: Correct application of the tourniquet

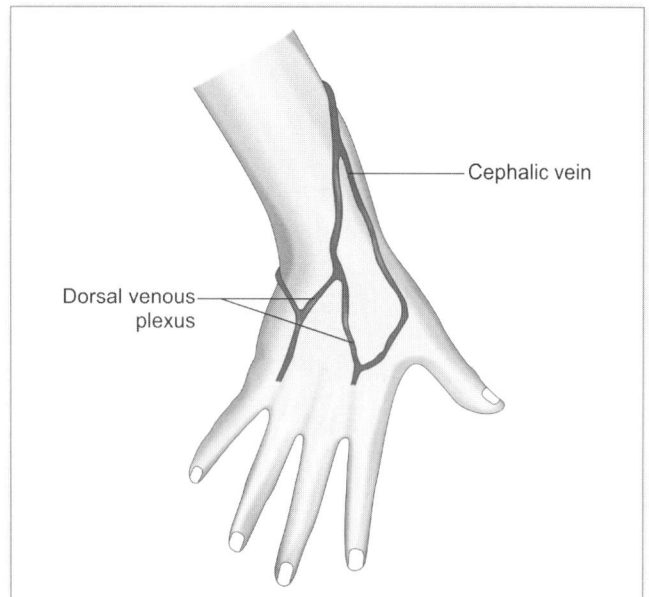

Fig. 11.2: Superficial veins of the hand dorsal venous plexus and cephalic vein

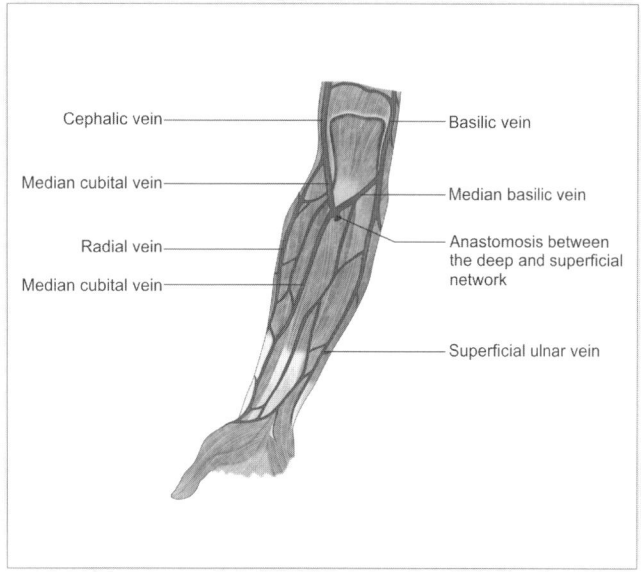

Fig. 11.3: Superficial veins of the forearm and of cubital fossa

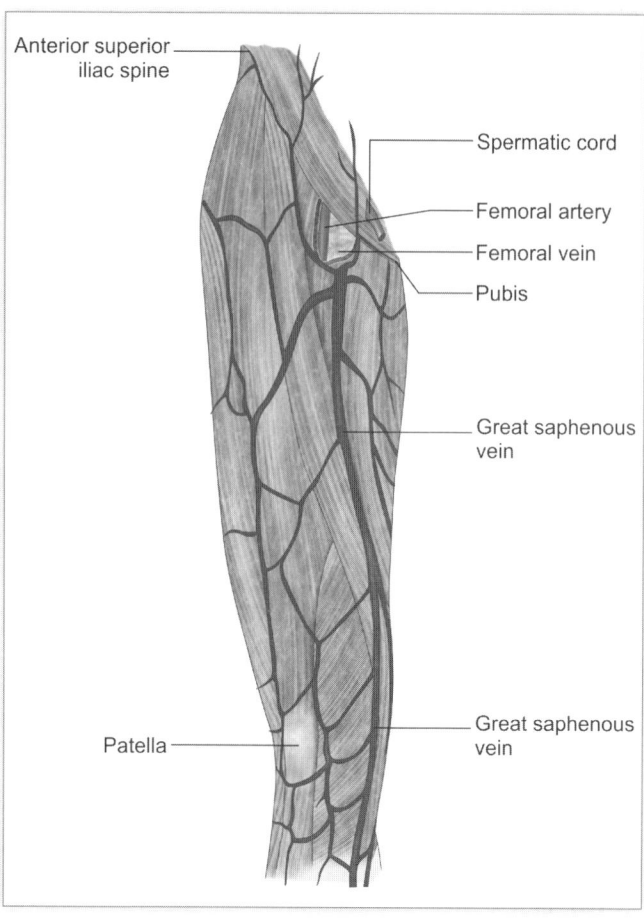

Fig. 11.4: Superficial veins of the thigh, anterior aspect

children) and containing 5 ml of isotonic saline; with the point of the needle held 1 centimetre distally to their own left index finger and 1–2 cm (depending on the patient's age) medially to it, the needle is inserted at an angle of 30° to the skin and to the course of the femoral artery; advancing slowly, the syringe is aspirated. An aspirate of dark blood will indicate access to the femoral vein. At this point the operator retracts the needle, connects the cannula to the intravenous line and opens the flow-regulator fully. Pressure of blood flow will push the vein walls apart and progression will be effortless.

VENOUS CUT DOWN

If the veins have collapsed and access to the femoral vein fails, use is made of surgical isolation (venous cutdown) of the great saphenous vein at the malleolus (Fig. 11.5).

The procedure is very simple: Allow the limb in which the vessel is to be isolated to hang over the side of the bed; apply a tourniquet at mid-thigh height and place the limb back onto the bed.

of the (preferably) left hand, palpates the femoral artery, identifying its course and, bearing in mind the mnemonic "NAVE" (nerve, artery, vein), (Fig. 11.4) will know that, by proceeding in a medial direction, the femoral vein is located medially to the artery, a finger's width (patient's finger) from it. This position is kept as a landmark.

In his/her right hand, the operator holds a syringe fitted with a peripheral venous catheter size G 14-16-18 (or 20 for

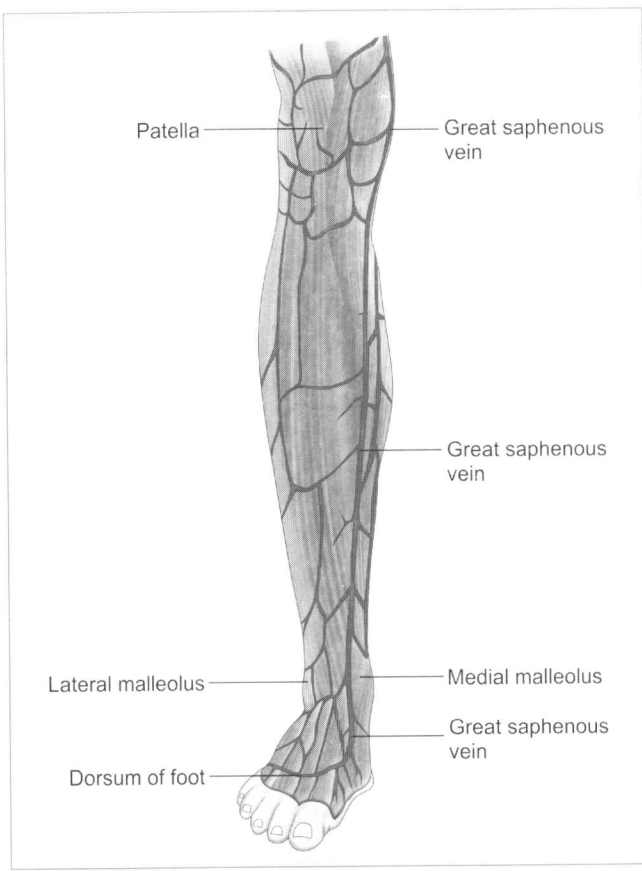

Fig. 11.5: Superficial veins of the leg, anterior aspect

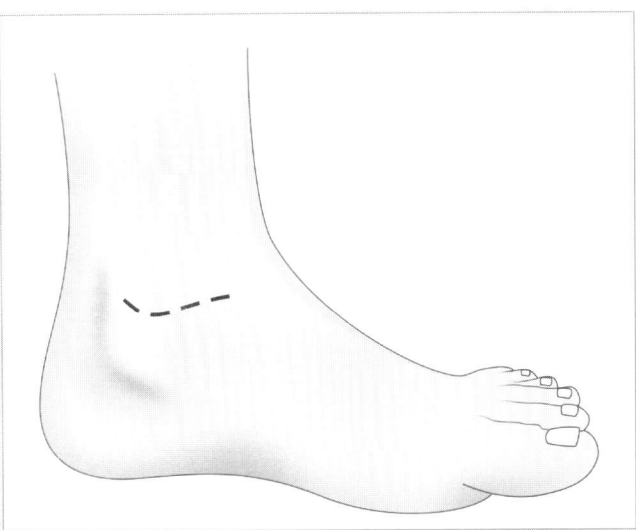

Fig. 11.6: Surgical preparation of the great saphenous vein; transverse incision 3 cm in width, performed two fingerbreadths (patient's finger) superior and anterior to the medial malleolus

MATERNAL INTENSIVE CARE

A patient in a normal state of health requires only 1500 ml of pre-operative hydration. A different approach is required for dehydrated patients in severe general condition, as with the majority of emergency C-sections in rural African hospitals.

Maternal intensive care, which should precede surgery, aims at improving the patient's general condition and maximizing her chances of survival. Time dedicated to intensive care is never wasted time; patients brought into the operating room in emergency conditions (excepting uterine rupture) and without adequate preparation react less well to operative stress, developing tissue hypoxia and organ malfunction.

Patients exhausted by intense pain and lack of sleep can be anxious, fearful, hard to manage, presenting a clinical picture generally described as "maternal stress".

This condition is characterised by water balance, acid base, electrolyte (hypernatremia) and caloric disorders and by infection of the birth canal.

Dehydration is always present, due to muscular activity without adequate intake of liquids. The skin is hot, dry, lacking tone; the lips are cracked; the tongue is dry; urine is highly concentrated and insufficient. When clinical signs of dehydration are present, water deficit will be around three litres.

A simple method for determining the degree of dehydration is the so-called *capillary refill* method: Squeeze a fingernail for five seconds and count the number of seconds it takes for the nail bed to return to its normal colour.

At the anatomical landmark of the great saphenous vein, "two (patient) fingerbreadths superior and anterior to the medial malleolus", make a transverse incision (Fig. 11.6) three centimetres in width. Identify the vein and isolate a length of it of two centimetres from the underlying fascia.

Two ligatures, one proximally and one distally, are inserted two cm apart (Fig.11.7A); the distal ligature (Fig. 11.7B) is tightened strongly, the proximal one loosely; applying traction to both (Fig. 11.7C) a V-shaped nick (to increase the surface area and facilitate the insertion of the intravenous catheter) is made on the surface of the vein. The intravenous catheter, already connected to the intravenous line and filled with solution (Fig. 11.7D), is inserted for a depth of 5-6 cm, the proximal ligature is now tightened strongly.

Use the sutures that close the incision to tie the cannula in place.

In the absence of an intravenous catheter, use the plastic tubing of a butterfly needle with the end cut on a bevel (Fig. 11.8).

Some authors suggest at this point the intravenous injection of a small quantity of local anaesthetic to reduce vasospasm following introduction of the catheter.

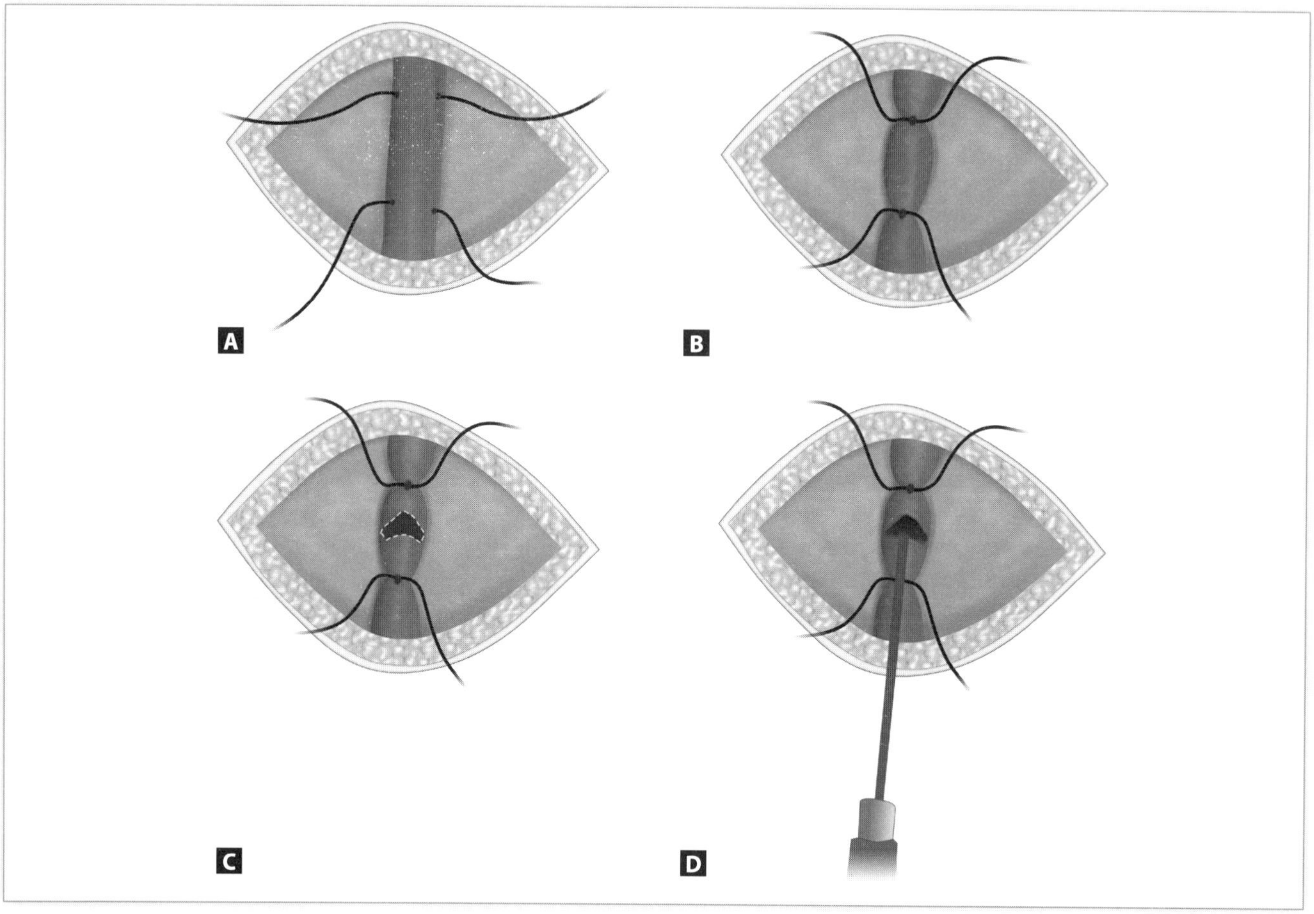

Fig. 11.7A to D: Having identified and isolated the vessel: (A) Two ligatures placed two centimetres apart are inserted under the vein; (B) The distal ligature is tightened; (C) The two ligatures are placed under traction and a V-shaped incision is made on the surface; (D) The cannula is inserted and the proximal ligature tightened

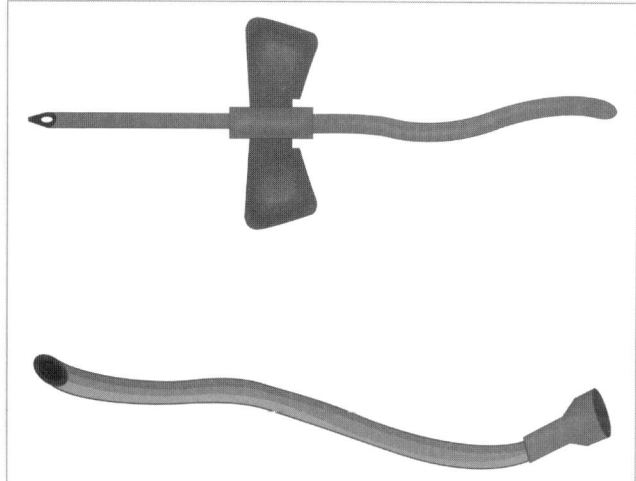

Fig. 11.8: Plastic tube of winged infusion needle with the distal end cut on a bevel

- If it takes less than 2 seconds, dehydration is slight and fluid loss is less than 5% of body-weight
- If between 3 and 4 seconds, dehydration is moderate
- If more than 5 seconds, fluid loss is 10% and the condition is severe (Table 11.1).

Metabolic acidosis is caused by the accumulation of lactic acid following uterine and muscular contraction, and by the presence of ketone bodies. Ketone bodies are an end-product of body fat metabolism, initiated to supply energy following insufficient caloric intake and glycogen depletion.

Clinical signs of ketoacidosis are a rapid heartbeat, rapid and deep breathing (respiratory alkalosis to compensate for the metabolic acidosis), fever, the presence of acetone in urine and dilatation of the colon as a consequence of the extracellular mobilisation of potassium. Dehydration exacerbates acidosis through the accumulation of anions in the body as a result of diuresis contraction.

Electrolyte imbalance: In order to rebalance the acidbase equilibrium, potassium is mobilised from the cells; this diminishes the contractile strength of smooth or involuntary muscle.

Fever: This is due to a break-down in the thermoregulatory function of sweating. It should be recalled, in this connection, that water has an extremely high specific heat capacity.

Table 11.1

Clinical manifestations of various degrees of dehydration

	Slight <5%	Moderate 5–10%	Severe 10%
Nervous system	Normal, restless	Confused	Lethargic, comatose
Mucosa	Moist	Dry	Chapped
Heart rate	Normal	Increased rate	Rapid
Capillary refill	<2 seconds	3–4 seconds	>5 seconds
Arterial pressure	Normal	Normal	Decreased
Respiratory rate	Normal	Normal	Increased rate
Diuresis	Normal	Decreased	Absent

The specific heat capacity of a substance is the number of calories needed to raise its temperature from 14.5°C to 15.5°C; this means that the number of calories lost through sweating is very high.

Infection of the birth canal: This is usually present when a prolonged labour has reached the stage of obstructed labour. It is not necessarily linked to vaginal examination but occurs spontaneously, in that the normal guest organisms of the vagina become pathogens and rupture of the membranes encourages ascending infections and amniotitis.

In advanced cases, the infection is supported by germs that create gases. Through palpation, one can feel emphysema of the uterus. If the foetus has been dead for sometime, the uterus may sometimes become tympanitic. Clinical signs are high fever, tachycardia and purulent, smelly vaginal secretion.

Terminal clinical signs are rapid hypotension, filiform pulse and a subnormal temperature.

Therapeutic Approach

Introductory remarks on physiology: Water is a fundamental constituent of the human body. It constitutes 65–60% of body mass in the adult female and 70–60% in the male. The water in our bodies is contained in two large compartments: The intracellular fluid compartment and the extracellular fluid compartment in a ratio of 2/3 and 1/3, respectively (Fig. 11.9).

For a woman weighing 65 kg, water represents 60% of body weight, amounting to approx. 36 litres distributed as follows: Intracellular compartment 2/3 of 60 = 36 litres; extracellular compartment 1/3 of 36 litres = 12 litres (Fig. 11.9).

The *intracellular compartment* constitutes that portion of fluid that hydrates the cells and partakes in metabolic processes; its composition in electrolytes, expressed in mEq, is represented in Table 11.2.

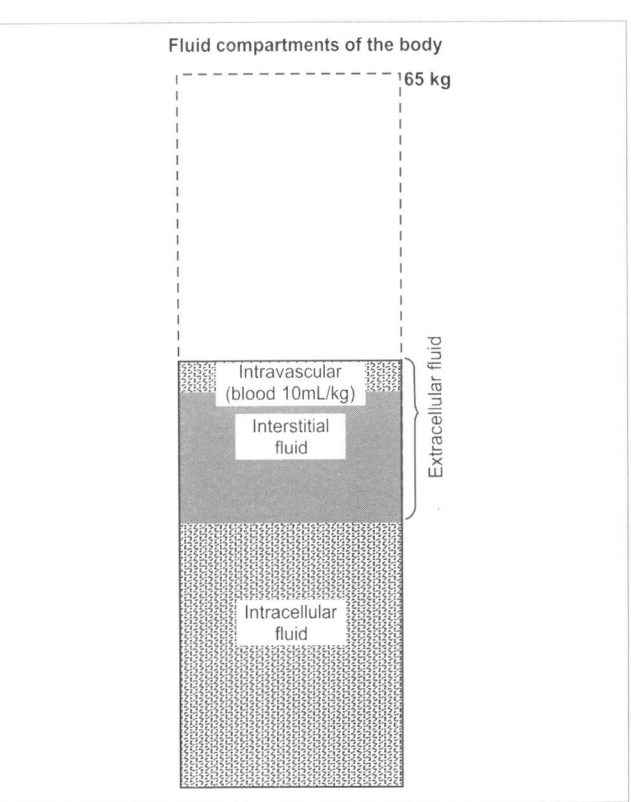

Fig. 11.9: Fluid compartments of the body

Table 11.2

Electrolyte composition of intracellular fluid

Na+	10	Cl–	2
K+	160	HCO3–	8
Mg++	35	HPO4–	140
		Proteins–	55

The *extracellular compartment*, containing 1/3 of the total fluid (12 l), comprises two sub-compartments: The interstitial compartment and the intravascular compartment in a ratio of ¾ and ¼, respectively. Thus, 9 litres (¾ of 12) are distributed in interstitial spaces and 3 litres (¼ of 12) in intravascular spaces.

The *interstitial compartment*, comprising the fluid film that bathe all of the cells, represents the intermediary between the intracellular compartment and intravascular space. Its amplitude bears a relation to the vast areas of cellular surfaces that require hydration and to the requirements of the consistency of the medium, which is achieved by subjecting the metabolites dissolved in it to super-abundant dilution so that they are not able to vary the composition of the medium in a metabolically significant way.

The composition of interstitial fluid, expressed in mEq, is set out in the Table 11.3.

The medium's consistency is also maintained by the continuous replacement of interstitial fluid. A crucial part in this process is played by the colloid osmotic pressure of plasma. If we recall from physiology that the hydrostatic pressure at the arteriolar end of the capillary is 30mmHg, while the interstitium is under a pressure of 20mmHg, we see how, within the vessels at the interstitium, a filtration mechanism is set up with fluid transition at 10mmHg.

Table 11.3
Electrolyte composition of interstitial fluid

Na+	145	Cl–	115
K+	4	HCO3–	30
Mg++	2	SO4–	2
Ca++	3	Organic acid ions–	5
		Proteins–	1

The transition of blood from the arteriolar to the venous end is characterised by two phenomena: A drop in hydrostatic pressure and a proportional increase in plasmatic proteins due to the escape of water at the arteriolar end. As a consequence of this increase the proteins develop an oncotic pressure of 25mmHg that will draw water back from the interstitium, whose hydrostatic pressure is at 15mmHg. The net result is the abstraction of an amount of fluid equalling the previous arteriolar outflow.

This fluid abstraction explains the following phenomena: Hypoproteinemic oedema, the fact that hypoproteinemia is associated with conditions of toxicity (due to failed replacement of interstitial fluid), and how the administration of protein in cases of hypoproteinemia is accompanied by hyperazotemia due, *not* to excessive catabolism but instead to the entry into circulation of nitrogenous residue compounds, present in great quantities in the interstitial fluid. The *intravascular space* comprises the water within the vascular bed and represents approx. ¼ of the extracellular compartment, therefore ¼ of 12 litres = 3 litres; its electrolyte composition is as follows (Table 11.4).

Table 11.4
Electrolyte composition of plasma

Na+	142	Cl–	103
K+	4	HCO3–	27
Mg++	3	SO4–	1
Ca++	5	Organic acid ions–	5
		Proteins–	16

Introduction to the Concept of Water Balance

Each day the body:
a. *Removes a certain quantity of water*, removal (water loss) occurs through:
   - The urinary tract—water elimination via the kidneys depend on water intake and on renal function. Where the latter is deficient, the amount of water per mOsm of substance removed increases; thus the water requirement increases just in order to remove catabolites
   - The non-renal pathway—extra-renal water loss is represented by:
   - Insensible water loss, amounting in an adult to 0.6 ml/kg/h. This has two components: Water vapour borne by exhaled air (approx. 400 ml in an adult), the exact amount is dependent on the one hand on the rate and depth of breathing and on the other on the temperature and dryness of inhaled air
   - Evaporation from the body's surface, which depends on body and environmental temperatures. Adolph et al. (1947) highlighted how in torrid climates this loss may total 5-6 litres/day
   - Faeces contain approx. 200 ml/day.
b. *Receives a certain input of liquids (intake)*. When intake is:
   - *Less than losses*, we have water deficit or dehydration
   - *Equal to losses*, we have water balance, or homeostasis
   - *Greater than losses*, we have water surfeit or hyperhydration (Table 11.5).

Table 11.5
Water balance

Intake less than losses	Dehydration	Hypertonic Isotonic Hypotonic
Intake equal to losses	Water balance	
Intake more than losses	Hyperhydration	Hypertonic Isotonic Hypotonic

Water Deficit or Dehydration

This pathological picture establishes itself when water losses exceed intake. Sodium, the main extracellular cation, is responsible for the water's tonicity; it clearly follows that losses can take on three characteristics due to the effects of water tonicity:
a. Loss of water and sodium whereby water loss predominates—here the tonicity of the medium increases with an osmolality above 290 mOsm; thus *dehydration is hypertonic*—as when it occurs during prolonged labour.

b. Loss of water and sodium in an isotonic ratio—here osmolality is equal at 290 mOsm; *dehydration is isotonic*.
c. Loss of water and sodium whereby sodium loss predominates—here osmolality is below 290 mOsm; *dehydration is hypotonic*.

The reason why sodium, which contributes only 48% of plasma osmolality, is held to be responsible for the tonicity of the medium can be explained as follows: Normal performance of vital processes requires ionic equilibrium—the sum of cations has to equal that of anions. To maintain electroneutrality, therefore, with each sodium variation (cation) a similar change of the same value takes place in chlorine (anion). Between them, the two are responsible for 96% of osmolality and their interdependence is so close that it's just as practical to refer to sodium alone.

Hypertonic Dehydration

The only clinical case we shall illustrate here is that of prolonged labour. With loss of water, or loss of water and sodium where water loss predominates, the resulting hypertonicity of the intravascular compartment draws water from the interstitium, which, having in turn become hypertonic draws water from and dehydrates the intracellular compartment. For this reason, hypertonic dehydration is referred to as cellular, global or essential dehydration. In terms of amplitude, the intravascular compartment remains normal due to the compensatory mechanisms described above, while dehydration of the interstitial and intracellular compartments is expressed by a drop in pressure and an increase in heart rate.

Hypertonic dehydration always accompanies prolonged labour, and is maintained by muscular activity without an adequate intake of liquid. This condition is particularly dangerous with obese patients (there is a growing obesity crisis in Africa) as 1 kg of fat contains 100 ml of water, while 1 kg of muscle contains 720 ml.

The patient complains of thirst; the skin is hot, dry, lacking tone; the lips are cracked; the tongue is dry; urine is highly concentrated and insufficient.

Fever is caused by the breakdown of the thermoregulatory function of sweating.

When these clinical signs of dehydration are present, there will be a deficit of approx. three litres.

The imminent operation contraindicates oral administration of fluids. Due to the predominating loss of water during a prolonged labour (cephalopelvic disproportion, obstructed labour), dehydration is hypertonic; correction with isotonic saline would further increase the tonicity of the intravascular compartment to the detriment of the interstitial and intracellular compartments.

For this reason, rehydration should be effected using a glucose 5% solution, with the first litre infused very rapidly.

As glucose 5% solution provides a caloric intake of just 200 calories per litre, 50 ml of dextrose 50% is injected via the intravenous line every half hour, after which the infusion is continued at full rate in an attempt to reduce damage to the endothelium caused by the hypertonicity of the medium. Often, however, this tactic fails to prevent thrombophlebitis.

When vomiting and effusive sweating are present, (loss of chloride anions), following at least 1500 ml of glucose 5% solution, administration of Hartmann's solution is indicated. This is to be preferred to isotonic saline, which can cause acidosis, as shown by the increase in plasma lactate levels (Ramanthan, 1983).

The quantity and composition of the solutions to be administered are determined by the clinical criteria described above, or by using venous pressure as a guide.

Measurement of venous pressure—We distinguish between:

Central venous pressure (CVP), which represents pressure at the right atrium (Sabathie, 1967). This varies between 3 and 10cm H2O, therefore values above 10 cm H2O are a sign of venous hypertension. To determine CVP a central venous pressure set is used, containing all the necessary equipment in a sterile condition. As such sets and the skills required are not always available in rural African hospitals; a good approximation is obtained by measuring pressure at the femoral blood vessels. If a three-way tap is available, one line leads to the infusion, the other is connected to a simply constructed manometer and the third is connected to the needle.

It is very easy to construct a rudimentary manometer: On the stand for the normal infusion, place a second intravenous drip of isotonic saline, whose intravenous line is connected to one of the tap ports. The line is filled and allowed to flow. After a few minutes, close the clamp up close to the bag and tape the line to the stand. Then cut the line just below the cut-off tap. The column of liquid will flow up to the where its internal pressure equals that of the venous blood. Now you can take a reading of the column height using a ruler, thus obtaining venous pressure expressed in cm H2O.

Mean venous pressure (Scebat et al. 1965) at the basilica or cephalic vein at the elbow.

In general this measurement varies between 4 and 15 cm of water.
- If a three-way tap is available, proceed as above
- If a three-way tap is *not* available, proceed as follows: An intravenous drip is connected to one arm (basilica or cephalic vein), which runs normally. Access the basilica or cephalic vein on the other arm. Using a large caliber peripheral venous catheter; connect to an intravenous drip of isotonic saline. Allow this to run, close the clamp and proceed as described above.

Peripheral venous pressure, measured at the peripheral veins in hands and feet, is of moderate clinical importance only.

Pre-operative hydration of the non-dehydrated patient: As explained above, Hartmann's solution (when available) is to be preferred to isotonic saline and 1500 ml should be administered.

Administration of Antibiotics

Antibiotic prophylaxis: There is a consolidated literature and a Cochrane review on the usefulness of antibiotic prophylaxis in C-section.
- Benzatylpenicillin (penicillin X) 4 mega I.V. or
- Ampicillin I.V. at a dosage of
- 1 gram, when the membranes are unbroken, or have been broken for less than six hours
- 2 grams, when the membranes have been broken for more than six hours.

Where labour has lasted over days or where the amniotic fluid is obviously infected, associate:
- Metronidazole 500 mg I.V.

Determination of Blood Group and of Haemoglobin

For postoperative checks, see Chapter 22.

BIBLIOGRAPHY

1. Domini E. Le basi della Terapia Infusionale. Verduci Ed. Scientifiche. Roma. 1990.
2. Laureng L, Gathala B. La pression veineuse centrale dans les etats de collapsus: ses limites. Atti della 44ª riunione della sac. It. Di Anestesia. Sez. Nord Italia, pag. 20, 1969.
3. Sabathie M. L'interet du controle de la pression veineuse en reanimation per et postoperatoire. Paris 1960.
4. Scebat ML, Acar J, Lenegre J, Slame R, Pequinot H. Quelle est le valeur de la mesure de la pression veneuse? Presse Medicale. 2013;73:1965.

CHAPTER 12

Anaesthesia

BASIC EQUIPMENT

- Door block, *anaesthesia data sheets* (Fig. 12.1) with pen attached (tied on). The chart records the patient's height and weight from which (Table 6.8) body surface area is derived as a guide for:
  - Administration of infusions
  - Correct dosage of medication.
- *Sphygmomanometer*
- *Stethoscope*
- *Self-inflating bag* (Ambu bag) *for adults* equipped with corrugated tubing for connection to oxygen concentrator or oxygen bottle
- *Self-inflating bag* (Ambu bag) for *paediatric* equipped with corrugated tubing for connection to oxygen concentrator or oxygen bottle
- *Guedel oropharyngeal airways* (various sizes)
- *Orotracheal tubes* of various sizes, furnished with:
  - connectors for Ambu bag
  - syringe for inflating pilot balloon on tube
  - pliers for blocking tube of pilot balloon
- *Tube introducer*
- *Laryngoscopes*, preferably two, with adequate supply of blades
- *Mucus suction catheter*
- *Nasogastric tube*
- Foot-operated or electric mucus suction pump
- *Pulse oximeter*
- *Oxygen*: dispensed by:
  - oxygen concentrator, a device capable of supplying medical oxygen from ambient air
  - oxygen bottle

BASIC MEDICATIONS

- Atropine: Commercially available package is of 1 mg/ml Dosage is 0.01–0.015 mg/kg body weight
  - Bupivacaine
  - Diazepam
  - Ephedrine
  - Ketamine (see section on the ketamine).
  - Lignocaine
  - Metoclopramide
  - Pethidine
  - Promethazine.

Preoperative fasting: (see previous Chapter).

PATIENT'S POSITION

For surgery, the operating table should meet the following requisites:

a. *Height:* A few centimetres below the surgeon's elbow, to allow adequate arm motion and smoothness of movement.

b. *Left lateral tilt of approx. 15°*: If the table will not allow this, a pillow or folded sheets should be placed below the patient's right buttock so that the uterus is pulled by gravity to lie on the left side. The reasoning behind this manoeuvre is to avoid *supine hypotensive syndrome* of the inferior vena cava or aortocaval compression syndrome that is to be observed in approx. 10% of parturients, characterized by marked maternal hypotension and fetal hypoxia (Holmes, 1960; Kerr, 1953).

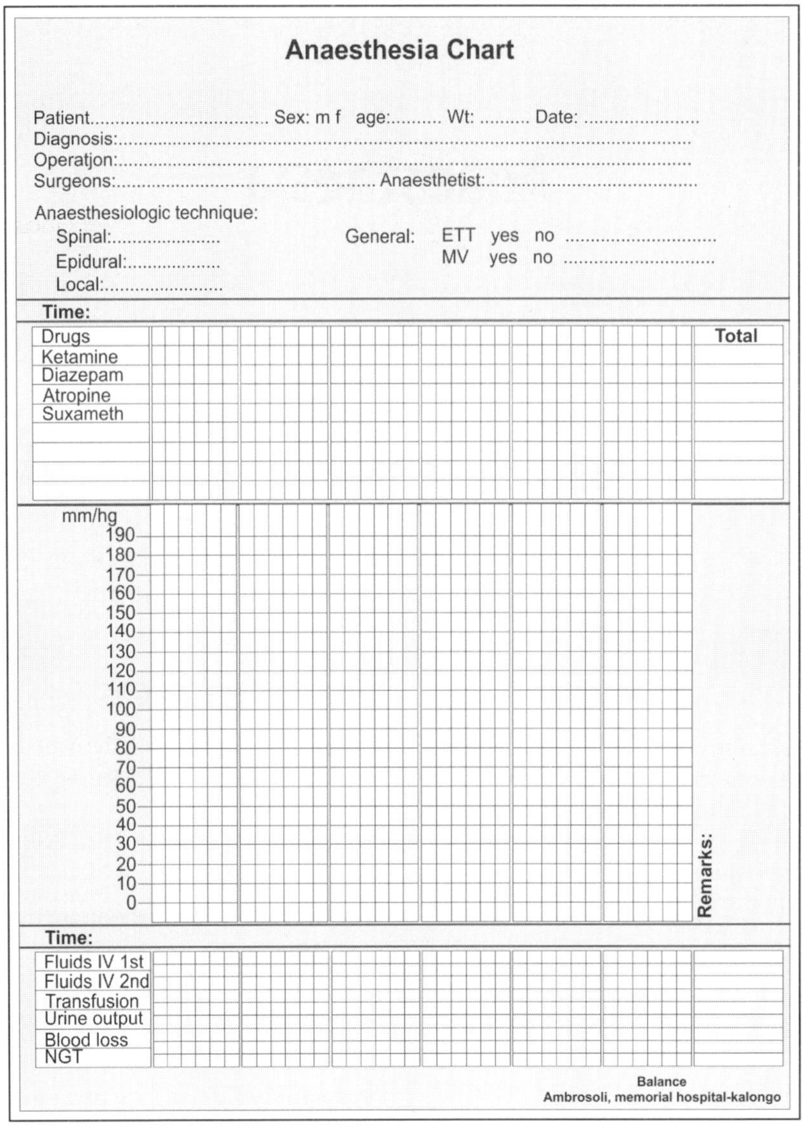

Anaesthesia Chart

Patient.................................... Sex: m f age:.......... Wt: .... Date: ....
Diagnosis:...
Operatjon:...
Surgeons:... Anaesthetist:..

Anaesthesiologic technique:
Spinal:...................... General: ETT yes no ....
Epidural:.................. MV yes no ....
Local:.......................

Time:

Drugs | Total
Ketamine
Diazepam
Atropine
Suxameth

mm/hg
190
180
170
160
150
140
130
120
110
100
90
80
70
60
50
40
30
20
10
0

Remarks:

Time:

Fluids IV 1st
Fluids IV 2nd
Transfusion
Urine output
Blood loss
NGT

Balance
Ambrosoli, memorial hospital-kalongo

Fig. 12.1: Anaesthesia data sheet

- *Pathogenesis of inferior vena cava syndrome*: In the supine position, the uterus exerts a compressive action on the inferior vena cava and on the aorta; venous pressure at the legs may reach 25 cm H_2O and the aortic calibre is reduced by 35–40%; cardiac output may be 20–30% lower in the supine patient than in the patient in a left lateral decubitus position.

The full-term parturient, when conscious, will automatically vary her bodily position to avoid compression of the aorta or of the vena cava by the gravid uterus. These adjustments do not occur in the anaesthetised patient, for which reason the uterus can exert a compressive action on these vessels, particularly on the vena cava, impeding venous return with a resulting reduction in cardiac output, a drop in arterial pressure, a reduction in uterine perfusion with a reduced supply of oxygen and various degrees of fatal compromise (reduction in fetal heart rate). Compensatory cardiovascular mechanisms include an increase in heart rate and vascular constriction of the peripheral vessels, but the latter is absent under general or spinal anaesthesia.

Without prompt intervention, death of the patient may soon follow.

Critical stages at which this syndrome can arise are:

- *On induction*: The patient is sweating, pale, dyspnoeic, restless, with a feeling of nausea and wanting to vomit; arterial pressure may still be normal; the heart rate is 140–160 bpm; overall symptomatology indicates that

the patient is compensating; induction would aggravate the symptoms.
- *In the course of the operation* and particularly when fundal pressure is applied to extract the foetus. The effects of pressure on the fundus upon extraction vary with their intensity and duration: From clinically insignificant effects on: cardiac output, systolic aortic flow time, heart rate and arterial pressure (Kim et al., 2002), to full-blown inferior vena cava syndrome and uterine rupture in an unscarred uterus (Pan et al., 2002).

A sudden drop in arterial pressure in the absence of haemorrhage indicates presence of the syndrome: prompt extraction of the foetus and exteriorisation of the uterus will remove the cause.

It may happen that inferior vena cava syndrome arises in conditions that permit neither leftward tilting of the operating table nor application of wedges (cushions or folded sheets) beneath the right gluteus region. An alternative (Kundra et al., 2007) is represented by leftward manual displacement of the uterine fundus from the midline by at least four centimetres by exerting energetic pressure on the right upper border of the uterus.

When performed routinely during spinal anaesthesia, this displacement appears more effective than left lateral decubitus position in preventing hypotension, which falls from 40% incidence to 4% and a mean fall in systolic blood pressure of just 20 mmHg compared to 29 mmHg for left lateral decubitus.

c. *A 10° downward tilt*: Anti-Trendelenburg position, for the following reasons:
   - *Avoids*, in the case of hyperbaric spinal anaesthesia, *upward diffusion of anaesthetic*, a frequent occurrence among parturients
   - The long axis of the uterus becomes straighter; the upper uterine segment is now at a higher level than the lower segment; the movement of retraction by the hand holding the fetal head becomes easier (Fig. 15.8) and the back of the hand no longer uses the lower edge of the lower uterine segment as a prop in extracting the head, a movement responsible for lacerating the lower uterine segment (a frequent beginner's error, explaining why C-sections performed by beginners are often bloodier than those by experts)
   - *Facilitates the flow of fluids*: (blood, amniotic fluid, washing liquids) into the paracolic gutters and the rectouterine pouch, enabling easier and more meticulous toilet of the abdominal cavity.

TYPES OF ANAESTHESIA

Maternal mortality during C. section attributable to anaesthesia-related causes (Hawkins, 1997) is 16.7 times higher under general than under local or regional anaesthesia. Risks to the mother under general anaesthesia are:

- *Intubation difficulties*: In approx. 5% of obstetric patients, incidence of failed intubation was 16 times higher than for non-gravid patients (Barnardo et. al 2000). It is useful here to assess Mallampati score.

Modified Mallampati score (Mallampati et al 1985):

Class 1: Soft palate, uvula, fauces, pillars visible

Class 2: Soft palate, uvula fauces, visible

Class 3: Soft palate, base of uvula visible

Class 4: Soft palate not visible.

- *Respiratory difficulty*: due to their reduced residual lung capacity and increased oxygen requirement (the foetus), parturients desaturate three times more quickly than non-pregnant women.
- *Inhalation of gastric contents.*

The most commonly employed anaesthesia techniques are:
a. *Conduction anaesthesia*: isobaric (subarachnoid) spinal anaesthesia potentiated hyperbaric (subarachnoid) spinal anaesthesia local anaesthesia
b. *General anaesthesia*: Ketamine
c. *Combined anaesthesia*: local + ketamine.

FUNDAMENTAL RULE

Before every anaesthesia intervention check:
- *Arterial pressure*: If, at the conclusion of preoperative hydration, the value for systolic pressure is below heart rate, do not use spinal anaesthesia; the risk of severe, pharmacologically incorrigible hypotension is very high. Ketamine is indicated here instead.

  Syst. press. 90, pulse 100: spinal anaesthesia is not indicated.

  Syst. press. 100, pulse 90, spinal anaesthesia is indicated.
- *Blood composition*: If the patient is anaemic (apart from the colour of the mucosa, capillary refill time is a useful indicator—if over 5 seconds, see previous Chapter), spinal anaesthesia is not indicated.

PREMEDICATION FOR ANAESTHESIA

Mandatory preanaesthesia steps:
1. Intravenous metoclopramide to prevent vomiting.
2. Preoperative hydration, indispensable in cases of spinal anaesthesia (see Chapter 6).
3. Premedication for anaesthesia: no type of anaesthesia can disregard premedication with diazepam (5–10 mg) and atropine (10–20 mg/kg), both in the same syringe, administered:
   - IM 3–15 minutes before elective C-section operations
   - IV on induction or anaesthesia in emergency C-sections.

MONITORING ANAESTHESIA

It is useful to have a pulse oximeter that enables assessment of oxygen saturation and heart rate; if unavailable, the assistant anaesthetist, while raising the chin with the fingers, can use the palm of the hand to evaluate frequency and depth of breathing.

A device often used in countries with limited resources is to attach a small cotton wad to the patient's nostril; frequency and magnitude of expansion of the cotton wad enable the anaesthetist to assess the patient's respiratory function.

SPINAL ANAESTHESIA (ISOBARIC SUBARACHNOID)

Spinal (subarachnoid) anaesthesia consists in injecting the anaesthetic directly into the subarachnoid space; the amount injected is 5–10 times inferior to the amount used in epidural anaesthesia. The most easily available anaesthetics are:

- *Lignocaine solution at 2%, without adrenaline, without dextrose:* Maximum dose is 3 mg/kg body weight; average dose for an adult is 200 mg. The drug is easily available and economically priced
- *Bupivacaine 0.5%*: Maximum dose is 2 mg/kg; it has a period of latency of approx. 15 minutes, but lasts longer—not a required characteristic in C-section. It costs four times as much as lignocaine; the drug is cited here for the sake of completeness.

Anaesthetic is *isobaric* when it has the same specific weight as cerebrospinal fluid; it is *hyperbaric* when its specific weight is greater. A hyperbaric form of the anaesthetic is obtained by suspending the drug in a 5% solution of dextrose.

The (subarachnoid) spinal anaesthesia described here uses *lignocaine at 2%, isobaric* (without dextrose), *without adrenaline.*

- *Indications*: Normal caesarean section for obstructed labour and in particular for preeclampsia and eclampsia, cases in which spinal anaesthesia is to be preferred to general as it induces vasodilation and, as *no hypertensive response to intubation is present*, there is no need to deal with a difficult intubation. In the presence of septic lesions at the site of anaesthesia, forego this technique; it should not be used due to a real danger of meningitis.
- *Advantages*: It is immediate; haematic levels of the drug in mother and foetus are one third of those for epidural anaesthesia (see above); better adaptation by the newborn to extrauterine life, as studied using the Early Neonatal Neurobehavioural score (see Chapter 26). At 15' scores for spinal and epidural anaesthesia are the same; after 2 hours more favourable for spinal and much higher than for general anaesthesia.
- *Disadvantages*: it is not always usable; a real risk of hypotension; it has short duration, from 60 to 90 minutes; the *postdural puncture headache* due to flow of cerebrospinal fluid, which may be avoided using finer needles.

- *Materials*: Place on a sterile cloth: A 2 ml syringe with normal local anaesthetic (0.5% lignocaine) connected to a winged needle, preferably large bore (for possible use also as an introducer); a second syringe containing 2 ml of 2% lignocaine or 2 ml of 0.5% bupivacaine and a spinal needle.

Method

The patient is seated with legs over the side of the bed, embracing a pillow, or is lying in left lateral decubitus position.

Disinfect the lumbar region with tincture of iodine; identify the injection site using as an anatomical landmark the line joining the two iliac crests, which cross the vertebral column in the interspace between L3 and L4, the usual site of infiltration.

The infiltration site is strictly the midline, where the thickness of the skin is much reduced.

To begin with infiltrate the skin and the subcutaneous tissue, overlaying the infiltration site, with a small amount of local anaesthetic then, with tip of the needle, scratch epidermis and dermis this to *preserve the honing of the anaesthesia needle*. As the ligamentum flavum is situated located at a at a depth of 2.5 cm, a simple method for gauging the depth is to connect the syringe filled with anaesthetic to a winged needle, preferably with a large bore, which having a length of 2.5 cm will facilitate assessment of the depth.

At this point:
- One can use the winged needle as an introducer:
- Pull out the winged needle; with the thumb, stretch the scratched area downwards and introduce the anaesthesia needle. The downward stretching of the skin enables a correct positioning of the needle.

Drawbacks

- *Hypotension*: Is a real risk and compels the monitoring of pressure and of heart rate every 2 minutes for the first 15 minutes. When present:
- Check the condition of the operating table,
  - Rapid hydration with one litre of crystalloid solution in 5 minutes
  - Administer oxygen
  - Ephedrine, at successive doses of 5 mg I.V., or 30 mg in 500 ml of dextrose
  - If ephedrine is not available, administer:
    » Adrenaline, one ampule (0.5 mg) diluted in 20 ml of isotonic saline, 1 ml at a time.
- *Upwards extension of the block,* when the mandatory, preliminary, condition *of 10° downwards tilt of the bed* is not met, the hyperbaric anaesthetic diffuses

upwards; when the block extends above the patient's umbilicus, her lower costal muscle will be paralysed and her respiration weakened, restlessness and breathing difficulties are observed.
- *Hypoxia*: Check; Respiratory assistance and, if necessary, intubate.

Local Anaesthesia (Combined)

Occasionally conditions arise in which no kind of anaesthesia (whether spinal or general) is available or practicable. Local anaesthesia is a simple and effective alternative (Mellor DJ, Bodenham, 1996) and, apparently, is better tolerated by parturients already in labour. It also has the advantage that bleeding is reduced, hypotension is not aggravated and it can, therefore, be usefully employed in 3rd semester haemorrhagic hypotension, in uterine rupture and eclampsia. A study recently conducted on eclamptic patients in Nigeria (Fyneface-Ogan S et. al, 2008) found in this technique a clear superiority in terms of maternal and fatal well-being: *"Local infiltrative anaesthesia appears to have a better maternal and perinatal outcome than general anaesthesia for eclamptic patients undergoing caesarean section".* Another great advantage of local anaesthesia is that the mother remains conscious, whereby the baby can be handed over as soon as it is extracted. Apart from occupying the mother, this serves to set up an immediate bond between mother and child. Among the contraindications we number: maternal obesity, intrauterine sepsis, non-collaborative patient.

With regard to premedication, there is disagreement among authors: some find premedication not indicated when there is a conflict between the well-being of the mother and that of the foetus. Given the rapid transition of the medication across the placental barrier, they recommend the administration of pethidine (50 mg) and promethazine (50 mg) directly into a vein or via intravenous drip following cutting of the umbilical cord, or as an alternative, an analgesic dose of ketamine (0.25 mg/kg). On the other hand, the mother may collaborate poorly and the foetus not be depressed. In this case, administration by direct intravenous infusion of pethidine and promethazine is indicated at the start of the operation as well as administration of diazepam 10 mg I.V., which, although it does transit the placental barrier, a single dose may be administered as it is unlikely to result in neonatal respiratory depression.

We proceed as follows:
- *Preoperative hydration*
- *Atropinisation*
- *Infiltration*: Using local anaesthetic
- *Lignocaine*: Easily available, it is economical and can be sterilised. Available in solutions of 1%, 1.5%, 2%, 4% and 10%, with or without adrenaline; the maximum adult dose is 3 mg/kg. For C-section, a 0.25% solution *with adrenaline* is used; the anaesthetic action lasts from 60 to 90 minutes.

Having a 2% solution available in 10ml ampules, by diluting the ampule in 70 ml of bi-distilled water or saline, we obtain a 0.250% solution. Approximately, one should not administer more than 100 ml.
- *Bupivacaine*: It is more expensive than lignocaine and has a longer duration of action, between 3 and 6 hours. The maximum adult dose is 2 mg/kg. For C-section, use it at a dilution of 0.25%. Adrenaline is not required. Do not administer more than 60 ml.

Method: The structures that generate pain when incised are the skin, the rectus sheath and the parietal peritoneum. The procedure consists in infiltrating, not the line of incision, but the areas situated on each side of it (Fig. 12.2). On both sides of the future site of incision, (2 cm out), on lines extending from the pubic symphysis to 5 cm above the umbilicus, using a 10 cm long needle which is held constantly parallel to the surface of the skin, a raised weal approx. 1 cm in height is produced with the local anaesthetic.

Let us recall that in the gravid patient at term, the abdominal wall is very thin and there is a high risk of perforating the peritoneum or the uterine wall; perforation is avoided only by meticulously holding the needle parallel to the skin surface (Fig. 12.3).

When anaesthesia is managed using local anaesthetics only, once the abdominal wall has been incised, it is

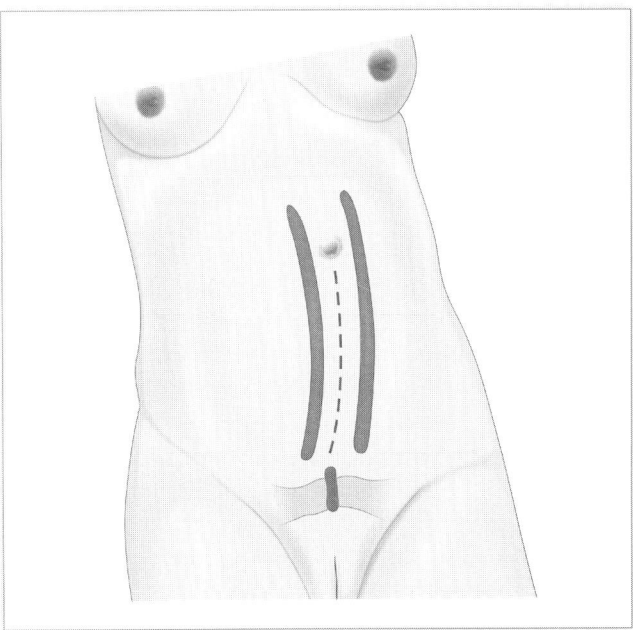

Fig. 12.2: Infiltration is not along the site of the laparotomy but on both sides of it at a distance of 1.5–2 cm. Infiltration is of the skin and the subcutaneous tissue and extends from the pubic symphysis up to 5 cm above the umbilicus, causing a raised weal approx. 1 cm high

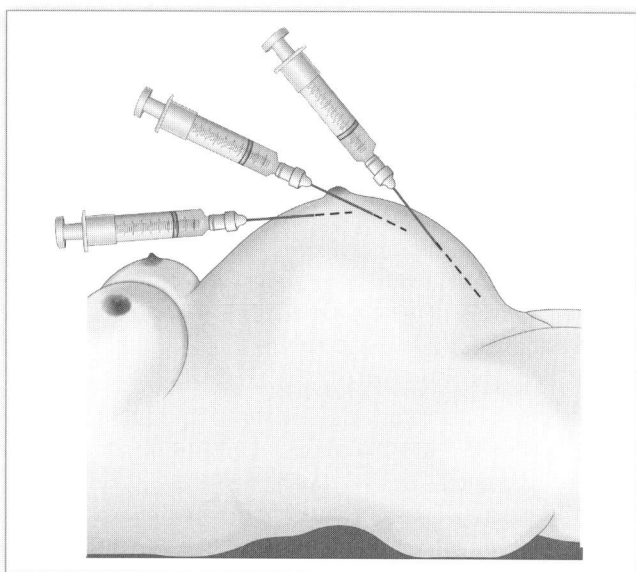

Fig. 12.3: The needle is held strictly parallel to the plane of the skin

advisable, when performing the hysterotomy, to infiltrate the visceral peritoneum (the operation will prove less painful). This time can be saved if the use of analgesics is planned; these can be:
- A reduced dose of ketamine (0.250 mg/kg) will enable extraction of the foetus, afterbirth and subsequent suturing of the uterus
- Pethidine (50 mg) and promethazine (50 mg); in cases of eclampsia pethidine (50 mg) and diazepam 5 mg.

GENERAL ANAESTHESIA

Ketamine

A derivate of phencyclidine, ketamine is an anaesthetic agent that has simultaneous analgesic, hypnotic and amnesic (short-term memory loss) effects. It induces a dissociative anaesthesia, a combination of deep analgesia and superficial sleep. Pharmacological product formats are of 10 mg/ml, 50 mg/ml and 100 mg/ml. storage is at room temperature.

Respiratory effects: When administered slowly, respiratory function remains unchanged and the pharyngeal and laryngeal reflexes (gagging and coughing) are maintained; salivary and tracheobronchial secretions are, however, increased and their inhalation is a real danger despite preservation of the protective reflexes. The bronchodilatory effects, due to direct action on airway smooth muscle or via an increase in catecholamine, make ketamine the anaesthetic of choice in asthmatic cases. Rapid administration may be followed by apnoea, which generally settles within a minute, but this may take longer when ketamine is administered simultaneously with other agents that induce respiratory depression, such as opioids. Its easy availability and lack of interference with respiratory function make ketamine the drug of choice in countries with limited resources, or where medical oxygen is hard or impossible to find.

Action on the circulatory system: Ketamine causes increases in arterial pressure and heart rate that are proportional to the dose administered. Maximum increment is generally reached within 2 minutes of administration; its effect on arterial pressure contraindicates the use of ketamine in preeclampsia or eclampsia. In elective caesarean sections, when administered at a dosage of 1 mg/kg, the increase in arterial pressure is not higher than a comparable dose of thiopentone. Ketamine has a myocardial depressant effect and is a vasodilator due to its direct action on the smooth muscle of blood vessels; haemodynamic stability is ensured by an increase in norepinephrine levels.

The property of bringing about a slight increase in heart rate and arterial pressure make it the drug of choice for third-trimester haemorrhages (abruption of a normally placed placenta, placenta previa) where vaginal accomplishment of the delivery is not advised.

Action on CNS: Hallucinations may occur, which may be reduced by administering benzodiazepine 0.15 mg/kg hour or 0.10 mg/kg intravenously.

Action on foetus: Ketamine passes rapidly through the placenta and within 1'37" of administration its concentration at the umbilical cord exceeds that in maternal blood; the peak is reached between 1'37" and 2'5" later. In practical terms, this means that *it is advisable to perform induction during preparation of the operating room*, thereby avoiding extraction of the foetus during the period of maximum ketamine concentration.

Analgesic effect: During postoperative recovery, where morphine is unavailable, ketamine may be administered at a dosage of 0.250 mg/kg, or I.V. by placing 50 mg of ketamine in a 500 ml intravenous drip, obtaining thereby a concentration of 0.1 mg/ml; the flow rate is 40–120 ml/h (13–40 drops per minute).

Conclusion: Ketamine is an anaesthetic of choice in countries with limited resources as it does not interfere with breathing, preserves the reflexes, does not require the administration of oxygen and its hypertensive action makes it ideal in cases of hypovolaemia.

Induction: This occurs at a dosage of 1–2 mg/kg body weight. If premedication has not been performed, ketamine is combined in the same syringe with one ampule of atropine, (1 mg with a vagolytic and antisialagogue action to reduce oral secretions). In order to avert apnoea, it is advisable to induce anaesthesia quite gradually, administering a third of the dose each minute.

At normal dosages, spontaneous respiration is not compromised, so when normal breathing activity is present, the administration of oxygen is not necessary.

Maintenance: occurs with fractioned doses of 0.5 mg/kg I.V., or by placing a 50 mg ampule in a 500 ml intravenous drip and regulating the flow according to the patient's degree of wakefulness; when breathing is spontaneous, the recommended dosage is 1 drop/kg/min (4 mg/kg/h).

If it is desirable to avoid the hypertensive effect of ketamine, oral premedication of clonidine (5 mg/kg) is administered. Clonidine is not recommended obstetrics.

BIBLIOGRAPHY

1. Bamigboye AA, Hofmeyr GJ. Local anaesthetic wound infiltration and abdominal nerves block during caesarean section for postoperative pain relief. Cochrane Database of Systematic Reviews. 2009; Issue 3. Art. No.: CD006954. DOI: 10.1002/14651858. CD006954. pub2.
2. Barnardo PD, Jemkins JG, Failed tracheal intubation in Obstetrics, a 6 year review in a UK region. Anaesthesia. 2000;55:685-94.
3. Dobson MB. Anaesthesia at the District Hospital. WHO Geneva 2000. Fyneface-Ogan S, Uzoigwe SA. Caesarean section outcome in eclam- ptic patients: a comparison of infiltration and general anaesthesia. West Afr J Med. 2008;27(4):250-4 (ISSN: 0189-160X).
4. Hahn MB, McQuillan PM, Sheplock GJ. Anestesia Loco Regionale. Mosby Doyma Italia; 1997.
5. Hawkins JL, Koonin LM, Palmer SK, Gibbs CP. Anesthesia related deaths during Obstetric Delivery in United States, 1979-1990. Anaesthesiology. 1997;86:277-84.
6. Holmes F. Incidence of supine hypotensive syndrome in late pregnancy. J Obst and Gynec Brit Comm. 1960;67,254.
7. Kerr MG, Scott DB, Samuel E. Studies of the inferior vena cava in late pregnancy. Obst and Gynec. 1953;1:371.
8. Kim TY, Ryu DH. The effect of fundal pressure at Caesarean section on maternal haemodynamics Anaesthesia. 2006;61(5):434-8.
9. King M. Primary Anaesthesia, Oxford Medical Pubbications, 1986. Kundra P, Khanna S, Ravishankar M. Manual displacement of uterus during caesarean section. Anaesth. 2007;62:460-5.
10. Mallampati SR, Gau SP, Gugino LD. A clinical sign to predict difficult intubation: a prospective study. Can Anaesth Soc J. 1985;32:429-34.
11. Mellor DJ, Bodenham A. Infiltration anaesthesia in the management of Caesarean section in a patient with a peripartum cardiomyopathy. Anaesthesia. 1966;51:409.
12. Pan HS, Huang LW, Hwang JL, Lee CY, Tsai YL, Cheng WC. Uterine rupture in an unscarred uterus after application of fundal pressure. A case report. J Reprod Med. 2002;47(12):1044-6.

CHAPTER 13

Laparotomies

REFRESHER OF SURGICAL ANATOMY OF THE ABDOMINAL WALL

Anterior Wall (Fig. 13.1)

Quadrilateral in shape, it is bordered superiorly by the xiphoid process and the costal arch, inferiorly by the pubic symphysis, and on each side by the lateral borders of the two rectus abdominis muscles.

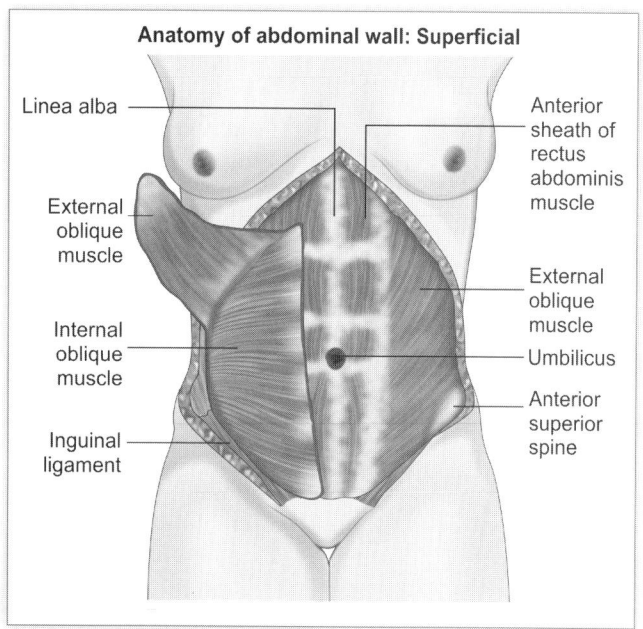

Fig. 13.1: Anterior abdominal wall (region), anterior aspect

Having incised the skin and the subcutaneous tissue, we find a muscular layer consisting of the rectus and pyramidalis muscles, enclosed by a whitish tendinous sheath.

The rectus muscles originate from the xiphoid process and the costal arches. Narrowing as they proceed caudally, they insert on the pubis. At intervals the rectus muscles are interrupted by three or four *tendinous inscriptions or intersections.* On the inferior portion, superficial to them and separated by a thin layer of connective tissue, are the triangular shaped *pyramidalis muscles* whose lower base inserts between the pubic symphysis and pubic tubercle. These muscles narrow cranially to insert on the linea alba at a point midway between symphysis and umbilicus.

The rectus and pyramidalis muscles are enclosed on each side by a fibrous sheath comprised of the aponeuroses of the three flat abdominal muscles, this sheath folds onto itself to form:

- *An anterior layer* comprising, above the umbilicus (Fig. 13.2), the aponeurosis of the external oblique and the anterior leaf of that of the internal oblique. Joining these below the umbilicus (Fig. 13.3) is the posterior leaf of the latter aponeurosis and that of the transversus abdominis
- *A posterior layer* comprising, *cranially to the umbilicus* (Fig. 13.2), the posterior leaf of the aponeurosis of the internal oblique muscle and the aponeurosis of the transversus abdominis, while caudally (Fig. 13.3), as the sheath of the internal oblique muscle does not fold, and to allow the superficial passage of the transversus abdominis aponeurosis the inferior part of the rectus muscles is separated from the underlying peritoneum by the *transversalis fascia* only. The latter originates from

LAPAROTOMIES

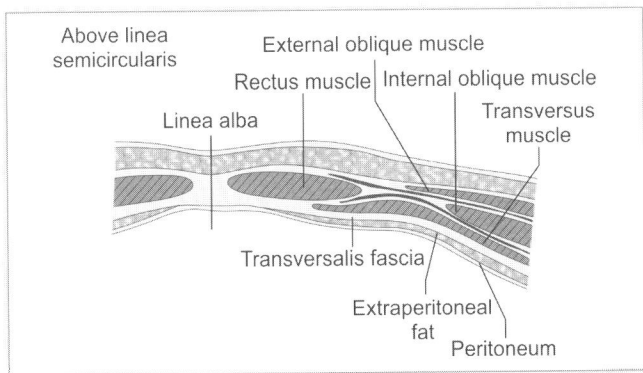

Fig. 13.2: Anterior abdominal wall (region), transverse section passing superiorly to the arcuate line, see text. The section includes both the muscle and the retromuscular layers

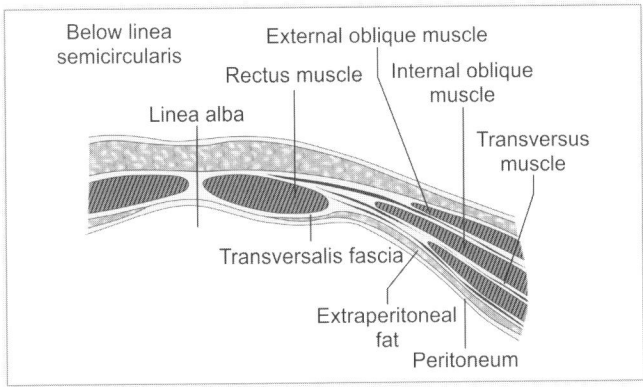

Fig. 13.3: Anterior abdominal wall (region), transverse section passing inferiorly to the arcuate line, see text. The section includes both the muscle and the retromuscular strata

the posterior leaf of the sheath enclosing the transversus abdominis.

The inferior border of the posterior leaf of the internal oblique aponeurosis follows a curved course: The semicircular or *arcuate line* (Fig. 13.4).

Having enclosed the rectus abdominis, the sheath joins up with its contralateral part on the midline to form a tendinous raphe, the *linea alba*.

Lateral Wall (Fig. 13.4)

The area comprised between the lateral border of the rectus muscles and the lateral border of the spinal muscles is divided into two regions: The larger, superior, is the *costo-iliac region*; inferior to it is the *inguino-abdominal region*. We shall describe the former only.

The costo-iliac region is limited anteriorly by the lateral border of the rectus muscle and posteriorly by the lateral border of the vertebral muscles; its superior limit is the costal arch and its inferior limit is a line passing from the anterior superior iliac spine to the lateral border of the rectus abdominis.

Deep to the superficial strata of skin and subcutaneous adipose tissue we find the first of the three flat abdominal muscles:

- The *external oblique muscle* originates from the lower seven or eight ribs and fans out anteriorly and inferomedially; its muscle fascicles terminate in a fibrous layer: The *aponeurosis of the external oblique*, quadrilateral in shape. Continuing in the direction of the fascicles, the aponeurosis inserts on the linea alba, pubis

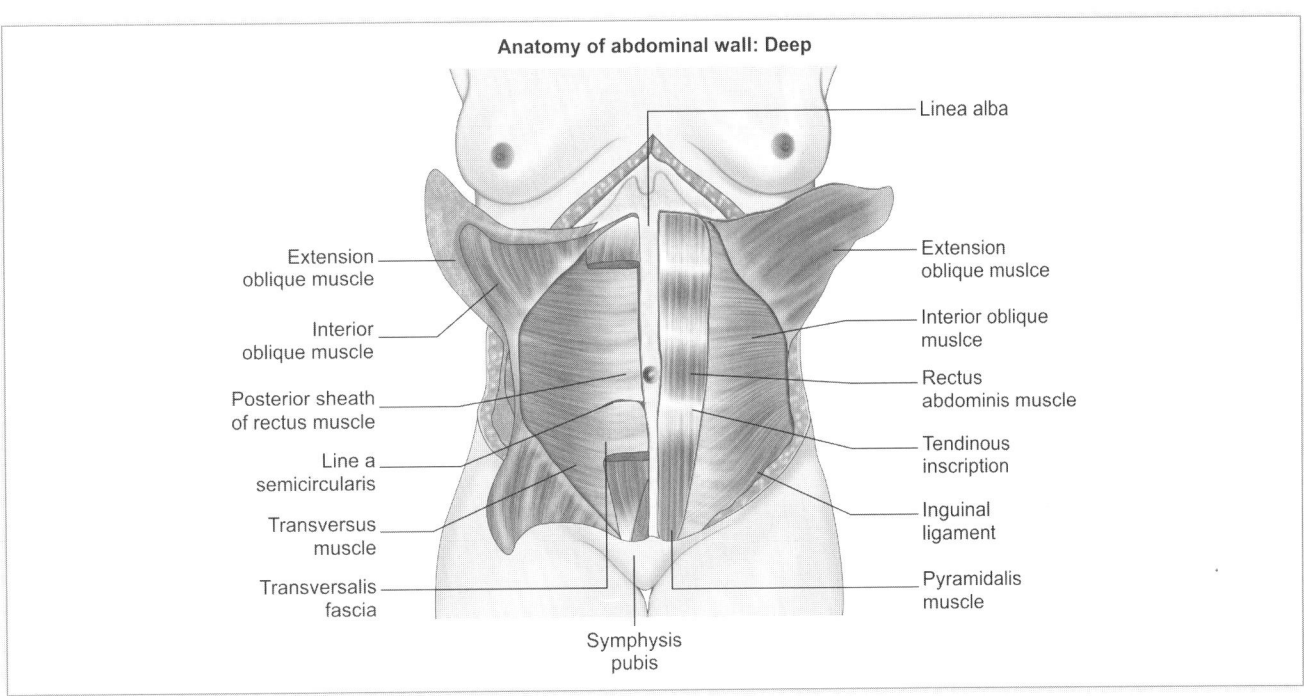

Fig. 13.4: Lateral abdominal wall (region), deep stratum. On right, section of rectus abdominis and of external oblique muscle. The arcuate line can be seen clearly

and inguinal ligament. Deep to the external oblique are:
- The *internal oblique muscle,* originates, via an aponeurosis, from the spinal processes of the lower two or three lumbar vertebrae, from the iliac crest and from the lateral third of the inguinal ligament, from where the fibres of its muscle fascicles follow a course perpendicular to those of the external oblique, terminating in a fibrous aponeurosis which, on joining the lateral border of the rectus muscle, splits into an anterior and a posterior leaf; this splitting is not present caudally to the umbilicus
- The *transversus abdominis,* deepest of the three flat muscles, originates from the costal cartilages of the lower six ribs, from the medial lip of the iliac crest and the lateral third of the inguinal ligament. The muscle fascicles converge into a broad aponeurosis: The *aponeurosis of the transversus abdominis.* As this approaches the linea alba, it crosses the rectus abdominis deeply in that muscle's superior two thirds and superficially in its inferior third. The inferior border of the posterior portion follows a curved course, with a caudal concavity: The *arcuate line* of the rectus sheath or *Douglas' fold.*

The three flat abdominal muscles are formed, then, of a fleshy part and a peripheral teninous part. They are in contact with each other, although divided by very fine fascia that are sometimes difficult to discern.

LAPAROTOMY

By the term laparotomy, we refer to the set of surgical procedures by which access is gained to the abdominal cavity.

In a caesarean section, the laparotomy has to facilitate execution of the hysterotomy and extraction of the foetus. As the type of hysterotomy varies in relation to clinical indications, uterine morphology and the degree of distension of the lower uterine segment, *it is therefore the hysterotomy that guides us towards the type of laparotomy.* Laparotomies may be either *vertical* or *transverse,* depending on the way this access is to be made.

Vertical Laparotomies

Vertical laparotomies (Fig. 13.5) can be midline or paramedian.
- *Midline laparotomies* (Fig. 13.6) are conducted along the linea alba and, according to their site and extension, are either subumbilical (Fig. 13.6A), supraumbilical (Fig. 13.6B) or xifo-pubic (Fig. 13.6 A+C+B)
- *Lateral laparotomies* (Fig. 13.5), conducted laterally to the linea alba, made longitudinally on the muscle, may be *paramedian, transrectal* or *pararectal,* along the lateral border of the rectus muscles. The most commonly used is an incision along the lateral border of the right rectus

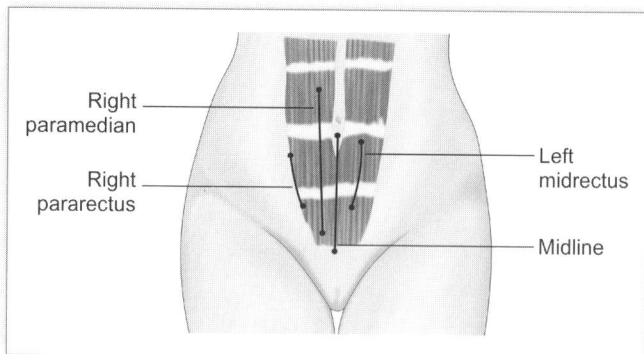

Fig. 13.5: Vertical laparotomy

abdominis according to Jalaguier. This is sometimes used in gynaecology but not in obstetrics.

In obstetrics, the *midline subumbilical laparotomy* (Fig. 13.6A), which extends along the midline from the pubis to the umbilicus is used. This is normally sufficient for obstetric requirements and offers the advantage of ease of execution, speed and, if greater investigation of the operative field is needed, it may be extended superiorly to the umbilicus. With *midline supra- and subumbilical laparotomy,* the incision contours the left side of the umbilicus to avoid cutting through the falciform ligament of the liver (Fig. 13.7). It is not aesthetically pleasing.

The incisions shown in Figure 13.8 represent incorrect laparotomy techniques for obstetric surgery.

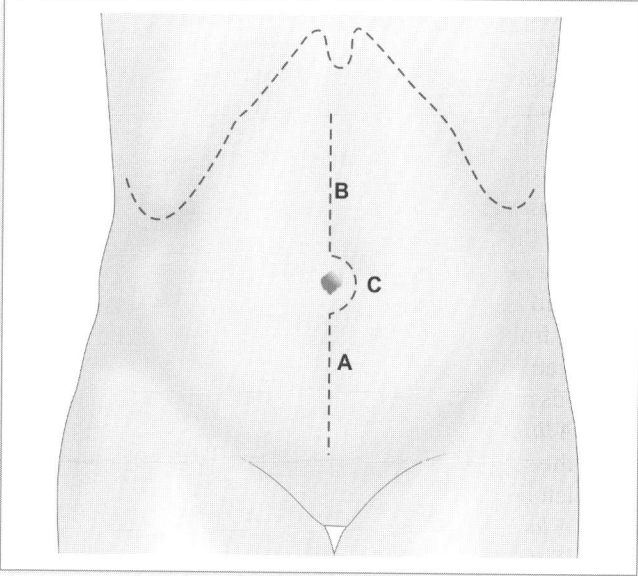

Fig. 13.6: Midline laparotomies, (A) Midline suprapubic-subumbilical; (B) Midline xifo-umbilical laparotomy; (ACB). Midline xifo-pubic laparotomy

LAPAROTOMIES

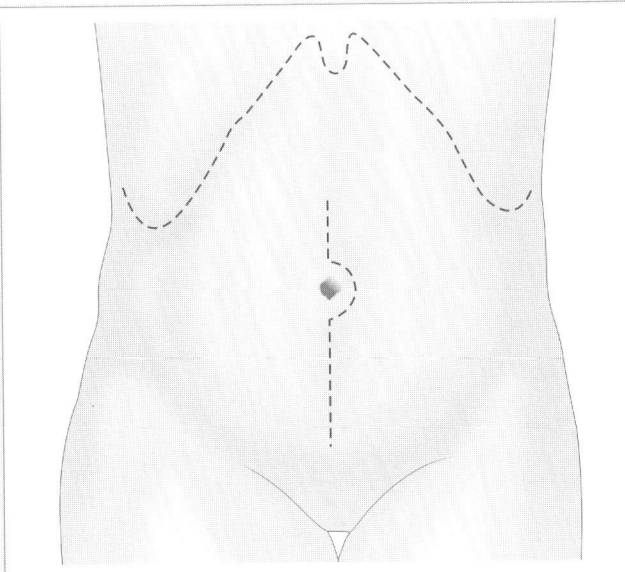

Fig. 13.7: A midline subumbilical laparotomy extended upwards by necessity, going around to the left of the umbilicus. The incision contours the umbilicus on the left to avoid damaging the falciform ligament

Midline Subumbilical Laparotomy

General Principles

The cutaneous incision (Fig. 13.6A) should proceed preferably in a cranial direction and stop at the inferior border of the umbilicus. There are two reasons for beginning the incision from below:
- The thickness of the abdominal wall gradually reduces as we move in a cranial direction. For this reason, beginning the incision from above makes it difficult to assess the precise thickness of the wall and incision of the underlying uterus is not infrequent
- *The distance between the umbilicus and pubic symphysis increases with advancing pregnancy*, going from 7 to 8 cm at the beginning of pregnancy to 14–15 cm at term. As the target is the lower uterine segment, the incision should be as inferior as possible and should therefore start from the mons pubis, extending—with the above precautions—in a cranial direction. Where the incision needs to be extended, this may be because:
  - *A little more space is required*: Leaving the skin intact, the superficial fascia may be incised, going around the left border of the umbilicus
  - *A lot more space is required*: A semicircular *incision* (Fig. 13.7) contouring on the left and at a distance of 1 cm the umbilicus is made on the skin and underlying tissues.

This incision will be facilitated as aesthetically more pleasing by putting, while incising, the area under tension with a forceps placed at 3 o'clock to the umbilicus.

Once the umbilicus is contoured, the incision is extended, as required, in a cranial direction, keeping strictly to the linea alba and caring not to incise the rectus muscles sheaths.

A full bladder, which it was not possible to catheterise
- A frequent occurence in obstructed labour—does not contraindicate a subumbilical laparotomy (see below).

Method

The forearm of the operating hand should always be parallel to the line of the incision; the scalpel is held like a violin bow and it is the index finger, which rests on the spine of the scalpel blade, that exerts and graduates pressure. The scalpel point is always directed towards the pubis (see also Fig. 13.8).

The incision is made with the belly of the blade, not with its point (especially in patients with little subcutaneous fat and when close to the umbilicus) In Figure 13.9 incorrect laparotomies are reproduced.

A right-handed surgeon stand on the left of the operating table and to stabilize the skin places the thumb and the index of his/her left hand on the mons pubis across the linea nigra (Fig. 13.10), stretches the skin downwards while with a coordinated movement, the scalpel proceeds in cranially (stopping close to the umbilicus). Make an incision through skin, subcutaneous layer and to the loose tissue over the linea alba; once reached clear from it the extraperitoneal fat with blunt dissection, securing the vessels if necessary, to a width of 2 cm on each side of the midline raphe. This manoeuvre is suggested in order to:
- Find the fascia more easily at the conclusion of the operation
- Avoid, at the closure of the fascia, inclusion of some adipose tissue which could jeopardise the quality of healing
- Allow, if the poor quality of the tissue so requires, use of a double-layered closure of the transversalis fascia, overlapping the edges: Imbrication (Figs 23.1 to 23.3).

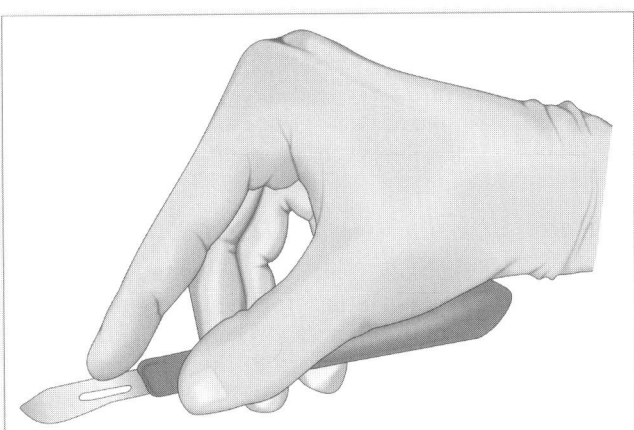

Fig. 13.8: Correct scalpel grip

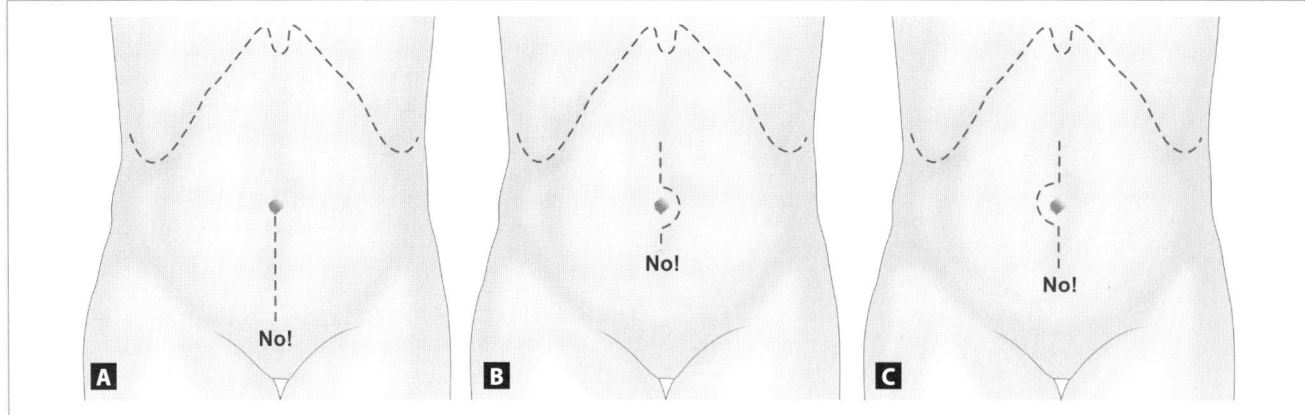

Fig. 13.9A to C: Incorrect laparotomies: From right to left (a) The incision does not begin at the mons pubis, making the available room poor; (B) The incision is too high and too short overall; the height will not allow sufficient exposure of the lower uterine segment; (C) The third incision is too high and goes around the umbilicus on the right

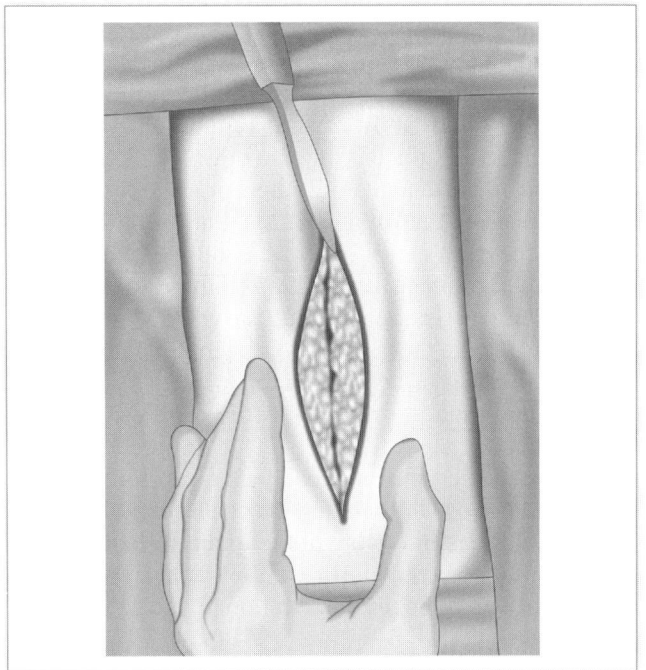

Fig. 13.10: Incision of skin and subcutaneous tissue, the (righthanded) operating surgeon stands on the left of the operating table. The incision starts from caudally, not cranially (at the umbilicus) where, due to thinness of the skin, there is a danger of damaging the underlying uterus

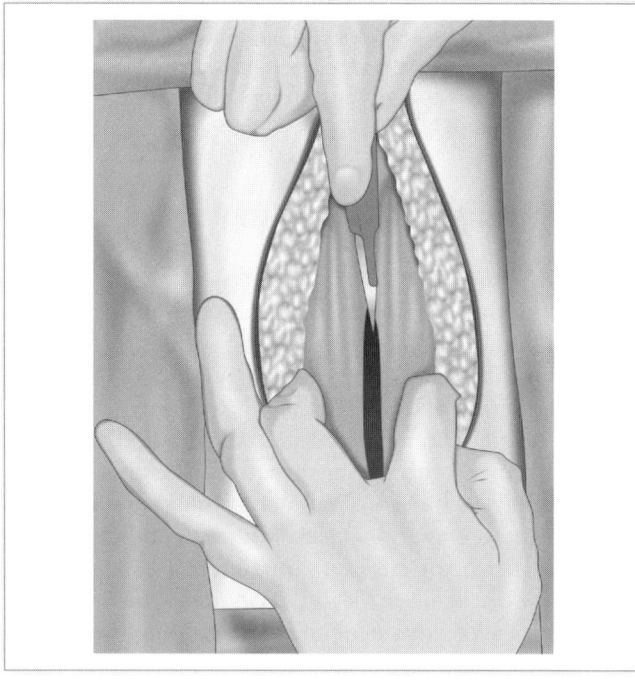

Fig. 13.11: Incision of the fascia along the linea alba. Extension, effected by sharp dissection, starts in the central part of the fascia

Incision of Superficial (Scarpa's) Fascia

a. *Incision of the linea alba:* Display the linea alba with its longitudinal line of decussating fibres and incise it directly in the midline for a short length (Fig. 13.11); the free borders are grasped with Kocher forceps, a Mayo scissors with curved blades and rounded tips is inserted, the tips pointing at the fascia undersurface; the scissors closed at their introduction, once inserted in order to detach the perimysium from the fascia, are opened, progression with tips closed.

The incision is extended down to the symphysis pubis (Fig. 13.12) and then upwards going just past the arcuate line. When the incision does not fall exactly on the midline raphe, but on one of the rectus sheaths, to identify which side of the midline raphe you are on, points of reference are as follow:
- The taught line between the umbilicus and the pubic symphysis
- The pyramidalis muscles
- The extraperitoneal fat and the peritoneum are exposed.

LAPAROTOMIES

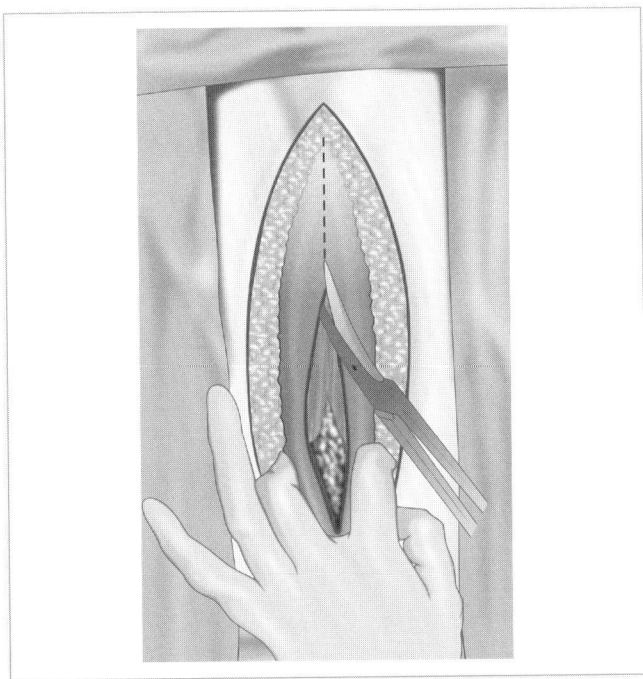

Fig. 13.12: Incision of the fascia is completed cranially and caudally using round-tipped scissors

b. *Incision laterally to the linea alba*: (seldom used) consists of incising the fascia for the required length on each side of and approx. 2 mm away from the linea alba, thereby obtaining a strip approx. 4 mm in width that is excised using scissors, thus exposing the medial borders of the two rectus muscles, whose separation is facilitated, as is their co-joining at the end of the operation. Separation of the muscles is lengthwise; (*the pyramidalis muscles are always left adhering to the fascia*).

Opening of the Transversalis Fascia and of the Peritoneum

The most frequent surgical accidents on opening are injuries to the bladder and to the gut. As preperitoneal adipose tissue does not allow sight of the underlying structures, it should be separated using the fingers until the transparent peritoneum is evident. As a general rule, opening should be performed as possible at the superior extent of exposure.

- *Prophylaxis of bladder damage*: With engagement of the presenting part, the bladder becomes an extrapelvic organ: The more urine it contains, the more space it occupies in the anterior abdominal wall. In cases of over distension of the LUS, where bladder catheterisation has been possible, a very simple means for locating the upper border of the bladder consists in pushing the balloon of a Foley urinary catheter upwards through the abdominal wall and identifying where it stops.

Should drainage using a soft catheter, while simultaneously pushing back the presenting part, had not proven possible, it is not advisable to persevere using more rigid catheters, due to the real danger of urethral damage. In this case the peritoneum should be opened high up. On where one should actually open the peritoneum and how far the incision should be extended, we have a series of anatomical landmarks which, if used correctly, will enable the surgeon to incise the peritoneum without fear. These landmarks are visible and tactile.

- *Visible landmarks*: The first tactic is, after separating the preperitoneal fat, to identify the uracus, which is a whitish cord originating from the bladder and joined just after its origin by two whitish forms: (Fig. 13.13) the *obliterated umbilical arteries*. Opening of the peritoneum is performed along the uracus, 4 cm from its origin on the

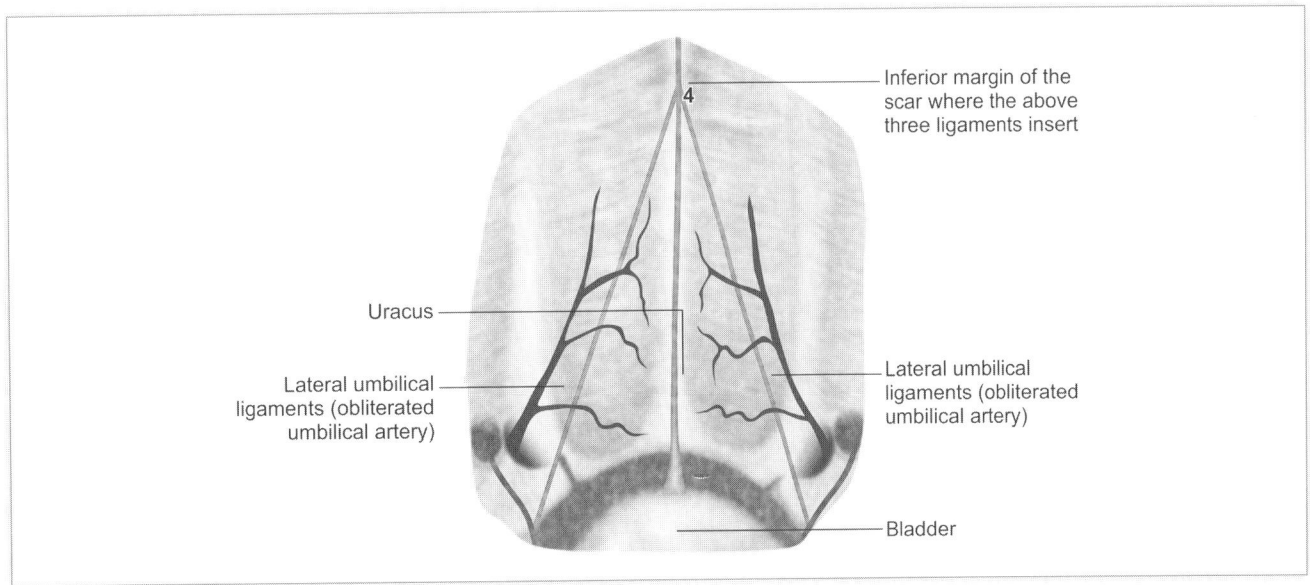

Fig. 13.13: Parietal peritoneum, posterior aspect

bladder According to some authors, as *uracus* serves a support action for the bladder, the two stumps should be reconnected at the end of operation. The correct manual procedure is as follows:

- Using two Volkman retractors, or using the three smallest fingers of the left hand, the operating surgeon and an assistant grasp the belly of the homolateral rectus abdominis (Figs 13.14 and 13.15) and simultaneously hook at the underlying peritoneum with their index fingers, stretching it in elevation. In this way, the peritoneum will raise in multiple transverse folds. Lift the peritoneum making it into a "tent" by holding it with forceps on either side of the midline. Squeeze the tent between the fingers and thumb To free any gut on the undersurface and make a small opening
- The opening may be made using scissors or scalpel; if we use scissors, we first apply pressure to one side of the fold only and check the other side for transparency and that no bladder or intestinal loop has been included
- Using a scalpel (Fig. 13.15), the incision should not be perpendicular but very oblique. The reason for this is, if there is damage to a small intestinal loop or to the bladder, the cut will not be vertical, but oblique, not too deep and easily repairable
- Having opened the peritoneum, the operating surgeon inserts two fingers into the cavity, ensures that there are no anatomical structures and, steadies the undersurface of the peritoneum with the index and middle finger and extends with scissors the

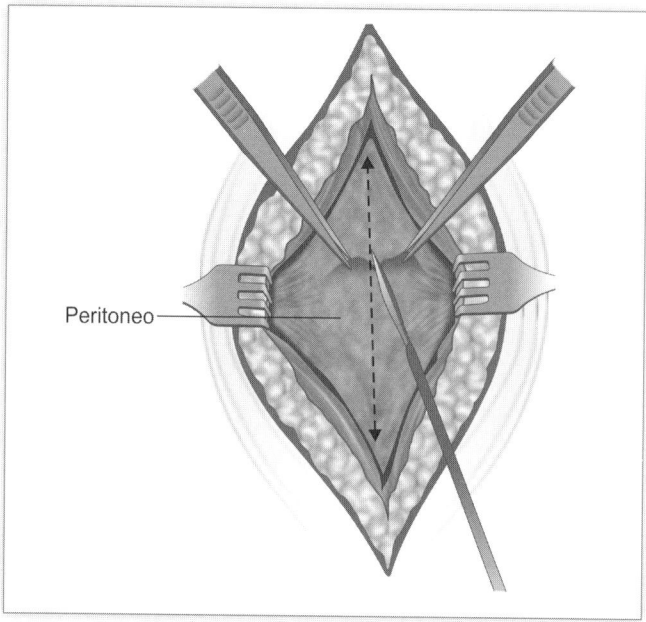

Fig. 13.15: Having identified the site of opening, a fold of peritoneum is elevated using two forceps, and cut in its central part; the line of cut is oblique

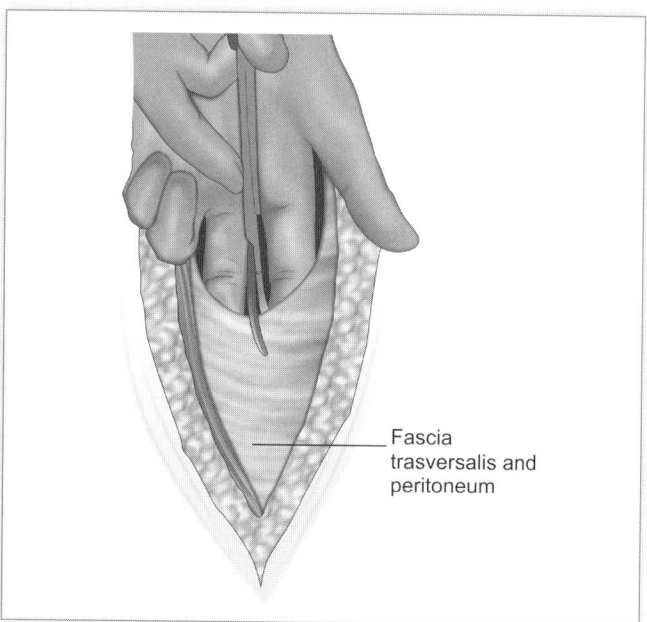

Fig. 13.16: Completing the celiotomy caudally

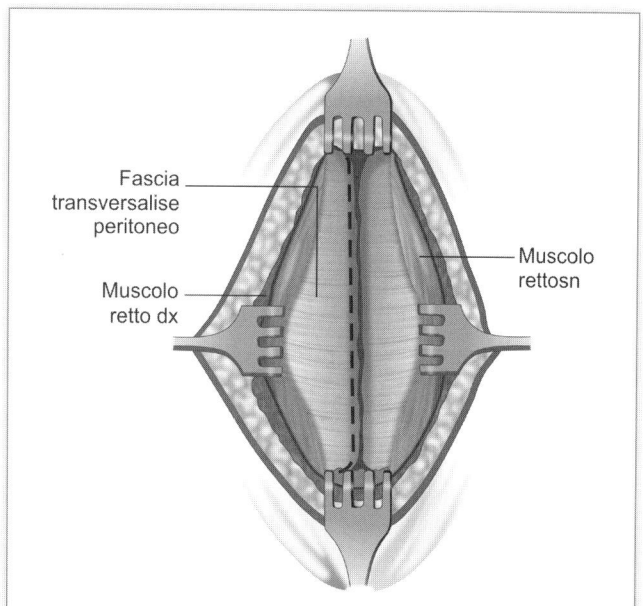

Fig. 13.14: The operating surgeon assistant retract the muscle bellies using Volkman retractors

peritoneal incision the full length of the wound, initially in a caudal direction (Fig. 13.16) and then in a cranial direction (Fig. 13.17) paying care that the scissors never overtake the fingertips. The following indications apply to how far the incision should extend caudally.

Transparency: With the peritoneum open, looking through the inferior strip of peritoneum, taking advantage of its

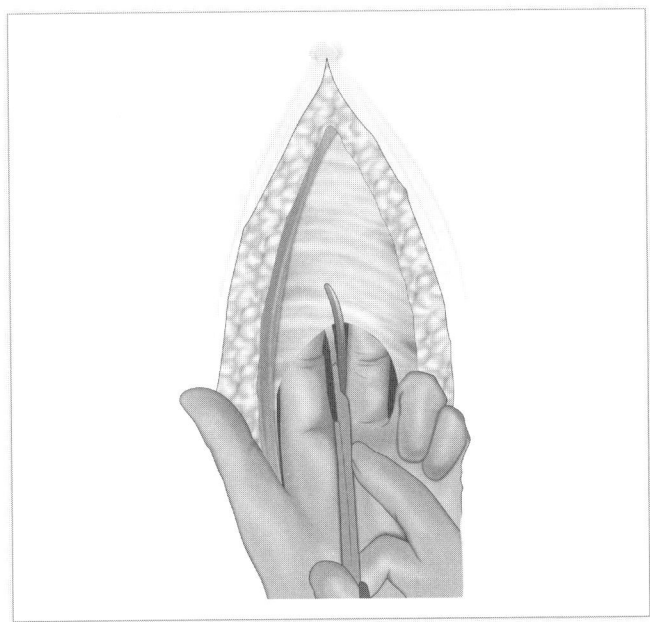

Fig. 13.17: Upward completion of the celiotomy; the volar faces of the two fingers are in contact with the undersurface of the peritoneum; the scissor tips never overtake the finger tips

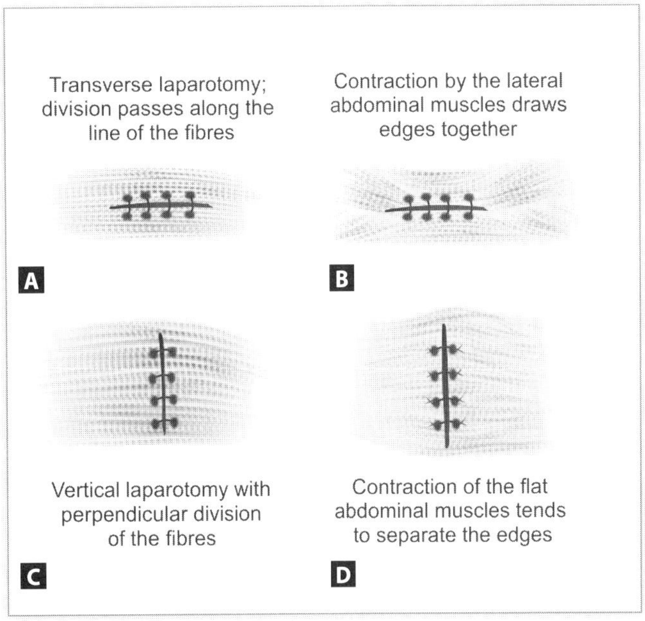

Fig. 13.18: Fibres of the rectus sheath fascia follow a horizontal course; (A) Transverse laparotomy; division passes along the line of the fibres; (B) Contraction by the lateral abdominal muscles draws edges together; (C) Vertical laparotomy with perpendicular division of the fibres; (D) Contraction of the flat abdominal muscles tends to separate the edges

transparency we see a translucent zone and an opaque, triangular central zone with the uracus arising from its apex: The location of the bladder. The incision is made to one of side of the translucent area.
- A signal that one is dangerously near to the bladder is given by perivesical fat.
  - Tactile landmarks: The apex of the bladder is easily identified by palpation.

Transverse Laparotomies

Most of these were introduced during the latter part of the 19th century and the beginning of the last century. Advantages leading to their rapid adoption were:
- *Infrequency of postoperative dehiscence*, then common with vertical laparotomies The intuition of the proposing authors was later confirmed by Sloan (1927), who was the first to demonstrate that the amount of stress to which the fascial edges are subjected by the transverse muscles of the abdomen is 30 times less with transverse laparotomies than in vertical laparotomy.

This derives from two anatomical factors:
- Division of the rectus sheath occurs (Fig. 13.18A) along the course of its fibres, thus a great many of them are separated rather than cut; the consequent functional anatomical damage is considerably reduced compared to vertical sections (Fig. 13.18C) and it can be repaired without compromising the strength of the fascia, which is the most important structure in avoiding possible postoperative dehiscence (see Fig. 19.1)
- As the incision into the aponeurosis is parallel to the lines of tension of the lateral abdominal muscles, when these contract following an increase in endoabdominal pressure, such as in response to movements of the trunk, coughing, vomiting or evacuation of the bowel, traction it is not exerted on the suture, subjecting it to pulling strain, as happens in vertical laparotomies (Fig. 13.18D), but it is exerted laterally, i.e. in the same direction as the incision, tending rather to draw the wound edges together (Fig. 13.18B). A study conducted by Hendrix et. al (2000) appears to cast doubt on the assumption that low transverse laparotomies are less prone to dehiscence
- *Reduced postoperative pain*, which allows better pulmonary ventilation. This is due to the fact that, as the surgical wound is away from the diaphragm, local pain does not aggravate respiratory movements and therefore does not inhibit breathing. The first studies on this issue go back to Elliot (1964), who found that maximum respiratory capacity is reduced by 15.2% in patients who underwent low transverse laparotomies against a 35% reduction in patients with vertical laparotomies
- *Postoperative ileus* is less common and of shorter duration
- *Aesthetic advantage*
- *Scar quality*: The cutaneous incision is paralell to Langer's lines of tension (1862), that is, in the direction

of the elastic collagenous fibres of the dermis. For this reason there will be minimal retraction of the skin edges and their realignment will be easier and more secure.

Laparotomy Site

This is located within the anterior triangle, an isosceles triangle (according to some a trapezium) whose base is the bis-iliac diameter and whose apex is the pubic symphysis (Fig. 13.19).

The anterior triangle bears a reasonable correspondence to the anterior segment (anterior pelvis) of the pelvic inlet and presents different characteristics according to differing pelvic types, from wide base and limited height (flat pelvis) to the smaller base and greater height of the android or anthropoid types.

The first description of a C-section conducted by means of a transverse laparotomy goes back to 1788; followed by Rapin (1894), Kustner (1896), Hartman (1900), Mackerodt (1905), Pfannenstiel (1907), Maylard (1907), Joel Cohen (1912) and Cherney (1943).

The techniques now listed are divided into two large groups according to whether or not access to the abdominal cavity involves transection of the rectus abdominis muscles. To the first group belong the laparotomies according to Pfannestiel, Joel Cohen (commonly used in the obstetric field) and Kustner; the second group comprises those of Mackenrodt-Maylard and Cherney, which are employed

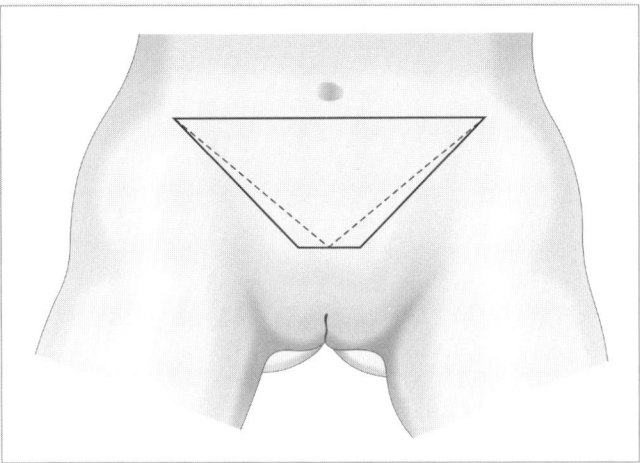

Fig. 13.19: Anterior triangle (or trapezium) of the pelvis

chiefly in gyneacology urology and in extra peritoneal CS (particularly Cherney) (Table 13.1).

Techniques not Involving Transection of the Rectus Muscles, but their Separation

- *Laparotomy incision according to Pfannenstiel:* (Figs 13.20C and 13.21). The cutaneous incision, curved and 12–14 cm in width, is performed 1–2 fingerbreadths above the pubic symphysis. Transverse incisions are made through skin, subcutaneous tissue and both

Table 13.1

Summary overview of the main transverse laparotomy techniques

Author	Skin site and direction of incision	Subcutis characteristics of incision	Fascia incision	Muscles	Traversalis fascia and peritoneum
Pfannenstiel	Pfannenstiel suprapubic curved	sharp dissection	transversal sharp dissection	digital separation	sharp dissection
Joel Cohen	interiliac to 3 fingerbreadths above symphysis straight	digital separation	sharp dissection blind technique	digital separation	digital separation
Kustner	suprapubic curved	sharp dissection	longitudinal	digital separation	vertical sharp dissection
Mackenrodt &Maylard	interiliac with caudal convexity (6 cm) from symphysis	sharp dissection	transverse	transverse incision	transverse incision
Cherney	suprapubic curved	transverse incision	transverse	disinsertion of rectus muscles from pubis	transverse

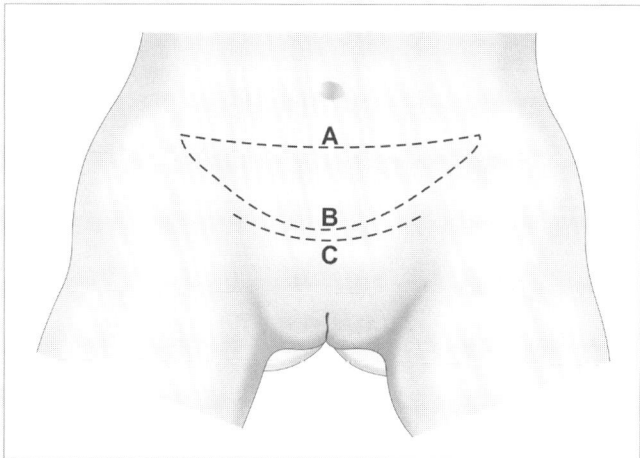

Fig. 13.20: Transverse laparotomies; (A) According to Joel Cohen; (B) According to Joel Cohen modified or according to Mackenrodt Maylard; (C) According to Pfannenstiel

anterior rectus sheaths. The distal and proximal flaps of the anterior rectus sheaths are retracted from the underlying muscles, which are separated along the midline. This exposes the posterior rectus sheaths, the transversalis fascia and peritoneum, which are then incised

- *Laparotomy incision according to Joel Cohen* (Fig. 13.20C) initially employed in hysterectomies, and subsequently used in C-sections.

We refer to the description of laparotomy as initially proposed by Joel Cohen (1912, 1972).

Transverse incision of the abdominal wall (Fig. 13.20A) between two points situated 2.5 cm inferomedially to the anterior superior iliac spines; the incision is mainly of the skin, not of the subcutaneous adipose tissue.

Across the midline, the subcutaneous tissue is tranversally incised and for a width of 5 cm the incision is deepened until the underlying fascia is reached, which is incised in turn, also transversely, across the midline, to a width of 2.5 cm.

The subcutaneous tissue is separated from the fascia by introducing curved scissors between the two, closed on their introduction, then opened, before progressing with tips closed.

Transverse expansion of the fascia incision using curved scissors; expansion of the space between the two rectus muscles using contrapposed index fingers, working first longitudinally and then transversely.

The peritoneum is opened as far as possible towards the cephalad end of the incision, to one side of the midline; separation is effected digitally; the opening is made transversely.

There are numerous variants of this technique: The rectilinear cutaneous incision varying in height from 3 to 8 cm (interiliac incision, Fig. 13.19A) above the pubic symphysis (3 fingerbreadths [patient's] above the symphysis according to NICE, Fig. 13.19B). Separation of the subcutaneous tissue is effected digitally. Having reached the fascia, a central eyelet is made with the scalpel and the opening is completed with scissors. Separation of the rectus abdominis muscles is effected with the fingers along the midline, initially in a longitudinal, then in a transverse direction. Opening of the peritoneum is made by separating it with the fingers, not by sharp dissection.

- *Laparotomy incision according to Kustner* (Fig. 13.22) transverse incision of skin and subcutaneous tissue as with the Pfannenstiel incision; the subcutaneous tissue is separated from the underlying fascia along a very extensive length to allow a vertical incision of the fascia along the midline; separation of the rectus muscles and longitudinal incision of the peritoneum follow. Not often used in obstetrics.

Techniques Involving Transection of the Rectus Abdominis Muscles

These are seldom used. Some literature relates to their employment in obstetrics and they are included here for the sake of completeness:

- *Mackenrodt and Maylard incision* (Fig. 13.20B): A transverse incision is made in the skin, subcutaneous

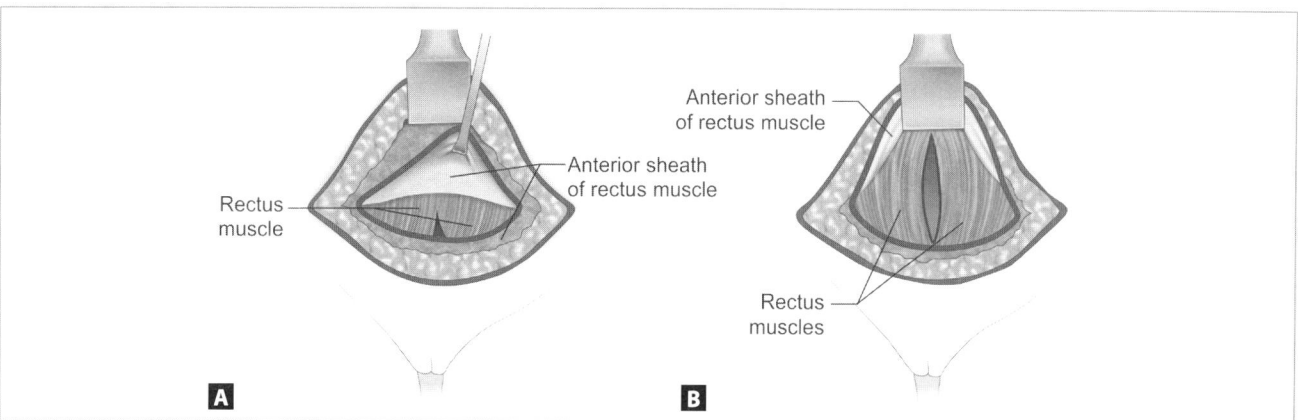

Fig. 13.21A and B: Low transverse laparotomy according to Pfannnenstiel; (A) Transverse section of the fascia; (B) Longitudinal separation of the rectus abdominis muscles

THE CAESAREAN SECTION

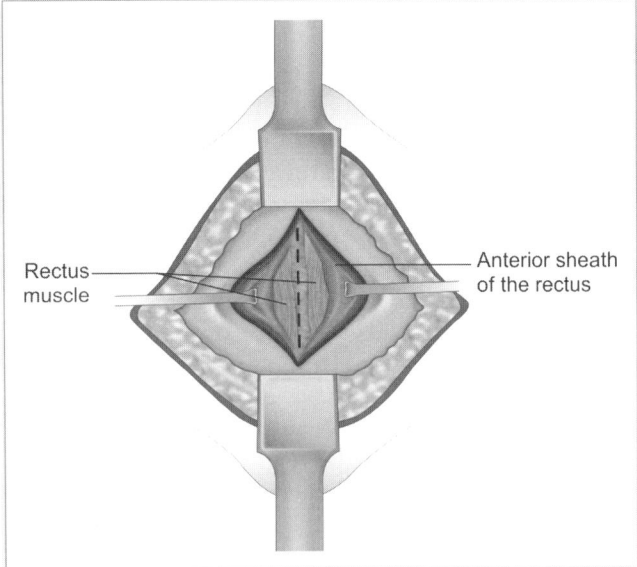

Fig. 13.22: Kustner laparotomy; transverse incision of the skin and subcutaneous tissue is followed by longitudinal incision of the fascia

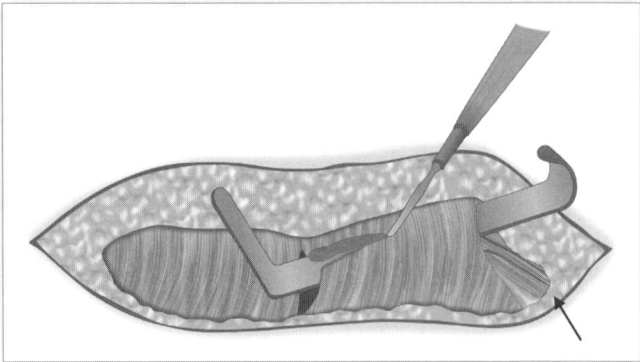

Fig. 13.23: Maylard low transverse laparotomy. Transection of the rectus muscles

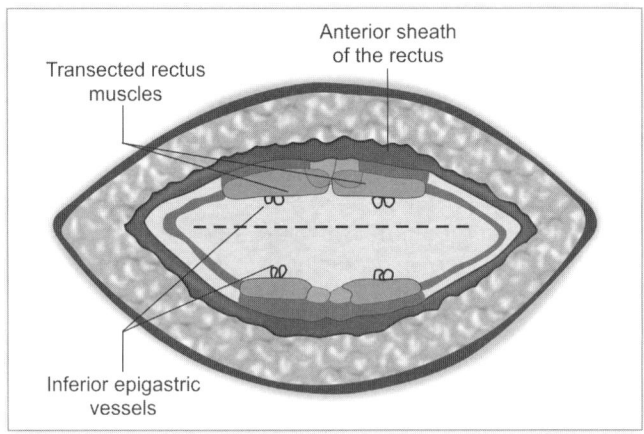

Fig. 13.24: Maylard low transverse laparotomy. Rectus muscles have been transected, transverse celiotom

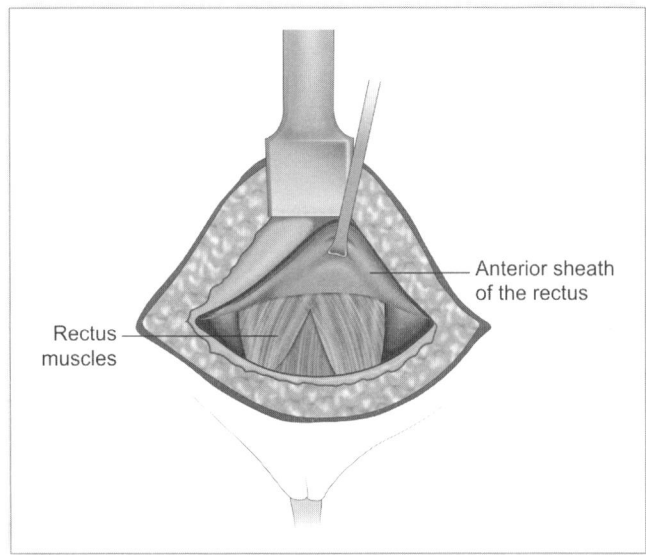

Fig. 13.25: Cherney low transverse laparotomy. The pyramidalis muscles can be seen. These are left in situ. The rectus muscle tendons are transected and disinserted from the pubis

tissue and the anterior rectus sheaths. The rectus muscles are transected transversely (Figs 13.23 and 13.24) using sharp dissection or cutting cautery. This is followed by ligation of the inferior epigastric vessels and incision of the transversalis fascia and peritoneum.

Cherney incision (Fig. 13.25): Skin, subcutaneous tissue and anterior rectus sheaths are incised transversely, as with the Pfannenstiel technique. The pyramidalis muscles are dissected free and sharply excised to expose the underlying *rectus tendons,* which are transected transversely 1-2 cm cranial to the superior edge of the pubic bone. *Rectus muscle should never be cut* thereby allowing their upward retraction. This is followed by incision of the transversalis fascia and peritoneum.

There is a vast literature comparing the various techniques; the parameters usually applied are duration of operation, haematocrit, postoperative pain and fever:
- *Time taken:* This depends on the requirements of the procedure: The timings for extracting a foetus whose head is not engaged are different to those for a foetus in obstructed labour. Irrespective of the technique used, the latter case has clear disadvantages in timing outcomes
- *Haematocrit:* This also depends on the time taken for extraction, for controlling haemorrhage (third and fourth stage of labour and hysterotomy haemostasis) as well as on the technical difficulty of the operation
- *Postoperative pain:* As a rule, this increases proportionately with the closeness of the laparotomy to the diaphragm, and is strictly linked to the technical difficulty of the operation
- *Fever:* Antibiotic prophylaxis (antibiotic I.V. on umbilical cord clamping) generally ensures apyretic postoperative

recovery. Fever is observed as a consequence of the operation when the uterine cavity becomes contaminated. However, in the tropics external causes, such as malaria, typhus or urinary and respiratory tract infections are frequent.

A recent critical Cochrane review (Mathai M, Hofmeyr GJ. 2007) finds that, in the short term, Joel Cohen laparotomies present advantages over Pfannenstiel in terms of operation duration and intraoperative blood loss. Postoperative recovery was also found to involve less postoperative pain, less frequent fever and a shorter hospitalization period. The study provides no information regarding severe complications, morbidity, mortality or long-term outcomes.

We believe, however, that *two parameters are missing* from all these studies:
- *The morphology of the pelvis or of the anterior pelvis* (in the case of combined forms). It is clear that a Joel Cohen incision in an android pelvis, with reduced biiliac diameter, is technically more complex than a Pfannenstiel incision with a flat pelvis
- *Indications for surgery*: In presence of a mechanical obstacle (cephalopelvic disproportion or obstructed labour) in which the lower uterine segment is overdistended, both a low transverse laparotomy (Pfannenstiel) and a high one (Joel Cohen) are contraindicated due to risk of injuring the bladder.

Procedure Followed by the Authors

In light of the foregoing, while employing, as indicated, the transverse laparotomy, we will not follow any one of the techniques described and rigidly codified above, but shall adapt the site and magnitude of the skin and fascia incision to the morphology of the pelvis and surgical indications.

Height and Site of Incision

a. *Skin and subcutaneous tissue:* This is made in an area of the anterior triangle or trapezium and is suited to the dimensions of the presenting part. The site and extension of the incision (Fig. 13.19) must be such as to allow the easy execution of the following stages (hysterotomy and extraction of the fetus), which is dependent on the depth of engagement of the presenting part and the extent of LUS over-distension, term under which three elements are included: *Elongation, distension, thinning* (see next Chapter).

In the case of *an obstructed labour* with a full bladder it has not proven possible to drain and with an overdistended lower uterine segment, it makes sense to opt for a vertical laparotomy right away, to avoid the real danger of bladder injury.

When the above conditions are not present, having selected the site for the incision, we suggest the following tactic: If right-handed the operating surgeon places their left hand (ulnar side towards the pubis) on the abdomen and pushes the skin downwards (Fig. 13.26). If one is not already present, this will form a subtle fold of skin, the *Bumm pelvic line*, which extends from one iliac spine to the other. With great frequency, the line of incision will coincide with this pelvic line. Now stretch the abdominal skin upwards and make the incision from left to right with the extension considered sufficient. The skin and Camper's fascia are incised along the whole extent (13–15 cm), while the subcutaneous tissue is cut only along the central part, where the incision deepens to Scarpa's fascia.

In the suprapubic and lateral inguinal region, Camper's fascia is a thin subcutaneous layer; it is very important that this is reidentified on closure as the application here of sutures will provide a good approximation of the skin edges.

Separation of the adipose tissue may be performed by sharp dissection or, as Joel Cohen proposes, by digital separation, which will help avoid injury to the inferior epigastric vessels and unnecessary haemorrhage. The inferior epigastric vessels, branches of the external iliac vessels, from which they originate below the inguinal ligament, proceed cranially, passing along the lateral border of the rectal sheath. At the level of the umbilicus, they anastomatise with the superior epigastric vessels. These medial terminal branches of the internal thoracic vessels are responsible for the "caput medusae" in portal hypertension.

b. *Fascia*: Adherence of subcutaneous tissue to the fascia is at its greatest at the linea alba, and *this adherence is exploited in identifying the linea alba.*

One proceeds as follows: The operating surgeon, if right-handed, using the left hand previously used first in

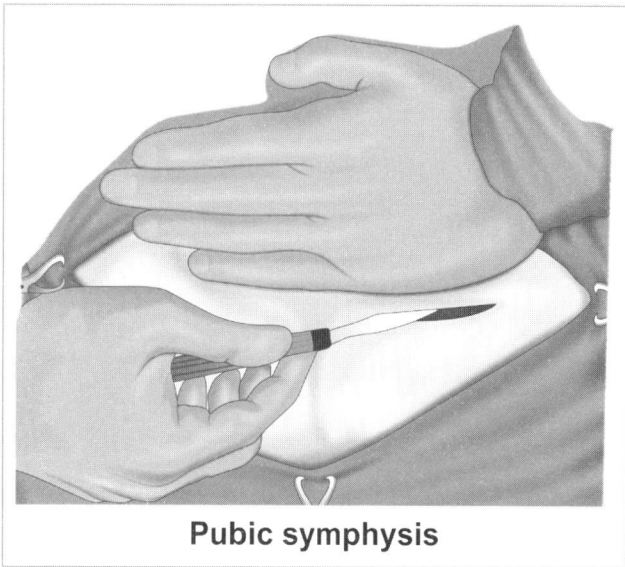

Fig. 13.26: Low transverse laparotomy; incision of skin and subcutaneous tissue follows the Bumm pelvic line

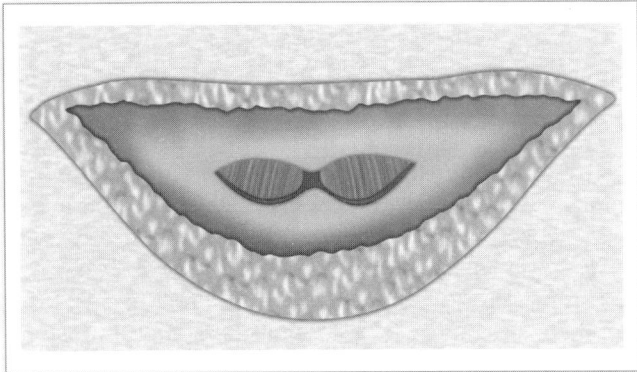

Fig. 13.27: Incision of the fascia, using sharp dissection, extending 3 cm on both sides of the linea alba; this produces a figure-eight shape

identifying *the Bumm line* and then in stretching the skin, now takes hold of the cephalad edge of the skin incision stretches and elevates it. The area of greatest adherence indicates the linea alba. Here, using the scalpel, a transverse incision 3 cm in length is made on each side (Fig. 13.27). This creates a horizontal figure-8, with the two loops joined in the middle by the linea alba. Kocher forceps are applied superiorly and inferiorly of the linea alba. From here, the subsequent stages are performed using.

- *Curved bladed mayo scissors with rounded tips*, are introduced *closed* (Fig. 13.28) and with the tips facing the fascia undersurface until the joint; having reached it, they return backwards in an open position, therefore bluntly detaching the fascia from the muscle (perimisium). Coming out at this point, they now incise, giving the incision a curved path with caudal convexity (Figs 13.29 and 13.30). Incision of the fascia should be between 16 and 18 cm.

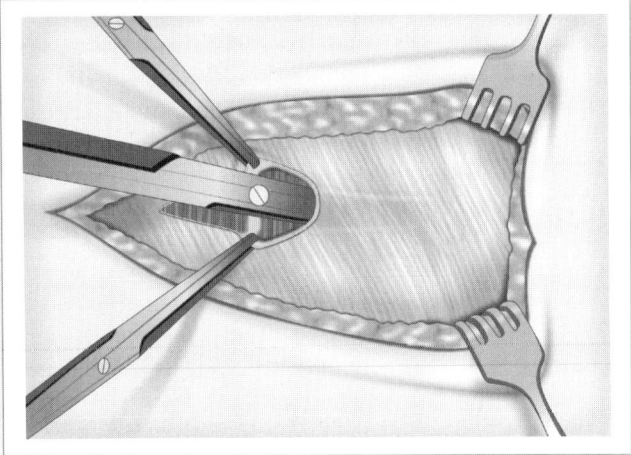

Fig. 13.28: The edges of the linea alba are grasped and elevated using two Kocher forceps. Each side is entered to the required depth using Mayo scissors, the tips facing the fascia undersurface. Here we see how the fascia is raised by the rounded tips of scissors

An incision made too low will not allow this length of incision and have the following two additional drawbacks:
- There is too restricted a space for extraction of the foetal head
- If too close to the pubis, the fascia could detach from the periosteum on suturing.

The authors carry out this manoeuvre incising all the way along the fascia with the belly of the scalpel (Figs 13.31 and 13.32).

Incision of the fascia is completed with its mobilization from the underlying rectus muscles. This is done as follows: Beginning from the inferior edge of the fascia, and while an assistant "tents" the fascia, elevating it with Kocher forceps, the surgeon grasps the central portion of the right hemisection, and elevating with force the cleavage plane (perimysium) of the fascia from the muscle will appear clearly, and this is extended using one or two fingers

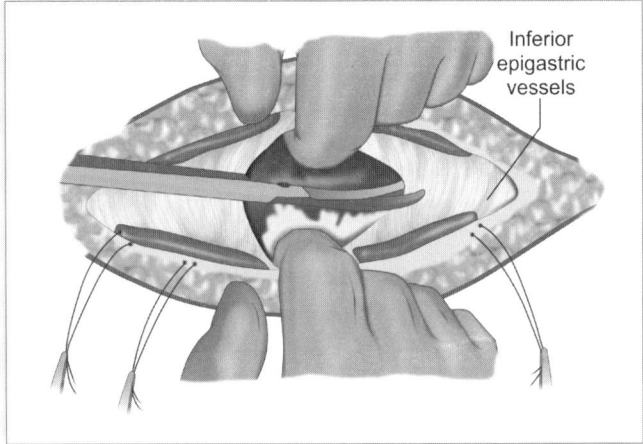

Fig. 13.29: Incision of the fascia: Observe how the back of the scissors is parallel to the inferior edge; the incision is curved

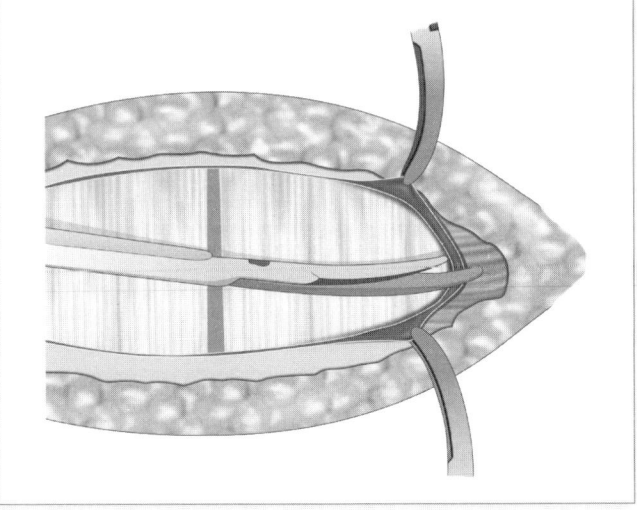

Fig. 13.30: Incision of the fascia is completed

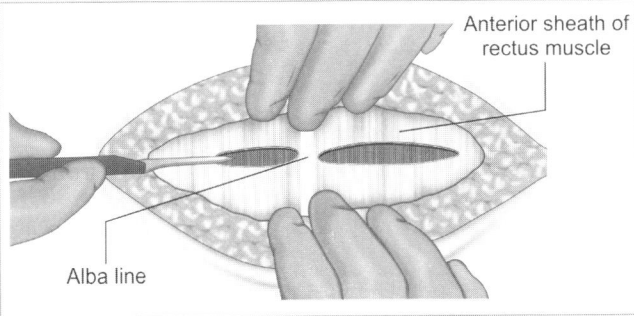

Fig. 13.31: Incision of the fascia by means of a scalpel

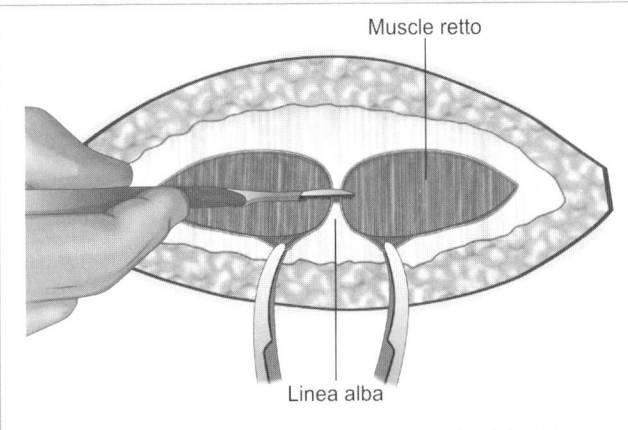

Fig. 13.32: Scalpel dissection of the fascia is completed

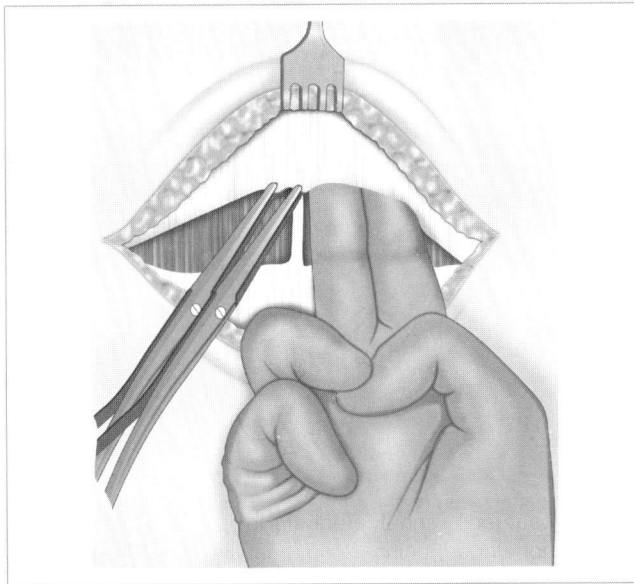

Fig. 13.33: Detachment of the muscle (perimysium) from the fascia in a lateromedial direction

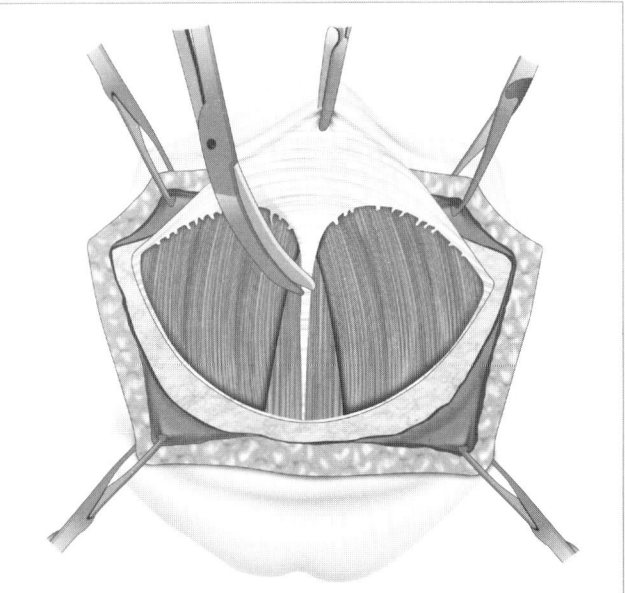

Fig. 13.34: Preparation of the pyramidalis muscles which here, for illustrative clarity, appear detached from the fascia

(Fig. 13.33) or sharp dissection in a lateromedial direction, stopping close to the lateral border of the pyramidalis muscle; the manoeuvre is completed contralaterally.

The index and middle fingers are introduced into each of the two freed spaces; an elevator traction is exerted and the pyramidalis muscles are divided from the underlying rectus muscles. This manoeuvre starts from the apex of their insertion on the underlying fascia (13.34) and proceeds caudally, paying care that dissection is distal to the point of contact between the two rectus sheaths.

This manoeuvre completed, the pyramidalis muscles will still adhere to the fascia and the medial borders of the rectus muscles will be clearly evident (Fig. 13.35).

Separation of the pyramidalis from the underlying rectus muscles is central to correctly accessing the abdominal cavity.

The same manoeuvre is performed on the superior edge (Fig. 13.36), paying care not to damage the *perforating vessels*. If this manoeuvre is performed correctly, the medial borders of the rectus muscles will be clearly evident for much of their extension (Fig. 13.35).

c. *Muscles*: Separation of the muscles, very easily done; performed lengthwise.
d. *Transversalis fascia and peritoneum*: The celiotomy can be either
   - *Transverse*: Using sharp dissection, it would be accompanied by less postoperative pain. When dissecting the uracus two points of reference should be applied to facilitate their matching on closure.
   - *Longitudinal,* Using sharp dissection (Fig. 13.13) or digital separation. This would leave the uracus

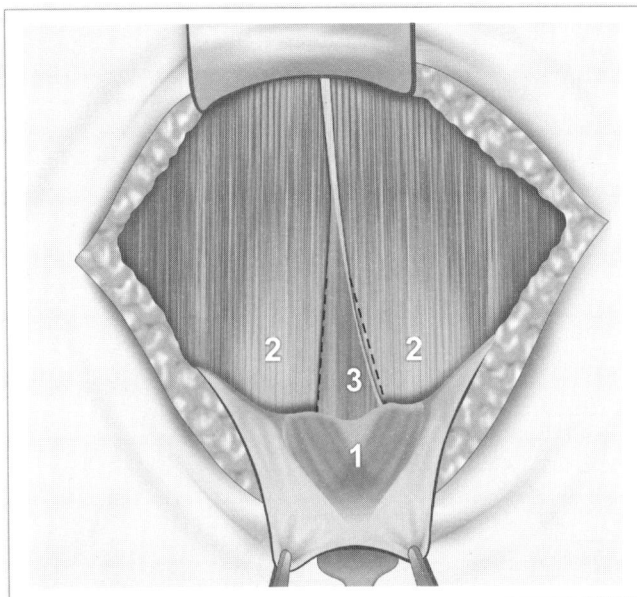

Fig. 13.35: Final view: The pyramidalis muscles (1) adhere to the fascia; note the triangular space (3) between the two recti (2), from where their division is begun in a vertical direction, starting from the inferior end

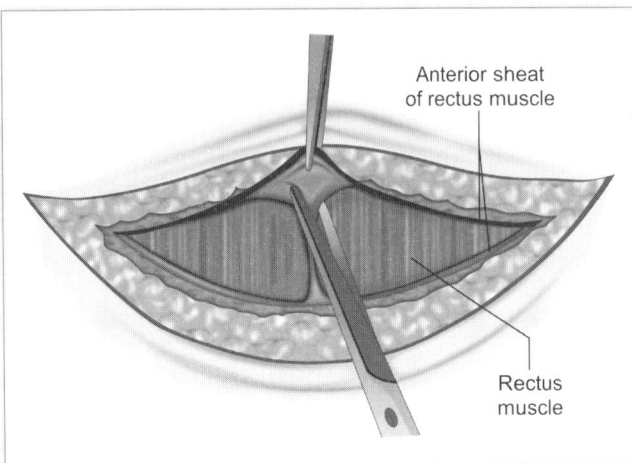

Fig. 13.36: Preparation of the superior edge of the fascia. Lateromedial detachment of muscles from the fascia (perimysium) has already been performed, paying care not to damage the perforating arteries. Dissection at the point where the rectal sheaths join

whole, with its supposed function of supporting the bladder. This is not possible using digital separation as described by Joel Cohen.

Having completed the laparotomy, some surgeons apply a suprapubic valve or an autostatic retractor, whose minimum aperture should be 12 cm (Allis test). The authors do not find these stages useful as, among other reasons, they impede correct execution of retropulsion of the presenting part.

Opening the Peritoneum in Presence of Widespread Adhesions

Widespread adhesions between the abdominal wall and the anterior wall of the uterus may already be suspected on abdominal palpation, due to:
- Characteristics of the laparotomic scar
- Lack of smoothness of flow of the skin over the underlying layers
- Reduced or absent mobility of the uterus, which retains its position
- The particular morphology of the uterus during contraction, and its changes in polarity.

If the adhesions are such that:
- They allow access to the abdominal cavity; lysis of the adhesions, where sharp dissection is required, should not be performed at the expense of the uterus, but incising liberally into the parietal peritoneum and transversalis fascia 2 cm from the edge of the adhesion. The reason for this is clear: Haemostasis is much easier for a peduncle with a flap of peritoneum than on the surface of the uterus
- They do not allow access to the abdominal cavity. This condition does not complicate, but rather simplifies the operation; it suffices to retract the bladder and to perform an enforced (denecessitate) *extraperitoneal C-section*. Having completed suturing, never attempt to remove the adhesions, which will reform, sometimes with unfavourable outcomes.

Isolation of the Site for the Hysterotomy

Ensure that the operating table is tilted downwards and that compresses are applied in the paracolic gutters.

In most cases of labour dystocia due to mechanical obstacle (cephalopelvic disproportion, obstructed labour, cervical or birth canal abnormalities), the patient arrives at the operating table with membranes already broken over many hours and with an infected uterine cavity. Indication is for an extraperitoneal C-section or the careful isolation of the hysterotomy site, iodinated swabbing of the cavity after third stages and visceral and parietal peritonisation accurate lavage of the pouch of Douglas, layered closure of the abdominal wall.

BIBLIOGRAPHY

1. Cherney LS. A modified transverse incision for low abdominal operations. Surg Gynecol Obstet. 1940;72:92.
2. Cherney LS. New trasverse low incision. California & West Med. 1943;59:215-8.
3. Chez RA, McDuff HC. The Pfannenstiel incision. Contemp Ob/Gyn. 1976;7:55.
4. Chez RA. Steps in performing the Maylard incision. Contemp Ob/Gyn. 1991;39.

5. Cohen SJ. Abdominal and vaginal hysterectomy, Allen and Mowbray, Oxford. 1972.
6. Hendrix SL, Schimp V, Martin J, Singh A, Kruger M, McNeeley SG. The legendary superior strength of the Pfannenstiel incision: a myth? A J Obst Gyn. 2000;182:1446-51.
7. Kustner O. Der suprasymphysare kreuzschnitt, eine methode der coeliotomie bei wenig umfanglichen affektioen der weiblichen beckenorgane. Monatsschr Geburtsh Gynakol. 1896;4:197.
8. Kustner O. Methodik der gynaekologischen Laparotomie. Verh Dtsch Ges Gynákol (9 Kongr). ix: 580, 1901.
9. Langer K. Zur Anatomie und Physiologie der Haut. II Die Spannung der cutis. S-B Akad. Wiss. Wien, math-nah. Kl 14, 133, 1862.
10. Mackenrodt A. Ergebnisse der Abdominalen Radikal-operation des Gebaermutterscheidenkrebses mittels Laparotomia hypogastrica. I Anatomie, Chirurgie und Klinik. Z. Geburtsh Gynaek. 1905;54:514.
11. Mathai M, Hofmeyr GJ. Abdominal surgical incisions for caesarean section. Cochrane Database Syst Rev. 2007; (1):CD004453.
12. Maylard AE. Direction of abdominal incision. Brit Med J. 1907;2:895.
13. Pfannenstiel J. Ueber die Vortheile des suprasymphysaren Fasienquerschnitt fuer die gynaekologischen Koeliotomien. Samml. Klin. Vortr. Leipzig, N. 268. Gyneaek: 97, 1735, 1907.
14. Sloan GA. A new upper abdominal incision. Surg Gynec Obst. 1927;45:678.

CHAPTER 14

The Various Types of Hysterotomy—Criteria of Choice

A caesarean section is assessed on the basis of the following:
- Correct clinical indication
- Suitability of the surgical technique employed. This is evaluated by considering the following:
a. *Short-term* outcomes regarding maternal morbidity and mortality and the well-being of the foetus. This is determined by:
   - Prompt diagnosis
   - Adequate preoperative preparation
   - Minimum time interval between the clinical indication for surgery and the operation itself
   - The appropriate technique of anaesthesia
   - Surgical technique non-injurious to birth canal (hysterotomy)
   - Careful hemostasis
   - Good approximation of edges, avoiding oozing surfaces
   - Careful toilet of the cavity.
b. *Long-term outcomes* regarding compatibility of the surgery with future pregnancies and labour; hysterotomy site and quality of suture are among the most important factors influencing the quality of long-term outcomes.

HYSTEROTOMY

A hysterotomy aims to access the uterine cavity for the purpose of extracting the foetus. Access may be either through a transverse or vertical hysterotomy. A close relationship between hysterotomy type and uterine rupture is known to exist; according to Bernestein (2000), the incidence is as follows:

Low transverse C-section 0.2–1.5%
Inverted T-shaped C-section 4–9%
Low vertical C-section 1–7%
Classic C-section (longitudinal incision on body) 4–9%.

Knowledge of these data should not influence the operating surgeon's choice of mode of access, which follows one *very clear rule*: «**extract the foetus while inflicting the minimum amount of damage on the birth canal**».

LOWER UTERINE SEGMENT

The lower uterine segment (LUS) (Fig. 14.1) is an anatomical and physiological entity that forms during pregnancy and retracts after it. The LUS is not clearly definable in anatomical terms, and some authors describe it simply as "that low, thin portion of the uterus which is interposed, in the latter stage of pregnancy, between the uterine corpus and os". It originates from the uterine isthmus and from the cervix, as is demonstrated by the presence of lower-segment C-section scars in the cervix.

In the primigravida, the LUS starts to form between the 3rd and 5th month, acquiring a specific physiognomy towards the 6th month. In a multipara, it forms later, sometimes at the onset of labour.

Process of formation: The main mechanism acting on the formation of the lower uterine segment is *intrauterine pressure* (Fig. 14.2).

The development of the ovum leads to a progressive increase in internal pressure (Fa) on the uterine wall and on the isthmus opposed by the contractive condition of the uterus (tonus). As the isthmus constitutes a point of least

THE VARIOUS TYPES OF HYSTEROTOMY—CRITERIA OF CHOICE

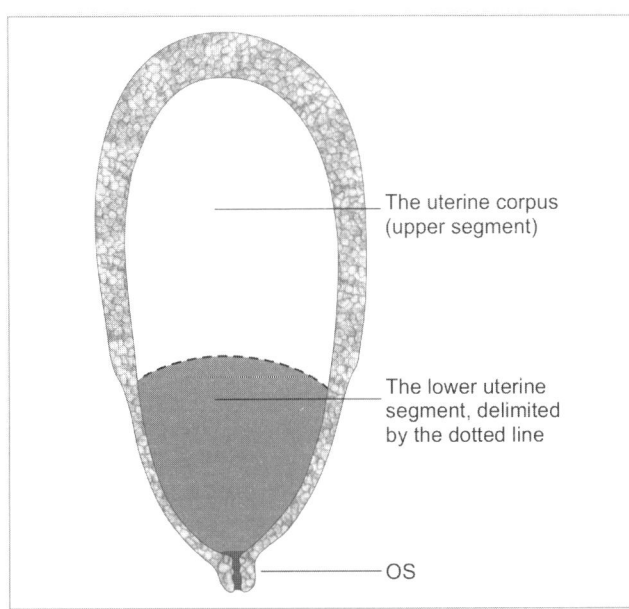

Fig. 14.1: Uterus

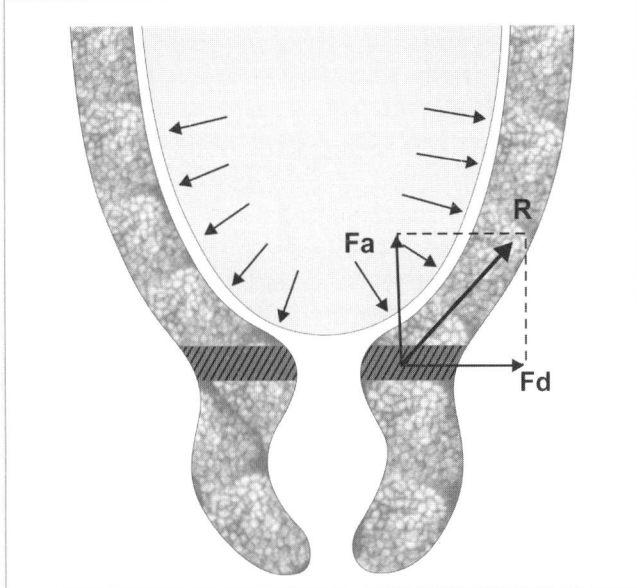

Fig. 14.2: Diagram showing the formation of the lower uterine segment (from P-Kamina, Anatomia Ginecologica ed Ostetrica. DEMI, Rome).
Abbreviation: Fa, uterine walls tone; Fd, dilatory force; R, resultant

resistance these two forces exert their action on: Dilatory force within it opposed by the uterine wall tone acting in cranial direction. The resultant (R) of these forces is an oblique lateral-cranial force on the isthmus, leading to its lengthening, which occurs as a process of thinning.

In the primigravida, at term of pregnancy, the LUS takes on a truncated cone structure with an upturned base. It features:
- *A superior border* corresponding to the point of close adherence of the peritoneum to the uterine wall, that is, the area of sudden change in thickness of the uterine wall
- *An inferior border* corresponding, before labour, to the internal uterine os
- *An anterior wall* which, at term of pregnancy, is broader and more convex compared to the posterior wall, measuring at its superior end 7–10 cm in height and 9–12 cm in breadth, dimensions that progressively reduce in a caudal direction. Thickness is between 3 and 5 mm.

Proceeding from the cephaloid end caudally, three futher zones can be identified:
- A short superior zone
- An intermediate zone
- An inferior zone, which is the thinnest, with a height of 2–4 cm. This is covered over by the bladder, which adheres loosely to begin with, but, proceeding caudally, its adherence becomes firm (this is the true inferior border of the uterine segment). Here a rich venous vascularisation appears with large tortuous veins that bleed profusely, if forcefully separated.

Because of its fineness and low vascularisation, the LUS is the site of choice for hysterotomy in a caesarean section.

During labour, the lower uterine segment takes on a funnel shape and accomodates the engagement and progress of the presenting part; the lateral borders of this funnel are represented by the ascending branches of the uterine arteries, which correspond, within some degree of approximation, to the lateral borders of the round ligaments. The inferior border of the LUS continues with the cervix to whose external border the vagina joins, forming together the soft parts of the birth canal.

It would appear evident that the hysterotomy:
- Should take place on a section of the LUS whose breadth is compatibile with the dimensions of the presenting part
- That the degree of distension of the LUS, which is in turn influenced by the patient's age, parity and any previous scarring or inflamatory phenomena, should be compatible with:
  – Insertion of the hand to a sufficient depth to grasp the most backwardly sloping portion of the presenting part
  – Retropulsion and extraction of the presenting part.

If these requirements are met, a transverse hysterotomy is indicated. If they are not met, it means that a critical point has been reached and there is a substantial risk, during delivery of the head of lateral extension of the hysterotomy with laceration of the LUS and/or injury of the uterine arteries and soft tissue of the birth canal. To prevent this from happening, traditional obstetrics (Kawawukume

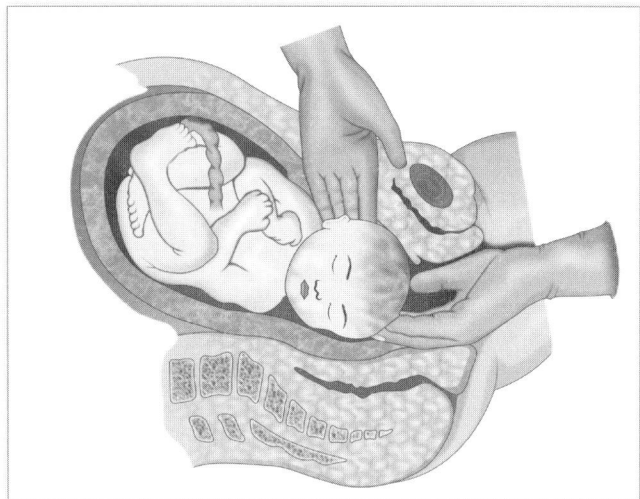

Fig. 14.3: Disengagement of the head using the "push from below" method

2001, Fasubae et al., 2002, Levy et al., 2005) provides for disengagement using:
- Pressure from below: *The push method* or *head first* (Fig. 14.3). This consists of asking an assistant to exert upward pressure through the vagina using a hand or fist against the presenting part to disloge it from the vagina; simultaneously, the operating surgeon, acting on the shoulders, exerts upward traction (Landesman manoeuvre, 1984), pressure must be applied during the interval between two contractions.

In the authors' experience, this is not a very reliable manoeuvre and is hazardous both because of the excessive pressure exerted on the foetal head and the stress on the birth canal.

- Upwards traction "the *pull method or feet first*". Access to the uterine cavity is made via a transverse hysterotomy or via a low vertical hysterotomy (Rosen et al., 1991, Kafali H, 2003), the latter is to be preferred as it is easier to perform, has less risk of extension of the hysterotomy, and risk of uterine rupture during subsequent pregnancies is the same as in low transverse hysterotomy. The obstetrician identifies a foetal foot and, applying traction to it, accomplishes *internal rotation* (reverse breech extraction) and extracts the foetus by the breech.

CRITERIA OF HYSTEROTOMY CHOICE

The problem arises of which criterion to use in determining a hysterotomy type; the method we use is as follows (Domini et al., 2006).

Having entered the abdominal cavity, the operating surgeon introduces no retractor or valve, but places the hand (palm towards uterus) between the pubic symphysis and the uterus (*uterus still intact*) and attempts to retract the presenting part applying pressure through the uterine wall.

If the manoeuvre:
a. *Succeeds*, retropulsion has occurred and the hysterotomy is transverse (Chapter 15), almost bloodless and foetal extraction is easy.
b. *Does not succeed*, its failure is an indication for a *lower/upper uterine segment transverse hysterotomy* (Chapter 15) with *reverse breech extraction of the foetus* (Domini and Guazzini, 2006).

With increasing frequency, the authors have been using the pull method, and access the uterine cavity via a *high transverse hysterotomy*, which they consider a reasonable and safe compromise between the (moderate) drawbacks of a low vertical hysterotomy and the dangers of a LUS transverse hysterotomy (see Chapter 15).

It may occur that a deeply impacted head prevents catheterization and that the bladder is full; this does not rule the manoeuvre out. The vesicouterine pouch is incised and the hand is inserted between bladder and uterus (palm towards uterus) and the manoeuvre is executed.

To the group of vertical hysterotomies we should add all those conditions, independent of engagement, which preclude or contraindicate access to the lower uterine segment (see Chapter 16).

BIBLIOGRAPHY

1. Blickstein I. Difficult delivery of the impacted head during caesarean section, intraoperative disengagement dystocia. J Perinat Med. 2004;32(6):465-9 (ISSN: 0300-5577).
2. Domini E, Guazzini S, Vicentini S, Urso M. Delivery of an impacted head at caesarean section. An easy and reliable manoeuvre to assess adequate and safe hysterotomy and to control bleeding. Gior It Ostet Ginec. 2006;28(5):207-8.
3. Fasubae OB, Ezechi OC, Orji EO, Ogunnyi SO. Delivery of the impacted head of the foetus at caesarean section after prolonged and obstructed labour, a randomized comparative study of the two methods. J Obstet Gynaec. 2002;22(4):375-8 (ISSN: 0144-3615).
4. Kafali H. Cesarean breech extraction for impacted fetal head in deep pelvis after a prolonged obstructed labour: A cesarean technique variation. The Internet Journal of Gynecology and Obstetrics. 2003;2(2).
5. Kawawukume EY. Caesarean section in developing countries. Best Pract Clin Obstet. Gynaecology 2001;15(1):165-78 (ISSN 1521-6934).
6. Levy R, Chernomoretz T, Appewlmanz Z, Levin D, Or Y, Hagay ZJ. Head pushing reverse breech extraction in case of impacted foetal head during Caesarean Section. Eur J Obst Gynaec Reprod Biol. 2005;121(1):24-6 (ISSN 0301-2115).
7. Rosa P. La structure du myomètre humain et sa signification fonctionelle. Bull. de la Féd. Soc. Gyn et Obst Langue franc. 1965;17(1):5-78.
8. Rosen MG, Dickinson JC, Westhoff CL. Vaginal birth after cesarean: A meta-analysis of morbidity and mortality. Obstet Gynecol. 1991;77:465.

CHAPTER 15

Transverse Hysterotomies

INTRODUCTION

There is universal consensus in current obstetric practice that a transverse hysterotomy (Fig. 15.1A) conducted on the lower uterine segment (LUS) is the option of choice. Not only is vertical hysterotomy (Figs 15.1B and C) never mentioned, it is abhorred.

From the previous chapter we recall that the LUS is shaped like a truncated funnel with a superior base (10–12 cm) and truncated apex (6–7 cm) facing caudally and 7 cm in height (Fig. 14.1).

Transverse hysterotomies are subdivided into:
- *Transperitoneal*
- *Extraperitoneal.*

TRANSVERSE TRANSPERITONEAL HYSTEROTOMIES

Numerous techniques have been proposed, of which we cite:

The Kehrer (1882) *transverse hysterotomy*, which involves the transverse incision and mobilization of a short flap of loose visceral peritoneum and reflection of the bladder (Fig. 15.2A). The hysterotomy is transverse. A shortcoming at the time was frequent lateral extension.

The Munro Kerr (1926) *lower segment curvilinear hysterotomy,* involves reflection of the bladder from the uterus (Fig. 15.3) to a depth as far as the point where it is inseparable from cervix. One centimetre superiorly to this point a semicircular hysterotomy is performed (Fig. 15.2B), distally to the Kehrer incision, but whose

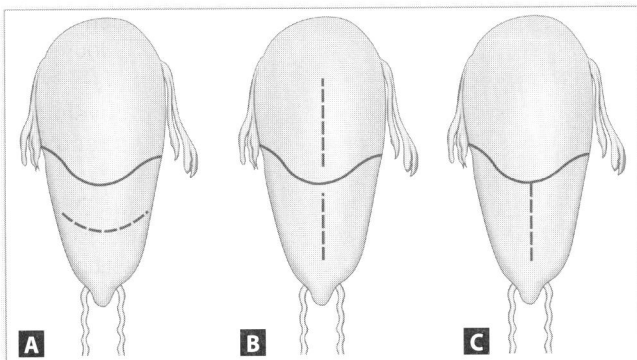

Fig. 15.1A to C: Various types of hysterotomy; (A) Lower-segment transverse hysterotomy; (B) Longitudinal hysterotomy on corpus or classic Sanger C-section; (C) Lower-segment hysterotomy

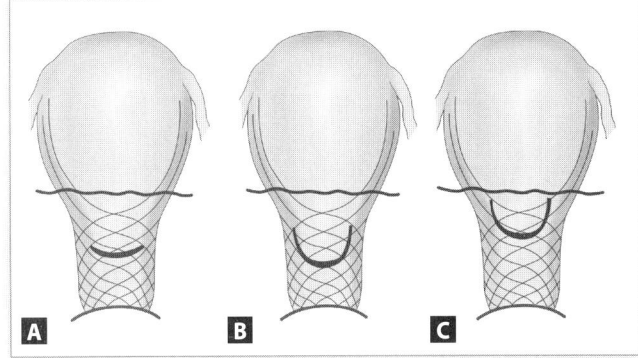

Fig. 15.2A to C: Transverse hysterotomies; (A) Kehrer transverse hysterotomy; (B) Munro Kerr hysterotomy; (C) High semicircular hysterotomy

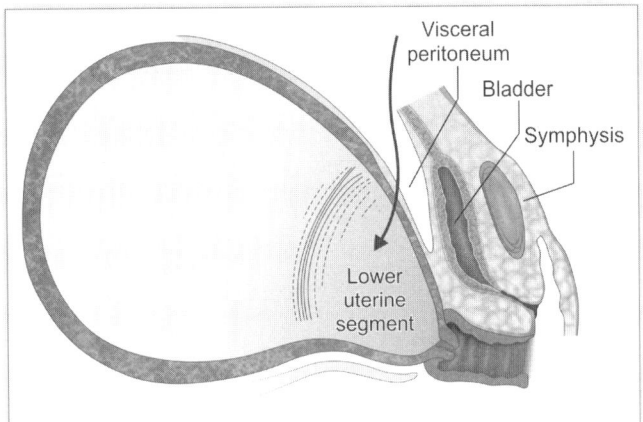

Fig. 15.3: Low transverse hysterotomy: Transverse incision and mobilization of the loose parietal peritoneum and reflection of the bladder. In this illustration, a Munro Kerr incision is made 1 cm superiorly to the area of maximum adherence of the bladder to the uterus

semicircular path permits possible upward, rather than lateral extension of the hysterotomy. Kerr already noted the hemorrhage risk associated with this procedure, but the technique was proposed during the pre-antibiotic era in which the obstetrician's objective was to ensure an extraperitoneal uterine incision and to avoid contamination of the abdominal cavity with the uterine contents as much as possible, thereby limiting the spread of infection and preventing adhesion of the uterus to the surrounding organs.

In case of infection, caudal traction on the cervix and its separation from the bladder allows drainage of the infection to occur vaginally. On healing, the bladder adheres perfectly to the uterus.

- *High semicircular hysterotomy* (Fig. 15.2C): Disadvantages linked to the Kerr technique led to a high semicircular hysterotomy, conducted 2–3 fingerbreadths superiorly to the bladder, which is reflected onto the uterus. This includes simultaneous incision both of the peritoneum and of the lower uterine segment.

We believe that the characteristics of a hysterotomy call for a *more precise definition than its height only* and that the extraction of the presenting part will be safer when a hysterotomy on the anterior face of the LUS meets the following requirements:

- *Site of incision* in an area of the LUS in which the space between the two round ligaments is compatibile with the dimensions of the head and at a distance from the most backwardly sloping portion of the presenting part, compatibile with the operating surgeon's hand
- *Symmetrical* to the two round ligaments; sometimes, due to dextroversion of the uterus, an incision that is symmetrical to the operative field is not so to the round ligaments and the hysterotomy extends leftwards, with laceration or incision of the ascending branch of the left uterine artery. Good obstetric technique would be to correct the dextroversion of the uterus before the hysterotomy
- *Strictly curvilinear*: In an elastic structure, the surface developed by a curved incision is greater than that by a rectilinear incision and in the event of an extension, this happens in a superior direction.

Degree of distension of the lower uterine segment, this is influenced by the age and parous status of the gravid patient and whether or not scar tissue is present, *compatible with subsequent strain constituted by*:

- Insertion of the hand between it (the LUS) and the presenting part
- Dimensions of the hand
- Portion of the hand that has to be introduced to reach the most backward-sloping area of the presenting part
- The manoeuvre of retropulsion and extraction.

TECHNIQUE USED BY THE AUTHORS

Hysterotomy

Having entered the abdominal cavity, the operating surgeon, using the round ligaments as a guide, ascertains whether there is torsion of the uterus (generally to the right) and, if required, takes measures to correct this; if this does not succeed, it is to be borne in mind on making the incision.

The surgeon performs the retropulsion manoeuvre keeping a grip on the presenting part, pushing it upwards towards an area where the breadth of the LUS is compatibile with the head dimensions. The scalpel is used to incise the anterior uterine wall (Fig. 15.4) at a point located 1 cm above the area of maximum convexity exerted by the head on the LUS and centrally to the two round ligaments; due to the internal compression, the incision will be almost bloodless.

At this point we strongly recommmend applying a reference stitch to both edges of the incision (see Fig. 15.22);

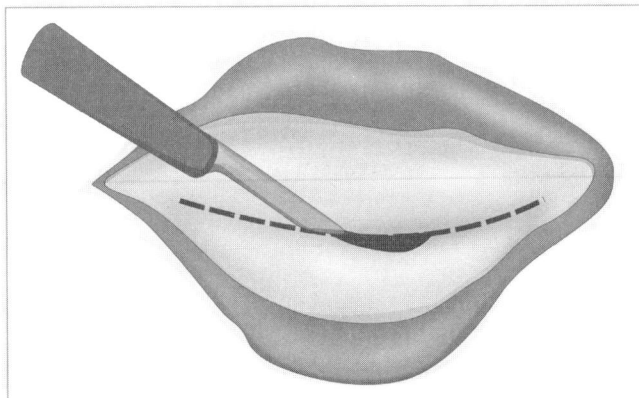

Fig. 15.4: Semicircular incision of the LUS. The first incision is made using the scalpel

at uterine suture, their traction and approximation will offer excellent matching of the edges.

It may happen that the LUS is overdistended and the site of the hysterotomy appears high. We point out that the *superior border* of the LUS is where the loose visceral peritoneum no longer slides along the anterior uterine wall, but remains firmly attached to it.

Again when confronted with an overdistended LUS, one can be unsure about the superior border of the bladder. To identify it, simply push the balloon of a Foley catheter upwards through the bladder wall and find point where it stops.

A full bladder that has proven impossible to drain does not contraindicate a low transverse hysterotomy. In this case, incise the vesicouterine fold (where this has not been done during the manoeuvre), load the bladder wth a suprapubic valve, individuate the future site of the hysterotomy and make the incision.

Extension and Morphology of the Hysterotomy (Curvilinear Path)

The main complications observed during hysterotomy are haemorrhaging of the incision surface or its lateral or caudal extension, with injury blood vessels.

In the statistics produced by WHO, death by hemorrhage during C-section is driven by a considerable percentage of cases of uncontrollable bleeding after lateral or caudal extension of the hysterotomy, either during expansion or on extraction of the presenting part.

While consensus exists that the hysterotomy should follow a curved line with a caudally directed concavity, there is no agreement on whether, once the initial hysterotomy has been executed, the incision should be expanded using the fingers or by sharp dissection.

Many authors (Magann, 2002; ACOG, 2002; NICE, 2004) recommended expansion using *blunt* (digital) *dissection* which is thought to involve less blood loss compared to *sharp dissection*.

Blunt expansion is achieved commonly when the operator pulls the index fingers apart from medial to lateral and cephalad at the same time (Fig. 15.5).

According to Cromi (2008) because circular and transversely running muscular bundles dominate the lower uterine segment, the uterine incision can be widened transversally by separating the surgeon's index fingers in the midline in a cephal-ad-caudad direction as well, resulting in less tissue trauma as dissection of the myometrium occurs along natural tissue planes.

An *extension* is defined as *any uterine wall defect*, either laterally into the uterine vasculature or vertically into the cervix or contractile uterus that *requires additional surgical steps to repair*.

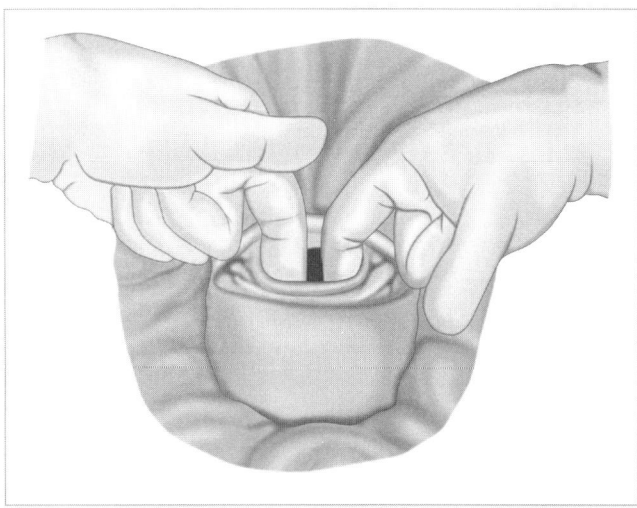

Fig. 15.5: Digital extension of the hysterotomy

Rodriguez (1994) and Hidar et al.(2007) found no difference between digital separation and sharp extension; Nazli (2004) is decidedly in favour of sharp dissection.

These two diverging guidances originate from very different clinical and geographical situations: Magann, ACOG and NICE express a Western experience, Nazli that of the kind of Obstetrics which is practiced in low resourced countries. Abalos (2004) points out that all the research on alternative techniques and materials in caesarean section is conducted in the West, where work environments and available resources are very different to those in countries with limited resources, where the population is not a "low risk population" and where gathering statistical data is inconceivable, for which reasons comparisons are not possible and findings not always applicable.

We believe that neither technique is better than the other, but that they each have very specific indications.

In a routine C-section, where the LUS still maintains its elasticity, expansion of the hysterotomy by means of digital separation is perfectly suitable. The elasticity of the myometrium makes up for the incomplete curvilinear incision and the manoeuvre is reasonably without haemorrhage.

But the condition of an LUS that has been overdistended due to a mechanical obstacle is very different: tissue elasticity has been used to its maximum, but not in a uniform way - stretching is greatest in the central part and least at the sides, with the distension curve showing an upward concavity (Fig. 15.6).

Under these conditions, digital separation is unlikely to succeed in imparting an upward curve to the hysterotomy: as the tissue has exhausted its elasticity, subsequent stress on the LUS due to insertion of the hand between it and the presenting part and operative delivery will cause a

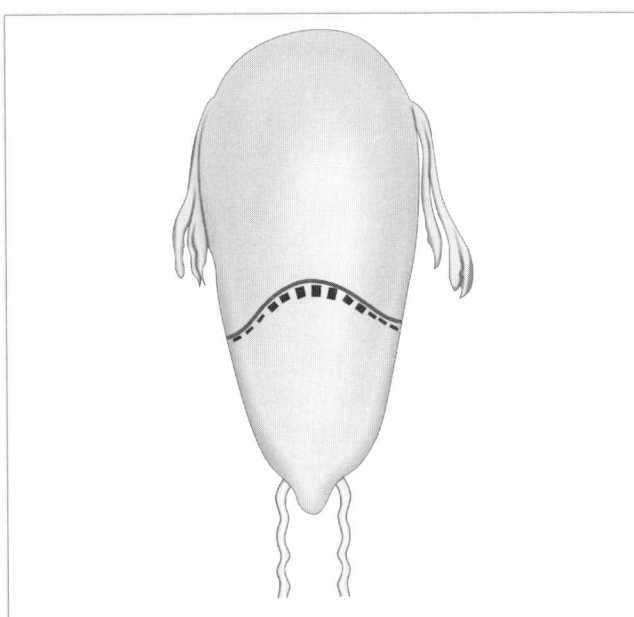

Fig. 15.6: Diagram of stress exerted on the LUS; it follows an upwardly concave curvilinear path. Stress is not uniform: At its maximum centrally, it decreases laterally. Digital divulsion follows the lines of strength (downwards)

laceration that will follow the line of stress - to the sides and caudad towards the cervix and vagina.

The authors although agreeing in finding digital extension perfectly acceptable when the LUS is not over distended, they routinely use *sharp dissection* (curved Mayo scissors with rounded tips): The curve of the scissors being parallel to that of the hysterotomy and the cut following a curvilinear path (Fig.15.7).

We believe that this makes the edges of the dissection clearer and improves their approximation on uterine suturing.

Delivery of the Foetus

The operating surgeon sets down any sharp instruments, introduces a free hand between the head and the lower uterine segment and proceeds until meeting the hand exerting external pressure, the fingers grasp and flex the head, which is retracted, gently lifted and delivered through the incision.

Possible Errors there are Two

a. *using the lower uterine segment as a prop:* this leads to catastrophic extension of the incision and may be obviated by checking that the operating table is tilted downwards and always keeping the forearm parallel to the axis of the uterus;

b. *force is exerted by the hand:* the sole function of the hand is to grasp and flex the head (Fig. 15.8); force is exerted by the arm and shoulder; the forearm is parallel to the uterus. Where the operating surgeon's arm is not strong enough, the solution is a simple one: the hand keeps its grip function and the surgeon moves his/her body weight in the opposite direction. Ideally they should know which side the foetal back is lying in order to carry out delivery of the head. Simultaneous gentle pressure on the fundus can facilitate expulsion of the head (Fig. 15.9), but fundal pressure should not be extended over time as it has haemodynamic effects on mother and foetus (Kim et al., 2006).

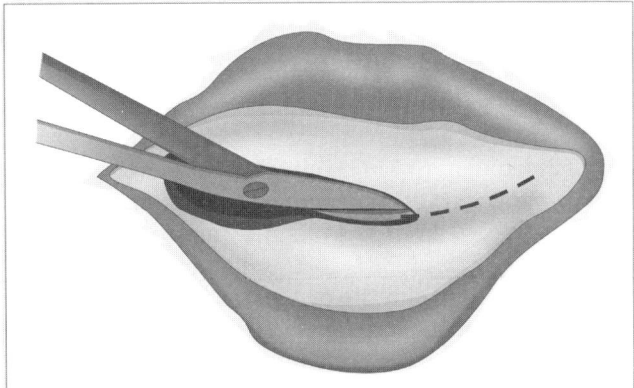

Fig. 15.7: Extension of hysterotomy using scissors. The incision follows a curvilinear path with inferior convexity

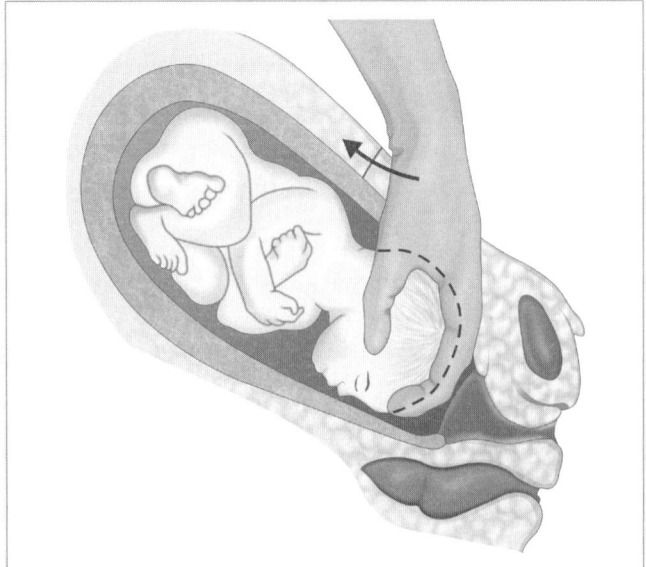

Fig. 15.8: Disengagement of the head: The forearm is parallel with the uterus' main axis; the hand exerts a gripping function only and should not use the inferior LUS margin as a prop during extraction. Force is exerted by the body, the shoulder and the arm

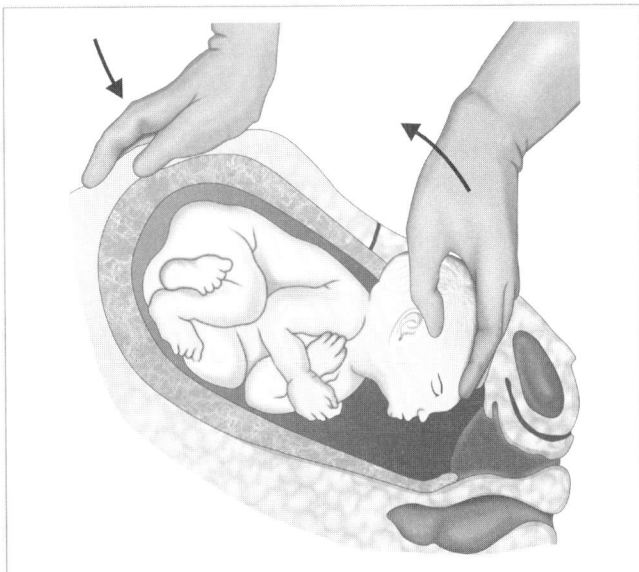

Fig. 15.9: Difficult operative delivery: Pressure on the fundus will facilitate flexion and delivery of the head

Difficult operative delivery: This may be linked to:
a. *Breadth of hysterotomy is incompatible with*:
   - the dimensions of the presenting part
   - a deeply impacted head
   - contraction ring action (see Chapter 3).

   A vertical incision in the central part of the superior edge of the hysterotomy (inverted T shaped incision) is recommended, to be preferably preceded by a similar cutaneous incision.
b. *Occipitoposterior rotation*, face presentation to the hysterotomy. The chin, which presents first, is grasped between thumb (placed on tongue Fig. 15.10) and forefinger and, by means of traction, is disengaged. Delivery of the head follows.
c. *Head high*: The head is high and does not spontaneously present to the hysterotomy, even under fundal pressure by the operating surgeon; in this case one proceeds with *version within the uterus*. A simple manoeuvre that always succeeds; identify head and back, follow the back down to the buttocks, having identified a leg, follow it distally to the foot, which, grasped, allows *version in uterus* and reverse breech delivery. There is no hurry as long as the foetus is attached to the placenta.
d. *Breech presentation*: extraction is performed following the same principles as a frank breech delivery, buttocks are extracted by hooking the groin with the index fingers; extraction of the lower limbs and trunk follows. Appearance of the inferior angles of the scapulae (scapulae visible) indicates the moment to deliver the shoulders using Lovset's manoeuvre. This is followed by delivery of the head; if difficulties are encountered, use a vertical incision of the upper edge; see above.
e. *Transverse position*: this indicates a *vertical hysterotomy*; where access to the uterine cavity is via a transverse hysterotomy, the shoulder is the largest part of the foetus to present first and very often the operating surgeon extracts the arm. Excluding a small foetus or polyhydramnios, operative delivery will be very difficult. A vertical incision is made to the central point of the upper edge of the hysterotomy (inverted-T incision).

Cord Clamping

The optimal timing for clamping the umbilical cord after birth has been a subject of controversy and debate; in 2009 Erikson-Owens stated "that *immediate clamping* is routine at caesarean section but lacks scientific evidence".

Physiologic studies in term infants have shown that a transfer from the placenta of approximately 80 ml of blood occurs by 1 minute after birth, reaching approximately 100 mL at 3 minutes after birth. On the assumption that gravity affects the volume of placental transfusion mandatory is holding the baby at least 20 cm below the level of the placenta, for 30–60 secs or more before clamping (*delayed cord clamping*).

This additional blood can supply extra iron, amounting to 40–50 mg/kg of body weight. This extra iron, combined with body iron (approximately 75 mg/kg of body weight) present at birth in a full-term newborn, may help prevent iron deficiency during the first year of life, poor iron stores can affect the developing brain,

Delayed cord clamping it is a safe, simple and low cost delivery procedure aimed at reducing iron deficiency anaemia in infants in developing countries; other associated neonatal benefits are a decreased incidence of intracranial haemorrhage in preterm infants. This applies also to vaginal delivery.

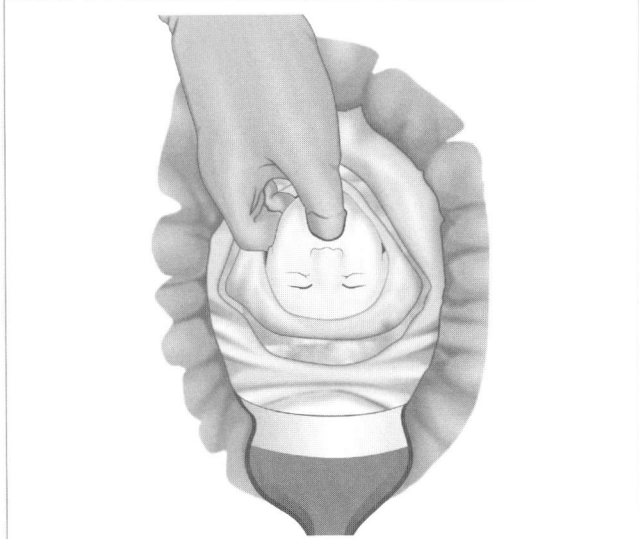

Fig. 15.10: Occipitoposterior position or face front presentation. The chin is grasped between thumb and index finger and extracted first

The authors' procedure varies according to circumstances:

Under normal conditions the baby is delivered and wrapped in the warm towel and held on the right side of the mother's thigh about 20 cm below the height of the incision. Sound procedure is covering the umbilical cord with a warm towel (the cord constricts with exposure to cold) while stimulating the baby to achieve adequate respiration prior to clamping; 40–60 seconds after delivery the cord is clamped and cut and the baby taken for resuscitation if necessary."

If the neonate is severely depressed with meconium-stained amniotic fluid the surgeon, to promote the outflow of fluid from the lungs and upper airways, as happens when the trunk in vaginal delivery progresses through the birth canal, holding the baby by the feet brings it to his own trunk and exert pressure on the thorax, clears the mouth and proceeds with *cord milking*, procedure which is strongly recommended in caesarean section for anterior placenta previa.

With low birth-weight babies, this manoeuvre is not advised or should be only partial to avoid overloading the circulation.

Concerns exist regarding universally adopting delayed umbilical cord clamping, which may jeopardize timely resuscitation efforts, if needed, especially in preterm infants. However, because the placenta continues to perform gas exchange after delivery, sick and preterm infants are likely to benefit most from additional blood volume derived from a delay in umbilical cord clamping. Another concern has been raised that delay in umbilical cord clamping increases the potential for excessive placental transfusion, which can lead to neonatal polycythemia, especially in the presence of risk factors for foetal polycythemia, such as maternal diabetes, severe intrauterine growth restriction, and high altitude.

With the baby delivered, the anaesthetist makes an I.V. injection of an oxytocin (ergometrine 0.4 mg, or oxytocin 5–10 I.U.)

■ HIGH TRANSVERSE HYSTEROTOMY (FIG. 15.2D)

The sole indication for this is obstructed labour with cephalic presentation.

In obstructed labour, the greatest danger comes from lateral and caudal extension of the hysterotomy during delivery *of the foetus* with injury to the uterine vessels and to the base of the broad ligament, with often uncontrollable hemorrhage (see Chapter 17 on how this haemorrhaging may be controlled).

Extension is sustained through stress exceeding the residual elasticity of an overdistended LUS following insertion of the operating surgeon's hand between the LUS and the deeply impacted presenting part. Predisposing factors are a hysterotomy that is inadequate in terms of *site* - where the breadth of the LUS is insufficient at that point for the dimensions of the head - and in terms of *morphology* - where the hysterotomy does not follow a curvilinear line with its ends pointing cephalad, for which reason the extension takes a caudad path.

The distension, mechanical obstruction (cephalopelvic disproportion or obstructed labour) imposes on the LUS, acts both cephalad and laterally, and so at its border with the upper segment, it will be 12–13 cm in breadth. This allows a very wide hysterotomy and ease of access for the hand that, identifying a foot, grasps it and, accomplishing a version *in utero*, extracts the baby by *reverse breech delivery*.

This is the manoeuvre widely employed by the authors, and which they consider a reasonable compromise between the disadvantages of a low vertical hysterotomy and the dangers of a transverse one. It is strongly recommended for its ease of execution, safety and good quality of uterine suturing (strictly in double-layer).

One difficulty it presents is that of matching two edges having differing thickness. For closure of the second layer, the authors prefer a continuous mattress suture.

Once fear of not finding a foot has been overcome, the procedure proves simple indeed.

Uterine Exteriorization

There is disagreement among obstetricians over the practice of exteriorising the uterus following operative delivery. Exteriorisation (Fig. 15.11) is a routine practice with us. In our opinion it offers better control of the uterus, easier suturing and a more precise assessment of blood loss,

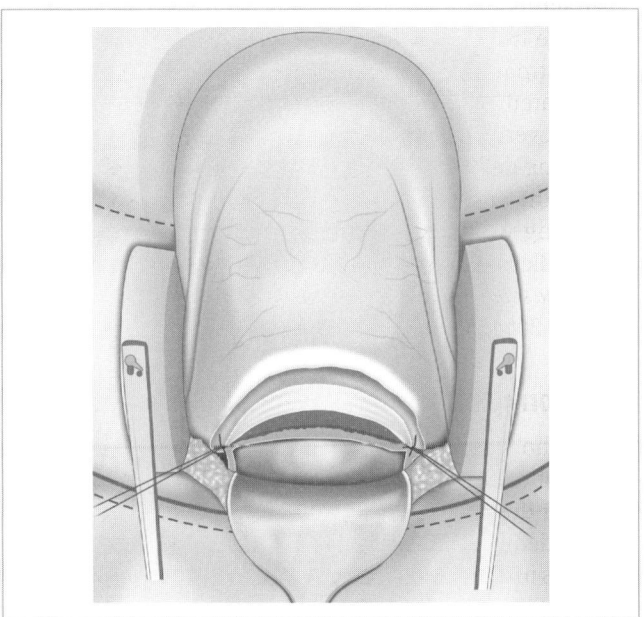

Fig. 15.11: Uterine exteriorization

which is reduced compared to the loss occurring when the uterus remains *in situ*. many studies have been made of the topic; the first (Hershley and Quilligan, 1978) was followed by many more (Combs et al., 1991; Magann et al., 1993; Magann et al. 1995; Edi-Osagie et al., 1998; Wahab et al., 1999). The reduction in blood loss could be ascribed to the reduction in capacity of the uterine blood vessels following their stretching (LaPlace's law) due to the exteriorizing and reduced congestion of the uterus. Finally, profuse bleeding can be more easily controlled using two-handed compression of the area of the hysterotomy (one hand on the posterior and one on the anterior parts of the LUS), by applying finger pressure on the uterine blood vessels, or by ligation of the ascending branches of the uterine arteries (Fig. 17.2).

A Cochrane review of the issue (Jakobs et al., 2004) found no significant differences between the two techniques (extra- or intra-abdominal repair). The first was associated with lower maternal morbidity, but with slightly longer period of hospitalisation.

Third Stage of Labour

We do not remove the placenta manually for two reasons:
- *Control of blood loss*: Rapid emptying of the uterus (foetus and amniotic fluid) is followed by a period of atony, whose duration is proportional to duration of labour, myometrial glycogen depletion and maternal acidemia and dehydration. During this period, hemostasis in the site of placental attachment, ensured by the plexiform network, does not occur, which will give us two sites of haemorrhage: The hysterotomy and the site of placental attachment.

In the tropics, anaemia due to malaria, malnutrition, intestinal parasites and maternal exhaustion due to repeated pregnancie is endemic. We should therefore take every measure to avoid blood loss.

Having delivered the fetus and leaving the placenta *in situ*, the operating surgeon commences uterine suture, during which the oxytocin will act and an almost bloodless third stage of labour will be observed.
- *Increased risk of inflammation*: Magann et al., 1995, Nice, 2004.

Hysterorraphy

The authors are aware that consensus is yet to be reached on whether uterine suturing should be performed using a single or double-layer. Critical reviews of the issue appear to have demonstrated a slightly higher percentage of uterine ruptures in low segment transverse hysterotomies repaired using a single layer (see also Chapter 10).

Using chromic surgical catgut N°1, Hauth et. al (1992) found significant differences in subsequent pregnancies in parturients in whom uterine suturing was conducted in a single layer compared to those receiving a double-layer. Similar findings were reached by Durnwald and Mercer (2003).

NICE finds that the efficacy of single-layer suturing has not been proven and recommends repair using double- layer. Bujold et al. (2002) found that in subsequent pregnancies, single-layer uterine suturing is four times more likely to encounter uterine rupture than double-layer. Gyamfi (2006) showed that the incidence of uterine ruptures in single-layer suturing is 8.6% against 1.3% for double-layer.

Statistical findings aside, we believe that the question could be reformulated in the light of the short- and long-term objectives the operating surgeon has set for the surgery.
- *In the short term*: Control of haemorrhage and closure of the hysterotomy; rapid reduction of the extension to the hysterotomy (from 10 to 3 cm in three days), remedying shortcomings in technique or in approximation of the edges
- *In the long term*: The quality of the scar is good when minimal is the structural and consequent functional subversion of the tissue where the scar has developed from; with reference to the uterus the required capacity is: Solidity, the ability to resist to the stress of distension which occurs during labour.

Diriment in this respect is the histological examination of a scar from a previous C-section: In large scars, muscle fibrocells invest the edges of the scar without crossing it; *it is in this site that*, in the event of uterine rupture (dehiscence), tissue disruption occurs, not within the scar.

In small-sized scars, muscle fibrocells bridge across the scar; there is minimal structural and functional subversion, so this is a solid, high-quality scar that does not interfere with the conduction (polarity) of uterine contractions, nor does it represent a risk factor of uterine rupture during a trial of labour.

Scar Quality and Extension

These are determined by:

a. *The amount of suture material utilised*: This is linked to the thickness of suturing material and the number of stitches or loops (in the case of continuous suture) that the operating surgeon uses in repairing a hysterotomy with an average width of approx. 10 cm. If the stitches are spaced 1 centimetre apart, on the fourth day (when the hysterotomy measures 4 cm) we will have one suture every 4 mm (crowding). We believe that a distance of not less than 12 mm between each stitch to be appropriate.

b. *Techique*: The function of interrupted or continuous suturing is to bring wound edged into apposition without inducing *ischemia*, which occurs and induces in fibrous tissue when the simple interrupted stitches or the loops

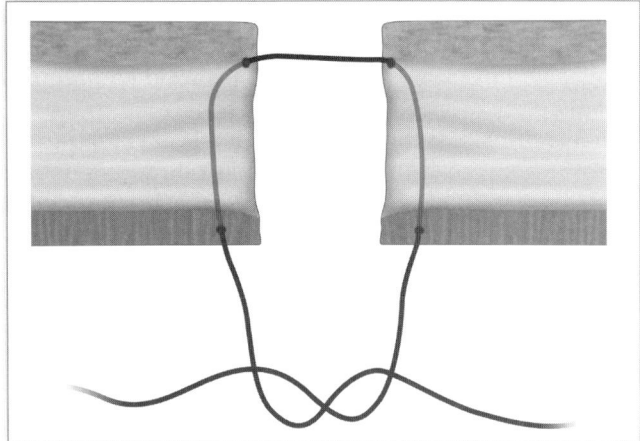

Fig. 15.12: Uterine closure using simple interrupted sutures Suturing technique follows the motto "in-out-out- in". The two ends are knotted inside the cavity, thereby reducing the amount of extraneous material in the myometrium

of simple or interlocked running sutures are too tight and strangulate the blood vessels.

When interrupted sutures are used, it is good practice to knot the stitch inside the cavity, thereby reducing the amount of extraneous material within the myometrium (Fig. 15.12).

c. *Quality of suturing material utilised*: Chromic catgut gives rise to larger quantity of scar tissue than do polyglycolic acid sutures. After forty days, the catgut stitch has been completely reabsorbed, but the suturing site is indicated by a dense mass of macrophages ringed by numerous lymphocites. This is not observed with sutures derived from polyglycolic acid or similar. The thread should preferably be monofilament and non-porous to avoid the capillary transmission of infections.

d. *Correct apposition of surfaces*: The different layers of myometrium have differing elasticity coefficients (higher in superficial, lower in deeper layers). When the hysterotomy is completed, retraction of the superficial layers is greater than in the deeper ones and the wound surface will take on the shape of a truncated V. Retraction does not occur uniformly on each hysterotomy edge: The superior edge undergoes less retraction, it follows a nearly vertical course, is shorter and thicker. The inferior edge undergoes greater retraction and is longer and thinner, so the two arms of the V-shape are not identical.

Resolution of the debate over whether the hysterotomy should be repaired using a single or double layer now passes to the operating surgeon. If the surgeon can guarantee that these two surfaces of varying thickness can be brought into contact using a single layer only, then single- layer uterine suturing is indicated. If the surgeon cannot guarantee this (and we cannot) then double-layer repair becomes advisable.

Our decision is also influenced by the long-term outcomes of incomplete approximation of the two edges: Excessive thinning of the LUS, down to a thickness of less than 1.6 mm at term of pregnancy is a major risk factor for uterine rupture (Asakura et al., 2000).

If, then, the choice is between starting the stitches from the outside, following the motto "out-in-in-out", or from the inside of the cavity, according to the motto "in-out-out- in", we follow the latter. The reason is simple, and is also to be found in the differing elasticity coefficients of myometrium and decidua.

Having been subjected to stress during delivery of the presenting part with an extension of the hysterotomy, the myometrium returns to its initial dimensions, once the stress is over. This is not the case with the decidua, whose lack of elasticity imposes a more extensive injury than that incurred by the more superficial myometrium.

If we wish to include the apex of the incision from the outside, we run the risk of moving too far laterally and damaging the uterine blood vessels, which mark the lateral border of the lower uterine segment. By starting the suture from inside, these vessels will be avoided, therefore the first stitches are "in-out-out-in" and the knotting occurs inside the cavity.

Irrespective of the way in which the first layer is executed, the problem arises of whether or not the decidua should be included in the suturing.

The principle that the decidua should not be included in the suture is currently under review. Yazicioglu et al. (2006) appear to have demonstrated that *not including it* compromises the quality of healing, "By selecting full-thickness suturing technique one may significantly lower the incidence of incomplete healing of the uterine incision after CS".

e. Suturing of the second layer can take place by means of an interlooking suture or using a mattress suture, which is especially indicated where the inferior edge is very thin, and which also offers the advantage that the suture material remains outside.

f. *sterile or infected wound surface.*

g. *patient's state of nutrition and circulation.*

METHOD USED BY THE AUTHORS

The authors use three continuous sutures to repair the hysterotomy (miometrium: double-layer, peritoneum: single layer) using N° 1 absorbable suturing material on atraumatic round-bodied needle.

Suture 1: The first suture (Fig. 15.13) starts from the edge opposite the operating surgeon. It is applied following the formula "in-out-out-in", followed by knotting and checking that the stitch includes myometrium and decidua equally

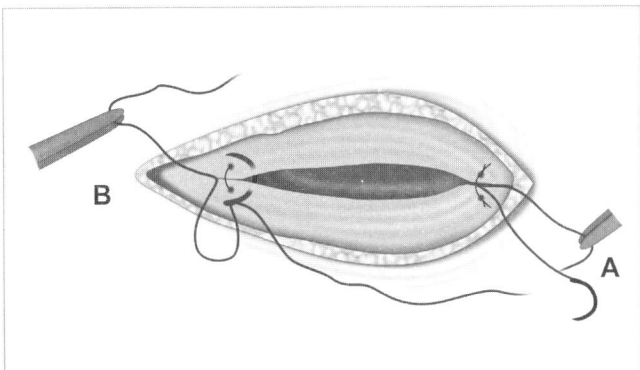

Fig. 15.13: Uterine suturing, first layer. The first suture, (A) begins from the opposite side to the operating surgeon and stops after the first stitch. A marker is attached to the tail end. The second suture, (B) begins from the operating surgeon's side and proceeds in an anteroposterior direction

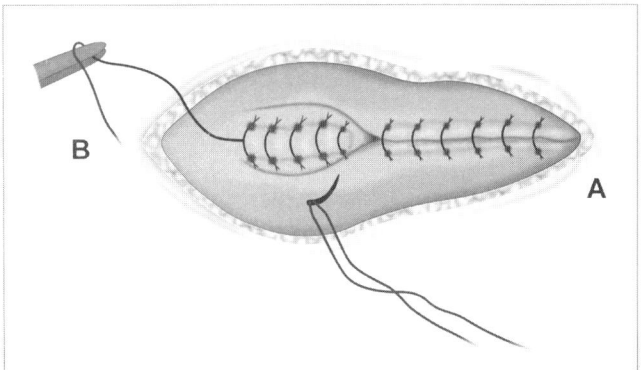

Fig. 15.15: Hysterotomy repair, second layer. The first suture: A now proceeds towards the operating surgeon and, on reaching angle B, is knotted with the marker of the second suture: A

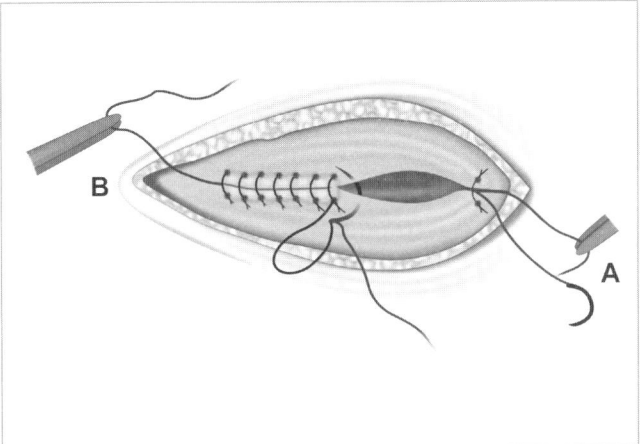

Fig. 15.14: Uterine suturing, first layer. The second suture: (B) proceeds towards the angle opposite the operating surgeon; once reached, it is consolidated with the marker (A)

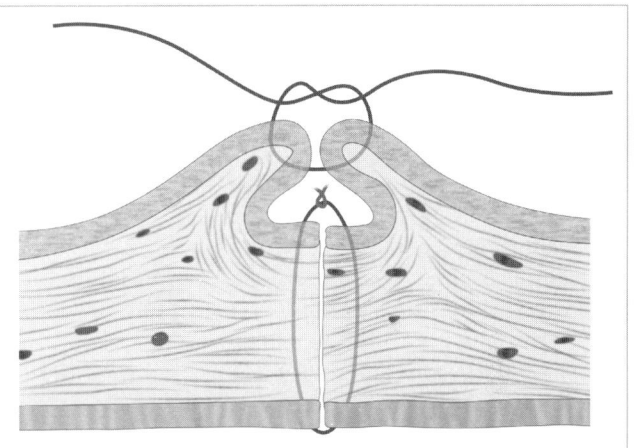

Fig. 15.16: In executing the second layer, extra care should be taken not to create a dead space, which could become a seat of infection difficult to control

and that there are no oozing areas. A tail at least 8 cm long is held with a forceps. The suture stops here.

Suture 2 starts from the operating surgeon side (Fig. 15.14), a tail, at least 8 cm long and held with a forceps, is left. The suture progresses in an anteroposterior direction reaching *suture 1* to whose tail is knotted: *The first layer is now completed.* The suture is not cut.

We precede suturing of the second layer with the following manoeuvre, which can be conducted only on an exteriorised uterus. The operating surgeon holds the uterus between both hands. The dominant hand, on the anterior uterine wall, has its fingers in contact, via surgical gauze soaked in saline, with the suturing. The other hand, on the posterior wall, with the fingers at the level of the suturing, exerts compression for a short time after which fingers and gauze are withdrawn. The suturing site and the edges of the hysterotomy to which the second layer are to be applied, will be clearly seen and bloodless.

This manoeuvre is very useful in cases of profuse bleeding from the hysterotomy. Compression protracted over one minute will render the edges bloodless and facilitate hemostasis. When executing the second layer, care should be taken not to create a little tunnel between the two layers (Fig. 15.16), in which serous fluids or blood can accumulate, an ideal pabulum for germs in a place hard for antibiotics to reach. An infection developing in this site will be hard to control and liable to compromise the quality of the suture, if not causing dehiscence.

Second layer: With suture 1 (Fig. 15.15A) we now start suturing proceeding in a postero-anterior direction until meeting the origin of *suture 2* (Fig. 15.15B), to whose tail is knotted. The suture is not cut. *Second layer repair is so completed.*

Visceral peritonisation, by means of a purse-string suture employing suture 1, begins at the surgeon's side; once completed a similar procedure is performed on the opposite edge and the suture procedure in a posterior anterior direction until the tail of the purse-string suture, on the surgeon's side, is reached and to it tied.

Peritoneal Closure

Peritoneal closure should meet two requirements:
a. *Prevent the spread of inflammation* from within the uterine cavity to the peritoneal cavity. The peritoneal property of preventing the spread of intrauterine inflammation to the abdominal cavity is well established and was, during the pre-antibiotic era, one of the motivating grounds for numerous C-section techniques, from that of Munro Kerr (partly extraperitoneal) to fully extraperitoneal techniques (Marshall, 1939; Ricci, 1942; Botella Llusia, 1949; Crichton, 1973). Still today, King's *Primary Surgery* recommends extraperitoneal C-section following Crichton (Fig. 15.24) in the presence of infection. Because of its simplicity, we strongly recommend this technique, which we describe, along with that of Botella Llusia, at the end of this Chapter.
The spread of inflammation to the abdominal cavity has immediate and delayed effects.
   - *Immediate* consequences include postoperative fever, potential ileus, dehiscence of uterine or laparotomic suture and poor quality of both the uterine and the laparotomic scar.

In the presence of severe intrauterine inflammation, some authors (us included), recommend preceding visceral closure of the peritoneum with meticulous lavage of the vesicouterine space using metronidazole solution and the placing of antibiotics in powder-form, as this is a difficult area to access for generally administered antibiotics and, apart from compromising the quality of healing, inflammation would be hard to control.
   - The *long-term* consequences include, in the case of subsequent labours, a *uterine scar* lacking stability (solidity) due to ample scar tissue that also represents an obstacle to uterine contractions, and a broad, thick *laparotomic scar* with an irregular border, adhering to the underlying tissue. These two clinical aspects are almost always present.

b. *Prevent adhesions between the uterine and abdominal wall*, which are especially tough and widespread in the case of concomitant infection. Not infrequently they impede subsequent pregnancy, the correct alignment during labour of the foetal axis with that of the birth canal, as well as being an obstacle to the normal propagation of the contraction wave (polarity) with contractile asymmetries of the uterus.

The authors are aware that there is as yet no resolution to the debate over whether (visceral or parietal) peritoneal closure should be carried out or not. This debate arose from a paper by Ellis and Heddle (1977), who hypothesized that these surgical steps were not indispensible. This paper gave rise to a long series of studies, some in favour (Elkins et al. 1987; Tulandi, 1988, Al Took 1999; Nather, 2001) and others against (Cheong et al., 2001; Myers et al., 2005). One of the arguments against peritoneal closure is the formation of adhesions, Buckman, (1976). Examining small-bowel obstructions arising after laparo-hysterectomy, Al Took (1999) found that 85% arose on visceral peritonealisation and the reamaining 15% on parietal peritonealisation. The argument that adhesions follow peritoneal closure could easily be turned back on its supporters: "it is not that peritoneal closure gave rise to adhesions, the contrary is the case: incomplete peritonealisation at that point is responsible for adhesions. Some of the arguments against peritoneal closure are ludicrous: the reduction of surgical time; a surgeon takes no more than three minutes to perform the two steps.

Myers et al. (2005) recently highlighted how percentages and extensions of adhesions are significantly greater in surgery where peritoneal closure has not been conducted, from which they conclude: "While preliminary, in the absence of any substantive benefit or published data regarding adhesion formation in cesarean section that contradict this finding, *the practice of nonclosure of visceral and parietal peritoneum at cesarean section should be questioned*".

We believe that the problem's solution is to be found in long-term outcomes.

The careful peritoneal closure (visceral and parietal) is a constant step in our operations. When we operate again on C-sections performed by us in the past, we sometimes find adhesions, but infrequent and never extensive, while these are always present and particularly extensive and stubborn when re-operating on patients in whom these stages were omitted (especially where non-closure was accompanied by inflammation). In the Tropics, most C-sections are performed as emergency surgery on women whose membranes have long since broken, with infected uterine cavity. Surgery is often performed in environments and with instrumentation whose sterility is not always perfectly guaranteed.

Intraoperative Measurement of the Obstetric Conjugate

Routine intraoperative measurement of the obstetric conjugate is an indispensible surgical step, as it often enables the discovery of previously undiagnosed pelvic abnormalities. Above all it offers precise determination of whether, in a subsequent pregnancy, trial of labour should be advised or an elective C-section, thereby avoiding the risk of uterine rupture (Adadevoh et al., 1989, van Dillen, 2007).

Indeed, we have found very restricted obstetric conjugates in some cases of uterine rupture that have come to our attention, which, if adequately assessed during a previous C-section, would have spared the patient's exposure to such a risk.

The manoeuvre is a very simple one: Having completed visceral peritoneal closure, the uterus is displaced to the right and, using a DeLee pelvimeter, or in its absence, forceps and a ruler, the distance is measured between the central part of the sacral promontory and the central point of the internal face of the pubic symphysis (Figs 15.17 and 15.18),

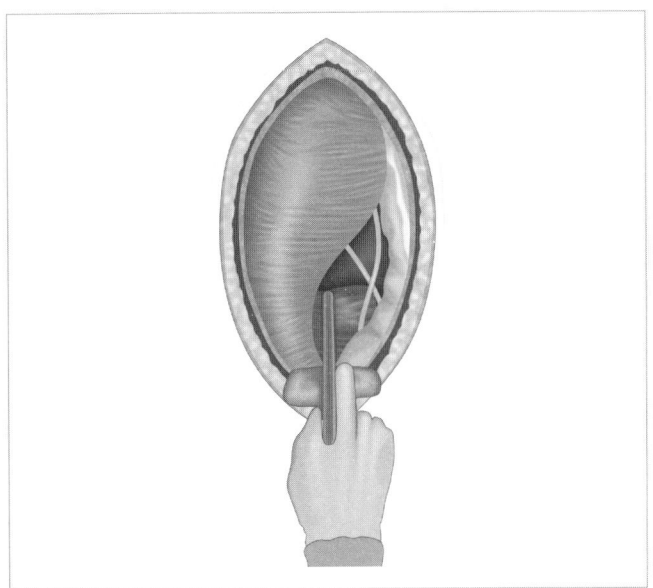

Fig. 15.17: Intraoperative measurement of the obstetric conjugate. Once the uterus has been replaced in the cavity and displaced to the right, a ruler is used to measure the distance between the promontory of the sacrum and the innermost point of symphysis posterior surface

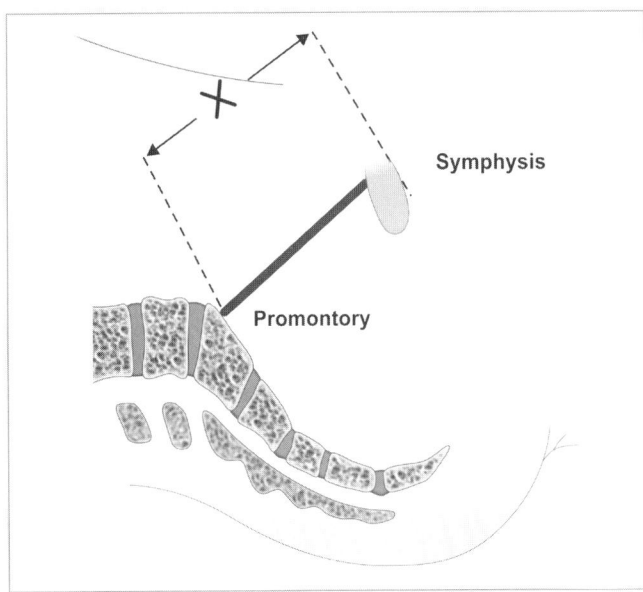

Fig. 15.18: See previous figure, saggital section

recording the value. One may be surprised by disagreements found between the obstetric conjugate as determined indirectly by vaginal exploration and that found intraoperatively (Domini et al., 2007).

Lavage of the Abdominal Cavity

About this step, too, there is disagreement: Some authors maintain that, given the excellent blood-absorbing capacity of peritoneum, lavage of the abdominal cavity is not necessary. Other authors recommend lavage using saline or low-molecular-weight dextran to prevent adhesions; yet others recommend, in the presence of inflammation, lavage with ampicillin, 2 grams, or with metronidazole.

Hillingam (2003), who conducted a critical review of the matter, considers lavage a ritual: "There are probably as many rituals in surgery as there are surgeons," and concludes that "Routine intra-abdominal irrigation at cesarean delivery *in a low-risk population* has no effect on postoperative maternal morbidity".

We routinely carry out careful cavity toilet and lavage using isotonic solutions as prophylaxis against adhesions, a *special attention is deserved to the pouch of Douglas;* in cases of inflammation, we add metronidazole solution.

In cases of severe dehydration, following careful cavity toilet, and in order to avoid circulatory overload, 500 ml of isotinic saline and 500 ml of glucose 5% solution may be left in the cavity, taking advantage of the peritoneum's capacity for absorption.

Bringing the Uterus Back in Line

This step precedes suturing of the abdominal wall; it consists in gathering the uterin fundus in the palm of one's hand, bringing it into contact with the pubic symphysis and keeping it in this position for some time. One will soon observe how a contraction occurs, which becomes constant over time.

Repositioning of the uterine axes, performed intraoperatively and during puerperium, should also be considered prophylactic against retroversion of the uterus, a frequent cause of secondary infertility.

EXTRAPERITONEAL TRANSVERSE HYSTEROTOMIES

These include a series of operations conceived during the pre-antibiotic era, which are still indicated under certain circumstances. Access to the LUS is made without access to the peritoneal cavity, thereby preventing its contamination by intrauterine inflammation.

Extraperitoneal C-sections may be:
- Elective
- Emergency.

Elective Extraperitoneal C-section

Occasional outcomes of C-section conducted in the presence of uterine infection, or of prolonged labour with membranes that have been broken over hours, are wound infection, peritonitis and paralytic ileus (often associated with pneumonia) and possibly fatal septic shock.

In a high percentage of cases, even meticulous observation of asepsis and antisepsis, careful surgical technique and hemostasis conducted under strictly aseptic conditions, meticulous toilet of the abdominal cavity and generous use of antibiotics do not prevent the above-mentioned complications, which are even more common in African rural hospitals.

Thus, arises the need to re-use surgical techniques that, in the West, belong pre antibiotic era. These include extraperitoneal C-section which, now as then, offers a way of saving a woman's life and fertility.

The observation that an extraperitoneal approach to the uterine cavity prevents the spread of inflammation from the uterus to the abdominal cavity provides further confirmation of the appropriateness of peritoneal closure during C-section. We would like to assure the reader that these techniques, like all the techniques described in this manual have been successfully tested by the authors, are simple and effective. We describe two technques:

a. *The Botella Llusia (1949) Hysterotomy*

A preliminary step is the bladder instillation of 150-200 ml methylene blue or gentian violet solution (Latzko, 1909). The laparotomy follows (see Chapter 13) Cherney incision with a transverse curvilinear incision of skin and fascia. The pyramidalis muscles (Fig. 15.19) are dissected free and

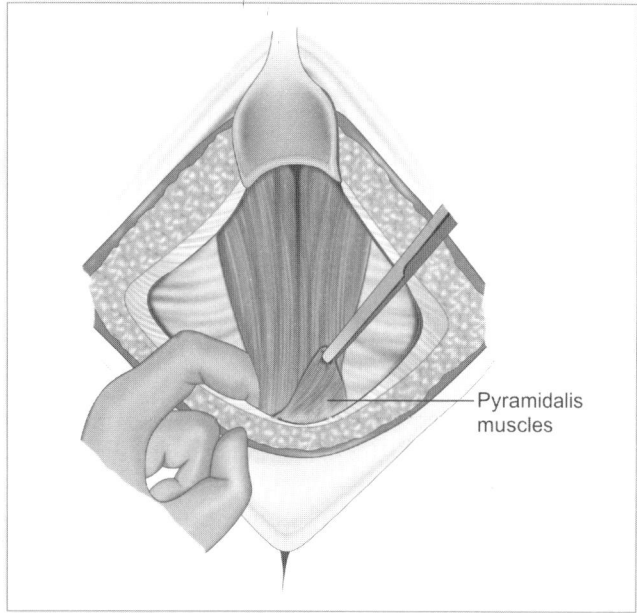

Fig. 15.19: Extraperitoneal C-section: Laparotomy according to Cherney—the pyramidalis muscles are separated from the recti

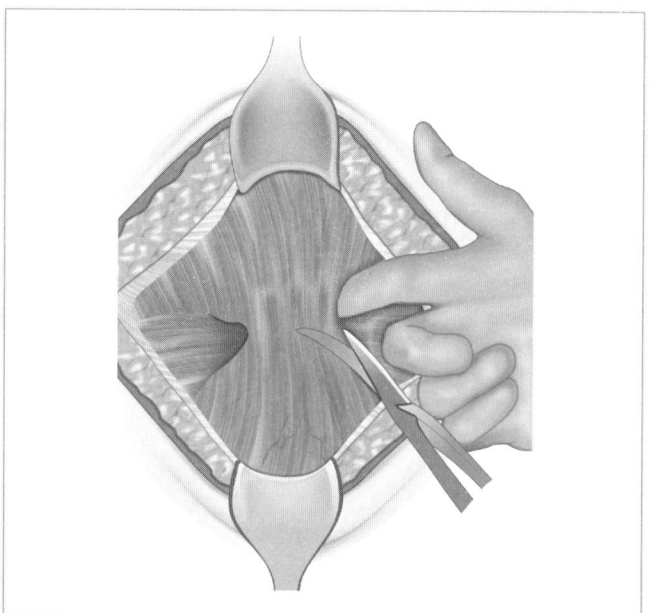

Fig. 15.20: Bladder mobilisation, sharp dissection of the area of greatest adherence of the bladder to the peritoneum

sharply excised to expose the underlying *rectus tendons*; with an index finger, a plane is developed between the fibrous tendons of the rectus muscle and the underlying transversalis fascia. Using a sharp no.10 scalpel blade, the rectus tendons are transected transversely 1-2 cm cranial to the superior edge of the pubic bone. *Rectus muscle should never be cut.*

Now follows mobilisation of the bladder from the LUS, which is initially performed by blunt and sharp dissection, proceeding lateromedially and in a cephalad direction, first on one side, then contralaterally, and finally by sharp dissection (Fig. 15.20).

We perform this in the following way: We grasp the bladder between thumb (on one side) and index and middle finger (on the other). Keeping our fingertips in contact with the LUS, we execute separation with simultaneous elevation by traction. Mobilisation is immediate and very easily done.

Having reached at the site of peritoneal reflection (from parietal to visceral) in proximity of the dome of the bladder, this is separated first upwards and then the bladder is separated downwards, thereby exposing a broad area of the LUS.

Having executed the initial hysterotomy (by sharp dissection, with a width of 2-3 cm), we apply a two stay sutures (Fig. 15.21) are inserted and the uterus is incised with a width of 2-3 cm, digital expansion follows (Fig. 15.22).

We believe the application of STAY sutures to be a very important step in that it enables identification of the wound edges and traction on them will reduce haemorrhage. The subsequent steps are those described for transverse hysterotomies. Closure is accomplished with 5-6 horizontal mattress sutures of permanent braided suture material

TRANSVERSE HYSTEROTOMIES

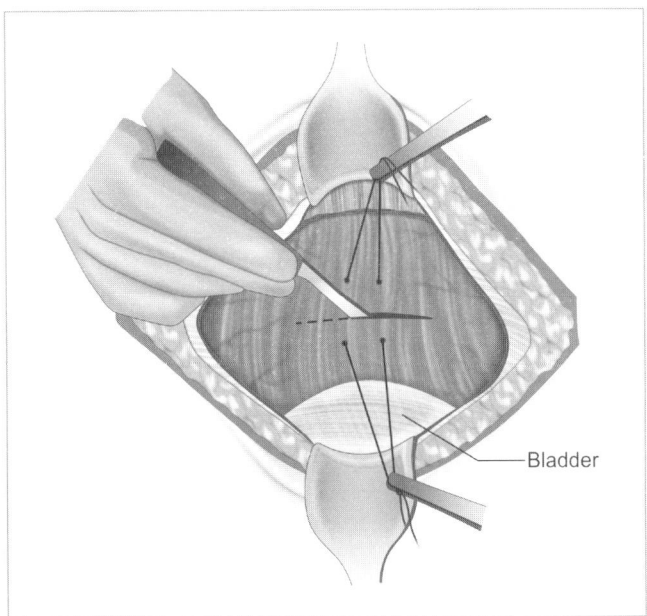

Fig. 15.21: Hysterotomy, application of reference stitches

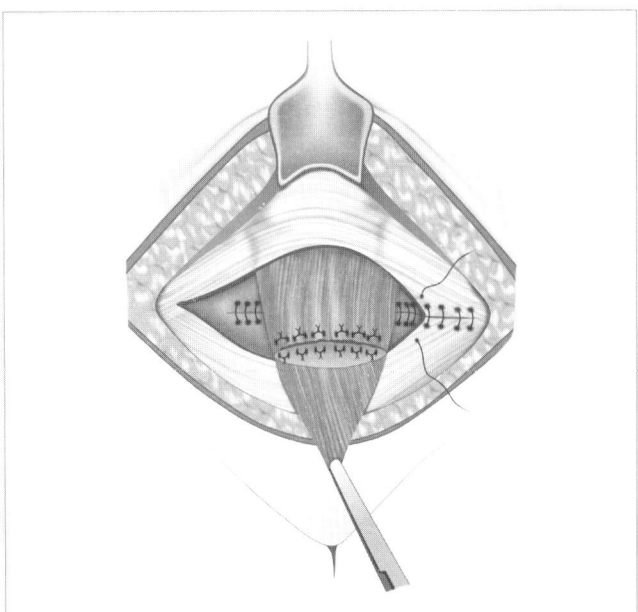

Fig. 15.23. Reinsertion of the rectus muscles to their attachment, while the pyramidalis muscles are kept under traction

retracted, latterally and caudad, from the overlying muscle planes.
- Having identified the uracus, forceps are applied close to its origin (Fig. 15.24A)
- Using traction on the forceps, the uracus and parietal peritoneum are placed under tension; both are dissected tranversely on both sides along a length of 3 cm (Fig. 15.24B)
- Again, energetic traction is exerted on the forceps to place the vesicouterine pouch under tension. This is incised transversely on both sides, to a width of 3 cm (Fig. 15.24C)
- The visceral peritoneum (which covers the LUS) is elevated as far as possible until the superior border of the LUS is reached (Fig. 15.24D)
- The parietal and visceral edges are sutured together; the peritoneal cavity is now closed once again (Fig. 15.17).

One has thereby exposed an ample portion of the LUS, on which one now proceeds as described for the Botella-Llusia technique.

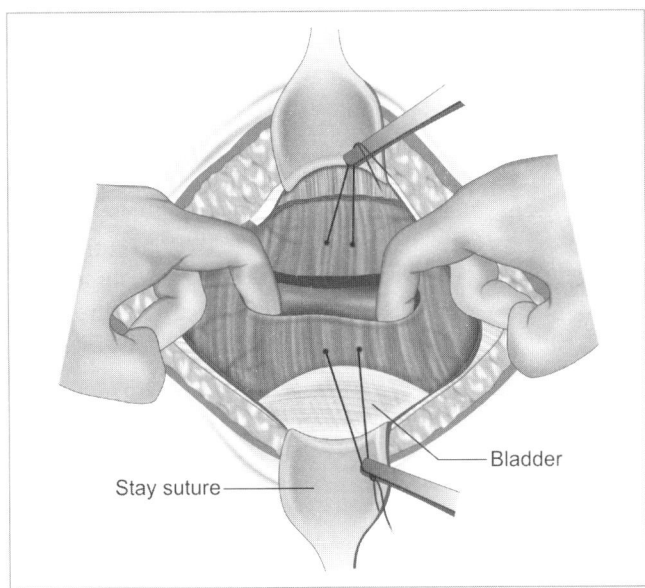

Fig. 15.22: Digital expansion of uterine incision. For the sake of clarity, pyramidalis muscles have not been shown

approximating the anterior rectus tendons to the intact distal anterior rectus fascia (Fig. 15.23).

b. *Crichton's Hysterotomy Technique (1974)*

Abdomen is entered through a subumbilical midline laparotomy.

The surgical steps are as follows: Incision of skin, subcutis and fascia; digital separation of the rectus muscles and identification of the transversalis fascia, which is extensively

Emergency Extraperitoneal C-section

Often, following a C-section in which peritoneal closure was not performed, extensive adhesions form between the uterine and the anterior abdominal walls, making it impossible to distinguish between the two planes. Here surgery is very simple if done in the following way.

In the case of a vertical laparotomy, by extending the cutaneous and fascia incision caudad (mons pubis) until the pubic symphysis is reached, it will be possible to identify the pyramidalis muscles, which, when separated, will indicate

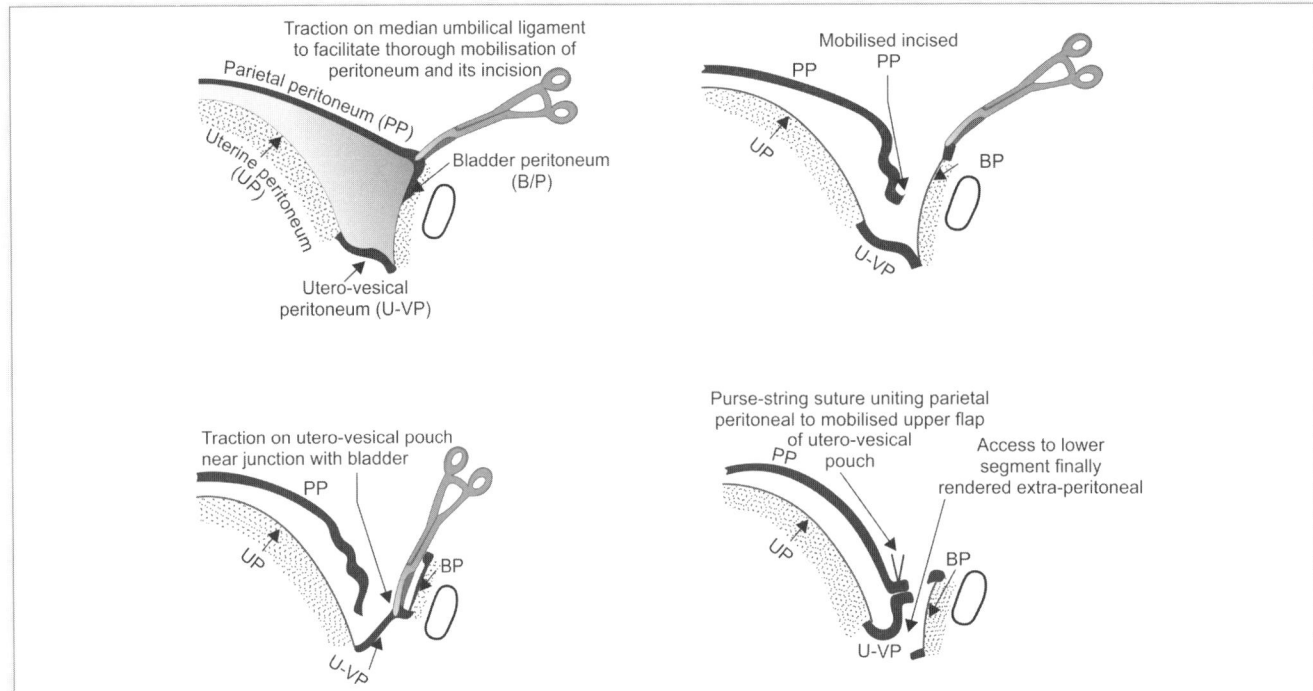

Fig. 15.24: Manner of handling peritoneum in simplified technique of extra-peritoneal caesar—Crichton, 1973

the site of attachment of the recti, which is always easily seen. At this point, proceeding cephalad and mediolaterally, the rectus muscles are from the underlying tissue until enough surface has been freed on which to execute the hysterotomy considered most suitable. This should be transverse by preference, as vertical incision of the LUS (following Opitz, see Chapter 16) has the disadvantage that it may extend caudally. Extraction of foetus and placenta is followed by double-layer closure.

Never attempt lysis of the adhesions; they would reform with the risk of intestinal obstructions.

Closure of the wall by anatomical planes; the patient may eat after a few hours.

BIBLIOGRAPHY

1. Abalos E. Alternative techniques and materials for caesarean section. RHL commentary (last revised: 3rd December 2004). The WHO Reproductive Health Library.
2. Adadevoh SWK, Hobbs C, Elkins TE. The relation of the true conjugate to the maternal height and obstetric performance in Ghanaians. Int J Gynecol Obstet. 1989; 28:243-51.
3. Al-Took S, Platt R, Tiflandi T. Adhesion-related small bowel obstruction after gynaecologic operations. Am J Obstet Gynecol. 1999;180:313-5.
4. Asakura H, Nakai A, Ishikawa G, Suzuki S, Araki T. Prediction of uterine dehiscence by measuring lower uterine segment thickness prior to onset of labour: evaluation by transvaginale ultrasonography. J Nippon Med Sch. 2000;67(5):352.
5. Bamigboye AA, Hofmeeyr GJ. Closure versus non closure of the peritoneum at caesarean section. Cochrane Database of Systematic Reviews. 2003, Issue 4, Art. n. CD000163. DOI: 10.1002/14651858. CD000163.
6. Botella Llusia J. Sobre una nueva técnica de cesárea extraperitoneal. Clin y Lab. 1949;48:259.
7. Buckman RF, Buckman PD, Hufnagel HN, Gerwin AS. A physiologic basis for the adhesion-free healing of deperitonealized surfaces. J Surg Res. 1976;21:67-76.
8. Bujold E, Bujold C, Hamilton EF, et al. The impact of a single-layer or double-layer closure on uterine rupture. Am J Obstet Gynecol. 2002;186:1326.
9. Chapman SJ, Owen J, Hauth JC. One versus two-layer closure of a low transverse cesarean: The next pregnancy. Obstet Gynecol. 1997;89:16.
10. Cheong YC, Bajekal N, Li TC. Peritoneal closure to close or not to close. Hum Reprod. 2001;16:1548-52.
11. Cherney LS. A modified transverse incision for low abdominal operations. Surg Gynecol Obstet. 1940;72:92.
12. Combs CA, Murphy EL, Laros RK. Factors associated with haemorrhage in Caesarean deliveries. Obstet Gynaec. 1991;77:77-82.
13. Crichton D. A Simple Technique of Extraperitoneal Lower Segment Caesarean Section. S Afr Med J. 1973;47:2011.
14. Cromi A, Ghezzi F, Di Naro E, Siesto G, Loverro G, Bolis P. Blunt expansion of the low transverse uterine incision at cesarean delivery: a randomized comparison of 2 techniques. Am J Obstet Gynecol. 2008;199:292-6.

15. Del Valle GO, Combs P, Qualls C, Curet LB. Does closure of Camper fascia reduce the incidence of post-caesarean superficial wound disruption? Obstet Gynecol. 1992;80: 1013-6.
16. Domini E, Guidi M, Guazzini S, Vicentini S. Misurazione intraoperatoria della coniugata ostetrica. Gior It Ost Ginec. 2007;29(8/9):283.84.
17. Edi-Osagie ECO, Hopkins RE, Ogbo V, Lockhaft-Cleff F, Ayeko L, Akpala WO, Mayers FN. Uterine exteriorisation at caesarean section, influence on maternal morbidity. Br J Obst Gynaecol. 1998;105:1070-8.
18. Elkins TE, Stovall TG. A histological evaluation of peritoneal injury and repair: implications for adhesions formation. Obstet Gynecol. 1987;70:225-8.
19. Ellis H, Heddle R. Does the peritoneum need to be closed at laparotomy? Br J Surg. 1977;64:733-6.
20. Harrigill KM, Miller HS, Haynes DE. The Effect of intra-abdominal irrigation at caesarean delivery on maternal morbidity; a randomized trial. Obstetrics and Gynecology, 2003;101(1):80-5.
21. Hauth JC, Owen J, Davis RO. Transverse uterine incision closure: one versus two layers. Am J Obstet Gynecol. 1992;167:1108.
22. Hershey DW, Quilligan EJ. Extra-abdominal uterine exteriorization at caesarean section. Obstet Gynaecol. 1978;52;189-92.
23. Hidar S, Jerbi M, Hafsa A, Slama A, Bibi M, Khairi H. The effect of uterine expansion at caesarean delivery on perioperative haemorrhaghe: a prospective randomised climnical trial. Rev Med Liege. 2007;62(4):235-8.
24. Hussain SA. Closure of subcutaneous fat: A prospective randomized trial. Br J Surg. 1990;77:107.
25. Jacobs-Jokhan D, Hofmeyr GJ. Extra-abdominal versus intra-abdominal repair of the uterine incision at caesarean section. Cochrane Database of Systematic Reviews 2004, Issue 4. Art. n. CD00085. DOI: 10.1002/14651858. CD00085.
26. Kehrer F. Ueber ein modifizierten verfahren bei Kaiserschnitt. Arch Gynaek. 1882;19:177.
27. Kerr Munro JM. The lower uterine segment incision in conservative Caesarean section. J Obstet Gynaecol Br Emp. 1921;28:475.
28. Kerr Munro JM. The technique of caesarean section, with special reference to the lower uterine segment incision. Am J Obst Gynecol. 1926;12:729.
29. Kerr Munro JM, Hendry J. Conservative caesarean section by the lower uterine segment incision. Surg Gynec Obstet. 1926;43:85.
30. Kerr JMM, Moir JC and Myerscouilh PR. Operative Obstetrics. London: Baillere, Tindall & Cassell; 1971.
31. Latzko W. Ueber extraperitonealen Kaiserschnitt. Zbl Gynaek. 1909;33:275.
32. Mackenrodt A. Die Radikaloperation des Gebärmutters-cheidenkrebses mit. Ausráumung des Beckens. Verh Dtsch Gynoekol ix: 139, 1901.
33. Magan EF, Dodson MK, Albert JR, Mc Curdy CM, Martin RW, Morrison JC. Blood loss at time of Caesarean section by method of placental removal and exteriorisation versus in situ repair of the uterine incision. Surg Gynaecol Obst, 1993;177;389-92.
34. Magan EF, Washburne JF, Harris RL, Bass JD, Duff WP, Morrison JC. Infectious morbidity, operative blood loss and length of the operative procedures after Caesarean delivery by method of placental removal and site of uterine repair. J Am Coll Surg. 1995;181:517-20.
35. Magann EF, Chauhan SP, Bufkin L, Field K, Roberts WE, Martin JN Jr. Intra-operative haemorrhage by blunt versus sharp expansion of the uterine incision at caesarean delivery: a randomized clinical trial. BJOG 2002;109(4):448-52.
36. Marshall CM. Caesarean Section Lower Segment Operation. Bristol. John Wright & Sons. 1939.
37. Mathai M, Hofmeyr GJ. Abdominal surgical incisions for caesarean section. Cochrane Database Syst Rev. 2007;(1) CD004453 (ISSN: 1469-493X).
38. Maylard AE. Direction of abdominal incisions. Br Med J. 1907;2:895.
39. Myers SA, Bennett T. Incidence of significant adhesions at repeat cesarean section and the relationship to method of prior peritoneal closure. J Reprod Med. 2005;50(9):659-62 (ISSN: 0024-7758).
40. Nather A, Zeisler H, Sam. CE, et al. Non-closure of peritoneum at cesarean delivery: Evaluation of the repeat cesarean sections. Wien Kfin Wochenschr. 2001;113: 451-4533.
41. Naumann RW, Hauth JC, Owen J. Subcutaneous tissue approximation in relation to wound disruption after cesarean delivery in obese women. Obstet Gynecol. 1995, 85(3):412-6.
42. Nazli Hameed, Mohammad Asghar Ali. Maternal blood loss by expansion of uterine incision at Cesarean Section - a comparison between sharp and blunt techniques. J Ayub Med Coll Abottabad. 2004;16(3):47-50.
43. NICE National Institute for Clinical Excellence; National Collaborating Centre for Women's and Children's Health. Caesarean section. London (UK). 2004;142 p. [688 references].
44. Ricci JV, Man JM. Principles of Extra-Peritoneal Caesarean Section. Philadelphia: Blakiston, 1942.
45. Rodriguez AI, Porter KB, O'Brien WF. Blunt versus sharp expansion of the uterine incision in low-segment transverse caesarean section. Am J Obstet Gynecol. 1994;171: 1022-5.
46. Tulandi T, Hum HS, Gelfand MM. Closure of laparotomy incisions with or without peritoneal suturing and second-look laparoscopy. Am J Obstet Gynecol. 1988;158:536-7.
47. Ueland K. Maternal cardiovascular dynamics VII Intrapartum blood volume changes. Am J Obstet Gynaec. 1976;126;671-7.
48. Wahab MA, Karantzis P, Eccersley PS, Russel LE, Thompson JW, Lindow SW. A randomized controlled study of uterine exteriorization and repair at caesarean section. Br J Obs Gynaec. 1999;9:913-6.
49. Yazicioglu F, Gökdogan A, Kelekci S, Aygün M, Savan K. Incomplete healing of the uterine incision after caesarean section: Is it preventable? Eur J Obstet Gynecol Reprod Biol. 2006;124(1):32-6 (ISSN: 0301-2115).

CHAPTER 16

Vertical Hysterotomies

A vertical hysterotomy involves accessing the uterine cavity and thereby extracting the foetus by means of a vertical incision in the anterior uterine wall.

INTRODUCTION

The assumption that any caesarean section (C-section) can be performed, irrespective of clinical indications, by means of a lower uterine segments (LUS) transverse hysterotomy is an assumption that can prove costly in the tropics and elsewhere.

There is still a specific clinical role for vertical hysterotomies, as a review of the literature demonstrates: Mc-Dermott (1996) reports 36 classic C-sections in the course of three years at Leeds Hospital and Chauhan et al. (2002) report 157 classic C-sections out of 37,863 deliveries over the decade 1990–2000, an incidence of 0.4%. St George et al. (2008) found 11 vertical C-sections over three years, and there are further such studies by Naef et al. (1995); Adair et al. (1996) and Martin et al. (1997).

Classically, vertical C-sections have been categorised, according to which part of the anterior uterine wall they affect, into:
- Lower-segment vertical C-section (Fig. 16.1) following Opitz (1911)
- C-section of the corpus, or classic C-section (Fig. 16.2) following Sänger (1882).

While useful from a training point of view, this classification does not fully reflect anatomical reality or current clinical requirements, it has been noted that:
- With ever increasing frequency, indications for C-section arise at an early stage of pregnancy (St. George 2008),

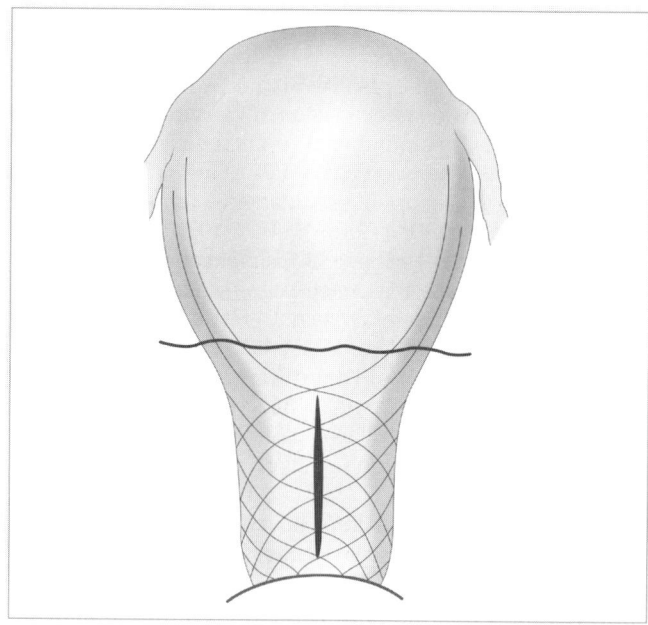

Fig. 16.1: Lower-segment vertical hysterotomy or Optiz C-section (strictly limited to the lower uterine segment)

including intrauterine growth retardation (IUGR), cases where prematurity is isolated or associated with oligohydramnios, transverse lie, breech presentation, constriction ring or LUS varicosity.

The incomplete development of the lower segment, at this gestational stage is incompatible with a transverse hysterotomy (danger of damage to uterine blood vessels). The alternative here is a vertical hysterotomy that, if

VERTICAL HYSTEROTOMIES

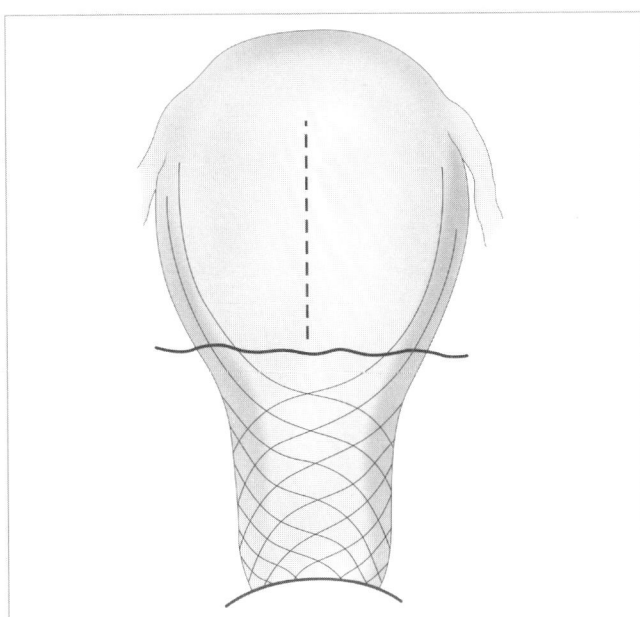

Fig. 16.2: Vertical hysterotomy of the corpus, or classic C-section following Sänger

LOW VERTICAL C-SECTION
(which does not reach the fundus)

Two vertical incisions are possible, depending on the gestational stage:
- A predominantly lower-segment C-section (Fig. 16.3)
- A lower-upper segment (corpus) C-section (Fig. 16.4).

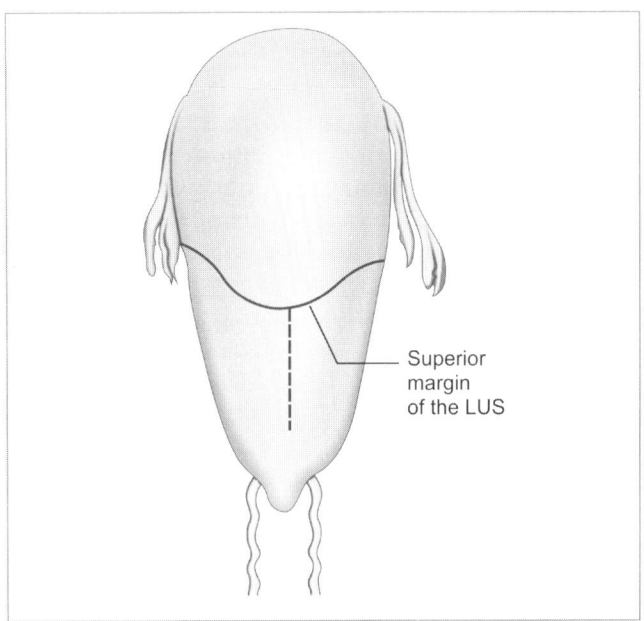

Fig. 16.3: A predominantly lower-segment C-section

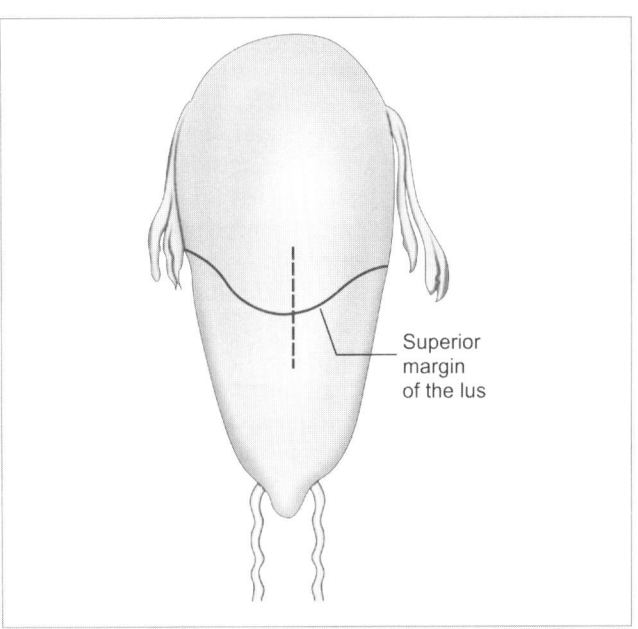

Fig. 16.4: Vertical C-section, body/lower-segment (Classic C-section)

limited exclusively to the LUS (Opitz), will often not provide sufficient space for extraction of the head without applying pressure to it (intracranial haemorrhages), making it indispensable that the anatomical limits of the LUS be crossed by extending the incision cranially;
- When faced, during labour, with a mechanical obstacle (cephalopelvic disproportion, obstructed labour), one may observe an increase in fundal thickness, a reduction of the surface area of the corpus and overdistension of the LUS. As a result, the area of upper-segment on which to perform the hysterotomy (Sänger) is extremely reduced, in order to avoid extending the incision up as far as the fundus, it becomes necessary to extend it caudally.

In light of the foregoing, it seems clear that lower-segment vertical C-sections are seldom possible. More frequently a cephalad extension (with lower-segment C-sections), or caudad extension (with corpus C-sections), becomes necessary.

Follow-up studies have shown that the incidence of uterine rupture in subsequent pregnancies is 3–4 times higher when the uterine fundus has been reached, than when it has not been reached by the incision.

We thus arrive at a revised classification of vertical hysterotomies:
- Low vertical C-section: the hysterotomy includes the lower uterine segment and also part of the upper segment (the uterine body), but does not reach the fundus
- High vertical C-section: The hysterotomy reaches the fundus.

PREDOMINANTLY LOWER-SEGEMENT C-SECTION
(Lower-segment vertical caesarean section)

According to Naef's (1995) classification, this should not extend more than 2 cm onto the superior uterine segment (uterine body).

The most common indications are: Intrauterine growth retardation in which prematurity is isolated or associated with oligoidramnios, transverse lie and breech presentation. Others are constriction ring or LUS varicosities.

Method

The abdominal cavity is entered via a vertical midline laparotomy (suprapubic-sub umbilical) preferable to a transverse laparotomy, as it offers more room for manoeuvre, the greatest ease of extension into the upper abdomen as well as the least blood loss, so that three essentials are reached: Accessibility, extensibility, security.

The visceral peritoneum is incised transversely approx. 4 cm from the vesical dome, to a width of 12 cm and bluntly reflected:
- Caudad as far as possible, together with the bladder, to the point of the bladder's maximum adhesion to the uterus (where vascularisation is very developed). Some authors recommend applying a retropubic valve to protect the bladder. We do not use this precaution as it impedes precise assessment of the distance to the bladder during incision, and reduces room for manoeuvre on extraction
- Cephalad, as far as possible until the area of maximum adherence is reached (superior margin of the LUS).

The area (Fig. 16.5) thereby attained, 12–14 cm in height (at term of pregnancy) is incised on the central section of the midline (Fig. 16.6). Subsequent extension, with rounded tips scissors, stops caudad 2–3 cm from the area of bladder adherence and cephalad at the superior margin of the LUS (Fig. 16.3); if necessity arises the incision may be further extended for a 2–3 cm depth into the upper segment (Fig. 16.3); amniotomy and delivery of the foetus follow. Once the uterus has been lifted and exteriorised from the abdominal cavity and the anaesthetist has administered an oxytocic (ergometrine 0, 4 mg IV or oxytocin) the third stage of labour occurs spontaneously. Suturing is done in two layers:
- First layer (Fig.16.7A): Start the first suture just beyond the inferior extremity of the incision, always following the "in - out - out-in" rule, tie the knot leaving a 6 cm long tail held with a forceps.

The second suture starts just beyond the superior extremity (Fig. 16.7B) of the incision, a knot is tied and a 6 cm long tail is left and held with forceps, the suturing progresses downwards with a simple (Fig. 16.8) or locked continuous suture, every bite including 2/3 of the thickness of the myometrium. It was previously thought that the decidua should not be included in the suture, but more recent studies (Yazicioglu et al., 2006) have found that its inclusion does not compromise suturing.

We point out that a continuous locked suture when it is done too tightly runs the risk of strangulation of the tissue blood supply and subsequent edge necrosis.

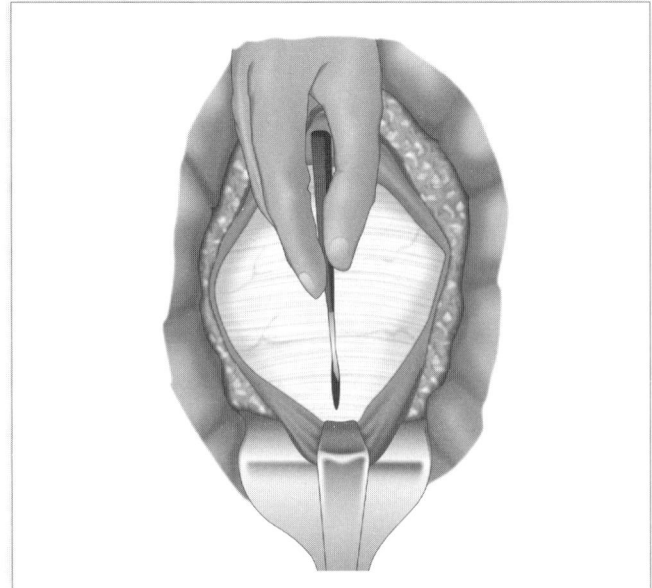

Fig. 16.5: A predominantly lower-segment C-section. Superiorly the peritoneum has been retracted as far as the area of maximum adherence to the myometrium, distally, the lower peritoneal and the bladder flap have been reflected as far as the point of maximum adherence to the uterus

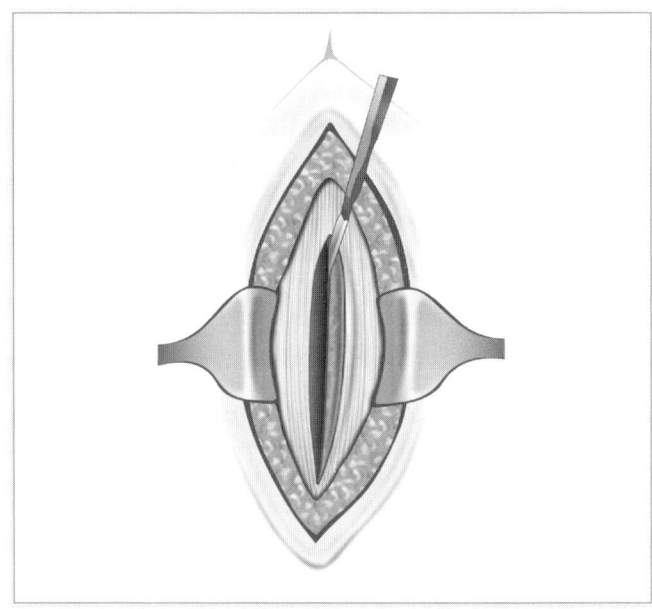

Fig. 16.6: The uterus is exposed and the incision begun on the lower part of the LUS, proceeds cephalad

VERTICAL HYSTEROTOMIES

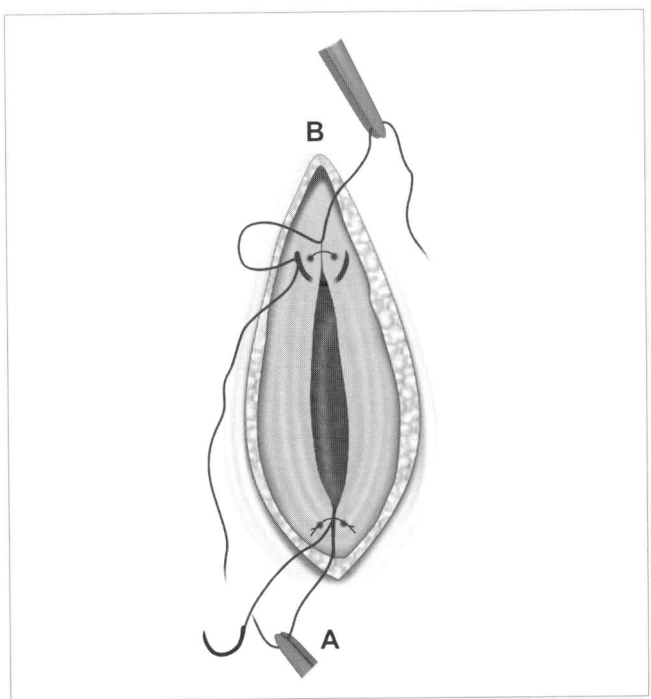

Fig. 16.7: First layer of uterine suturing. (A) The first suture begins from inferior corner and ends after the first stitch; (B) The second suture begins from the superior corner and proceeds caudally

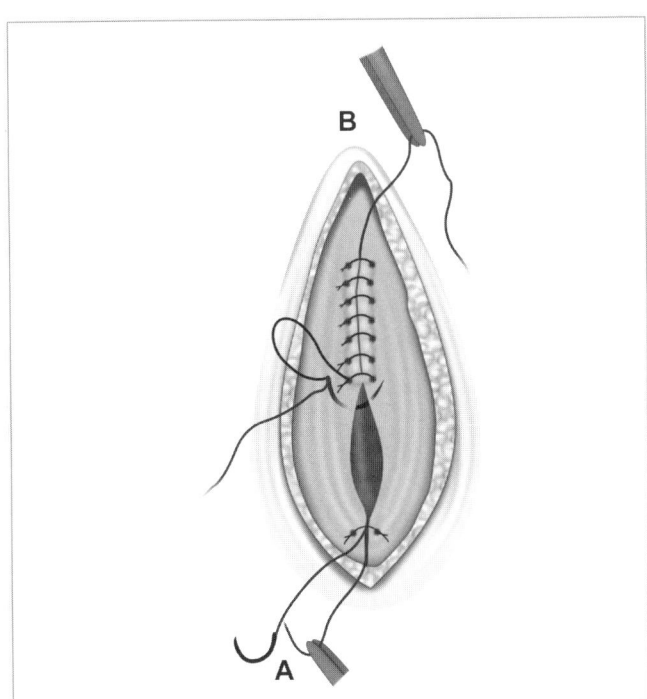

Fig. 16.8: First layer of uterine suturing. The second suture (B) proceeds caudally and, on reaching the inferior corner, is knotted with the marker (A)

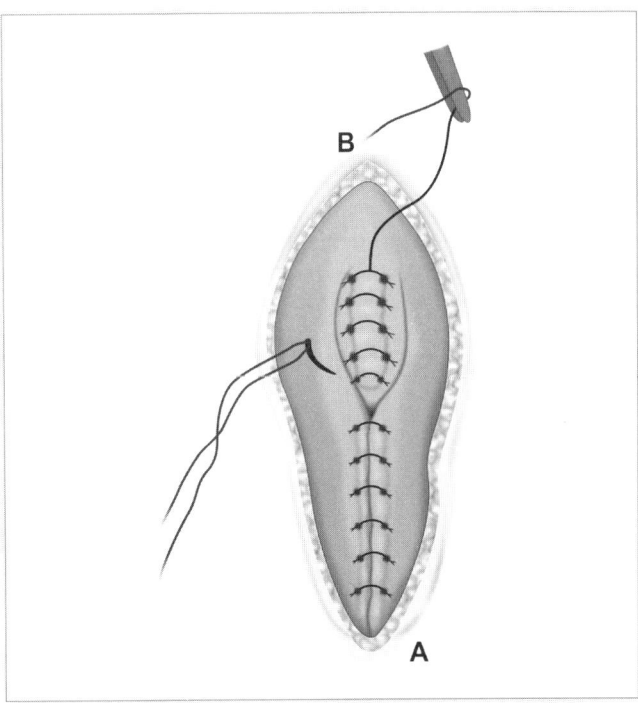

Fig. 16.9: Uterine suturing, second layer. The first suture, (A) now proceeds cephalad and, on reaching the superior end, is tied to marker (B)

Once the inferior angle has been reached the thread is tied to the tail—held with the forceps—of the first suture, both are now held with a forceps.
- Second layer, employing the first suture (Fig. 16.9), proceeds cephalad, with the features described above and, once reached the superior edge, it is tied to the tail of the second suture.

This is followed by visceral peritoneal closure.

VERTICAL CORPUS/LOWER-SEGMENT C-SECTION

See Figure 16.4.

Indications

Mechanical obstacle during labour (cephalopelvic disproportion or obstructed labour); extensive varicosities over LUS, previous vertical C-section, previous repair of a vesicovaginal fistula.

Method

Abdomen is entered through a midline vertical laparotomy (suprapubic—subumbilical) which, contouring on the left the umbilicus can be easily extended to the upper abdomen.

Transverse incision of the peritoneum and its caudad mobilisation, stopping close to the area of maximum vascularization and adherence of the bladder to the LUS.

A vertical midline incision, at least 12 cm long, is made in the anterior wall of the uterus follows very specific rules:
- The point of the scalpel is never used: Always use its rounded belly
- The incision always begins from the inferior end, (Fig. 16.4), keeping a distance of approx. 2 cm from the area of maximum adhesion of the bladder to the LUS
- The incision occurs in steps; after a first incision by the scalpel, wait a few moments and observe the spontaneous separation of the edges if this is not complete, execute a second, and perhaps a third cut, the latter using scissors with rounded tips.

The biggest drawback is when, during delivery, there is a cephalad or caudad extension of the incision; the second event is more dangerous than the former, hence the rule "the delivery manoeuvres must always bear on the superior end and never on the inferior end".

This rule is easily followed in cases of cephalic presentation; the feet are easy to find and the flexibility of the trunk facilitate breech delivery of the foetus (Fig. 16.7).

In a breech presentation, however, attempts to extract the head almost invariably result in extension of the incision towards the fundus. The following manoeuvre is recommended: Firstly, one arm is freed, then the other, and then caudad traction is exerted on them while the head is simultaneously flexed forwards; this will make it possible to flex the trunk, thus facilitating extraction of the remaining part of the foetus' body.

This is followed by exteriorisation of the uterus, concomitant administration of oxytocics and suturing, during which an almost bloodless third stage of labour occurs.

With regard to uterine suturing, the consensus is that should take place in three layers.

The guiding principle here is: When repairing a vertical hysterotomy, approximation of the edges should not be effected by the operating surgeon tugging on the thread, but through pressure applied to the edges by the assistant. Therefore, the suturing should serve to maintain the position attained.

We shall illustrate how this may be executed.

a. Simple interrupted suture for the first layer and continuous sutures for the remaining two.
   - First layer, simple interrupted suture: Generally a semi-circular Mayo needle with round tip, with the tip starting from inside and then "in-out-out-in" offers good grip on the tissue and when the suture dissolves, the knot will fall inside the uterine cavity, thereby reducing the amount of extraneous material within the myometrium (Fig. 15.12).

Each bite should at least include ½ of the thickness of the myometrium.

We recommend that suturing proceeds from the ends towards the middle, alternating stiches between the two ends. Starting from one end, place the next stitch at the other end, the third close to the first and alternating in this way until reaching the centre. The final two or three sutures are knotted in one go.

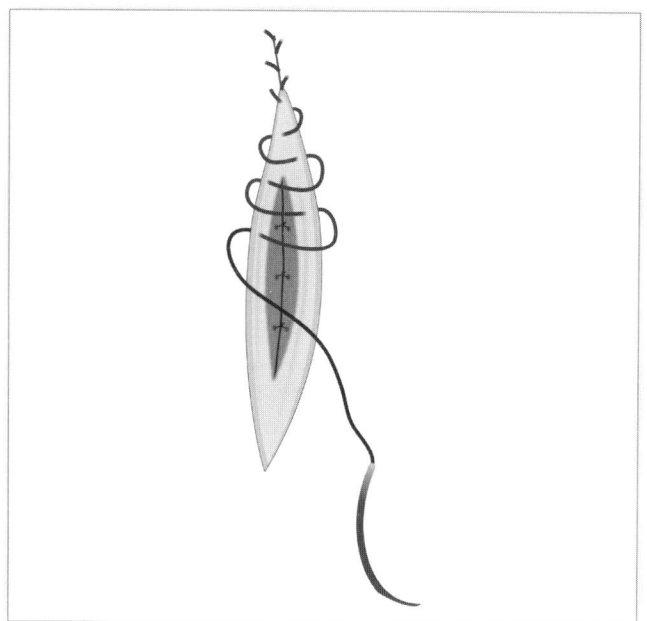

Fig. 16.10: Uterine suturing, third layer The inverting suture is effective in avoiding oozing surfaces which could give rise to adhesions

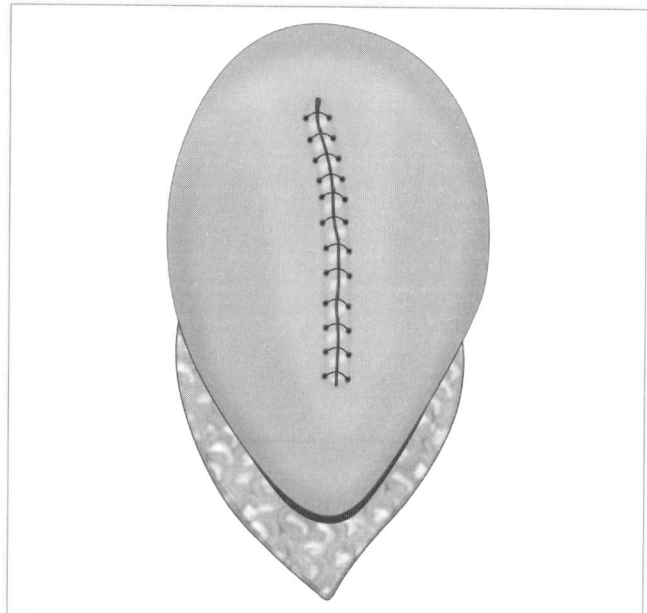

Fig. 16.11: Uterine suturing, third layer. The suture is complete: Final view

It may happen that, during extraction of the foetus, the hysterotomy extends caudally, making it difficult to visualize its apex, in such cases one is tempted to exert traction on the uterus, which is generally inadvisable; by grasping the dome of the blade with a ring forceps and elevating it, the apex will be perfectly visualized thus facilitating placing the suture.

Cases such as this justify the 'in-out-out-in' application of sutures; it helps avoid possible inclusion of the bladder in the suture, which may happen with an 'out-in-in-out' procedure.

The tail of the distal stitch is not cut off, but left 6 cm long to allow tying of the second suture.
- Second layer is executed using continuous suturing as in Figure 16.8B, starting at the superior end (thereby enabling one to check whether or not haemostasis has been effective). Bites of tissue up to one or two millimetres below the uterine surface should be included; approximation of the wound edges will be facilitated if the assistant exerts pressure on them from outside
- The third layer aims to leave a well peritonealized surface to prevent adhesion and an inverting running suture is here recommended. An anchor stitch is inserted at the superior angle and the closure of the uterus is done with an inverting suture which pierces each wound edge from outwards within (Figs 16.10 and 16.11).

b. Continuous suturing for all three layers
   – First layer: Apply the first suture on the inferior angle, always following the 'in-out-out-in' principle. Do not cut the trailing suture and leave a 6 cm long tail hold it with a forceps (Fig. 16.7A).

Start suturing from the superior edge (in-out-out-in); tie it; do not cut off the tail, but apply a marker to it (Fig. 16.7B); continue with a continuous suture (Fig. 16.8), either simple or interlocking, which should include 2/3 of the thickness of the myometrium, including the decidua, contrary to traditional recommendations. Having completed the suture down to the inferior edge, the thread is tied to the tail of the first suture.
   – The second layer proceeds cephalad, with the features described above, (Fig. 16.9)
   – The third layer is done with an inverting suture.

This is followed by the manœuvres described for transverse hysterotomies and wall closure (Chapter 19).

BIBLIOGRAPHY

1. Adair CD, Sanchez-Ramos L, Whitaker D, et al. Trial of labour in patients with a previous lower uterine vertical caesarean section. Am J Obstet Gynecol. 1996;174(3):966-70.
2. Chauhan SP, Magann EF, Wiggs CD, et al. Pregnancy after classic cesarean delivery. Obstet Gynecol. 2002;100 (5 Pt 1):946-50.
3. Macdermott RIJ. Classical caesarean section-long term morbidity. Journal of Obstetrics and Gynaecology. 1995;15(6):379-81.
4. Martin JN, Perry KG, Roberts WE, Meydrech EF. The case for trial of labour in the patient with a prior low-segment vertical caesarean incision. Am J Obstet Gynecol. 1997;177(1):144-8.
5. Naef RW 3rd, Ray MA, Chauhan SP, et al. Trial of labor after cesarean delivery with a lower-segment, vertical uterine incision: is it safe? Am J Obstet Gynecol. 1995;172(6):1666-73; discussion 1673-4.
6. Opitz E. Zur Technik des Kaiserschnittes. Zbl. Gynaek, 1911;35:970.
7. Sänger M. Der Kaiserschnitt bei Uterus-fibromen. Arch Gynaek. 1882;19:370.
8. St George L, Kuah KB. Low vertical uterine incision in caesarean section. Australian and New Zealand Journal of Obstetrics and Gynaecology. 2008;27(1):10-3.

CHAPTER 17

Management of Intraoperative Complications

CONTROL OF HAEMORRHAGE

Incontrollable uterine haemorrhages during a Caesarean section (C-section) represent an obstetrician's nightmare; standard procedures suggested for their control are as follows:
- Ligation of the internal iliac arteries
- Subtotal hysterectomy.

The former has only a modest efficacy (60%) and is often beyond the surgical skills of the obstetrician; the latter is often poorly accepted by populations, particularly in the case of a primigravida, whose lack of reproductive ability can make her a real outcast of her community.

In this chapter, we shall offer the obstetrician an alternative approach to this problem and illustrate the criteria that have guided our clinical practice in managing this emergency. This approach has been developed over almost a lifetime of experience in the Tropics and in countries of limited resources.

A more rational approach consists in instituting clinical practice that is suited to the site type of haemorrhage.

Haemorrhages may Originate

a. *From the wound edges of the hysterotomy* executed in a normal site, where the ends of the incision are equidistant from the round ligaments. The cause is identified as *uterine atony* or *abnormal vascularisation*.
b. *From a hysterotomy that*, having failed to account for dextroversion of the uterus, is performed symmetrically to the operative field but not midway between the two round ligaments and the uterine blood vessels lateral to them. For this reason the incision *has expanded beyond the left round ligament*, damaging the adjoining vessels. This uterine haemorrhage is typical for beginner obstetricians and is a reproach to whoever failed to warn them of this possibility. So our first golden rule is:
The ends of the hysterotomy should be the equidistant from the two round ligaments, and not come closer than 1 cm to them. To this end, the operating surgeon should ensure there has been no dextroversion, or, if there has, should take it into account.
c. *From a hysterotomy that has failed to take into account the thinning of the LUS and the degree to which the presenting part has engaged*, so that, during extraction, the hysterotomy extends. Extension most often occurs along a lateral edge (mainly to the left) and reaching the base of the broad ligament, or it may be central. This provides our second golden rule: *A lower-segment transverse hysterotomy has precise indications: When these are met and a difficult extraction is expected, it is better to extend the incision using Mayo scissors (curved with rounded tips), imparting a cephalad direction to the edges.* This precaution will tend to direct any expansion of the hysterotomy upwards, where potential haemorrhages are more easily controllable (Eisenkop 1982).
d. *From an abnormal placenta* (placenta previa) or from an intrinsic pathology (placenta adhaerens, accreta, percreta).

The cause of most haemorrhages is to be found in obstetric practices that have not assessed the clinical picture with precision, examples of this are as follows:

a. A laparotomy not proportionate to the presentation and position of the fetus.
b. A hysterotomy:
   - That has failed to take into account for the dextroversion of the uterus
   - It is not proportionate to the degree of engagement or to the degree of distension of the lower uterine segment with resulting tearing of the latter during delivery of the foetus.

We may conclude that control of obstetric haemorrhages is attained through two points:
- *Prophylaxis*: That is, adequate obstetric clinical practice
- *Surgical control of haemorrhages*.

Prophylaxis

- *Adequate obstetric clinical practice*: The informing principles have been stated above
- *Prophylactic ligation* of the ascending branches of the uterine arteries is indicated in gynaecological surgery: Myomectomy, metroplasty and hysterectomy.

This is difficult, if not impossible to perform in C-sections before the foetus has been extracted. The ascending branch is easy to identify. As illustrated by Couvelaire (1913), it is located where the artery ceases to be mobile and becomes attached to the uterine border, in an area superior to the bifurcation of the uterine artery and 3 cm from the ureters. Ligation is performed here (difficult to execute before extraction of the foetus).

Surgical Control of Haemorrhages

This is effected by means of:
- *Identifying the site of haemorrhage.*

The first, essential step involves exteriorising the uterus (Fig. 15.11), this manoeuvre brings about stretching of the ascending branches of the uterine arteries, a reduction of their calibre and therefore a significant reduction in their capacity. It also allows manual haemostatic operations to be conducted once the site of haemorrhage has been identified, ahead of effecting definitive haemostasis.

Haemorrhages can originate:

a. From the *edges of a hysterotomy incision* that has kept its original dimensions.
b. From a *lateral extension of a hysterotomy*, affecting the uterine blood vessels.
c. From the *(central or lateral) caudad extension* of a hysterotomy.
d. From the area of insertion of a placenta that is abnormal in terms of:
   - *Site* (placenta previa) in the LUS in which reduced reaction by the decidua can be observed
   - An *intrinsic pathology* (adherent placenta, placenta accreta or percreta).

HAEMOSTATIC PROCEDURES

If the haemorrhage originates.

From the Edges of a Hysterotomy

That has maintained its original dimensions: *Once uterine suturing has been completed,*

a. Place a gauze soaked in isotonic saline onto the suture and use the four fingers to exert pressure on it, while seeking to mould its edges (to flatten them) while the other hand is placed on the posterior surface of the uterus at the suture site, exerting compression for two to three minutes. In most cases, haemostasis will ensue. You can then see a translucent pink area at the hysterotomy edges, which indicates the surface of the myometrium, merging into a reddish, irregular area that is the dissected wall. Applying sutures onto the smooth surface will almost certainly gain control of the haemorrhage.

If the inferior LUS flap is too thin, and you are concerned that it might get torn during suturing, use a horizontal continuous mattress suture instead of the continuous over and over one.

If just one bleeding point still remains, perform haemostasis with a single U-shaped interrupted stitch.

b. If the above does not attain the desired effect, turning your back on the patient, bring into the palm of your hand the distal part of the uterus and exert a pressure between thumb and index, 2 cm distal to hysterotomy, to the lateral borders of the uterus and the blood vessels running parallel to it and continue exerting pressure for some minutes.

If even by this manoeuvre haemorrhage control is not gained, proceed without hesitation to ligation of the ascending branches of the uterine artery, as described in the paragraph on uterine devascularisation.

From Downwards and Central Expansion of Hysterotomy Lower Margin

Crucial is to assess how deep the tear has extended, the instinctive reaction to put it into evidence by lifting the uterus seldom proves effective. It is enough to apply one or two ring forceps to bladder dome and to lift this cephalad; the edges of the tear will then be clearly visible.

Repair is done with single interrupted stitches that strictly follow the "in - out - out-in" rule.

From a Lateral Extension of a Hysterotomy Affecting the Uterine Blood Vessels

If the tear does not extend deeply to involve the broad ligament, proceed with ligation of the ascending branches of the uterine artery, as described in the paragraph below.

UTERINE DEVASCULARISATION

The ligation of the ascending braches of the uterine arteries in the control of otherwise incontrollable uterine haemorrhages was first proposed by Waters (1952), and taken up by Tsirulnikov (1979), who introduced the procedure of "*uterine devascularization?*"

A complete devascularisation involves ligation of the ascending branches of the uterine arteries associated to the ligation of uterine branch of the ovarian artery and of the Sampson's artery (round ligament), resulting in 3 ligations on each side.

Uterine devascularisation (Fig. 17.1) has undergone two-fold development:
- *In its site*: Tsirulnikov proposed that ligation of the uterine artery pedicle before its bifurcation (ascending and descending branch) running the risk of ligating the ureters; currently, as also recommended by WHO, ligation of the ascending branch only is preferable. He also proposed a different site for ligation of the uterine branch of the ovarian artery
- *In its method of execution*: This has become progressive, having noted the superfluity of ligating all three vessels when two or three ligations proved sufficient. This consists in a stepwise reduction of uterine vascularisation, starting:
- From the ascending branch of the uterine arteries alone, which provide 60% of uterine vascularisation. This step alone has an 80–96% success rate, therefore higher than ligation of the internal iliac division of the hypogastric arteries (60%). There is a rich literature on the subject (Fahmy, 1987; O'Leary, 1995; Salvai et al., 2002, WHO, 2004).

If the ligation is performed with a single interrupted stitch using absorbable suturing material, it is followed (O'Leary, 1980, 1995) by uterine artery recanalisation; reproductive function is not impaired and moving on to ligation of the uterine branch of the ovarian artery, unilaterally or bilaterally, and finally on to the round ligament (Sampson artery).

Ligation of the ascending branch of the uterine artery: The operation is easily performed; it consists in transfixing the uterus (Fig. 17.2(1)) from the anterior to its posterior wall (avoiding the round ligament and the infundibulopelvic ligament at a point located *2 cm inferior to the hysterotomy and 3 cm medial to the uterine border (2x3 rule)*, preferably using a half-circle round-bodied Mayo needle, mounted with (N° 1–2); absorbable suturing material. The generally available atraumatic needles are not as suitable, as they tend to be sized too small for the thickness of the uterus.

One proceeds as follows bilaterally: the exteriorized uterus is rested on the pubis; grasp the round ligament and the infundibulopelvic ligament between thumb and forefinger; elevate them by a few centimetres and identify, by its transparency, an avascular area in the underlying peritoneum. Transfix through this and, through the myometrium from anterior to posterior 2 cm below the hysterotomy and 3 cm medial to the uterine border, tie tightly.

If haemorrhaging is profuse and you are not very sure of your technical ability, place curved (but not toothed) Klemmer forceps on the above-mentioned point, including the round and infundibulopelvic ligaments. When this is ready, transfix the uterus at a point inferior to the Klemmer forceps, which you remove. Lift the ligamentous and vascular peduncle and transfix the underlying peritoneum in an avascular area. Now tie tightly.

The uterus will soon turn pallid: It will present fibrillating contractions followed by a persistent contraction.

If haemostasis has not been achieved, proceed (Fig. 17.2(2)) with ligation, either mono- or bilaterally, of the uterine branch of the ovarian artery (immediately inferior to the uterine insertion of the utero-ovarian ligament). In our experience, bilateral ligation has been required in two

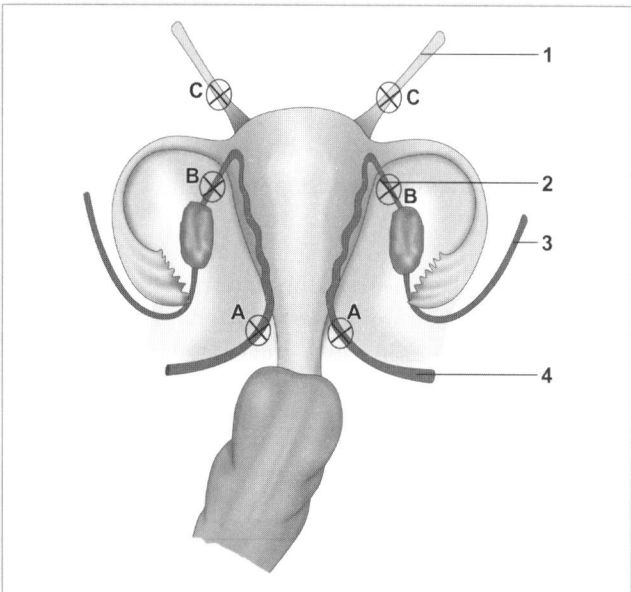

Fig. 17.1: Uterine devascularisation following Tsirulnikov: (A) Ligation of uterine blood vessels in the area where the peduncle is still mobile, not far enough away from the ureter; (B) Ligation of the ovarian branch of the uterine artery at the level of the central portion of the infundibulopelvic ligament; (C) Ligation of the Sampson artery of the round ligament

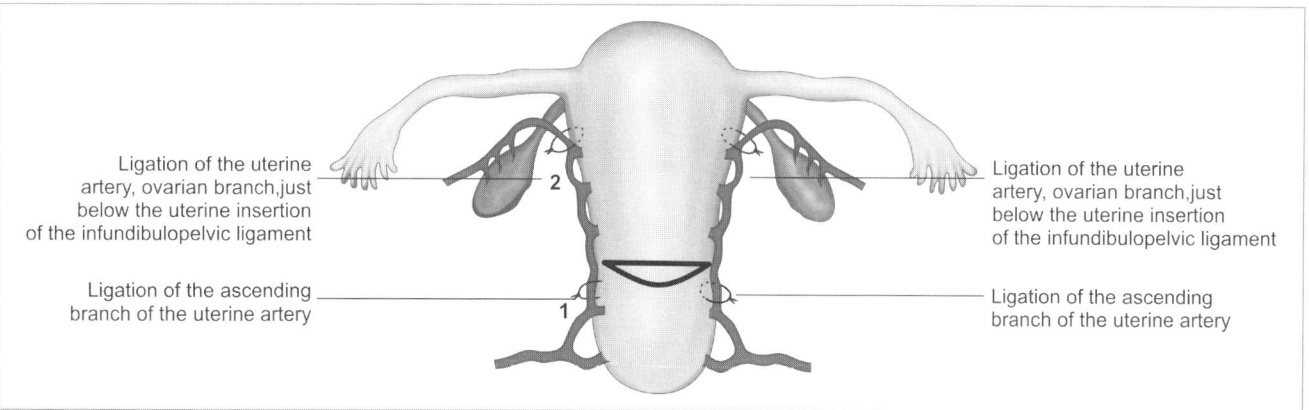

Fig. 17.2: Uterine devascularisation

cases only. Finally, proceed to the round ligament and the Sampson artery.

N.B. The instrument box should always contain long and curved Klemmer forceps and two curved, half-circle round-bodied needle points (Mayo needles).

Forceps on the uterine artery: Circumstances sometimes arise in which it is not possible to ligate the uterine arteries. In this curved Klemmer forceps (not Kocher forceps) are applied to the uterine arteries. The operation is completed and the abdomen is closed, leaving the forceps jutting out of the abdominal wall. On the 3rd–4th day these are easily removed (in our experience of two cases, which turned out well).

From a Lateral Extension of the Hysterotomy, which Advances to the Broad Ligament

From which the haemorrhage originates. Treatment for this eventuality has also been codified. Proceed as follows:
- Lift the uterus cephalad and laterally to the side opposite the haemorrhaging
- Forcipressure is applied to the artery; dissection and ligation of the homolateral round ligament. This will facilitate preparation of the anterior fold of the broad ligament
- Grasp between thumb and forefinger the base of the broad ligament, exert a pressure on it, and proceed in a medio-lateral direction until the haemorrhage is controlled Apply here ring forceps (never Kocher forceps) and clamp them, applying a maximum of two notches on the rack. Now you are faced with one of two choices:
  - *Leave the forceps in place*: The two manoeuvres: The upward and lateral stretching of the uterus combined with elevation and compression of the broad ligament, should have distanced the ureter. If it is clamped by the forceps over 24–36 hours, no damage will be incurred (a renal echography is useful and reassuring here). The forceps will be removed after 2 days
  - *Apply a second ring forceps laterally to the first*, which are slowly removed, and try to identify and to ligate the damaged vessel. Where this does not succeed, replace the forceps in their original position, from where they will be removed on the second day. Never use Kocher forceps on the base of the broad ligament (we have said this already, and repeat it here), nor attempt to place haemostatic sutures haphazardly. The majority of injuries to the ureter result from such actions (see paragraph on ureteric injuries below).

Haemorrhage not Controlled Through Uterine Devascularization

Generally, these haemorrhages originate from the LUS, site of attachment of a placenta previa, Uterine devascularisation will have no effect on this, as this part of the uterus is supplied mainly by the uterine artery, descending branch whose ligation via laparotomy is difficult.

This haemorrhaging may either be:
a. *Contained:* Haemostasis being easily attained by applying figure-of-eight sutures to the haemorrhaging area.
b. *Extensive* over a sizeable anterior or posterior area of the lower uterine segment.

When haemorrhaging is profuse, do not despair; it can be brought under control using two manoeuvres that could be used consecutively.
- Having identified the site of bleeding (anterior or posterior part of the LUS), using absorbable suturing material N° 1 or 2 mounted on a round-bodied atraumatic needle, the first suture is inserted 1 cm above the site of haemorrhage; proceed downwards with simple over and over or locked continuous sutures, each horizontal loop

1 cm apart, from the margin of the area of haemorrhage, if too extensive a second suture is passed. Tighten each suture as you proceed, using the thread to exert traction in a cephalad direction until control of the haemorrhage is attained. Generally, 3-4 rounds are enough

- If you are not completely satisfied with the result obtained, a decisive alternative is available: Transvaginal clamping of the descending branches of the uterine arteries *(Domini, Guidi, Guazzini, 2006)*.

If you find these operations too complex, use the "brace-suture" technique (B-Lynch, 1997).

Managing Haemorrhages by the B-Lynch Technique

Indications are intractable haemorrhage (uterine atony, placenta previa) during or subsequent to a C-section or vaginal delivery.

The author reports highly favourable outcomes and no influence on subsequent pregnancies (see literature).

For the sake of completeness, we report this technique, which we have observed but have never found occasion to use.

The procedure is performed under general anaesthesia, generally using ketamine due to its action on arterial pressure. The patient is catheterised, at a moderate Trendelenburg inclination, and placed in the Lloyd Davies position (lithotomy position) for access to the vagina to check the control of bleeding.

Access to the abdominal cavity is via the laparotomy used for the C-section (in cases of haemorrhage following a C-section) or by lower transverse laparotomy.

Re-opening of the visceral peritoneum (in the case of a prior C-section) or opening of the vesico-uterine pouch and caudad reflection of the bladder.

Removal of the uterine sutures of lower-segment transverse hysterotomy.

The uterus is exteriorised; the uterine cavity is evacuated of blood clots and examined. The external surface of the uterus is examined in search of bleeding points. If none are found, bi-manual compression of the uterus is performed to check whether the technique could be successful. If bleeding is controlled in this way, the technique is applied.

- The hysterotomy has not yet been sutured
- Using a curved 70 mm round-bodied hand suturing needle on which a 2 0 chromic catgut suture is mounted: penetrate the uterine cavity at a point 3 cm inferior to the lower edge of the hysterotomy and 3 cm from the lateral border (Fig. 17.3(1)):

Leave the cavity: 3 cm proximally to the upper edge of the incision and 4 cm from the lateral border; feed the thread down the entire anterior face of the uterus (Fig. 17.3(2)) and

Puncture the fundus anteroposteriorly: 3-4 cm from its superior border (Fig. 17.3(3)), bringing us to the posterior face of the uterus (Fig. 17.4(1)),

Bring the needle into the uterine cavity through the posterior wall at the same level as the superior anterior exit point (Fig. 17.4(2)). The thread is run transversely and

Leaves the cavity close to the contralateral border at a point 3 cm proximal to the upper edge of the hysterotomy and 4 cm from the lateral boundary of the uterus (Fig. 17.4(3)). The needle is now passed cephalad along the posterior wall (Fig. 17.4(4)) and *punctures the fundus posteroanteriorly*, 3-4 cm from its border; this brings us to the anterior surface of the uterus (Fig. 17.3.(4)).

Enter the uterine cavity at a point 3 cm proximally to the upper edge of the uterine incision and 4 cm from the lateral border (Fig. 17.3(5)).

Leave the cavity at a point 3 cm inferior to the lower edge of the hysterotomy and 3 cm from the lateral border of the uterus (Fig. 17.3(6)).

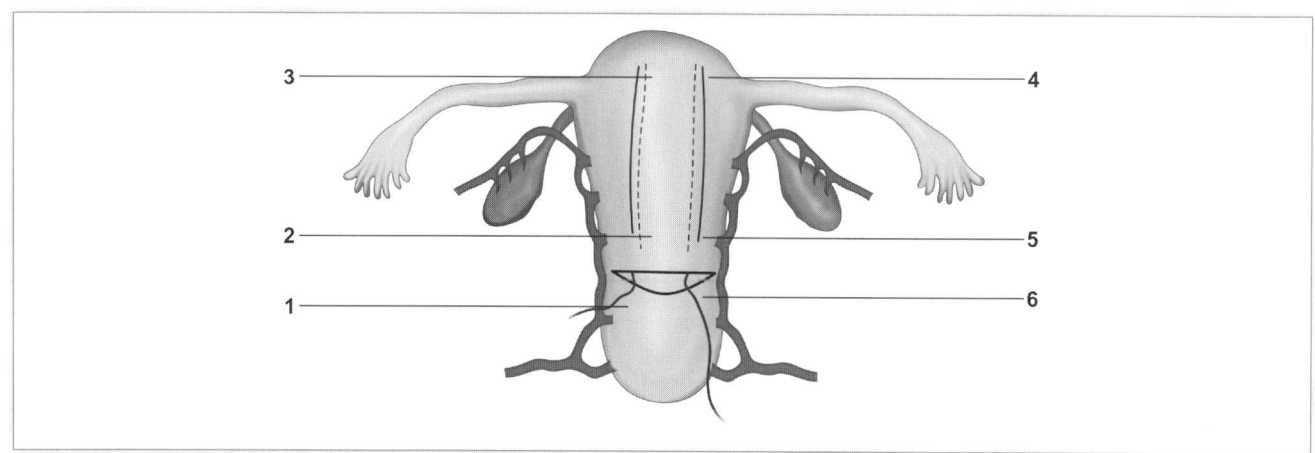

Fig. 17.3: Managing uterine bleeding using the B-Lynch technique: Anterior view of uterus. This apprach is suggested for a surgeon standing on the patient's right hand side

MANAGEMENT OF INTRAOPERATIVE COMPLICATIONS

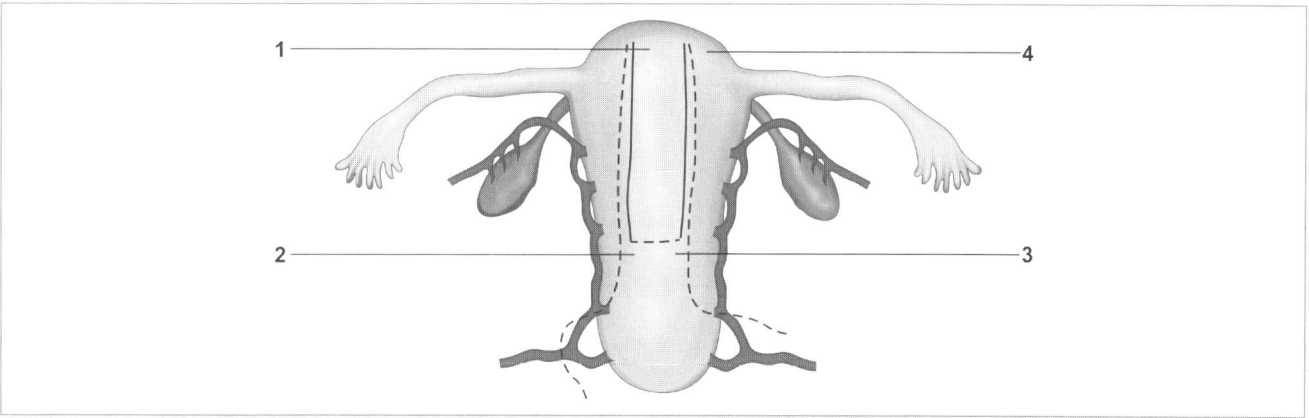

Fig. 17.4: Managing uterine bleeding using the B-Lynch technique: Posterior view of uterus

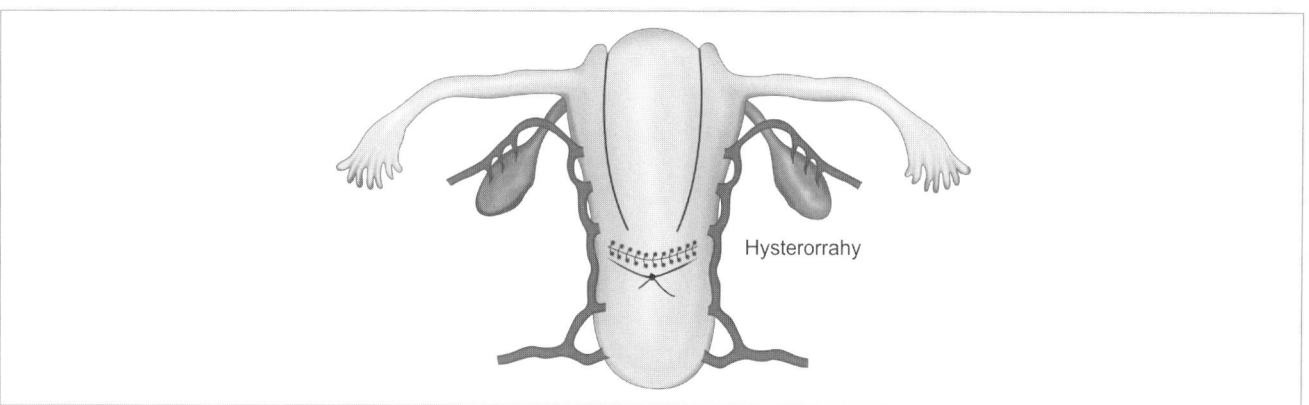

Fig. 17.5: Managing uterine bleeding using the B-Lynch technique: Anterior view of uterus

Repair of the uterine incision: The operating surgeon exerts traction on the strands while the assistant compresses the fundus. The uterus will be compressed and the two strands of the suture are knotted (Fig. 17.5).

In view of the optimal results obtained:
- By *stepwise uterine devascularisation* if haemorrhage presents during a C-section
- By *transvaginal clamping of the uterine blood vessels*, as a prophylactic haemostatic operation in C-sections for placenta previa (Domini et al., 2008) or as therapeutic operation in post-partum haemorrhages (Guidi, 2008), The Authors have some concern regarding the use of this procedure, particularly for *post partum haemorrhages* due to:
- The *waste of precious time* in preparing for the operation and transfer to theatre
- The disproportion of inflicting a hysterotomy on an anaesthetised patient for the sole purpose of applying a suturing thread.

Should transvaginal clamping prove insufficient, a laparotomy need provide for devascularization only.

Injuries of the Lower Uterine Segment that are Difficult to Visualize

As noted above, it suffices to apply one or two ring forceps to the bladder and to lift this cephalad; the edges of the tear will then be clearly visible. Repair is effected by means of interrupted sutures that strictly follow the 'in-out-out-in' procedure, or by continuous suturing that starts from within the uterus.

INJURY TO THE URINARY TRACT

Bladder Injury

Incidence and Risk Factors

Incidence varies depending on country and historical period: Qatar 0.08% (Douleh, 2006); Mexico 0.087% (Urueta, 2009); United States 0.28% (Phipps, 2005); Saudi Arabia 0.44% (Rahman, 2009); Pakistan 0.5% (Ghazi, 2008).

Risk factors
- *Prior C-section* is the principal risk factor (Urueta 63%; Phipps 67%; Rahman 81%, Dauleh 93.8%); 3.82% of repeat C-sections are complicated by a bladder injury (Rahman, 2009)
- The *degree of urgency* (foetal distress, placenta previa) is another factor that puts the patient at risk of bladder injury. In Douleh's study sample, this value was 75%. Similar values were reported by Faricy (1978); Rajasekar (1997) and Yossepowitch (2004).

Type of laparotomy: Bladder injuries during midline laparotomies are found to have an incidence 6 times as high as those reported for lower-segment transverse laparotomies. In our opinion, this finding should be interpreted in light of the indication for a midline laparotomy, which is expectation of a difficult operative delivery due to cephalopelvic disproportion. Here very commonly it is not possible to catheterise a full bladder, leading to a higher likelihood of injury to it (see Chapter 13).
- Adhesions from prior laparotomies.

Site

The following sites may be affected:
a. The dome of the bladder 60%–93% of cases according to the literature (Douleh, Phipps, Farcy).
b. The posterior bladder wall.

Dimensions: Injuries measuring 1 cm are very rare; those between 2 and 6 cm constitute 60% of cases; the remaining 30% are over 6 cm in size.

Pathogenesis

a. *Dome of the bladder*: This is found with a slight prevalence among primigravidae in the presence of cephalopelvic disproportion or obstructed labour. The injury may occur:
   - *On opening the peritoneum*: An overdistended bladder becomes an extrapelvic organ. If, on grounds of urgency or due to the organ's overdistension, tactile or visual anatomical landmarks for the bladder—perivesical fat and the uracus—are not appraised, it becomes possible to injure the bladder (see Chapter on laparotomies)
   - *During preparation of the vesical peritoneal flap* during a hysterotomy in which, due to over distension of the LUS, it was not possible to identify the superior border of the bladder clearly. In this case help is provided by pushing the bulb of a Foley catheter through the bladder wall; this will advance as far cephalad as the dome of bladder.
b. The *posterior bladder wall*: These occur during lysis of adhesions between the bladder and the lower uterine segment following a prior C-section, or following uterine rupture.

Diagnosis

This is generally immediate and offers the advantage that the bladder, having been emptied by the cystotomy, reassumes its normal dimensions and tone, allowing:
- Easier identification of the peritoneum, which, if the injury is to the dome, is now opened at a more cephalad level
- Better identification of the borders, when the posterior bladder has been involved.

Prophylaxis

- Clinical practice by the obstetrician, even when faced with an emergency situation, should be such as to limit the possibility of injury to the bladder (Thomson, 1997). When bladder distension almost reaches the umbilicus, two approaches may be adopted:
  - Puncture the bladder with a fine needle to empty it. If an aspiration tube is attached to the needle, emptying is quicker. If this procedure is considered too dangerous:
  - Skin and fascia incisions are extended cephalad, contouring the umbilicus to its left and, proceeding vertically for 4–5 cm; the peritoneum is now opened and the bladder is retracted using a valve.

Where adhesions are present between bladder and LUS, if these prove obdurate following an initial attempt to mobilise the bladder, it is advisable not to persevere as this can lead to profuse bleeding, *injury of the bladder* or LUS, this is because adhesions are often accompanied by thinness of the lower uterine segment. Here, ignore the bladder injury and make a uterine incision 1–2 cm superior to the injury. Deliver the foetus, exteriorise the uterus and apply haemostatic sutures to the corners of the uterine incision.

Diagnosis

Diagnosis of a bladder injury may occur
- *Before operative delivery of the foetus*: As extraction of the foetus is the indication for surgery, once a suitable site for opening the peritoneum or for the hysterotomy has been located, foetal extraction and exteriorisation of the uterus should precede any repair operation
- *After operative delivery*.

Therapy

Repair of bladder injury precedes repair of the lower uterine segment, of the hysterotomy site or of an incision wound laceration.

Repair of the Bladder Dome

The steps are as follows:
- Apply haemostatic sutures to the corners of the uterine incision

- Apply two stay stitches or two Allis forceps approx. 0.5 cm from the end of the bladder injury
- Mobilise bladder from the lower uterine segment, leaving a free margin of not less than 3 cm

A simple cystotomy is normally repaired in two to three layers consisting of:

a. Interrupted sutures: the first sero-muscolar layer (Fig. 17.6) is closed with N° 3 absorbable suture mounted on a round-bodied needle (half circle), the second (Fig. 17.7) with interrupted inverting sutures (Lambert's suture).
b. Continuous sutures, with the first layer consisting of a simple running closure of the mucosa with a 3-0 absorbable suture mounted on a round-bodied needle (Davis JD. 1999); the use of permanent suture, especially silk, is contraindicated, as it can serve as an impetus for stone formation(Morrow FK et al., 1974). The second layer may be closed with a running imbricating stitch using either 2-0 or 3-0 absorbable suture to include the submucosa and muscularis.

Repair of Posterior Bladder Wall

Once an unplanned cystotomy is recognized, the first step should be to thoroughly examine the defect to determine the extent of the injury. An important consideration is to determine whether the trigone or ureters have been affected by the cystotomy but the majority of the bladder injuries that occur during the time of caesarean occur at the dome or at the posterior wall and are easily repaired with a layered closure. If there is concern whether there may have been urethral involvement in the injury, then the obstetrician may consider having the anaesthesiologist inject 40 mg of indigo carmine into the patient's IV to examine for extravasation of dye proximal to the bladder, which would suggest ureteral injury.

Repair of the posterior bladder wall can be slightly more difficult than repairs to the dome, but by following the procedure set out here you should avoid the two major complications of injuries to the posterior bladder wall, which are vesicouterine fistula, first described by Youssef (1957)

- Hence the name "Youssef's syndrome" – and vesicovaginal fistula.

We should recall how the surgeon's motto: "Identify the structures and repair them" is facilitated by the presence of the catheter bulb. If you have trouble identifying margins of the bladder injury, traction on the lower uterine segment or on its edges will enable you to expose the damaged area to it along its whole extension. Now isolate the area with a closely-packed tamponade and apply stay sutures.

If the edges of the injury are clear, start suturing promptly, otherwise rectify them. Repair in two to three layers as above, the sutures should not be interlocking, nor overtightened (it should not give rise to ischemia) strangulating the blood vessels.

If you think you are getting close to the orifice of one or both ureters, do not run the risk of including them in the suture. Catheterise them using a ureteral catheter, which should always be available in the operating room. If such a catheter is not available, one could use:

- A winged scalp vein needle set from which the needle has been removed and the end cut on a bevel; these are to be preferred for their length
- A cannula-needle from which the trocar has been removed.

In order to confirm bladder integrity, one may back fill the bladder with sterile milk or methylene blue dye. Two advantages of using the former material are that it is readily available on labour and delivery, and it does not stain tissue

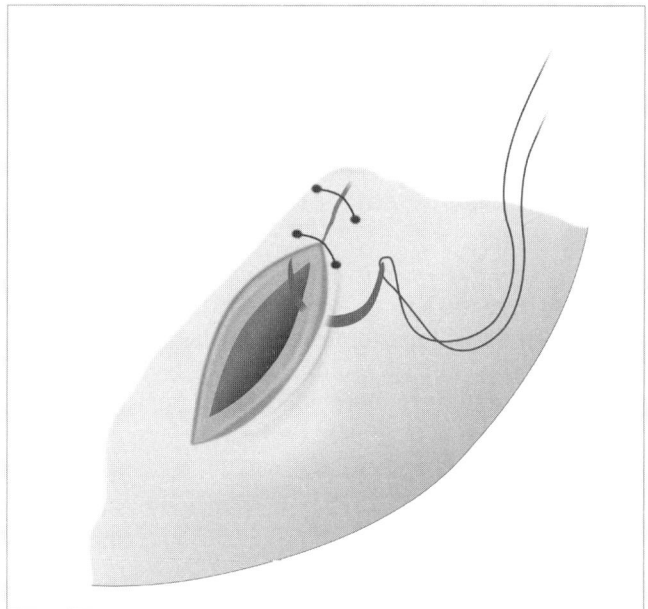

Fig. 17.6: Repair of a bladder injury using single interrupted sutures; first layer seromuscular sutures

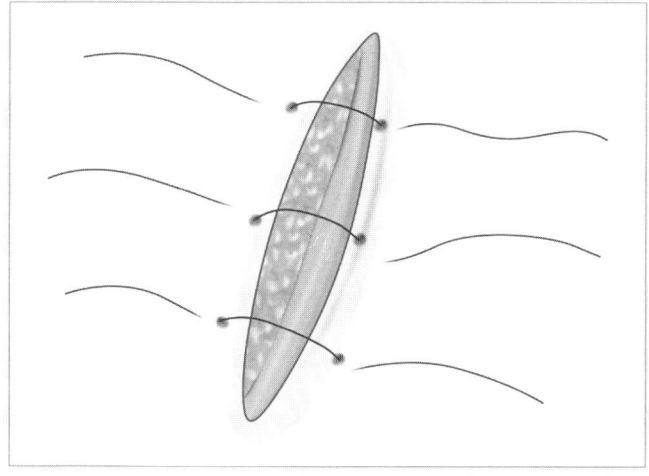

Fig. 17.7: Repair of a bladder injury using interrupted sutures; second layer, Glover's sutures

like methylene blue, which may limit one to detect the presence of a recurrent leak.

After bladder integrity is confirmed, if the serosal margins can be approximated. A third running stitch of absorbable suture may be placed. Bladder should be continuously drained with the use of a Foley catheter for at least 7–10 days postoperatively.

Check that it isn't obstructed by blood clots, and instruct the patient to assess bladder distension and to inform the nurse or doctor promptly when full. The patient should drink at least four litres of water per day.

Injuries to the Ureter

Injuries to the ureter during C-section are a rare eventuality (0.02%); they occur:
- Mainly following a ligation carried out to control bleeding deriving from an extension of the hysterotomy (from uterine rupture) either laterally towards the base of the broad ligament, or centrally towards the vagina (Gortzak, 2001)
- In a smaller number of cases, these injuries damage the ureters directly (Eisenkop, 1982; Rajasekar, 1997).

Most authors (Thomas, 1994; Hankins, 1995; Ghazi, 2008) agree that, due to dextroversion of the uterus, the left ureter is the one most often affected; others, (Eisenkop and Rajasekar), dispute this hypothesis.

Prophylaxis

Good surgical preparation includes knowledge of the risk factors and an ability to anticipate and prevent every injury; the following recommendations have been made:
- Clinical practice by the surgeon, even when faced with an emergency situation, should be such to limit the possibility of injury to the urinary tract (Thomson, 1997)
- Particular attention should be paid when opening the visceral peritoneum and in preparation of the visceral flap with dissection of the bladder from the LUS (Faricy, 1978; Davis, 1999; Hema, 2001)
- Each end of the uterine incision should always point upwards (Eisenkop, 1982)
- In controlling bleeding, compression is to be preferred to haemostatic sutures applied haphazardly (Feeney, 1959; Daly, 1988; Simm, 2005).

Diagnosis

This may be intraoperative or postoperative:
- *Intraoperative*: Should one suspect resection or ligation of the ureter, it is important to inject a dye intravenously (5 ml of indigo carmine or 5 ml of methylene blue). Where resection has occurred, diffusion of the dye will be seen at the incision site; if ligation has occurred, a cystotomy will be necessary to observe elimination of dyestuff from the vesicoureteral junction. If doubt persists, the corresponding ureter should be cannulated
- *Post-operative*: Postoperative recovery following a complicated C-section should be followed with particular attention (Nielson, 1984), the clinical picture will vary according to whether ligature or resection has occurred. In the first case prevailing symptoms will be pain at the costovertebral angle corresponding to the injury, unexpected fever and persistent oliguria. Renal U/S will identify hydronephrosis. Where resection has occurred: Fever, abdominal distension which may be accompanied by ileus, haematuria and watery secretion from the genitals.

In these cases it is good practice to consult a general surgeon or urologist.

Ureteral Reimplantation

This is a reasonably simple piece of surgery: It includes preliminary steps and actual implant technique.

Preliminary Steps

These include:
- *Ligation of the vesicoureteral stump*: This is performed only where the stump is very short; if it is very long, terminoterminal anastomosis should be considered with the proxymal ureteric stump.

If short, the stump is elevated using surgical forceps and forceps pressure is applied to the base (forcipressure); this is ligated using simple 2.0 catgut

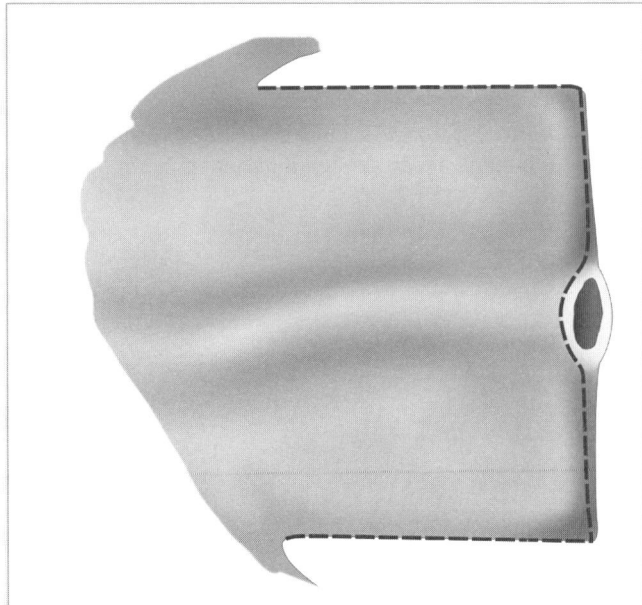

Fig. 17.8: Preparation of the proximal part of the ureter: The peritoneum is preserved bilaterally for a width of 2 cm. The portion of the ureter covered in peritoneum is its dorsal side

MANAGEMENT OF INTRAOPERATIVE COMPLICATIONS

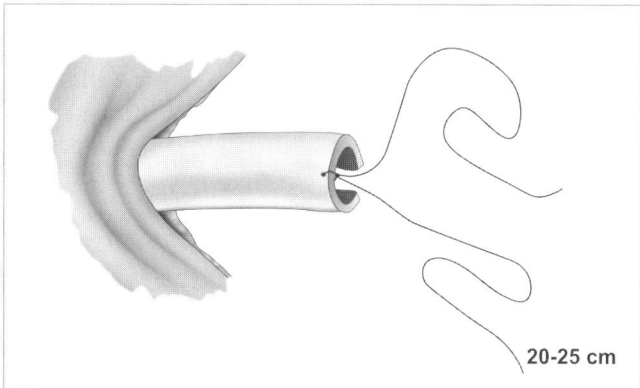

Fig. 17.9: Reimplantation of ureter: Blind technique (Ljubljana technique) to the dorsal side of the ureter. A tension suture is applied; the two strands are approx. 20–25 cm long

- *Identification and preparation of the ureter*: Having identified the resected end of the ureter, this end is isolated and elevated bluntly, preserving the peritoneum for a width of at least 2 cm bilaterally (Fig. 17.8). Any small haemorrhages present are controlled using swabs soaked in isotonic saline
- In the ureter's area of maximum adhesion to the peritoneum, (dorsal border), using an atraumatic round-bodied needle, (0 chromic catgut), we apply a fully penetrating tension suture 3 mm from the end. This is knotted with one throw only, leaving at least 20 cm long, ends which are held with a forceps (Fig. 17.9)
- *Filling the bladder with 200 ml of isotonic saline:* This will enable identification of the most suitable site for reimplantation, which:
  a. Can be reached without tension; this may occur either:
    » *Spontaneously* or
    » *Following mobilisation,* the vesicolysis begins (Fig. 17.10) from the pubic symphysis, executed with a flat hand inserted below the rectus abdominis muscles. The bladder dome is then grasped using ring forceps and stretched towards the side of the resected ureter, isolating the bladder from the peritoneum and from the contralateral loose connective tissue.
  b. If it *cannot be reached*, one should consider termino-terminal anastomosis or an ureterocutaneostomy.

Having identified the site for the implant, preferably a point covered with peritoneum, we apply two stay sutures 2 cm apart, including the muscle.

The bladder can be reached from the ureter without tension (spontaneously or following vesicolysis).
We propose two techniques, both very simple:
- *Reimplantation, blind technique*
- *Reimplantation, open technique.*

Reimplantation, Blind Technique

This is the technique standardly utilised by the Ljubljana School; we suggest using it first - then if difficulties arise, we move on to the next (open technique).

Materials Required

- A rabbeted (grooved) curved probe (Fig. 17.11); the bend is 3.5 cm from its end
- Free needles, lancet point (3/8) or needles with a crescent-shaped line, long.

Method

Using a long narrow scalpel, the bladder is incised vertically (some authors recommend an oblique incision) in the space between the two tension sutures. With the scalpel left in place, the bladder is drained and, when empty, the scalpel is replaced by forceps, whose jaws we divaricate once they have entered the bladder (widening the breach) to introduce the rabbeted probe, whose groove points ventrally. This advances until its bend coincides with the cystotomy.

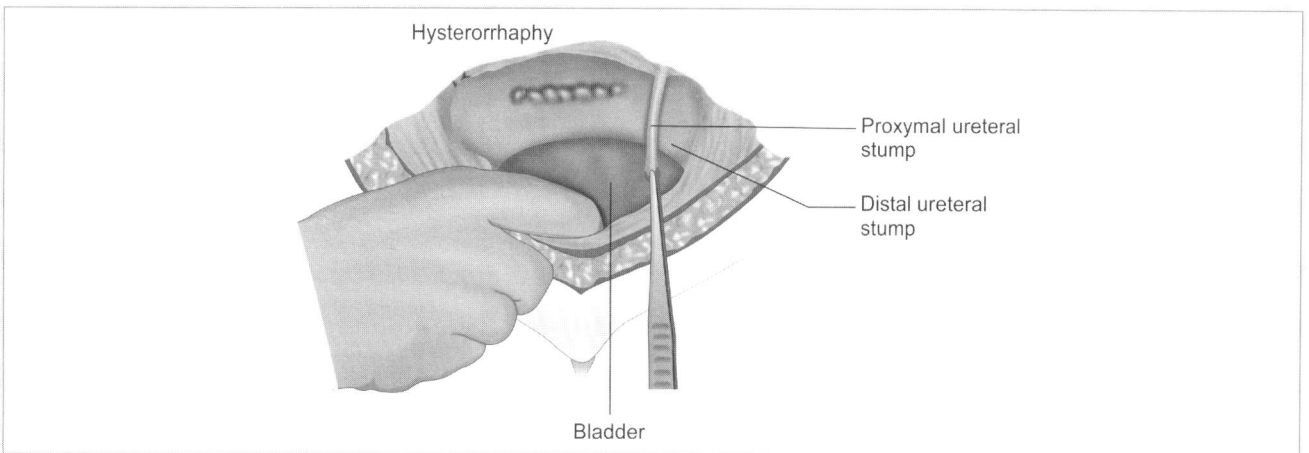

Fig. 17.10: Vesicolysis: Reimplantation of ureter following subtotal hysterectomy for uterine rupture

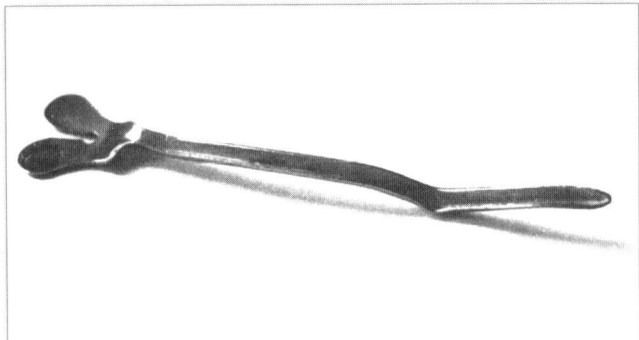

Fig. 17.11: Rabbeted probe with 130° bend 3.5 cm from end

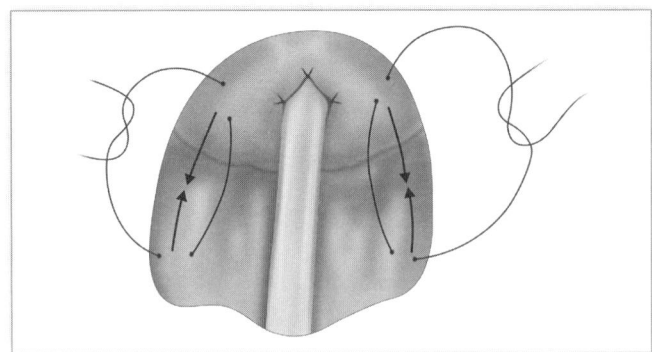

Fig. 17.13: Load-easing sutures for the ureter implant; the bladder is anchored to a nearby solid structure

We position the ureter, checking it has not been twisted back on itself, and on the ventral face (the face opposite that covered by peritoneum, where we applied the suture), only if certain that the blind technique is to be used, we make a 5 mm incision.

Now we mount one of the lancet-point needles with one of the strands from the ureter suture and, letting it run along the guide, whose point exerts pressure on the needle's point of insertion, (3 cm from the cystotomy), it is brought out again and forceps are applied to the thread. The second needle is mounted and, using the probe as a guide, it runs down and exits (3 cm from the cystotomy) approx. 5 mm laterally to the first.

We allow the ureter to slide along the probe until it enters the cavity by means of traction exerted on the threads from outside. Once the ureter has penetrated into the bladder and has reached its definitive position, the threads are tied (Fig. 17.12).

Now follows anchoring of the ureter to the cystotomy incision (3-4 sutures) using simple 3 0 chromic catgut, starting from the posterior angle (Fig. 17.12).

Load easing sutures are recommended to avoid tension on the sutures connecting the ureter to the bladder. These may be:

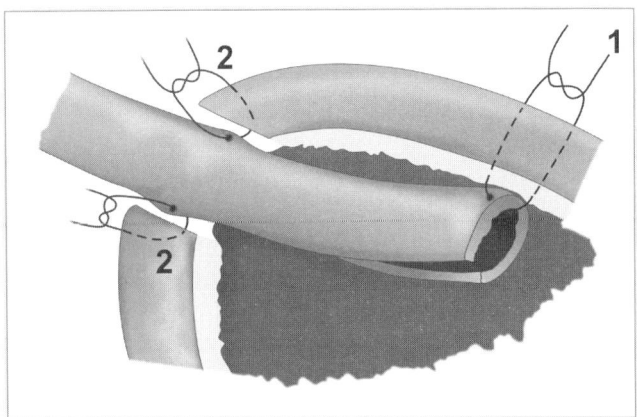

Fig. 17.12: With assistance from the stay sutures, the ureter is introduced into the bladder, advancing 3.5 cm; 1. The stay sutures, brought outside the bladder 5 mm apart, are tied

- Applied bilaterally at the entry of the ureter into the bladder, 2 cm apart; a suture is applied to include the bladder (muscularis included) and any strong structure nearby and the two strands are tied (Fig. 17.13). It may happen that no solid structures are available, or that the operating surgeon is uncertain where to apply the sutures. In this case an equally effective procedure is:
- Apply appositional sutures to the bladder (Fig. 17.14A and B), embedding the ureter in a hollow.

Omission to perform one of these two latter steps correctly can jeopardise the operation.

Reimplantation, Open Technique

This technique is to be used when difficulties are encountered or anticipated using the method above.

- Having identified the implant site, a stay suture is applied to the ureter; the 5 mm incision on the ventral side of the ureter is not made
- The assistant raises with two Allis forceps the anterior wall of the bladder to the midline (Fig. 17.15). The surgeon:
  - Incises the bladder wall between the forceps, allows the bladder to drain, applies two small dilators (Fig. 17.16) and identifies the trigone of the bladder and the vesicoureteral junction
  - Introduces curved forceps into the bladder and uses the points to exert pressure in the area identified for the reimplantation. The jaws are opened slightly and the external wall is incised from outside; the divaricated forceps tips now protrude on the external face of the bladder
  - Using the open forceps jaws and pulling on the tension suture thread, the ureter is introduced into the bladder and secured as shown in Figure 17.17
  - Closure of the cystotomy and reinforcement of the ureter at its entry into the bladder
  - Load-easing sutures are applied for the ureter (Fig. 17.18).

MANAGEMENT OF INTRAOPERATIVE COMPLICATIONS

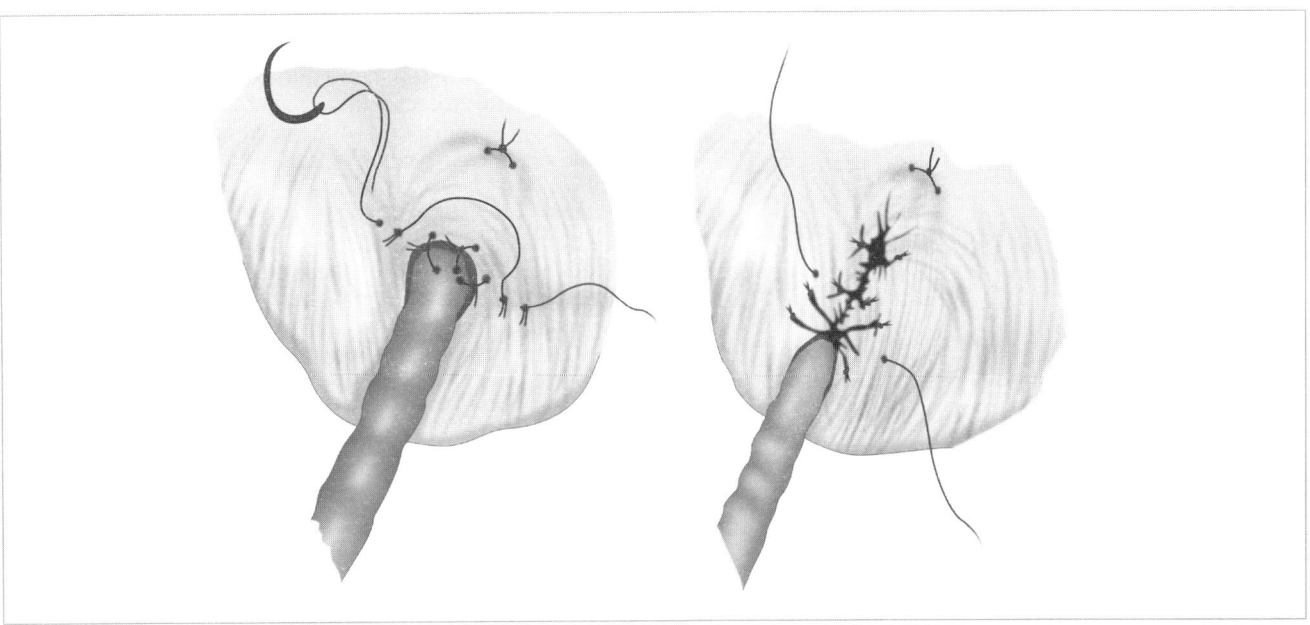

Fig. 17.14: Load-easing sutures for the ureter implant applied by embedding its point of entry: **A.** first suture, **B.** subsequent sutures, final view Care should be taken that the embedding does create kinking or stenosis of the ureter

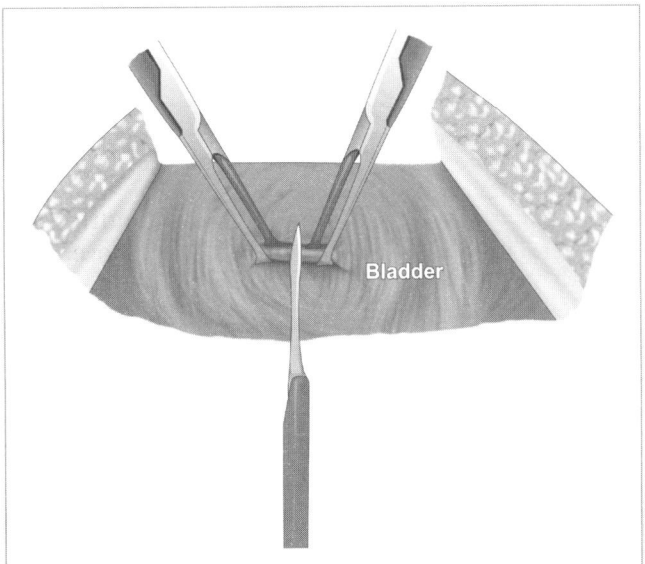

Fig. 17.15: Forceps and scalpel used to make an oblique incision in the bladder. Access is gained for the ureter to the inside of the bladder by divaricating the jaws of a pair of forceps. No longitudinal incision has been made to the ventral side of the urete

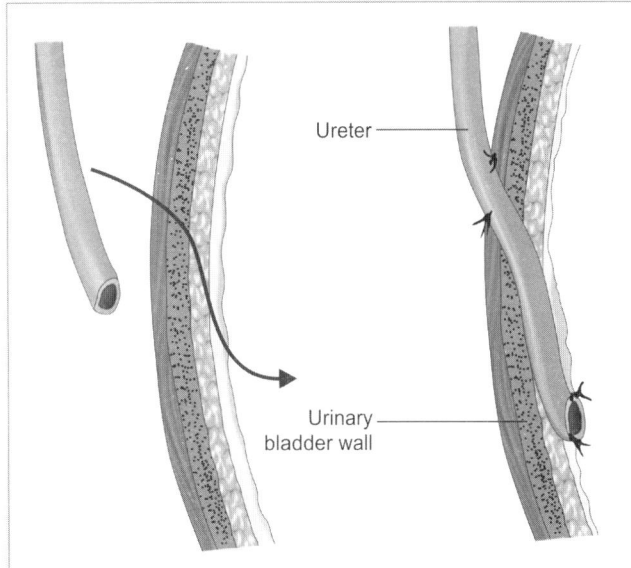

Fig. 17.16: The oblique, intraparietal route taken by the ureter has an anti-reflux function

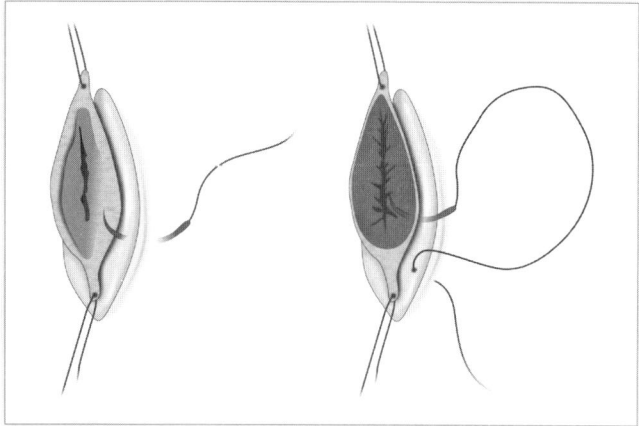

Fig. 17.17: The dorsal side of the ureter is sutured to the superior margin of the cystotomy; the ventral margin is sutured to the inferior margin of the cystotomy. Suturing is completed

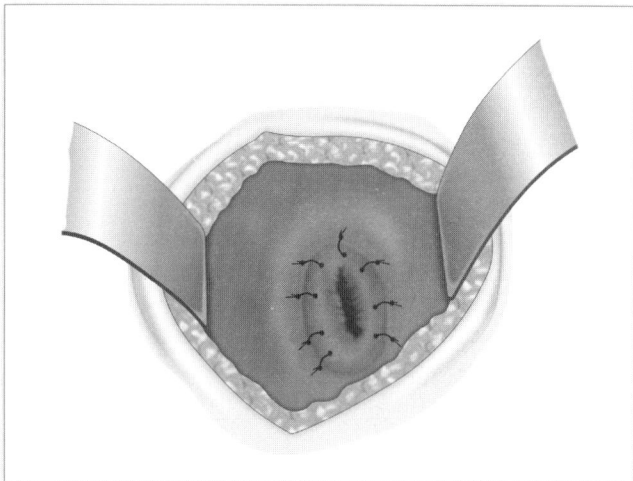

Fig. 17.18: Suturing has been completed

BIBLIOGRAPHY

1. B-Lynch C. The B-Lynch surgical technique for the control of massive post partum haemorrhage: an alternative to hysterectomy? Br J Obst Gynaec. 1997;104:372-5.
2. Couvelaire A. Introduction à la chirurgie uterine obstetricale. Steinheil, Paris, 1913.
3. Dauleh W, Al Sakka M, Shahata M. Urinary Tract Injuries During Caesarean Section. Qatar Medical Journal. 2006;15(2):18-23.
4. Daly JW, Higgings KA. Injury to the ureter during gynaecologic surgical procedures. Surg Gynecol Obstet. 1988;167:19-22.
5. Domini E, Timon D. Manuale di Ostetricia e Ginecologia Tropicale. 342-345. CIC Edizioni Internazionali, Roma, 1990.
6. Domini E, Guidi M, Guazzini S, Vicentini S. Preoperative transvaginale clamping of uterine arteries descending branches; a safe and reliable method to prevent from profuse bleeding during Caesarean Section for Central placenta previa. A preliminary report. G It Ostet Ginec. 2008;30(5):179-80.
7. Domini E, Guazzini S, Orlotti C. Uterine devascularization. G It Ostet Ginec. 2006:28(9):425.27.
8. Eisenkop SM, Richman R, Platt LD. Urinary tract injury during caesarean section. Obstet Gynecol. 1982;60:591.
9. Faricy PO, Augspurger RR, Kaufman JM. Bladder injuries associated with caesarean section. J Urol. 1978;120:762-3.
10. Feeney JK. Injury to the ureter in gynaecologic and obstetric operation. Ir J Med Sci. 1959;399:126-30.
11. Ghazi A, Iqbal P, Saddique M. Bladder and ureteric injuries during obstetric and gynaecologic procedures. Pakistan J Surg. 2008;24:54-6.
12. Gortzak UI, Walfisch A, Gortzak Y, Katz M, Major M, Hallak M. Accidental vaginal incision during caesarean section. A report of four cases. J Reprod Med. 2001;46:1017-20.
13. Hankins GDV, Clark SL, Cunningham FG, et al. Operative Obstetrics. Norwalk, Appleton & Lange. 1995. pp. 517-27.
14. Hema KR, Johanson RB. Techniques of performing caesarean section. Baillieve's Clin obstet Gyencol. 2001;15:17-47.
15. O' Leary JA. Uterine artery ligation in the control of postcaesarean haemorrhage. J Reprod Med Mar. 1995;40(3):189-93.
16. Phipps MG, Watabe B, Clemons JL, Weitzen S, Myers DL. Risk factors for bladder injury during cesarean delivery. Obstet Gynecol. 2005;105(1):156-60.
17. Porcaro AB, Zicari M, Zecchini Antoniolli S, Pianon R, Monaco C, Migliorini F, Longo M, Comunale L. Vesicouterine fistulas following cesarean section: report on a case, review and update of the literature. Int Urol Nephrol. 2002;34(3):335-44.
18. Rahman MS, Turki Gasem, Al Suleiman SA, Al Jama Fathia E, Sameera Burshaid, Rahman Jessica. Bladder injuries during cesarean section in a University Hospital: a 25-year review. Arch Gynec Ob. 2009;279:349-52.
19. Rajasekar D, Hall M. Urinary tract injuries during intervention. Br J Obstet Gynaecol. 1997;104:731-4.
20. Salvai J, Schmidt MH, Guilbert M, Martino A. Vascular ligation for severe obstetrical haemorrhage review of the literature. J Gynecol Obstet Biol Reprod (Paris). 2002;31(17):629-39.
21. Simm A, Ramoutar P. Caesarean Section: Techniques and complications. Current obstet and gynecol. 2005;15:80-6.
22. Thomas DP, Burgess NA, Gower RL, et al. Ureteric injury at caesarean section. Br J Urol. 1994;74:122-3.
23. Tsirulnikov MSJ. Gyn Obst Biol Repr. 1979;8:751.
24. Tsirulnikov Verspyk E, Resh B, Sergent E, Marpeau L. Surgical uterine devascularization for placenta accreta, immediate and long term follow up. Acta Obstet Gynecol. Stand. 2005;84(5):444-7.
25. Urueta JA, Mares MB, Gorbea Chávez V, Velázquez Valassi B. Risk factors for bladder injuries during cesarean section. Actas Urológicas Españolas July / August 2009.
26. Waters EG. Surgical Management of posrpartum haemorrhage with particular reference to ligation of uterine arteries. Am J Obstet Gynecol. 1952;64:1143-8.
27. Yossepowitch O, Baniel J, Livne PM. Urological injuries during caesarean section: intraoperative diagnosis and management. J Urol. 2004;172:196-9.
28. Youssef AF. Ménurie (urines mélangées du sang de règles) en tant que complication de la césarienne basse. Am J Obst Gyn. 1957;73(4):759-67 (Bibliogr.).
29. Youssef AF. Gynecological urology. Thomas, edit., Springfield (111), USA 1960. pp.679-94.

CHAPTER 18

Tubal Sterilization

Tubal sterilization refers here to a voluntary and permanent birth control intervention by means of interrupting the continuity of the fallopian tubes by their clamping and ligation, or by excision of a section of them.

INDICATIONS

These are subdivided in classic and elective.

Classic Indications

These are the indications envisaged by classic obstetrics, such as:
- *Maternal causes*: Cardiopathy, diabetes, lung disease
- *Uterine causes*: Following a longitudinal caesarean section (C-section), uterine rupture, repeated C-sections.

While recourse to tubal sterilisation is justified by maternal pathology, it is becoming less and less so in cases of classic C-section, repeated C-sections and uterine rupture; what may be impaired by such operations:
- *Is not the ability to conceive and to bring a pregnancy to term*—Scar dehiscence (silent rupture during pregnancy) represents a minimal percentage, while rupture during labour has a clear statistical profile
- *But rather the ability to give birth vaginally*—which is easily made up for by elective C-section.

Let us now move on to the classic indications for tubal sterilization.

Vertical Hysterotomy

A vertical hysterotomy *is not* of itself an indication for tubal sterilization. In our chapter on vertical hysterotomies we highlighted how, according to whether or not the fundus is affected by the incision, the previous classification of lower *and upper segment (corpus) vertical C-sections* had been replaced with that of *low and high vertical C section.*

There is an 8–10% (12% Rosen et al., 1991; ACOG 1999) of uterine ruptures among parturients admitted to labour, whose previous delivery had been via a high vertical hysterotomy; this means that 90–92% of these women succeed in vaginal delivery.

Furthermore, scar weakness is determined not just by the type of hysterotomy, but by the surgical terrain on which the operation was performed. In the wound healing process, a highly significant role is played by:

a. *Patient's age and parity*: Routine indications for a vertical hysterotomy are celaphopelvic disproportion or obstructed labour; conditions frequently found among very young primigravidae.

We know that the pelvis completes its development at around 18–20 years, for which reason performing tubal sterilisation on a 14–16 year-old following a vertical hysterotomy is a questionable procedure, indicative of poor obstetric training. It deprives a young woman, at the start of her life, of the future ability to be a mother, possibly making her a social outcast.

b. *Surgical terrain* on which the hysterotomy is performed: Anaemic, malnourished, septic.
c. *Degree of sterility* of the conditions in which the operation is conducted.
d. *Method utilised*: Haemostasis, proper apposition of edges.
e. *Amount and quality of the suture material used.*
f. *Postoperative recovery*, fever.

If all these indications are heeded, the scar will be sound and, once a certain period of time (two years) has passed, will allow another pregnancy.

Repeat C-sections

One of the rules commonly followed in obstetrics is tubal sterilisation after the third C-section. In this connection Roberts (1991) wrote a paper "Where is the evidence".

We all have found ourselves performing a 3rd, 4th and even 5th C-section on patients who have withheld their consent for tubal sterilisation, without observing any particular abnormalities in the uterus. This observation is supported by van Dillen's (2007) study in a semi-rural hospital in Namibia, which reports 2nd, 3rd, 4th and subsequent C-sections without encountering abnormal events.

It is advisable to rectify the edges of the uterine incision (removing scar tissue) before uterine suture.

Reproductive ability is of extreme importance in the Tropics, and every decision affecting it should be discussed with the patient and her family, perhaps agreeing that the second part of a subsequent pregnancy should be spent close to the hospital.

Generally, African hospital have nearby 'Waiting Homes' or 'Shelters', where non-bedridden parturients ('floor cases') stay ahead of labour.

Uterine Ruptures

We refer the reader to Chapter 21.

Elective Indications

These involve the patient's express consent, with some limitations.

Never carry out a C-section for the sole purpose of performing tubal sterilisation:
- A wife's consent should be corroborated by written agreement of the husband and/or family
- If a woman is still young and has just two or three children, present counter-arguments. A common occurrence is that at 30–35 years of age, when the children are grown up, mothers return seeking new pregnancies, now no longer possible.

If a C-section candidate is determinate, never perform it during operation, but defer it to some time later as it is not uncommon for a surgeon, during a C-section, to miss anomalies in the examination of the new born child that may indicate death during its first days of life.

Before proceeding, one month later, with sterilization by mini laparotomy, always check that the child has survived.

If the patient has many living children and appears exhausted by her many pregnancies, do not hesitate to interrupt tubal patency during the C-section, if C-section is indicated.

Complications

These have an incidence of 1–4% and are subdivided into:
- *Immediate* (postoperative)
- *Late-onset*—which are further subdivided into:
  a. *Post-tubal syndrome* (Shain et al., 1985; Rulin et al. 1989), characterised by dysmenorrhoea, menorrhagia, cycle irregularity and pelvic pain.
  b. *Sterilisation failure:* The first large-scale study of this issue was conducted by Thomas (1953). Reviewing 35,000 sterilisations, it highlighted a failure rate of 0.5%, which Garb (1957) found to be 0.4%.

In a nationwide study carried out in the United States, (1989), CDC units monitored patients over a 5-year postoperative follow-up, with a high control rate (85%). This found a higher failture rate, of 0.8%. These findings were accepted by ACOG, who in 1991 admitted that, while over 99% of women who have undergone this operation do not get pregnant, the procedure does not guarantee sterility. The findings of a second study, which appeared in 2002, did not diverge significantly.

The percentage of failures (subsequent pregnancies) varies with:
- *Stage at which the operation is performed*: One of the earliest studies (Prystowsky, 1955) demonstrated how the ratio of failures is 1:57 when sterilisation is effected during a C-section, against a ratio of 1:340 when it is performed during puerperium, following a vaginal delivery
- *Method used*
- *Ratio between intrauterine and extrauterine pregnancies:* The percentage of ectopic pregnancies varies according to method used. The safest methods are found to be spring clamps and rings. Mono- or bipolar coagulation, which could give rise to a tubal fistula, are found to have double the failure rate of Pomeroy tubal ligation. No data are available for the Madlener technique.

Method

- *The Madlener technique for tubal sterilisation*: This method, first used in 1910 and described in 1919, occludes the tube by means of double compression held in place by a ligature. In Madlener's own words: "The operator grasps the tube in the mid-portion, where it is most mobile and elevates it to angulate at approximately 90° [forming a loop]. A crushing clamp is then applied so as to encounter the tube obliquely along with a small portion of the mesosalpinx". By opening and closing the Kocher or Klemmer forceps a few times, "closed tight so that the tissue is surely crushed paper thin. The crushing clamp is then removed and a thin thread ligature [non-absorbable] is placed in the groove". The ligature is not cut, the tube is elevated once more and forceps applied across its axis, 5 mm inferiorly to the previous ligation. The crushing action is repeated and the ligature, again non-absorbable, is knotted once again; the loop is not resected.

This is the procedure followed by the authors.

- *Pomeroy tubal sterilisation*: Conceived by Pomeroy in 1919, this method was first described by his students, (Bishops, E. Nelms, W.) in 1930. The technique effects sterilisation by means of separation of two tubal ends and their occlusion through fibrosis.

The tube (Fig. 18.1) is elevated in its mid-portion using Allis forceps. A figure-of-eight suture in No. 0 chromic catgut, is placed around the loop (Fig. 18.2) and tied. The loop is resected (Fig. 18.3) above the ligature. The catgut will be absorbed after some time, and the two ends of the cut tube have become sealed off and widely separate (Fig. 18.4).

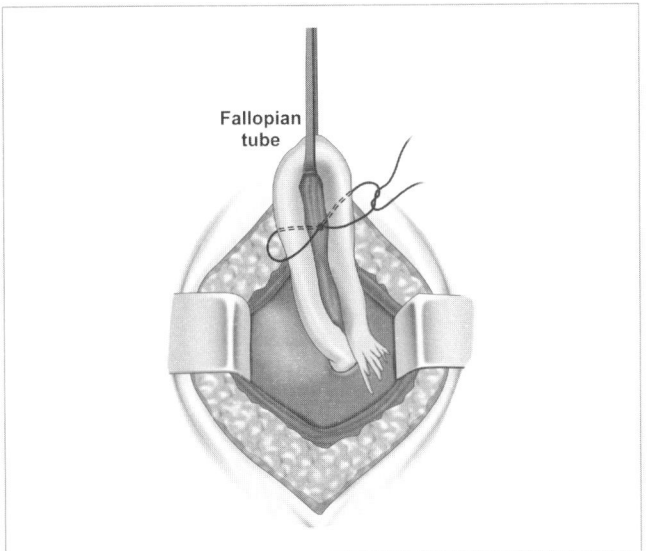

Fig. 18.1: 1 Pomeroy tubal sterilization the tube is elevated near the middle with an Allis forceps, a figure of 8 ligature is placed 5 mm below the apex of the loop

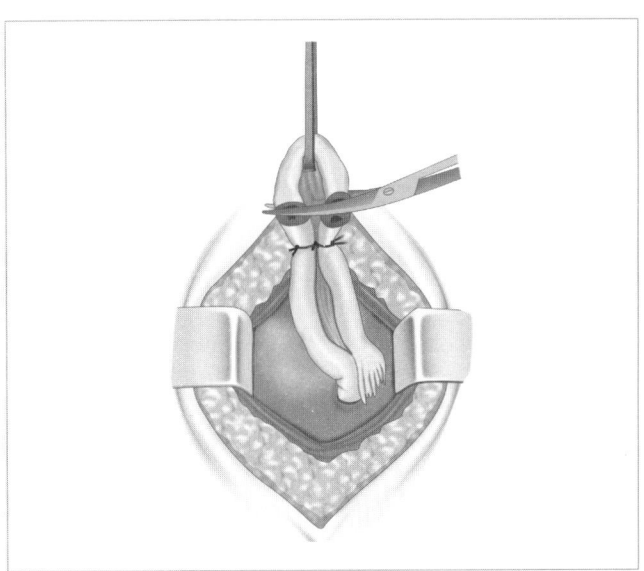

Fig. 18.3: Pomeroy tubal sterilization: The loop of tube above ligature is cut off with scissors

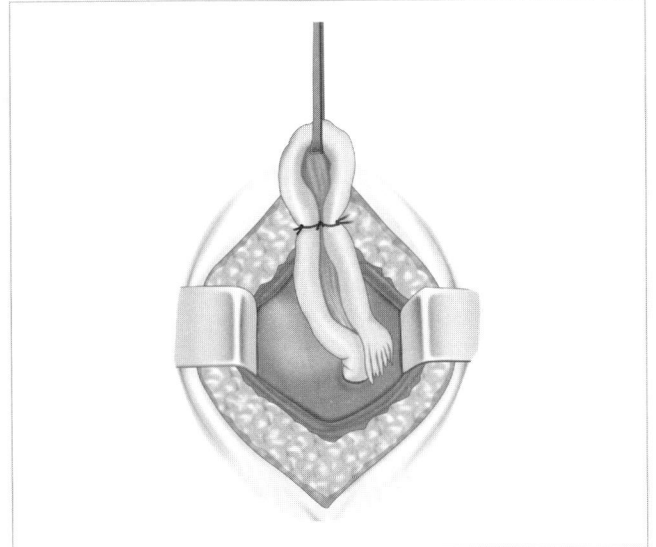

Fig. 18.2: Pomeroy tubal sterilization: The ligature is firmly but gently tied

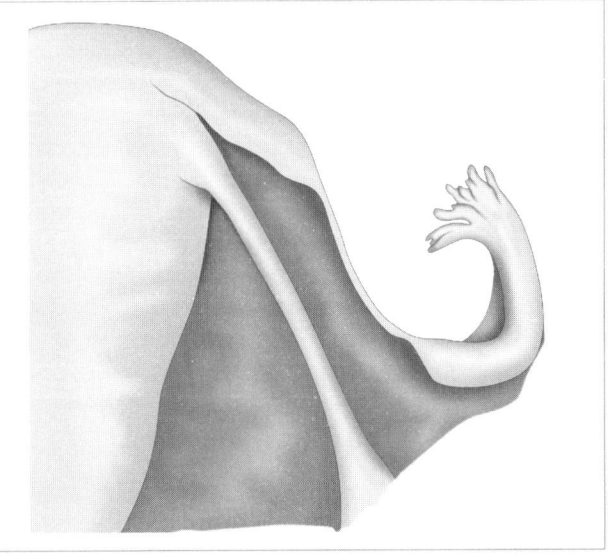

Fig. 18.4: Pomeroy tubal sterilization, long-term outcome: The two ends of the cut have become sealed off and widely apart

BIBLIOGRAPHY

1. Bishops E, Nelms W. A simple method of tubal sterilisation. New York State J Medicine. 1930;30:214-6.
2. Centers for Disease Control and Prevention. Fact Sheet: Risk of Ectopic Pregnancy after Tubal Sterilization, August 6, 2002.
3. Dillen van J, Meguid T, Petrova V, Roosmalen van J. Caesarean section in a semi-rural hospital in Northern Namibia. BMC Pregnancy Childbirth. 2007;7:2.
4. Madlener M. Ueber sterilisierende Operationen an den Tuben Zbl F Gynak. 1919;43:380-4.
5. Phillips JM. American Association of Gynaecologic Laparoscopists 1979 Membership Survey. J Reprod Med. 1981;26:529.
6. Prystowsky H, Eaastman NJ. Puerperal tubal sterilization. Report of 1830 cases. JAMA. 1955;158:463.
7. Roberts, Lawrence W. Elective section after two sections- Where is the evidence?. Br J Obst Gynaec. 1991;98:1199-202.
8. Rulin MC. Changes in menstrual symptoms among sterilized and comparison women, a prospective study. Obstet Gynaec. 1989;74:149.
9. Shain RN. Menstrual pattern change 1 year after sterilization: result of a controlled, prospective study. Fertil Steril. 1989;52:192.

CHAPTER 19

Abdominal Wall Closure

This is the final step in every laparotomy; correct execution and good final outcome presuppose knowledge of the healing mechanisms for surgical wounds and of the factors that may interfere with them.

PHYSIOLOGICAL INTRODUCTION OF WOUND HEALING

Stimulated by the surgical incision, wound repair occurs in four overlapping phases: Haemostasis, inflammation, proliferation and maturation (Waldrop et al., 2000, Chin et al., 2005).

Haemostasis: Characterised by the aggregation of platelets, from their *degranulation*, substances that act on the wound are released, these include: PDGF (platelet derived growth factor), which in turn activates TGF (transforming growth factor beta), PAF (platelet activating factor), fibronectin and seratonin. Concomitantly, coagulation mechanisms are activated, with fibrin supporting recruitment to the wound site of leukocytes, neutrophil granulocytes and monocytes that remove devitalised tissue and bacteria. The monocytes promote the proliferation of fibroblasts and neovascularisation.

Within 24 hours, epithelial cells are migrating towards the wound from surrounding healthy tissue. Within 24–48 hours, effective protection against germs and bacteria has been re-established and over 5 days the skin has resumed a normal appearance.

Inflammation: Macrophages, cellular lysis and neutrophils provide a source of cytokines and growth factors, which are essential for the normal healing process.

Proliferation: The formation of granulation tissue, filling the space between the two oozing surfaces, begins on the third postoperative day and continues over many weeks.

Maturation: This commences on the seventh postoperative day and continues over an year (Waqer et al., 2005; West et al., 2005). It is characterised by the migrazione of fibroblasts, that starts 48 hours after the incision and peaks after 7 days. Fibroblasts provide for collagen synthesis, which is usually completed within a month, and for subsequent remodelling, characterised by interweaving of fibres, which lasts for an year, ensuring that the wound is increasingly able to withstand tensile loads. The wound's tensile strength, compared to that of healthy tissue, is 20% at 3 weeks, 60% at 4 months and reaches a maximum after an year, although it will never equal that of the original healthy tissue. The scar remains red and prominent for approximately 8 weeks and then, as the collagen remodels, it retracts and the erythema abates.

The lines of force acting on the wound edges originate from surrounding healthy tissue and the underlying muscles. As the tensile strength of scar tissue is less than that of normal tissue, once the sutures have been removed, the wound edges will tend to pull apart if the incised surface lies perpendicular to these lines of force; but the wound will suffer no deformation and the edges will tend to stay together if the incision is parallel to these lines of force.

As described, the healing process requires two essential conditions:

a. *That the wound edges are kept in stable contact*: The suturing is responsible for this;

b. *That factors liable to interfere with nomal healing processes are absent*: This requires an adequate supply of oxygen (that the suture is not tied too tightly as to induce *ischaemia*), normal blood sugar levels and the absence of toxic or septic factors that reduce the synthesising ability of collagen and the bactericidal powers of the neutrophils (Smith M et al., 1967; Fleischer GM. et al., 2000).

REPAIR OF A VERTICAL LAPAROTOMY WOUND

Guiding Principles

There are various schools of thought about how to repair a laparotomic wound—whether to suture each anatomical plane in layered closure or to use a single-layer suture (mass closure), and what suture material to use.

Layered Closure following Anatomical Layers

Some authors (including ourselves) believe that each layer of the abdominal wall has its function and that the best way to ensure correct healing is to follow these layers, using inert sutures of suitable size and tension for each layer, after having removed any scar tissue to obtain well vascularized edges with normal repair capacity.

Parietal peritoneum

The peritoneum covers two functions—to prevent from adhesions and spread of infections. The spread of infection to the abdominal wall, with resulting *dehiscence of the wound* itself is a frequent occurence following septic abdominal surgery.

One open question is whether or not to close the peritoneum.

Repair to a peritoneal defect is mainly effected by macrophages present in the peritoneal fluid and to a lesser extent through concomitant centripetal diffusion of mesothelial factors from the surrounding areas, analogously to the action of epithelial cells in the case of a skin injury. Another mechanism is stem-cell transformation (Ellis, 1971). Within 3–4 days, the area is indistinguishable from the surrounding peritoneum.

According to some authors (Karipineni et al., 1976; Ellis & Heddle, 1977; Kapur et al., 1979; McFadden & Peacock, 1983; Pietrantoni et al., 1990), this speed of repair to peritoneal defects renders surgical repair superfluous; omission of peritoneal closure is thought not to predispose to adhesions nor to influence wound strength or dehiscence.

Supporters of peritoneal suturing believe that *the speed of repair to the peritoneum is proof of the importance of peritoneal integrity.*

A further advantage of non-closure is thought to derive from a reduction in operating times. "Neither the visceral nor the parietal peritoneum should be sutured at CS because this reduces operating time and the need for postoperative analgesia, and improves maternal satisfaction" (NICE, 2004).

All the evidence and case samples cited so far refer to Western countries where a septic C-section is a rare occurence, where sterility of instrumentation and good quality sutures are guaranteed. These conditions are not always present in resource-poor countries. Given the non-existence of literature concerning the peritoneal closure/non-closure debate for the latter group of countries, we can refer only to our own experience. This shows how widespread adhesions between the abdominal peritoneal wall and the anterior uterine wall are almost constantly the consequence of operations in which peritoneal closure has not been performed, and how adhesions can be widespread and tenacious enough to render the anatomical layers indistinguishable.

Adhesions can also be observed following laparotomies and C-sections in which peritoneal closure has been performed, but they are then more moderate in extent and lysis is easier (always by sharp, not blunt dissection).

The hypothesis that non-closure does not lead to an increase in adhesions has recently been questioned (Myers et al., 2005; Cheong et al., 2006), who assigned the following 'adhesion score':

1. No adhesion.
2. Adhesions present; lysis not necessary or very easy.
3. Extensive, tough adhesions that impede uterine exteriorisation; lysis is necessary.
4. Adhesions whose lysis is required (intestinal occlusion) before a repeat caesarean section.

They used these criteria to classify adhesions encountered in subsequent C-sections. Severe adhesions (Classes 3 and 4) were found in 17 out of 40 patients (21% of cases examined) in which peritoneal closure had been omitted, but in only 1 out of the 18 cases in which peritoneal closure had been performed. This led to a conclusion that peritoneal closure is advisable: *"In the absence of any substantive benefit or published data regarding adhesion formation in caesarean section that contradict this finding, the practice of non-closure of visceral and parietal peritoneum at cesarean section should be questioned."*

Method used by the authors (Fig. 19.1). Closure of the parietal peritoneum is performed using non-interlocking continuous suturing (No 2/0, 3/0 catgut or vycril). We start with *reperitonealization of the bladder flap* with a purse string suture which begins 3 cm laterally from the bladder dome and once reached it continues beyond for a further 3 cm.

To prevent from adhesions, the peritoneum edges have to be everted (face outwards the abdominal cavity), for this reason the purse string suture proceeds from the extraperitoneal surface to the intraperitoneal one and

ABDOMINAL WALL CLOSURE

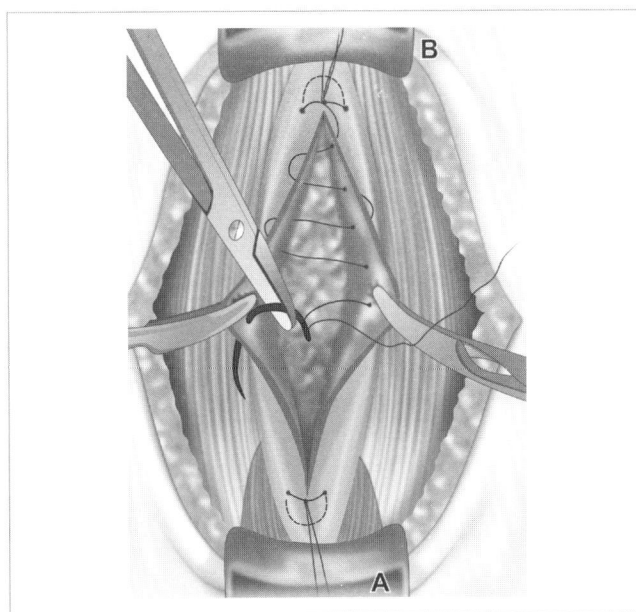

Fig. 19.1: Repair of a longitudinal celiotomy. (A) Inferior peritoneal end; (B) Superior peritoneal end. The repair starts from A using a half purse-string suture that takes in 6 cm of peritoneum; the half purse-string is knotted and a 6–8 cm tail is left. B is then included in a half purse-string suture, which is knotted and the suture proceeds caudad, including the transversalis fascia

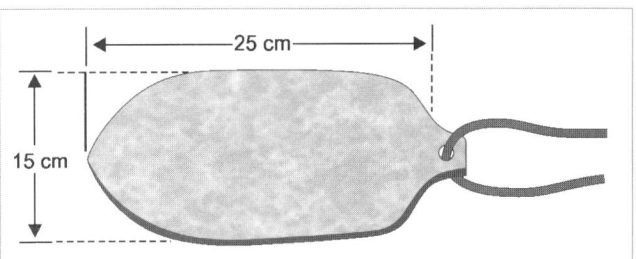

Fig. 19.2: Fish-shaped viscera retainer

progresses similarly to the last bite where it goes the other way: from the intraperitoneal surface to the extraperitoneal one; the two ends are tied together and a long tail left.

Starting now from the superior end, as the peritoneum cannot withstand mechanical stress, we anchor the suture to the posterior fascia of the rectus abdominis muscle sheath and proceed caudad with an *everting continuous suture* until meeting the tail of the inferior purse string suture; the two ends are tied together.

If the celiotomy is transverse we begin by suturing the wound-end closest to us (purse string suture) following the same procedure described above as first, then with the opposite one. The two ends are tied together.

If you have difficulty with:
- *Accessing the lateral peritoneal margins*—apply a pean clamp to the superior end of the peritoneum that covers the bladder. Traction in the direction opposite to that of the edge you want to locate will expose the peritoneum, to which a pean clamp is applied—preferably not to the free edge, but to a fold (which has more strength - Emmet's technique);
- *Accessing the superior peritoneal margin*—use your dominant hand (right hand if you are right-handed) to grasp the superior end of the laparotomic wound with your thumb inside the cavity and the four fingers outside; using the four fingers as a pivot, rotate the abdominal

flap externally. This will expose the borders of the rectus abdominis sheath and the end of the peritoneum, which you can now suture. Always leave a long tail (8–10 cm), which can be used to tie the suture at each throw in case of dilated small gut loops;
- *Closure of the peritoneum*—due to the presence of dilated intestinal loops. We recommend three methods in order of increasing severity:
  - Apply two Kocher forceps to the fascia and exert strong upward traction; this movement should provide useful space. Remember that in closing the peritoneum, you should be concentrating on each suture as it happens; if you leave a long tail, each throw can be tied
  - Insert a spatula or a 'fish' (Fig. 19.2) between the intestinal loops and the peritoneum. Such a 'fish' can easily be cut from a car inner-tube and as rubber can be sterilised
  - By spraying the intestinal loops with 10 mL of local anaesthetic without adrenaline, combined with 20 mL of isotonic solution, you will be surprised how well this helps.

Apposition of the muscle bellies

Integrity of the anterior abdominal wall is essential for developing the endoabdominal pressure indispensible for such functions as defecation, urination, vomiting, childbirth and in lifting loads.

The muscular columns of this wall are the rectus abdominis muscles. Inserted on the pubis, they lower the thorax and ribs by flexing the thorax against the pelvis. They thus serve both as expiratory and flexor muscles of the thorax, presenting a *dorsally directed concavity*, which is straightened as they contract, thereby compressing the viscera and developing endoabdominal pressure.

Diastasis recti (separation of the two rectus abdominis muscles in the midline at the linea alba) is a frequent post partum and post laparotomy occurrence, clinically manifest during contraction.

Failure to correct a pre-existing diastasis, or lack of apposition between the rectus muscles when their sheaths have been opened has the following consequences:
- *Short-term*: endoabdominal pressure is exerted directly on the fascia, predisposing to wound dehiscence;

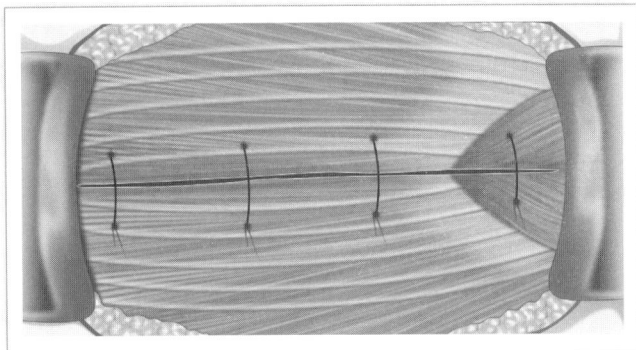

Fig. 19.3: Repair of a laparotomic wound following anatomical strata; myorrhaphy of the rectus muscles using single interrupted sutures

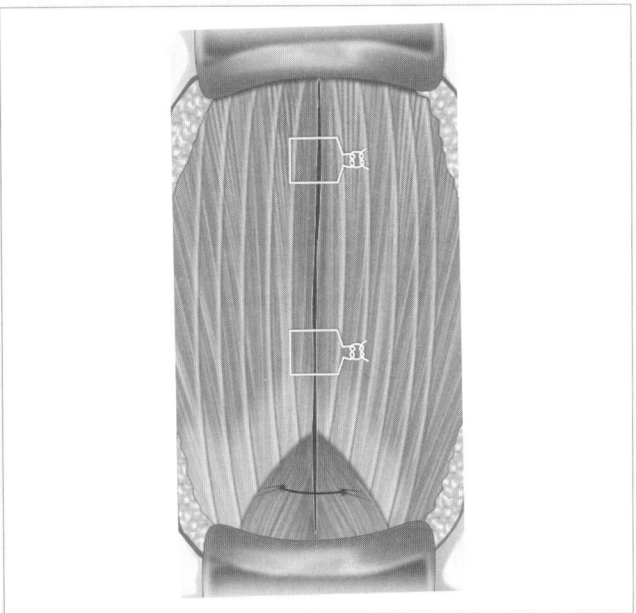

Fig. 19.4: Repair of a laparotomic wound following anatomical strata; myorrhaphy of the rectus muscles using U-sutures and square knots

- *Medium- and long-term:* diastasis recti may entail:
  - Reduction in endoabdominal pressure (30%), reduced ability to lift heavy loads (15%) and difficulty (38%) raising oneself from a supine position
  - Abdominal pain (47%) when endoabdominal pressure builds up protrusion of abdominal contents (42%) ventral hernia.

Additively, these factors reduce a mother's ability to work, which is felt especially in resource-poor countries, where following childbirth, women are expected to carry the child, gather firewood, carry water and provide meals.

Apposition of the muscle bellies may be effected:
- Using single interrupted sutures (Fig. 19.3)
- Using (Fig. 19.4) two U-shaped sutures tied using a square knot (two doubled knots)
- Using continuous suturing along the medial edges of the recti.

Closure of the fascia

It is the fascia that, among the abdominal wall layers: skin, subcutaneous tissue, fascia, muscle and peritoneum, that effects containment of the viscera.

The *holding capacity of a suture*, apart from the intrinsic characteristics of the tissue in which it is placed, depends on three further variables:

a. *The direction of the fibres in which the suture is applied*: Sutures applied orthogonally have a firmer bite. From a histological viewpoint, the fascia comprises three layers, from superficial to deep these are: *lamina fibrae obliquae, lamina fibrae traversae* and *lamina fibrae irregularium*. In all of these fibres, it is the transverse orientation that predominates (Fig. 13.17), so that, when making:
   - *A vertical incision* (midline laparotomy), the suture is exposed to lateral stresses whenever the abdominal wall muscles contract, which will tend to drive the wound edges apart
   - *A transverse incision*, which runs in the direction of the fibres. Each contraction here approximates the fibres and therefore the wound edges (see the section on transverse laparotomies in Chapter 13 and Fig. 13.18A and B).

Just as the stresses exerted on the suture will vary with its relationship to the fibres, so too will the suture technique vary.

b. *The distance from the wound edge* at which the suture is applied.
c. *The amount of tissue* included in the bite.

Fascia repair may be effected using continuous or interrupted suturing.

Continuous Suturing

Jenkins (1976) was the first to examine the problem of stress and suture strength from a mechanical point of view. Mathematical operations on his results derived the '*one-centimetre rule*' that sutures should be placed 1 cm from the fascia edge and that the gap between one suture and the next should be 1 cm (Fig. 19.5). This entails an optimal ratio of 4:1 between the length of suture thread used and the length of the surgical wound. The adoption of this rule has led to a dramatic fall in wound dehiscence and ventral hernias. Even when the suture is of the fascia only, this 1-centimetre rule should not be changed, as sutures placed too closely together have been associated with higher incidence of wound-infection (Israelson et al., 1993) due to the presence of extraneous material, while placing sutures further apart would not ensure constant contact between the wound edges, necessary for good healing. Subsequently, Kendall (1991) and Varshney et al.

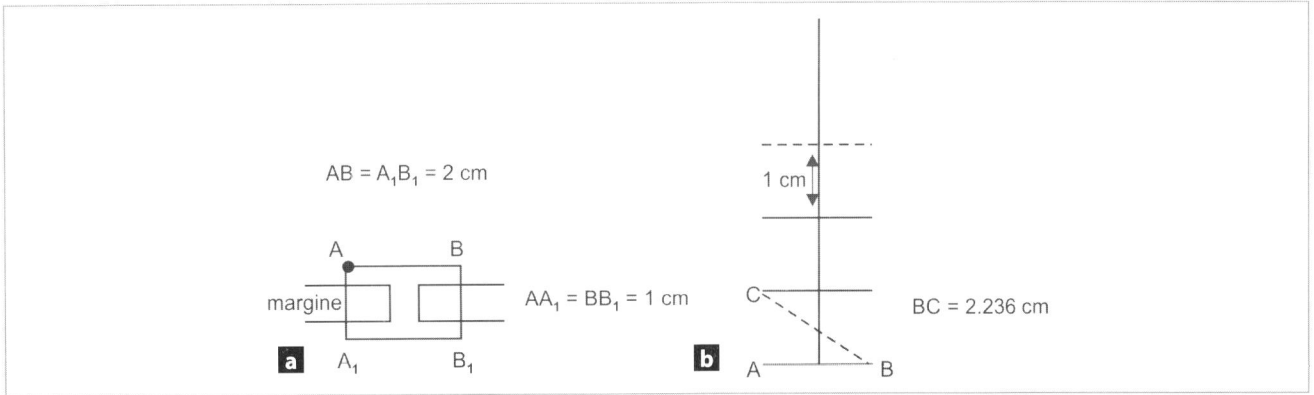

Fig. 19.5: Repair of a laparotomic wound following the anatomic layers. Joining the fascia using continuous suturing, Jenkins' rule. (a) AB, suture straddling the fascia edges at distance AB = 2 cm; (b) If sutures are 1 cm apart, the throw from B to C is 2.236 cm in length. Therefore, the length of thread required for one stitch is 2 + 2.236 = 4.236 cm, which becomes 4 cm when the thread is pulled

(1999) have held that greater suture holding strength can be derived from including in the bite a portion of muscle to a depth of 1 cm. This leads to an optimal ratio of 6:1 between suture thread length and length of surgical wound.

Method

- *Continuous suturing:* Some authors recommend two simple continuous sutures starting from the wound ends and meeting in the middle. Whether or not throws should be simple or interlocking is a matter of debate. We point out that the overriding function of a lock-stitch suture is not - contrary to popular belief - haemostasis, but prevention of wound puckering, which is possible as continuous sutures pull on each other
- *Method used by the authors*: Despite its many advantages, continuous suturing presents the sole drawback that suture fastness can be endangered by the failure of a single throw. The suturing technique we use combines the advantages of the interrupted suture with those of continuous suturing. The suture comprises two continuous sutures that start from the wound ends and meet in the middle. If we examine an individual stitch; starting from a corner, it is passed 'in - out - out-in' and is knotted *internally* (subfascially), leaving a tail approximately 10 cm long. The following stitch is 1 cm away, passes in-out-out-in and is again knotted. Proceeding in this way, until reaching the mid-point of the suture, one then starts from the opposite wound-end: the two sutures meet in the middle and are knotted.

Interrupted Sutures

The 'one-centimetre rule' can also be applied to interrupted suture. However, the incidence of dehiscence and ventral hernia is higher among wounds repaired using interrupted sutures than for those repaired by continuous suturing. This derives from the fact that sutures undergo two directions of stress: Transverse and longitudinal. In cases of abdominal distension, the latter stresses may cause wounds to lengthen by up to 30% (Jenkins, 1976). It seems clear that an interrupted suture can cope with transverse stresses, keeping contact between the wound surfaces, but cannot deal with longitudinal stresses, or maintain contact in the gaps between two sutures, while a continuous suture can.

A second reason could be (Whipple and Elliott) the overtightening of sutures, which occurs more frequently in interrupted suturing. Tissue strangulation could lead to ischaemic necrosis, lessening the ability of tissue to withstand stress, in comparison to tissue where the wound edges were simply approximated.

Single-layer Closure (Mass Stitching)

With the terms 'mass closure' or 'mass stitching' we refer to suturing that includes all strata: Fascia, muscle, and peritoneum in one operation. Mass closure can be effected by means of interrupted or continuous suturing.
- *Interrupted sutures:* These may be simple or (preferably) Smead Jones sutures, of which two variants exist (Figs 19.6 and 19.7). According to Sivam (1995), these offer better results in emergency laparotomies
- *Simple or interlocking continuous sutures:* These are found to have the following advantages (Chow, 1995): Strength and less time required to execute compared to layered closure, they also leave no dead spaces between each layer.

Closure of Subcutaneous Layer and of Skin

Subcutaneous tissue and camper's fascia

There are opposing views on whether the subcutaneous layer ought to be sutured. Some authors (Stark, 1992)

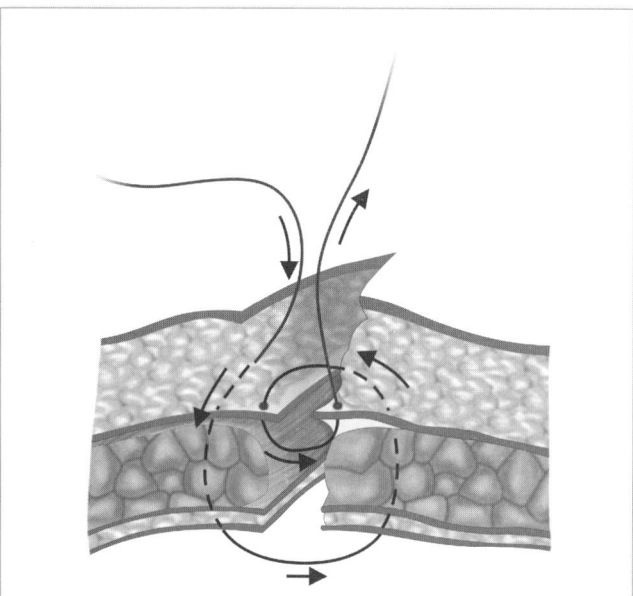

Fig. 19.6: Single-layer closure of laparotomic wound using interrupted sutures. Smead-Jones I Suture: Initial throws both include: Fascia, muscle and peritoneum. The loop is completed with a fresh bite into the fascia

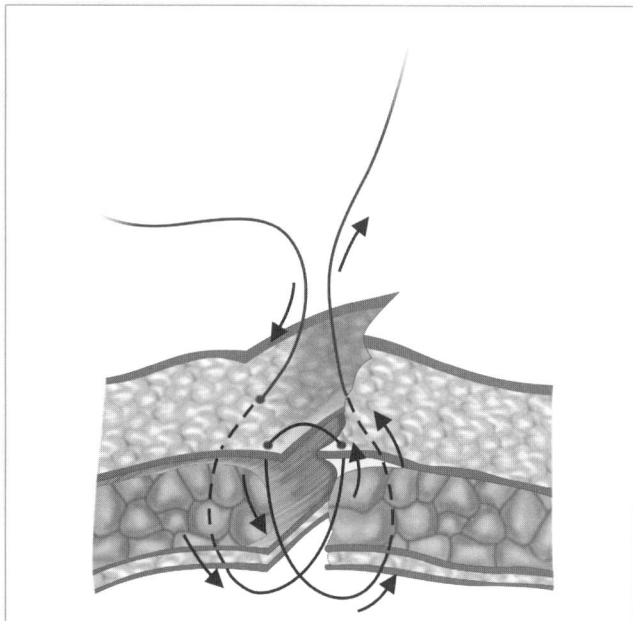

Fig. 19.7: Single-layer closure of laparotomic wound using interrupted sutures. Smead-Jones II Suture: On entry, the stitch passes through fascia, muscle and peritoneum, whence, across the space between the two peritoneal and rectus muscle flaps, it passes directly to the contralateral fascia, then back to the homolateral fascia, after which it passes back through contralateral peritoneum, muscle and fascia

maintain that suturing should never take place, while others (Nauman et al., 1997) hold it advisable to suture the subcutis when its thickness is greater than 2 cm.

Our practice is to suture *always* Camper's fascia with interrupted sutures: This prevents the spread of infections from the skin to deeper strata (some authors maintain the opposite), and it facilitates the subsequent apposition of skin margins. Omission of suturing has been associated with the formation of seroma or haematoma and to promote superficial wound dehiscence, especially in pregnancies where featuring high levels of tissue vascularization and oedema (Hussain, 1990; Del Valle et al., 1992).

Suturing is always preceded by debridement of the subcutaneous tissue and wound using tincture of iodine.

We do not suture Camper's fascia in septic surgical procedures.

Skin

Skin repair techniques vary according to whether or not the wound is infected.

a. If *the wound is not infected*, the surgeon may choose:
   – Simple interrupted sutures or Donati sutures. The latter offer good apposition of edges
   – Continuous suturing that may be subcuticular or external mattress suturing; nylon is the ideal material (5 knots, alternating).

   According to some authors, it is not advisable to use continuous suturing in the Tropics in that any drainage of pus sacs or hematoma could compromise the fastness of the internal suturing.

b. If *the wound is infected,* it is judicious to position three or four apposition sutures on the skin, "delayed primary suture", and to proceed with wound repair only when the inflammation is under control (Diminick, 1988).

Load-easing or Deep Tension or Retention Sutures

Following septic sugical procedures in obese or malnourished patients in which difficult re-canalisation and/or healing is foreseen, it is advisable to avoid excessive stress on the fascia by placing load easing or *deep tension sutures*.

All abdominal layers are held together without tension, the sutures take the tension off the wound edges.

Before initiating closure of the abdominal wall, simple or U-sutures in nonabsorbable material—nylon monofilament is indicated—are applied 2 cm from the wound edges (Fig. 19.9). These may:

- *Include all of the layers of the abdominal wall,* but exclude the peritoneum (Fig. 19.8A) or include it (Fig. 19.8B)
- *Be simple* (Fig. 19.8B) or *double* following Smead Jones (Figs 19.6, 19.7 and 19.9)
- *Be single* and knotted individually (Figs 19.10 and 19.11), *or double* (Figs 19.12A to C) *or U-shaped sutures* (Fig. 19.14).

ABDOMINAL WALL CLOSURE

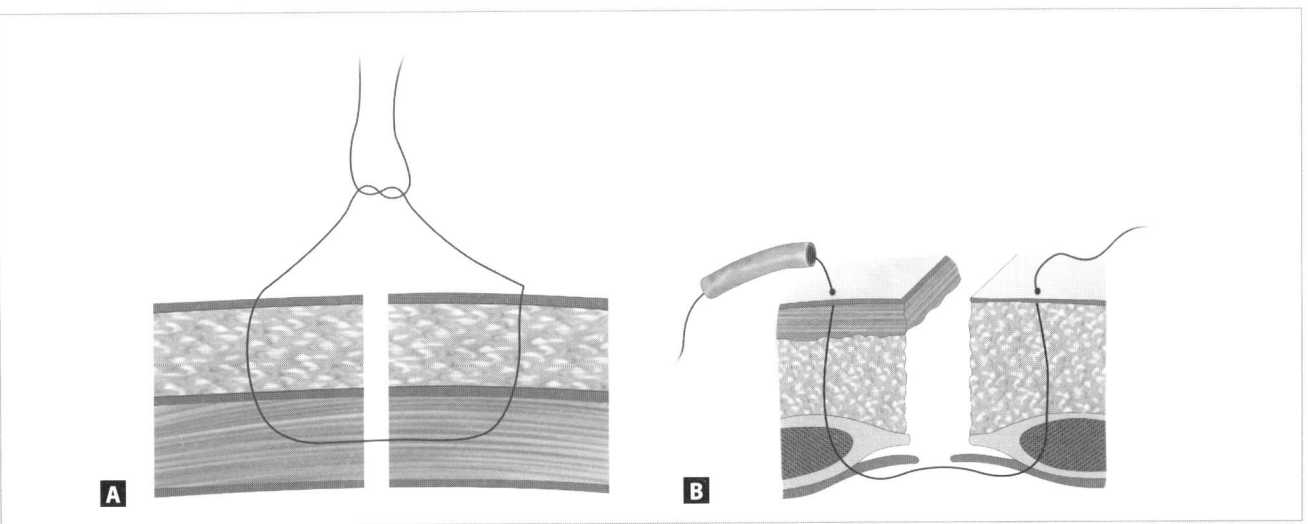

Fig. 19.8: (A) Deep load easing or tension suture that does not include the peritoneum; (B) Deep tension suture that includes the peritoneum

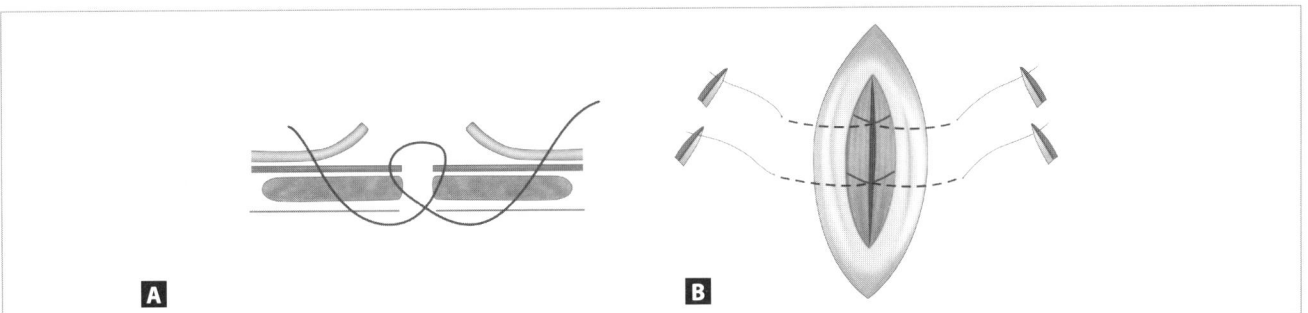

Fig. 19.9: (A) Saggital section; (B) Anterior view. Double deep tension suture reminiscent of the Smead Jones variant II, from which it differs in that it starts and finishes above the skin

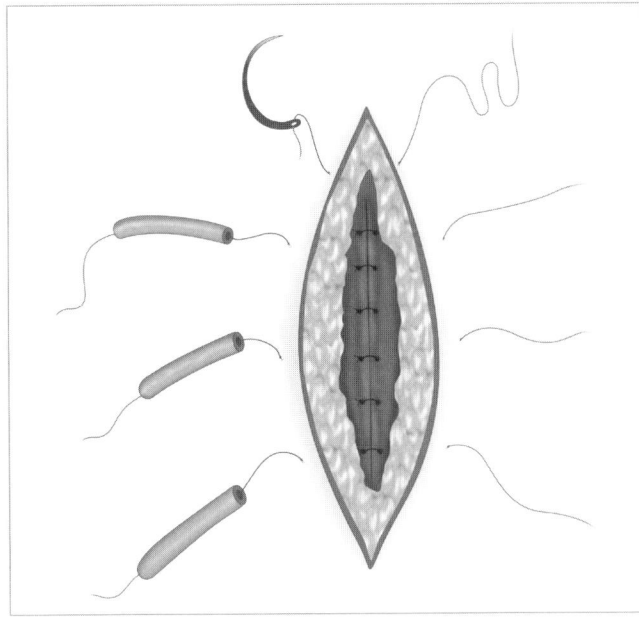

Fig. 19.10: Single deep tension sutures

Having closed the abdominal wall, the sutures are tied together, starting from the central suture (Fig. 19.12B). Here, it is important to avoid direct contact between knot and skin as the stress would soon cause a decubitus wound on the underlying skin and the progressive embedding of the suture itself, undermining its support function.

In order to avoid this, segments of intravenous line, 1.5 cm in length, are interposed between knot and skin and the superficial throws are passed over these (Figs 19.8B; 19.10 to 19.12). An alternative are small rolls of gauze.

If available a platelet in plastic material (Fig. 19.13) can be used to distribute the stress of the abdominal wall. Sutures should not be tied under tension. Generally, three deep tension sutures will suffice; these are removed on the 14th postoperative day.

REPAIR OF A TRANSVERSE LAPAROTOMY WOUND

This may be performed either following the anatomical strat or by mass closure.

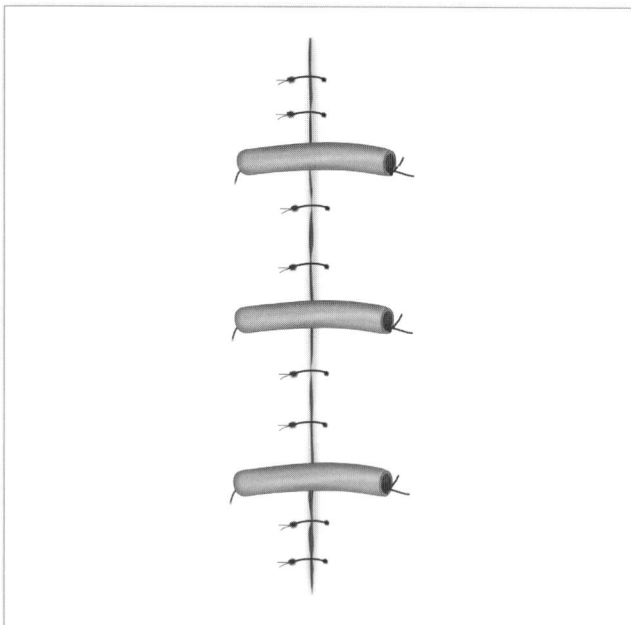

Fig. 19.11: Single deep tension sutures individually knotted

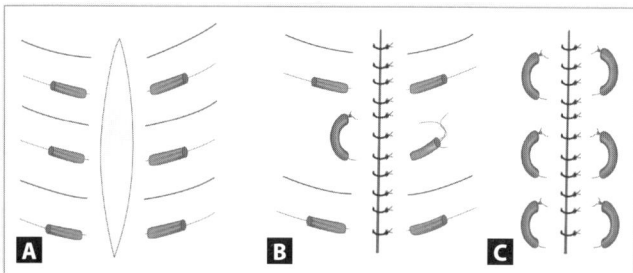

Fig. 19.12: (A) Single; (B) Tied in pairs; (C) Final view

Layered Closure following Anatomical Strata

a. *Parietal peritoneum*

See the relevant section above on repair of a vertical laparotomy.

b. *Apposition of the muscle bellies*

The integrity and mutual adherence of the rectus muscle sheaths enables these muscles to act synergically, which is indispensible for their ability to develop endoabdominal pressure (see previous section).

Subumbilical laparotomies, particularly if transverse, entail discontinuity of these rectus abdominis sheaths and their diastasis under contraction.

Reconstruction of the muscle layer is therefore an indispensable step in abdominal wall closure.

As it is not possible to reconstruct the sheaths, the muscles are approximated by applying sutures to the muscle tissue itself.

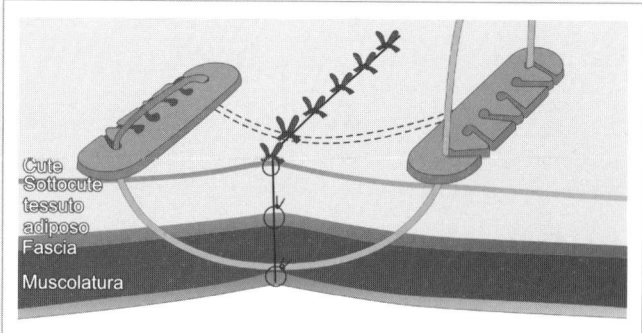

Fig. 19.13: Deep tension sutures to avoid skin decubitus wounds from the suture and its embedding. A platelet of plastic is interposed between skin and thread. If this device is not available, segments of intravenous line will do the same job (Figs 19.8B, 19.10 to 19.12)

Muscle tissue has a limited ability to withstand suturing and will lacerate under both the longitudinal and transverse stresses exerted by stitches. To avoid this, it is indispensible that the muscle is anchored to a rigid suture that can bear the load. If it is not possible to use the overlying fascia for this, the suture should be applied directly onto the muscle belly (see previous section).

Omitting to approximate the muscle bellies, associated with non-closure of the peritoneum (Stark's technique) consitutes, in our opinion, a technical error. It allows endoabdominal pressure, now no longer directed vertically by the rectus muscles, to act directly on the fascia, which sometimes leads to dehiscence and evisceration (Fourmié et al., 2008).

We proceed as follows: We think that three sutures —inferior, superior and one intermediate, suffice to reconstruct the muscle layer.

- *Inferior suture*: (Fig. 19.14) A round-bodied needle mounted with (N° 1 or 0) absorbable thread starts from the deep portion of the distal end of a rectus muscle (including approximately 1/3 in the bite). The suture emerges and punctures (for anchorage) both the pyramidalis muscles (which should always be left adhering to the fascia); it punctures from external to internally the distal end of the contralateral muscle. The strands are knotted and reconstruction is complete.
- *Superior suture*: The surgeon grips the belly of the far rectus abdominis and stretches it caudad. At the highest accessible point the following suture is applied: Starting from the muscle's internal aspect and including approximately 1.5–2 cm in the bite, it emerges, punturing the fascia at the point where the sheath was originally inserted. The surgeon grasps the controlateral muscle belly and stretches it caudad, puncturing it from the outside inwards. The two suture strands are knotted and reconstruction is complete.

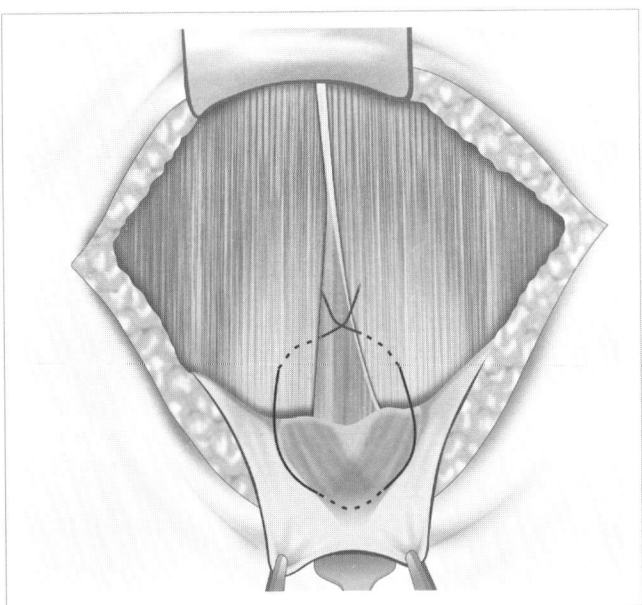

Fig. 19.14: Myorrhaphy of the pyramidalis muscles to the rectus muscles

- *Intermediate suture*: If considered necessary, a U-shaped suture is applied as described above. With a width of 1 cm, it is knotted using a square knot, or using a continuous suture that runs along the medial borders of the rectus muscles, connecting them.
  c. *Closure of the fascia*
  As the incision has followed the direction of its fibres and, as shown in Figure 19.5, each contraction will tend to approximate the wound edges. Suturing of the fascia is performed using a continuous suture. The authors's technique: We start by reconstructing the wound end on the surgeon's side; a cutting needle is used with the point starting from the deep aspect of the fascia and including both sheaths, following an 'in-out-out-in' path. We knot, apply a second suture to secure the end and knot this, leaving a long tail held with a forceps.
  We now proceed similarly with reconstruction of the opposite wound end. Continuous suturing is continued with two closely spaced sutures at the linea alba level, whch is the site of maximum tension on the fascia. Suturing proceeds until it reaches the surgeon's end and the two tails are tied together.
  d. *Subcutaneous tissue and Camper's fascia*
  The reader is refered to the paragraph in the previous section. This suturing is not performed with septic surgical procedures.
  e. *Skin*
  The reader is referred to the previous section. Some authors (Stark) use three sutures; according to Donati, apposition of the edges using an Allis clamp for 15 minutes suffices.

BIBLIOGRAPHY

1. Chin G, Diegelman R, Schultz G. Cellular and molecular regulation of wound healing. In Wound healing. Edited by: Falabella A, Kirschner R, Boca Roton FL. Taylor, Francis Group; 2005. pp.17-37.
2. Chow KK. Il Taglio Cesareo. CIC Edizioni internazionali, Roma 1990.
3. Del Valle GO, Combs P, Qualls C, Curet LB. Does closure of Camper fascia reduce the incidence of post-caesarean superficial wound disruption? Obstet Gynecol 1992;80:1013-6.
4. Diminick AR Ann. Delayed wound closure: indications and technique. Emerg Med. 1988;17:1303.
5. Ellis H. The cause and prevention of postoperative intraperitoneal adhesions. Surg Gynecol Obstet. 1971;133: 497-511.
6. Ellis HJ, Heddle R. Does the peritoneum need to be closed at laparotomy? Br J Surg. 1977;64:733-6.
7. Fleischer GM, Rennert A, Ruehmer M. Infected abdominal wound and burst abdomen. Chirurg. 2000;71(7):754-62.
8. Fourmié A, Madzou S, Sentilhes L, Descamps P. Two observations of evisceration after caesarean section performed according the so called Stark procedure. Gynecol Obstet Fertil. 2008;36(12):1211-3.
9. Holtz G. Adhesion induction by suture of varying tissue reactivity and calibre. Int J Fertil. 1982;27:134-5.
10. SA. Closure of subcutaneous fat: A prospective randomized trial. Br J Surg. 1990;77:107.
11. Kapur BML, Daneswar A, Chopra P. Evaluation of peritoneal closure at laparotomy. Am J Surg. 1979;137:650-2.
12. Karipineni RC, Wilk PJ, Danese CA. The role of the peritoneum in the healing of abdominal incisions. Surg Gynecol Obstet. 1976;142:729-30.
13. Kendall SWH, Brennan TC, Guillou PJ. Suture length to wound length ratio and the integrity of midline and lateral paramedian incision. Br J Surg. 1976;78:705-7.
14. Jenkins TPN. The burst abdominal wound: A mechanical approach. Br J Surg. 1976;63:705-7.
15. Israelson LA, Jonsson T. Suture length to wound length ratio and healing of midline laparotomy incisions. Br J Surg. 1993;80:1284-86.
16. Israelson LA, Jonsson T, Knutson A. Suture technique and wound healing in midline laparotomy incisions. Eur J Surg. 1996;162:605-9.
17. McFadden PM, Peacock EE. Preperitoneal abdominal wound repair: Incidence of dehiscence. Am J Surg. 1983;145:213-4.
18. Myers SA, Bennett TL. Incidence of significant adhesions at repeat cesarean section and the relationship to method of prior peritoneal closure. J Reprod Med. 2005;50(9):659-62.
19. Naumann RW, Hauth JC, Owen J. Subcutaneous tissue approximation in relation to wound disruption after cesarean delivery in obese women. Obstet Gynecol. 1995;85(3): 412-6.
20. NICE - National Institute for Clinical Excellence National Collaborating Centre for Women's and Children's Health. Caesarean section. London (UK): 2004 Apr. 142 p. [688 references].

21. Pietrantoni M. The efficacy of whether to suture the parietal peritoneum with vertical incisions at caesarean section. Surgical Forum. 1990;41:487.
22. Pollock AV, Greenall MJ, Evans M. Single layer mass closure of major laparotomies by continuous suturing. J R Soc Med. 1979;72(12):889-93.
23. Sivam NS, Suresh S, Hadke MS, Kate V, Ananthakrishnan N. Results of the Smead-Jones technique of closure of vertical midline incisions for emergency laparotomiesa prospective study of 403 patients. Trop Gastroenterol. 1995;16(4):62-7.
24. Smith M, Enquist IF. A quantitative study of impaired healing resulting from infection. Surg Gynec Obstet. 1967;125:965-7.
25. Stark M. Adhesion-free caesarean section. World J Surg. 1992;17:419.
26. Stark M. Technique of caesarean section: The Misgav Ladach method. Women's Health Today. The proceedings of the XIV World Congress of Gynecology and Obstetrics, Montreal September 1994. New York: Parthenon Publishing Group 1994: 81-85.
27. Varshney S, Manek P, Johnson CD. Six-fold suture: Wound length ratio for abdominal closure. Ann R Coll Surg Engl. 1999;81(5):333-6.
28. Waldrop J, Doughty. Wound healing physiology. In: Acute and chronic wounds: Nursing management. Edited by: Bryant R. St. Louis: Mosby; 2000. pp.17-39.
29. Waqer S, Malik Z, Razzaq A, et al. Frequency and risk factors for wound dehiscence/burst abdomen in midline laparotomies. Journal Ayub Med Coll. 2005;17(4):70-3.
30. West J, Gimbel M. Acute surgical and traumatic wound healing. In: Acute and chronic wounds: Nursing management. Edited by: Brayant. St. Louis: Mosby; 2005. pp.189-96.

CHAPTER 20

Perimortem and Postmortem Caesarean Delivery

Outcome for the foetus (foetal well-being) when caesarean delivery begins within 4 minutes of cessation of maternal cardiac activity, with extraction of the foetus within 5 minutes, differs from outcomes where extraction does not occur within these time constraints (Weber CE 1971). This observation led Katz (1986) to revise the concept of postmortem Caesarean section (C-section), stating that two clinical entities can be identified under this general heading:
- *Perimortem caesarean delivery*, begun within 4 minutes of asystolia, with operative delivery within 5 minutes
- *Postmortem caesarean delivery*, occurring outside the above time constraints.

Similar good foetal outcomes were subsequently observed in C-sections performed on patients in a critical or moribund conditions; frequently it was found that surgery not only did not result in exacerbation of patient's condition, but sometimes improved it, particularly when the critical condition was a circulatory and respiratory collapse due to embolism.

C-sections performed on patients in critical or terminal conditions have thus been revised from interventions that could further deteriorate maternal conditions to being a life-saving procedure for the mother, a view now accepted and recommended by the American Heart Association (Barando et al., 2000).

These patients, too, have been included in the perimortem caesarean delivery group, leading to a re-definition of the concept:

"By *perimortem caesarean delivery*, we mean operative delivery via laparotomy effected in a gravid patient in the third trimester of gestation under critical or terminal conditions, or within the first four minutes of cardiac arrest, with extraction of the foetus by the 5th minute".

Whitten (2000) found a 62.5% survival rate for neonates, neurologically healthy, when the C-section was performed in the time limits described.

Subsequent critical observations and a literature review conducted over 20 years confirmed this hypotheses (Katz et al., 2005).

PHYSIOPATHOLOGY

When a caesarean section is performed within 4 minutes of maternal cardiac arrest, removal of the foetus and externalisation of the uterus bring about two kinds of benefits:

Cardiocirculatory System

a. In 90% of term parturients, a 30% reduction in cardiac output is observed in the supine position, due to compressive effects exerted by the gravid uterus on the inferior vena cava.
b. Uteroplacental perfusion accounts for 30% of cardiac output (Dildy et al., 1995) and this volume of blood can now be directed to other regions.
   The result is that in a term parturient, removal of the foetus leads to an increase of 30–80% in cardiac output (DePace et al., 1982) which, associated with resuscitation, is able to guarantee sufficient bloodflow to the CNS.
c. A whole series of studies highlights how chest compression and resuscitation are more effective after

delivery (DePace et al., 1982) and are facilitated by the fact that they may be performed on the patient in the supine decubitus position.

Respiratory System

At term of pregnancy a 20% reduction in residual functional capacity is observed, with a resulting reduction in oxygen reserves and a more rapid development of anoxia following apnoea (Katz VL, 1986): These conditions are removed by foetal extraction.

In association with resuscitation measures, these benefits may lead to improvement in cardiocirculatory condition and be capable of maintaining adequate circulation to the central nervous system and resulting preservation of its functions during arrest.

From the above it is apparent how prompt and appropriate intervention greatly increases the survival chances of both mother and foetus (DePace et al., 1982) even when we consider that today different causes lead to maternal death compared those prevalent in the past.

An epidemological study conducted by Katz (1986) found that, in the last centrury causes of maternal death in pregnancy were mainly chronic and based on infections, while currently they are acute and mainly of cardiorespiratory aetiology.

This distinction highlights how different the clinical conditions are of neonates born to mothers who die following a chronic, debilitating, infectious disease, compared to the condition of neonates born to mothers who have died after an acute cardiocirculatory event.

INDICATIONS

- *Adequate gestational age*: This is roughly defined, lacking other means, by the fundal height. There is unanimous consensus (Ritter JW, 1961; Arthur RK, 1978; De- Pace NL et al., 1982; Katz VL et al., 1986; Strong TH Jr et al., 1989; Whitten M. et al., 2000) that the pregnancy should not be less than 26 weeks old. This is because the operation would be unlikely to benefit the foetus in the absence of adequate neonatal resuscitation facilities, nor would it benefit the mother, as the effects of pregnancy on the cardiovascular system are less pronounced before the 28th week, so the mother would not derive the same benefit as with a pregnancy nearing term
- *Short time interval between cardiac arrest and operation*: Foetuses extracted within 5 minutes of maternal asystolia do not generally present neurological complications. Lopez-Zeno JA et al. (1990) report a case of a foetus delivered without neurological complications 25 minutes after maternal death
- *Adequacy of resuscitation measures* during the interval between arrest and surgery

- *There is no need to check for foetal heartbeat*, as this would be a waste of precious time.

METHOD

Resuscitation operations *should not be interrupted* during surgery.
- *Preliminary operative steps*: Catheterisation of the bladder, disinfection and draping of the abdomen are cut out
- A slight Trendelenburg position, to promote return of venous blood from the inferior limbs, once the foetus has been extracted and the womb exteriorised
- *Access to the abdominal cavity* is effected via a midline subumbilical laparotomy
- *Access to the uterine cavity*, is effected, according to gestational age and the surgeon's skill, via a low semicircular or vertical hysterotomy.

It should be borne in mind that the ultimate surgical objective is to save the mother's life: Surgical technique should be proportionate to avoiding injuries to the mother (bladder and intestine) or to the foetus.

After operative delivery, the foetus is held (by the feet) sloping down from the mother and the umbilical cord milked before being clamped to increase foetal blood volume.

Once the neonate has been removed:
- A blood sample is taken from the umbilical cord for hematological testing, thereby avoiding the need to source the neonate
- A section of cord is clamped at each end and kept for blood gas analysis; the blood it contains will remain stable for approx. 60 minutes
- *Uterine exteriorisation* from the abdominal cavity
- *If resuscitation measures succeed*, haemostasis should be performed with care and the hysterotomy and laparotomic wounds adequately repaired. Antibiotic therapy
- *If resuscitation measures do not succeed*, repair of the hysterotomy and laparotomic wounds will have an aesthetic purpose only.

BIBLIOGRAPHY

1. Arthur RK. Postmortem cesarean section. Am J Obstet Gynecol. 1978;132(2):175-9.
2. Barnado PO, Jenkins JG. Failed intubation in Obsttetrics, a 6 years review in a UK region. Anaesthesia. 2000;55: 690-4.
3. Cunningham FG, MacDonald PC, Gant NF, et al. Eds. Williams Obstetrics. 20th ed. Stamford, Conn: Appleton & Lange; 1997. p. 404.
4. DePace NL, Betesh JS, Kotler MN. Postmortem cesarean section with recovery of both mother and offspring. JAMA. 1982;248(8):971-3.

5. Dildy GA, Clark SL. Cardiac arrest during pregnancy. Obstet Gynecol Clin North Am. 1995;22(2):303-14.
6. Katz VL, Dotters DJ, Droegemueller W. Perimortem caesarean delivery. Obstetrics & Gynaecology. 1986;68:571-6.
7. Katz V, Balderston K, DeFreest M. Perimortem cesarean delivery: were our assumptions correct? Am J Obstet Gynecol. 2005;192(6):1916-20.
8. Lopez-Zeno JA, Carlo WA, O"Grady JP, Fanaroff AA. Infant survival following delayed postmortem cesarean delivery. Obstet Gynecol. 1990;76(5 Pt 2):991.
9. Marx GF. Cardiopulmonary resuscitation of late-pregnant women. Anesthesiology. 1982;56(2):156.
10. Ritter JW. Postmortem cesarean section. JAMA. 1961;175:715-6.
11. Strong TH Jr, Lowe RA. Perimortem cesarean section. Am J Emerg Med. 1989;7(5):489-94.
12. Weber CE. Postmortem cesarean section: review of the literature and case reports. Am J Obstet Gynecol. 1971;110(2):158-65.
13. Whitten M, Irvine LM. Postmortem and perimortem caesarean section: what are the indications?. J R Soc Med. 2000;93(1):6-9.
14. Why mothers die? 2000-2002. Confidential Enquiry into Child and Maternal Health RCOG Press, 2004.

CHAPTER 21

Uterine Rupture

By *uterine rupture* we refer to a full-thickness disruption of the uterine wall that also involves the overlying visceral peritoneum (uterine serosa) subsequent to stress sustained through contraction of the myometrium, through overdistension of the uterus due to increase in its content (multiple pregnancies, polyhydramnios), through obstetric measures or through traumatic events.

This event, which may occur during pregnancy or during labour, includes two clinical situations, which vary according to age, parity, aetiology, pathogenesis, clinical picture, type of surgery planned and final outcome:
- *Rupture of native (unscarred) uterus*
- *Rupture of scarred uterus.*

Complications of uterine rupture are haemorrhage, shock, amniotic fluid embolism, disseminated intravascular coagulation, postoperative infection and ureteric damage. When the patient survives she is often infertile and sterile.

Uterine rupture is among the leading causes of maternal and perinatal death (Faleimu, 1990).

UTERINE RUPTURE DURING PREGNANCY

Rupture of Native (Unscarred) Uterus

By rupture of a native uterus we mean discontinuity throughout the whole thickness of the uterine wall. This may or may not be associated with the overlaying serous membrane.

It is a rare occurence during pregnancy (Taylor et al., 1979). A study by Gardeil (Ireland, 1994) found 1 rupture out of 30,764 pregnancies (0.0033%), no ruptures among 21,998 primigravidae and just 2 (0.0051%) among multigravidae. The event was found to be more frequent by a meta-analysis (1976-1998) of 7 large-scale studies totaling 1,108,660 deliveries, with 7,440 spontaneous ruptures, equivalent to 0.013%.

Incidence is higher in low-resourced countries: Schrinsky and Benson (1978) put it at 1: 920 (0.11%); the same authors found that ruptures during pregancy make up 14% of total ruptures, the remaining 86% are observed during labour. Ruptures correlate positively with:
- *Violent abdominal trauma* during fights, followed by road accidents, particularly when the victim is wearing a seat belt
- *Multiparity*, (see below) particularly if associated with polyhydramnios or multiple pregnancies
- *Placenta accreta and percreta.*

Rupture of Scarred Uterus

Uterine rupture should be distinguished from *uterine scar dehiscence*. The latter, in contrast to frank uterine rupture, involves the disruption and separation with very limited bleeding of a pre-existing uterine scar without affecting the overlaying peritoneum and seldom results in major maternal or foetal complications. It is often observed following intercourse. For a definition of uterine rupture, the reader is refered to the opening paragraph of this Chapter.

Among the causes, we mention the following:
- *Scar to uterus following a hysterotomy* (C-section, myomectomy, metroplasty), perforation, curettage extending beyond the base layer of the endometrium.

Wall distension, sustained through a single or multiple pregnancy, leads to a gradual thinning and dehiscence of the scar. An LUS thickness of 1.7 mm, according to Asakura (2000), or of 2 mm (according to Gotoh, 2001), found within a week of delivery, represents a critical point, below which rupture of the uterus becomes highly likely.

Other possibilities are represented by low placenta insertion with infiltration and dissociation of scar tissue, placenta accreta, gestational trophoblastic disease, choriocarcinoma or uterine horn pregnancy.

From the point of view of symptomatology, this event may occur unnoticed and within just a few hours one will observe a progressive worsening of the patient's general condition. It may also be clinically unexpressed: An occasional finding during the course of a Caesarean section is that the LUS appears reduced to a very fine flap of tissue, which may also be absent and the uterine cavity breach is covered by the peritoneum only, through which amniotic fluid can be seen.

UTERINE RUPTURE DURING LABOUR

The data on general incidence are quite uniform across the Western World: 1: 8434 (0.012%) deliveries, while they vary across resource-poor countries: 1:92 (Diab, Yemen, 2005); 1:110 (Gessessev, Ethiopia, 2002; Khan et al. Pakistan, 2002); 1:112 (Chuni, Nepal, 2006); 1:135 deliveries (Onwuhafua et al., Nigeria, 1998); 1:425 (Lama et al., Kenya, 1991) 1:489 (Yalda, Iraq, 2009); 1.851 (Saleem, 2000, Kuwait); 1:866 (van der Merwe, South Africa, 1987); 1: 6331 (Chen et al., Singapore, 1995).

Ratios between the different forms also differ. When data are available, the second form (scarred uterus) clearly predominates in Western countries and in centres of excellence in resource-poor countries, where they otherwise tend to be in equilibrium, with slight predomination by one or the other: Prior scar 36% (Yalda, Iraq, 2009); 41.5% (Ekpo, Nigeria, 2000); 51% (Al Saleem, Kuwait 2000), 52.8% (van der Merwe, South Africa, 1987).

Data stemming from centres of excellence in resource-poor countries do not reflect healthcare realities on the ground, as there is a great divide between these centres, which are able to collect and statistically process data, and the rural hospitals, health centres and villages where most deliveries take place. Care is provided in the villages by traditional midwives.

The presence of statistical data indicates that a given population is able to access healthcare facilities; the finding that a high percentage of uterine ruptures are observed in cases of prior C-section indicates that the women in question have had at least two opportunities to access a hospital facility.

Absence of data indicates:
- That the healthcare facility is very often not capable of recognising and treating pathological events (uterine ruptures), of processing their incidence and transmitting the relevant data to the Health Ministry or to scientific associations
- That the population has no access to healthcare facilities.

The percentage of women who cannot even access these facilities: Rural hospitals, health centres, is very high (Sundari 1992, Chipangwi 1992), for which reason care during delivery is provided in the villages by "traditional midwives, whose hazardous practices can lead to uterine rupture, sepsis, and shock". Uterine rupture is believed to be a common occurence and rural areas, mainly affecting primigravidae under 20 years old, a statistic that contrasts sharply, as we shall see, with those derived from large urban centres.

In the absence, then, of precise data and to trace the actual proportions of this phenomenon in these areas, where the obstetrician often has to work, we must refer to WHO statistics.

1. According to WHO data, approx. 5.2% of the population will become pregnant in the course of a year, and 9.2% of these pregnancies do not progress. Therefore, term pregnancies occur in 4.72% of the population.
2. Recent WHO statistics highlight how, in Sub-Saharan Africa, during pregnancy or labour, 15% of parturients will develop a complication requiring qualified medical assistance, and that a caesarean section percentage among these of between 6% and 15% would indicate good obstetric practice.
3. The 15% of parturients who do not receive this assistance will face:
   - Death (Table 21.1): By haemorrhage 26%, sepsis 22%, obstructed delivery 13%, eclampsia, 6%
   - Severe disabilities 33%; of these, the most feared are pelvic floor injuries, vesical and vaginal rectal fistulas, lower limb disabilities due to lesions of the sacral plexus, chronic anemia, chronic pelvic pain, depression and maternal exhaustion.

The percentage of obstructed labour uterine rupture is therefore 15:100x13 = 1.95% of the 15% of parturients who do not receive qualified medical assistance, predominantly among primigravidae, a figure in line with the findings from Yemen and Zambia.

High as it is, this percentage still appears an underestimate. This may be better understood by analysing the obstacles standing in the way of accessing and accomplishing delivery in these centres.

Such 'delays' come under three main headings:
- *Do it at home*: Management of the birth is often entrusted to traditional midwives, who are often unable to distinguish between cephalopelvic disproportion, obstructed delivery or a delay in the advancement of labour, and administer herbal remedies orally or in the vagina, which have analgesic or uterotonic effects with resulting hypertonicity, uterine rupture and foetal death (Veal, 1992).

Often the mother and mother-in-law, who have often given birth to many children, are the ones to decide about transportation to the local hospital. They are often against the idea, believing that the delay in labour is due to cowardice of the parturient, who is often extremely young. Thinking she does not want to push for fear of pain, they inflict blows on her
- *Getting there*: Difficulty in finding the money for the transport, or in finding any means of transport, which may sometimes be a simple bicycle with a seat mounted on a rack, on which the woman in labour is placed. Concerns over safety: Journeying by day, and especially by night, through areas of high insecurity
- *In the hospital*: In numerous hospitals, the admission criterion runs: "no money, no admission". Even once inside, there may be difficulties finding an obstetrician, a doctor, drugs, infusions...

Maternal Mortality
Table 21.1
Incidence of maternal mortality

Authors	Year	Country	Percentage
Zelop	1993	United States	0%
Castaneda	2000	Mexico	0%
Khan	2004	Pakistan	0%
Diab	2005	Yemen	1,7%
Lema et al.	1991	Kenya	2,1%
Al Saleem	2000	Kuwait	3,3%
Bujold	2002	Canada	4,2%
Yalda	2009	Irak	5,0%
Van der Merwe*	1987	South Africa	5,6%*
Onwuhafua	1998	Nigeria	22,0%
Gessessev	2002	Ethiopia	24,0%

(*) among primigravidae only.

In the West, maternal mortality following rupture of the uterus varies between 0% and 1%, while it is between 5% and 10% in resource-poor countries (Shipp et al., 2002).

Death rates vary according to whether the uterus is unscarred or scarred: All maternal deaths belong to the former group, wth percentages varying between 8.5% (van der Merwe) and 15% (Golan). Onwuhafue and Al Saleem report no deaths among the scarred group.

The datum showing low or absent mortality among scarred uteruses indicates that the woman has had the opportunity to access a healthcare facility (during a prior pregnancy and during the reported pregnancy) capable of performing a C-section and of processing the relevant statistics.

The high percentage of ruptures among non-scarred uteruses indicates a population in which access to the hospital has been preceded in most cases by a protracted labour in a village or in an outlying healthcare centre.

Foetal Mortality

Incidence of foetal mortality is reported in Table 21.2.

Table 21.2
Incidence of foetal mortality from hospital case records

Author	Year	Country	Percentage
Chen	1995	Singapore	7.4%
Ofir	2003	Israele	10,3%
Lema	1991	Kenya	60%
Yalda	2009	Irak	62%
Nahum	2008	*	74%
Mishra	2006	Nepal	94%

(*) *summarises data from three low-resourced countries*

Risk Factors

Risk factors include pelvic morphology and size, to which are added categories of gravidae among whom risk of uterine rupture is greater than the statistically accepted norm of 1:200 deliveries (0,5%) in the low-resourced countries.

These are pregnancies following:
- Numerous prior C-sections
- Classic C-section
- Low vertical C-section
- Low transverse C-section with single-layer hysterorrhaphy
- Low transverse C-section on abnormal uterus
- Prior C-section not preceded or followed by a vaginal delivery
- Prior C-section in which labour has been induced or enhanced by uterotonic agents
- Interval between current pregnancy and prior C-section less than 2 years
- Pregnancy with foetus over 4,000 grams following a C-section
- Prior myomectomy by laparoscopy or laparotomy.

These gravidae require careful attention during labour and rapid access to an operating room should be preplanned.

Aetiopathogenesis of Rupture in Unscarred and Scarred Uteri

Uterine rupture during labour occurs as a result of stresses sustained through:
- *Contractions of the myometrium*
- *Obstetric manoeuvres.*

Uterine rupture following contractions of the myometrium that are spontaneous, induced or supported by uterotonic agents, or the presence of a mechanical obstacle, such as:
- Abnormal foetal lie: Oblique or transverse
- Lack of alignment between major axis of foetus and that of the birth canal
- Cephalopelvic disproportion, obstructed labour
- Birth canal anomalies;
  - Ovarian or pelvic tumour; uterine fibroma previa
  - Modifications in the soft tissues of the birth canal, as may occur through traditional practices: Infibulation or sterility therapies using stinging herbal pessaries or scalding
  - Stenosis or rigidity of the uterine cervix, uterovaginal septum
  - Sexually transmitted infections with fibroses such as: Lymphogranuloma venereum, granuloma inguinale, bilharziasis and stenosing carcinomas.

The mechanisms by which the uterus responds to a mechanical obstacle are to increase the force and frequency of contractions; this can culminate in *uterine tetany* (extremely prolonged uterine contractions that may be life threatening to the foetus).

a. *Increase in the power of contractions* as explained in Chapter 3, the uterus can be divided into two functional sections: The upper part or *corpus,* which is the active, contractile and retractile segment, and the lower, passive segment, which is easily distended. Due to the action of contraction/retraction, the uterine cavity, shaped like a truncated cone, gradually reduces, causing the presenting part to advance.

When faced with an obstacle, the functionally predominant fundus continues its action and, due to its progressive shortening, the cavity gradually changes in shape, from truncated cone to circle. Once this cricitcal point has been reached, the propulsive function of the contractions breaks down, while their compressive effect continues (see Chapter. 3). The fundus continues with its retracting action, and its inferior border, where it meets the now overdistended LUS, retracts away from it. This leads to a reduction in the height of the uterine fundus, overdistension and pain in the LUS and a depression between the two parts in the formation of Bandl's retraction ring. These constitute the clinical manifestation of a mechanical obstacle during labour.

Distension of the LUS proceeds until a critical point is exceeded and laceration occurs at the point of greatest stress (Fig. 15.6). A co-factor in laceration is *ischaemia* due to distension and compression exerted by the presenting part (A similar process may be observed in other parts of the uterus: At the borders, corpus, fundus and posterior wall.)

In some cases, the so-called *arrested labour* is observed and the critical point is not reached.

b. *Increase in the frequency of the contractions*: Six contractions every ten minutes, noticed during two consecutive observations, which may lead to *tetany*, which is functionally ineffective but may severely compromise placental gas exchange.

The *contractile activity of the myometrium* may be *spontaneous or sustained by uterotonic agents.*

Oxytocin augmentation, oxytocin administered:
- *In normal dosages*, but whose utilisation is contraindicated by pelvic index (Bishop's pelvic scoring system) <9, or parity >5 or by a prior hysterotomy
- *In dosages not corresponding to the physiology of contractions.*
  Misoprostol.
  Breech extraction.

Uterine Rupture following Obstetrical Manoeuvres

- *During external version*, performed by a poorly skilled person and under anaesthesia
- *During internal cephalic-podalic version* in the case of a second twin
- Following excessive fundal pressure or due to heavy pushes by the patient, where inadequate pelvic dimension has been disregarded
- In problematic forceps application
- Violent rupture during obstetric handling, such as breech extraction under incomplete dilation
- During destructive operations (craniotomy), during protracted labour, with an overdistended LUS
- In vacuum extractions performed on incompletely dilated cervix following prior LUS transverse C-section; in these cases, the uterine scar is subject to double stresses: Cephalad, by action of the uterus, and caudad, by action of the head and suction cap.

The following events may act upon:

Unscarred uterus

In the West, incidence of rupture for an unscarred uterus is very low, while it is high in low-resourced countries.

Pre-disposing factors are as follows:
- In the *West*, first pregnancy at advanced age, short stature, male sex at birth, prostaglandin-induced labour
- In *low-resourced countries*, a substantial role is played by:
  - *Physiological immaturity,* (which makes the teenager vulnerable to pregnancy complication); the pelvis completes its development only towards the 18th–20th years, for which reason, if pregnancy occurs

earlier, she often observe labour complicated by cephalopelvic disproportion or by obstructed labour. Incidence increases with decreasing age
- *Parity*: At-risk groups are primigravidae, particularly when young (for the reasons stated above), and the multiparous with a parity of 4 (Mokgokong & Marivate, 1976), above 4 (Schrinsky & Benson, 1978) or above 5 (Golan, 1980; Al Saleem, 2000, Khan Pakistan, 2003). The multiparous appear to be at greater risk than the primagravidae, with a ratio of 94% against 6%. This figure we treat with a lot of caution, for the reasons stated above.

Factors predisposing the multiparous patient to uterine rupture can be traced to variations, across the pregnancies, of the fibrous tissue/muscle tissue ratio with increase of the former which leads to reduced myometrial tone, responsible for the more frequent foetal lie anomalies observed among them (see Chapter 6). In association with a concomitant deficit in the rectus abdominis muscles tone, the uterus is displaced ventrally, leading to a 'pendulous abdomen' (anterior uterine obliquity), in which the major foetal and uterine axes do not coincide with that of the birth canal, so the expulsive force vector is directed against the promontory. Hence, the posterior wall of the lower uterine segment and of the vagina encounter the main thrust of pressure from the foetal head, with frequent ruptures.
- *Hypokinesia in labour*, requiring uterotonic agents
- *Low socioeconomic status and educational level*
- *Low pregnancy BMI*, which is lower in the economic deprived group
- *Lack of visits to obstetric outpatient clinic.*

Scarred uterus

A scarred uterine may have been sustained through:

Prior C-section: Uterine rupture following a C-section represents a serious responsibility for:
a. *The obstetrician who performed it*. Its causes may be intraoperative and postoperative.

Intraoperative causes, concern:
- Type of hysterotomy, which becomes more relevant as we move from lower-segment transverse hysterotomy, through low hysterotomy with an intraoperative vertical supplementary incision in the superior edge (inverted-T shape hysterotomy) and low vertical hysterotomy (C-section which does not reach the fundus), to a classic C-section that reaches the fundus
- Type of hysterorrhaphy: Single layer suturing has a higher percentage of dehiscence
- Whether or not peritoneal closure is performed. Adhesions between the anterior uterine wall and the abdominal wall may cause anomalies in foetal presentation or anomalies in uterine contraction (polarity)
- Suture material utilized
- Lack of intraoperative assessment of the obstetric conjugate, a very important parameter when advising the patient on whether trial of labour or elective C-section is more suitable in a subsequent pregnancy (See chapter 15 and Fig. 15.17, 18).

Postoperative causes concern:
- Course of fever.
b. *The Hospital administration*, which failed to provide for a preferential pathway (or financial support) for the following pregnancies.

Myomectomy (see risk factors).

Overdistension of the uterine wall during prior deliveries, as in the case of inadequate pelvic dimension, with the myometrium squeezed against the bony wall and scar formation.

Laceration of the uterine cervix with scar formation, occurring during prior pregnancies, either spontaneously or resulting from obstetric handling. Due to their reduced elasticity, these may extend cephalad during dilation and affect the uterine artery.

Uterine cavity curettage, which has extended beyond the functional and base strata of the endometrium.

Uterine perforation.

Pathological Anatomy

The direction of a uterine laceration is perpendicular to the line of maximum tension. Uterine rupture is defined according to:
a. *Site*
- The *lower uterine segment* (Fig. 21.1) is the regular site for uterine rupture: 47% (Khan, Pakistam, 2002); 57.4%

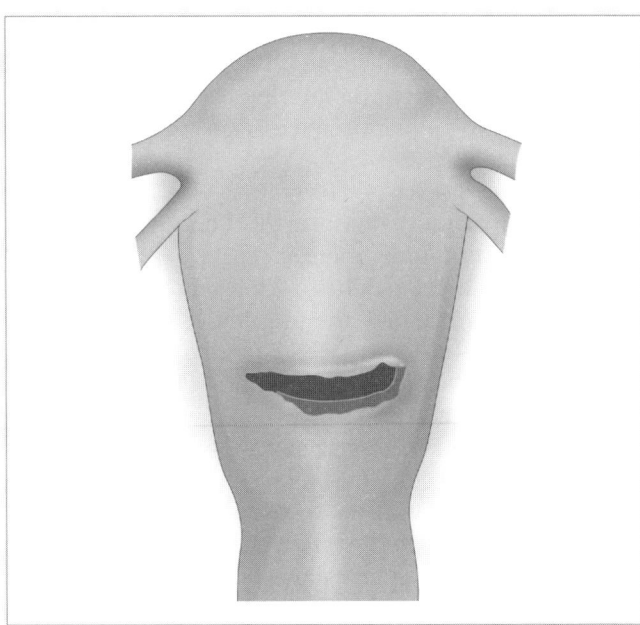

Fig. 21.1: Limited rupture to lower uterine segment: Horizontal development

(Gessessev, Ethiopia, 2002). Generally, the rupture is horizontal and located at the superior border
- *Left lateral border* (Figs 21.2 and 21.3) as a consequence of uterine dextroversion: 23.5% (Khan, Pakistan) 24% (Gessessev, Ethiopia, 2002)
- *Fundus*, 20.6% Khan, Pakistan
- *Right lateral border*: 5.6% (Gessessev, Ethiopia, 2002), 8.8% (Khan, Pakistam, 2002)
- *Corpus*: (Fig. 21.4) 5.6% (Gessessev, Ethiopia, 2002), 6% (Khan, Pakistan, 2002). This is often seen in a pregnancy following a classic C-section, a metroplasty, myomectomy or following trauma injuries
- *Posterior wall* (Fig. 21.5)
- *Multiple lesions of the corpus.*

The prognosis (mortality rate) varies according to the site affected. The most ominous outcomes are for multiple lesions (3:12 or 25%), followed by posterior wall (2:16 or 13%), left lateral border (15:183, 8.2%), lower uterine segment (2:49, 4%).

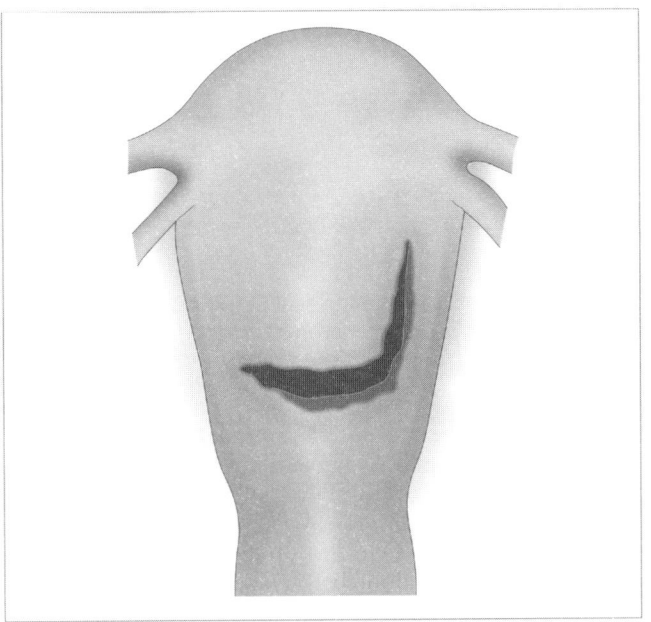

Fig. 21.2: Rupture of the lower uterine segment with cephalad extension

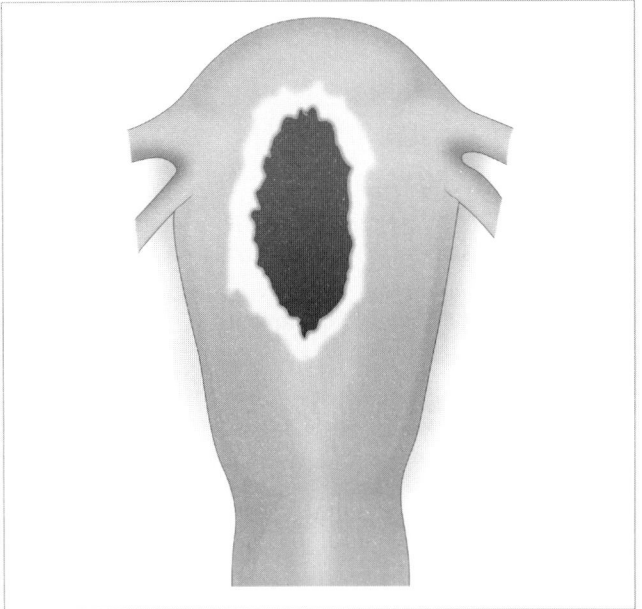

Fig. 21.4: Complete rupture occuring on the scar of a vertical hysterotomy

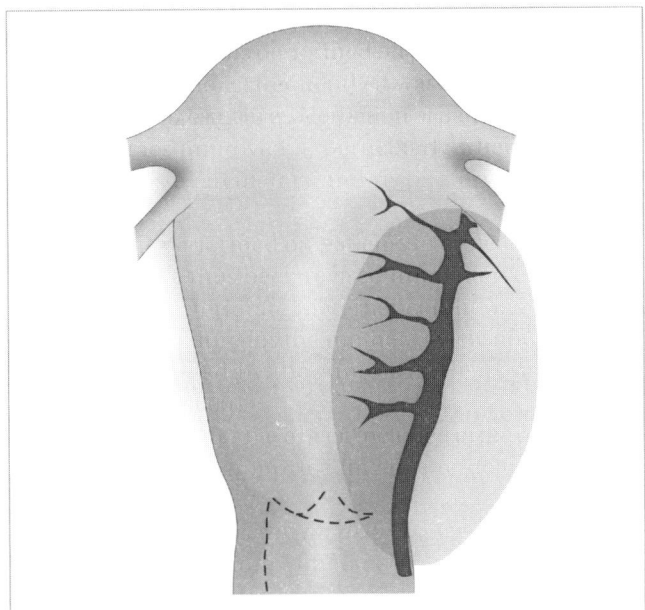

Fig. 21.3: Partia rupture of the left lateral border: Haematoma has penetrated through the two folds of the broad ligament

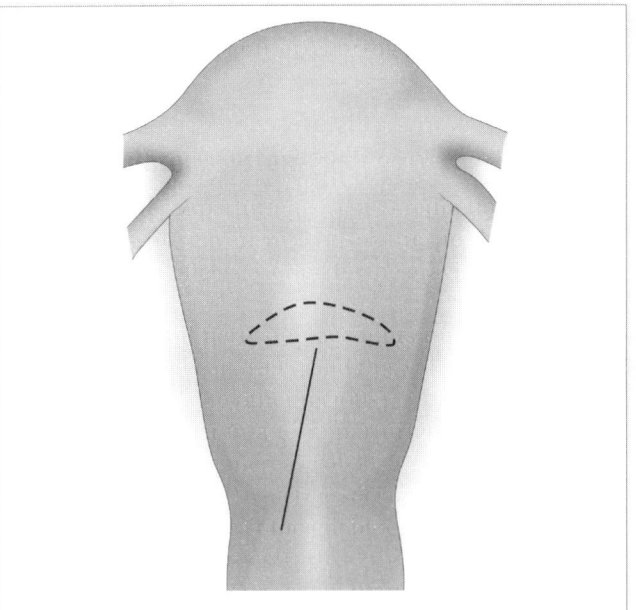

Fig. 21.5: Rupture of the posterior uterine segment, typical in multiparous patients with anterior obliquity

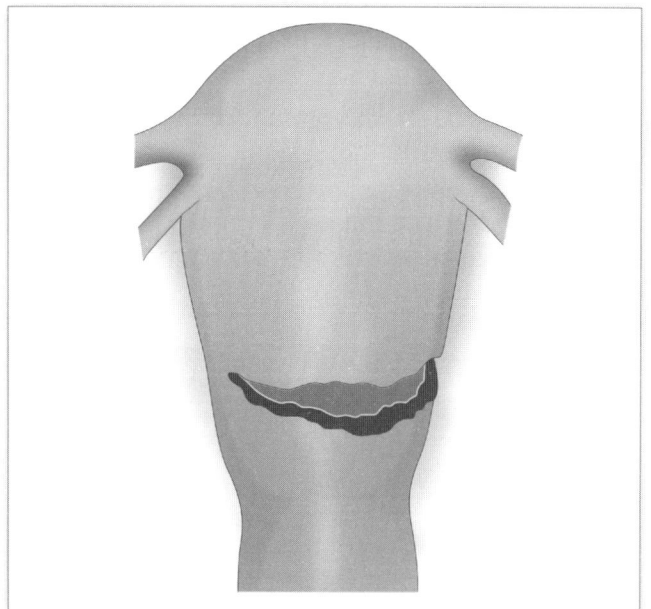

Fig. 21.6: *Partial* uterine rupture: The lesion, developing horizontally, initially affected the anterior LUS; it extended to the left border and posterior face

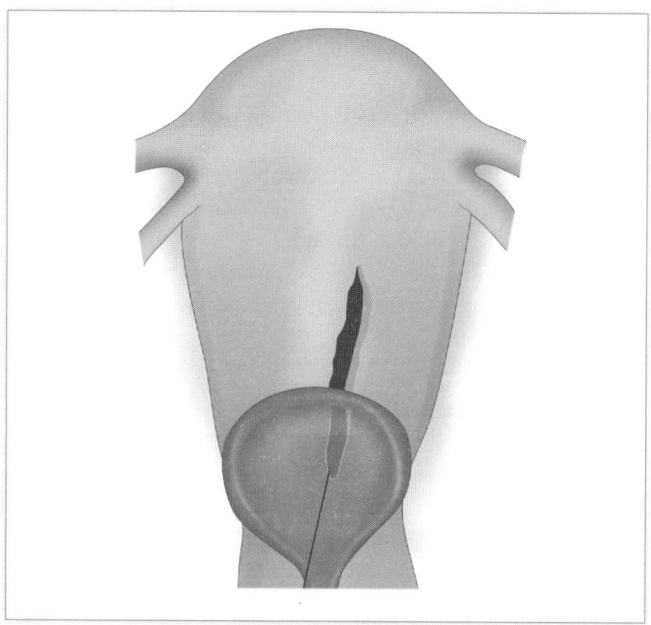

Fig. 21.7: *Complicated* uterine rupture; The posterior bladder wall has been affected

b. *Partial or total extension*, depending on the surface area affected (Fig. 21.6).
c. *Involvement of the peritoneum*: Solutions of continuity are subdivided into:
   – *Incomplete*, when the overlying peritoneum is not affected. If this is sustained by the lower uterine segment, the foetus is not expelled into cavity and the prognosis is more auspicious. When the left lateral wall is affected, the laceration is generally longitudinal and occurs at the broad ligament; foetus and blood create a passage between the two folds of the ligament, therby giving rise to a tumefaction of unclear definition (Fig. 21.3)
   – *Complete*, when the overlying peritoneum is also affected by the solution of continuity. Foetus and placenta are often expelled into the abdominal cavity and the uterine corpus retracts.
d. *Involvement of neighbouring organs*:
   – *Non-complicated or complicated*, according to whether neighbouring organs are affected. Rupture of the anterior wall is often associated with rupture of the bladder (Fig. 21.7). However, ureteral, intestinal and uterine cervix lesions may also occur, generally resulting from a prior lateral laceration with scar formation. Cervix laceration is often associated with concomitant colporrhexis, rupture of the vaginal vault.

Injuries to the Bladder

These may occur as a consequence of uterine rupture or during surgical handling (incidental bladder injuries).

- Lydon-Rochelle et al. (2001) found an incidence of 8%, compared to 1.2% among women who had not suffered uterine rupture
- Shipp et al. (2002) found an incidence of 18% (5:28) among pregnancies following a low transverse hysterotomy
- Kieser and Baskett (2002) report a cystotomy incidence of 17% (3:18) among women who had suffered rupture of the uterus
- Leung et al. found a 7% incidence of secondary bladder injuries following rupture and of 12% incidental injuries during surgical handling. Total incidence is 19%.

For methods of repairing injuries to the bladder and ureter, we refer the reader to Chapter 16.

Symptomatology

The clinical picture of uterine rupture during labour may be broken down into two stages.
a. *Prodromal stage*
   – The parturient has facial pallor; she is anxious; the heart rate often shows arrhythmia; she groans, feels she is near death and that something is about to break
   – Contractions are painful; *pain precedes the contraction*
   – Contraction intensity increases
   – Contraction frequency increases (>6 contractions every 10 minutes, over two consecutive observations), which may lead to *uterine tetany*
   – The round ligaments, particularly the left one (in the case of dextroversion of the uterus), are stretched and painful
   – The lower uterine segment is overdistended and extremely painful

- Appearance and upward progress of the retraction ring; the more quickly it moves cephalad, the closer is uterine rupture
- On examining the pelvis, the presenting part (head, shoulder) appears overriding in the superior pelvic strait
- Foetal distress (86%) anomalous foetal heart rate and prolonged late decelerations (Rodriguez, 1989)
- Rising vaginal fornices.

b. *Uterine rupture*
- Pain from rupture: The patient screams and says something has broken in her abdomen
- Collapse resulting from vagal hypertonia and anaemia; hypotension; the patient no longer groans and is in a state of calm
- Sudden arrest of contractions
- Profuse genital haemorrhage (37% of cases)
- Abundant haematuria, suggesting rupture of uterus and of the bladder.

Rupture of a low cervical scar generally occurs during labour but without any clearly identifiable signs or symptoms. For this reason, delivery may advance until the expulsion of a normal foetus.

Diagnosis

Directions towards the diagnosis of uterine rupture should give prevalance to the symptoms of mother and foetus over abdominal signs, as the latter vary according to whether rupture affects a scarred or unscarred uterus, whether it is a complete or incomplete rupture, and whether a large vessel is affected.

Uterine rupture may occur unnoticed, especially during trial of labour with a prior hysterotomy (C-section) or following obstetric handling to extract the foetus under anaesthesia.

The advisability of prompt diagnosis stems from:
- *Maternal prognosis* in uterine rupture varies with whether it was diagnosed before or after delivery (Mokgokong et al., 1976). In the first case maternal mortality is 4.5%; this rises to 10.4% in the second
- *Foetal well-being*: The time interval between rupture and birth, during which a foetus may be extracted without neurological sequelae is between 10 and 37 minutes (Miller, 1997; Zelop, 1999, Shipp, 2002).

Because of the short time available, it is advisable, to identify at-risk patients on admission, to start the partogram and be ready to identify the first signs of rupture and prepare for surgical rapid completion of delivery.

Uterine rupture may be diagnosed during labour or following delivery.

Diagnosis of Uterine Rupture during Labour

Maternal Symptomatology

- *Intact uterus*: The sequence of symptoms is intense abdominal pain (46%) at the moment of rupture; tachycardia, hypotension, pallour (31.7%) haemorrhage (31.7%) and shock that intensify progressively
- *Scarred uterus*: Here the symptomatology is more nuanced, with less pain at the moment of rupture, often limited to an area of pelvic tenderness. The general phenomena of shock, tachycardia and hypotension are not as accentuated. Rupture may occasionally go unnoticed and be diagnosed after delivery.

Foetal Symptomatology

Prolonged late decelerations preceding rupture are followed by brady-arrhythmias and subsequent disappearance of the foetal heart sounds.

Abdominal and Pelvic Clinical Picture

In complete rupture with foetal extrusion into the abdominal cavity, the foetal parts may be identified directly below the abdominal wall; the uterine corpus is retracted and contracted. Where a large vessel has concomitantly been ruptured, distension of the abdomen will be noticed and reduced tone of the abdominal wall, typical of haemoperitoneum, which may easily be confirmed by paracentesis.

Incomplete rupture: The laceration, usually longitudinal, occurs along the lateral wall, generally the left wall, at the broad ligament. The foetus and the blood create a passage between the two leaves of the ligament, therby giving rise to a tumefaction of unclear definition, which may also be palpated through the abdominal wall.

Upon vaginal exploration, blood loss via the genitals and haematuria, if there has been concomitant lesion of the bladder. The presenting part (head or shoulder), which was previously squeezed or wedged in the superior strait, can now be pushed back.

Diagnosis of Uterine Rupture following Delivery

25% of patient deaths occur among patients whose uterine rupture was not diagnosed after delivery.

Rupture of a scarred uterus (lower-segment scar or low cervical scar) generally occurs during labour. However, clearly identifiable signs and symptoms are sometimes absent. For this reason, delivery may advance until the expulsion of a normal foetus, followed by deterioration in the general condition of the mother, who complains only of severe pelvic pain.

Abdominal palpation is not very significant and precious time is often lost because the rupture is not diagnosed on examination. Thus we have the rule: *Every puerperium that contines to lose blood after delivery, or is in shock, must be carefully assessed for signs of rupture.* Or, better still: "*After every delivery following a hysterotomy or obstetric manoeuvre, conduct an exploration of the uterine cavity, which is easily accessible through the amply patent cervix*" (Silberstein, 2003).

In incomplete uterine ruptures, a tumefaction can be observed outlining one of the uterine borders, which may resemble a full bladder (Fig. 21.8A). A useful differential diagnosis is catheterisation of the bladder (Fig. 21.8B), if the swelling persists, it is compatible with hematoma of the broad ligament.

If in doubt, act swiftly: *Women are not killed by laparotomies but by the failure to perform one.*

When rupture of the uterus occurs *in a village or in an outlying medical centre*, if rupture is accompanied by resection of a large vessel, death follows after a short time and there will not be time to get the patient to a hospital. Where a large vessel is not involved, the patient will be referred to the hospital by the village or medical centre only after protracted labour has been followed by uterine rupture.

In such cases, the clinical picture, dominated by sepsis and dehydration, will depend on the site and extent of the rupture and on the amount of time between rupture and hospitalisation.

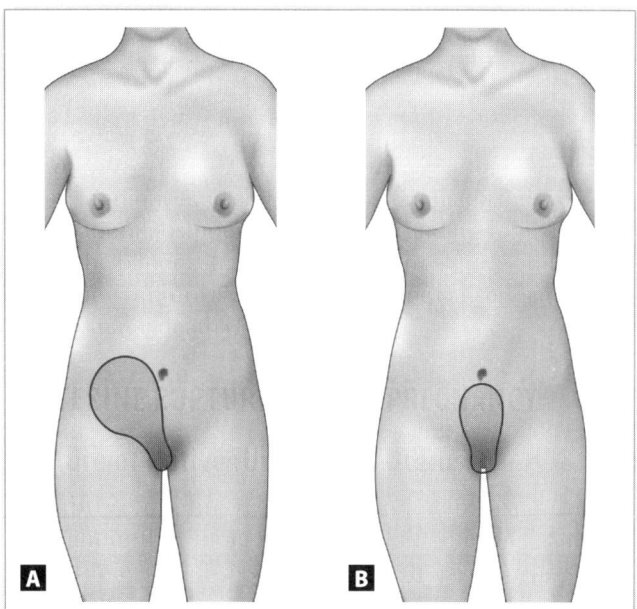

Fig. 21.8A and B: Differential diagnosis of a tumefaction that surrounds the uterine borders without clearly defined margins (more commonly on the left): (A) Swelling; (B) The swelling is no longer salient after catheterising the bladder.

To the sequence of symptoms already described should be added the patient's foetor, caused by dehydration and putrid discharge from the genitals, and the patient's anxious state (in which a prominent role is played by hypernatremia through dehydration). A blood count will show higher than normal haemoglobin values due to haemoconcentration.

Therapy

Never attempt a vaginal completion of delivery where uterine rupture is suspected.

Surgical practice with uterine rupture will vary with:

- *The location where the event occurred*, whether in hospital or outside; if within the hospital, practice takes on the characteristics of an emergency operation for possible section of a large vessel. Preparation follows the procedure described in Chapter 11: Indwelling bladder catheterization (where possible); general anaesthesia using Ketamine, which is to be preferred; where general deterioration has progressed, local anaesthesia may be used with the administration of Ketamine on extraction. When the patient arrives from outside, resuscitation measures precede the operation

- *The site and extent of rupture*: The operation is started, bearing in mind that, in the event of complete rupture with broken membranes, the cavity will generally be heavily contaminated. Septic shock should therefore always be considered, with prophylaxis and adequate therapy initiated promptly. Catheterise the bladder, where possible. A thorough lavage of the abdominal wall using soap and water, followed by disinfection, precede access to the abdominal cavity, which is performed by midline supra and subumbilical laparotomy that contours the umbilicus on its left side. The inferior edge of the skin incision should almost reach the mons pubis. It is essential that the laparotomy wound edges be protected against contamination from the abdominal cavity as far as is possible. If rupture has occurred in the village, or in hospital following many hours of labour with broken membranes, the cavity will be highly septic.

A full bladder never constitutes an obstacle to laparotomy. One proceeds as follows: After opening the fascia, urine may be removed using a syringe, or the bladder may be retracted. For opening the peritoneum to access the abdominal cavity, the uracus offers an optimal anatomical landmark. Once open, the foetus is removed and urinary catheterisation performed.

Having accessed the abdominal cavity, if significant haemoperitoneum is present, and if blood supplies are not available, where rupture is recent and the cavity only slightly contaminated, autotransfusion may be considered. In war surgery, blood from a haemoperitoneum is routinely transfused, even when contaminated; results are decidedly superior to non-transfusion.

Even while adhering to Lawson's (2003) principle, *that repairing a uterus should be preferred to hysterectomy*, the possibilities of doing so are higher for ruptures of scarred than for unscarred uteri (70% of scarred uterine ruptures against 14% of unscarred, van der Merwe, 1987).

Operation type should be selected according to:
- Site of rupture (Fig. 21.9)
- Type of rupture (Fig. 21.9)
- Extent of rupture (Fig. 21.9)
- Haemorrhage
- General condition of the mother
- Attitude of the mother and family members to future pregnancies.

Conserving surgery depends on the site and estension of the laceration and on the mental attitude of the surgeon; it could be performed where the following requirements are met:
- Transverse laceration on the LUS
- Laceration limited to the lower uterine segment; not extending to the broad ligament, paracolpium or cervix
- Easily controllable haemorrhage
- Good general condition of mother
- Wish for future pregnancies
- No clinical or laboratory signs of coagulopathy in progress.

Conservative Management

The *repair* procedure is:
- *Technically undemanding*
- *Safe* (Kelly, 1998): If the patient has understood that she will have to spend the latter months of her next pregnancy close to a hospital and undergo an elective C-section, and if the hospital has set up preferential referrals for hospitalising and assisting these women. Having met these conditions, Kelly (1998) reports case records from an Ethiopian rural hospital in which, out of 245 ruptures, the uterus was conserved in 238 women. It was possible to follow 111 of these over 6 years, 3 months, and between them they brought 117 neonates into the world by elective C-section: Mother and child doing well. Such is current orientation—in sharp contrast with past convictions that uterine rupture in low-resourced countries represented in any case the end of the patient's reproductive life, to the extent that conservative surgery was accompanied by tube ligation as an indispensible complementary step.

In the case of *complete rupture* with expulsion of the foetus, once foetus and placenta have been removed, one proceeds to exteriorisation of the uterus, rapid lavage of the abdominal cavity, isolation of the surgical field and assessment of the extension of the tear.

To ease the delivery of the foetus and of the placenta the tear should be extended in the least dangerous (for the mother) direction, usually: Midline, avoiding injury to the bladder, ureters and uterine blood vessels.

Having extracted the foetus, the uterus is exteriorized from abdominal cavity.

Having exteriorised the uterus, repair is preceded by refreshing of the wound edges.

Over the course of our career, we have experimented with various repair techniques. The simplest and at the same time the most effective is, in our view, effected in two layers and seeks to include the minimum amount of suture material in the wound.

The first layer (Fig. 15.12) comprises *interrupted sutures* that start inside the uterine cavity, approx. 0.5 cm from the wound edge. These trace a semi-circle through the myometrium and emerge 2 mm from the surface; they then follow a reverse path. Knotting is effected inside the cavity. There are two reasons for this kind of suturing: Approximation of the edges is better, and the knot, which is the main part of the suture material, is no longer within the myometrium, but in the cavity, where it falls and is expelled. Suturing starts each wound end, applying the sutures in alternation, to meet up in the middle.

With vertical lesions of the lower uterine segment or of the posterior wall that deepen in a caudad direction, the suturing described above is the preferred technique to avoid damaging a vessel or including a ureter. Interrupted suturing starts as described from within the uterus, proceeding cephalad from the inferior edge.

The second layer is an external mattress suture, or a Gallagher suture.

Some authors (including us in the past) recommended applying a drain between the broad ligament and vagina,

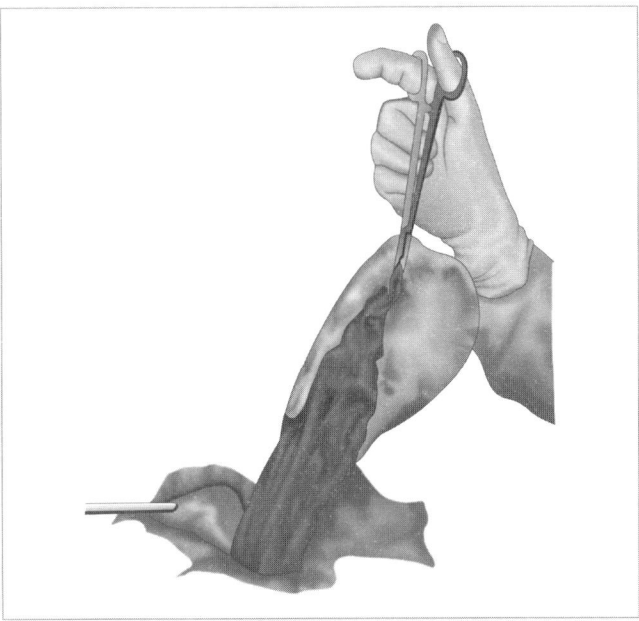

Fig. 21.9: Complete uterine rupture affecting the left lateral border and uterine cervix

passing through the laceration to the myometrium. We no longer share this approach: If the drain is soft and small in diameter, compression exerted by involution will prevent drainage, but if it is too large and rigid, a point of least resistance will remain in the scar after its removal. This represents a danger in a subsequent pregnancy.

With a laceration of the uterine cervix extending into the vagina, excessive traction on the uterine borders will not achieve much. Applying two ring forceps to the bladder and pulling it cephalad will allow the edges of the laceration to be exposed, with good visualisation.

When faced with a *haemorrhage*, the following rule applies:
a. If the laceration does not extend to the broad ligament, stepwise uterine devascularisation, as described in Chapter 17, will be effective. We do not recommend ligation of the internal iliac artery: This is an operation not within the scope of all surgeons and certainly less effective than the procedure described in this section.
b. When faced with haematoma of the broad ligament, or with a laceration extending to its base, stretch the uterus cephalad (this manoeuvre will displace the ureter inferiorly) and from the side opposite to the lesion, apply ring forceps from the side where the haemorrhage originates to the base of the broad ligament, at the lateral border of the uterus. If bleeding continues, apply forceps laterally to these and continue in this way until bleeding stops. Remove previous forceps, clamp the ring forceps by one rack only, or two at most. This will compress the vessel but not the ureter if it has been included. Check bleeding and proceed with clamping, resection and ligation of the *homolateral round ligament* and open its anterior leaf, which will offer a much larger operational area. Proceed with ligation of the vessel (atraumatic round-bodied needles). If you are concerned that you are not able to ensure haemostasis, do not worry; leave the forceps *in situ* and close the laparotomic wound. The haemostatic forceps will be removed on the following day through the laparotomy. In the worst-case scenario if the ureter has been clamped, hydronephrosis may develop, but the patient will be alive.

Never apply Kocher forceps, as these can permanently damage the ureter.

Destructive Surgery

Injuries to the uterus may be incompatible with subsequent pregnancies, while environmental factors could make destructive surgery unadvisable: Here perform a repair followed by tubal sterilisation. Destructive surgery consists in a sub-total hysterectomy. This is the only possible intervention as, during dilation and flattening, the cervix of the dilated, flattend an soft uterus has lost the anatomical identity and substance that facilitate its identification and removal in a non-gravid uterus. Destructive surgery is preceded by approximate reconstruction of the viscera by suturing, aimed at providing orientation for the surgeon. The vascular peduncles are included in a double bite.

The steps are as follows:
- CRL (clamping, resection, ligation) at the uterine extremities of annexes and round ligaments
- Preparation of the bladder and peritoneum
- CRL of the uterine blood vessels
- Wedge resection of the anterior and posterior walls of the uterus, a few centimetres superior to vessel ligation, and removal of uterus. The wedge incision will facilitate approximation of the margins; a high amputation will not withstand pelvic strain with resulting prolapse, a common observation among women in resource-poor countries, who undertake heavy work
- Double-layered uterine suture.

Data from the literature is extremely contradictory (Table. 21.3): Percentages of `(subtotal) hysterectomies vary considerably with author, year and country.

Closure

The final step is visceral peritoneal closure, measurement of the obstetric conjugate (in the case of conserving surgery without tubal sterilisation), abdominal lavage with metronidazole solution, positioning of patient in anti trendelenburg position to promote drainage of lavage fluid, careful toilet of the paracolic gutters and of the pouch of Douglas and, if necessary, realignment of the uterus.

- Insertion of a surgical drain (device connecting a cavity with the external environment), sourcing the most sloping part of the recto-uterine pouch (pouch of Douglas). In case of a very septic procedure, to this would be added a second, subdiaphragmatic, drain to prevent a subdiaphragmatic abscess or perihepatitis: *Fitz-Hugh-Curtis syndrome,* sustained by inflammation of the peritoneal fluid through its continuous clockwise circulation.

A drain should never be included in a repair to a laparotomic suture. With a sole drainage, access to the abdominal cavity is via an incision on the right pararectal line, at varying levels, taking care not to include any arterial vessels in the incision site.

If the operation is highly septic, the drain sourcing the recto-uterine pouch should have *left pararectal access* and the subdiaphragmatic drain should have *right pararectal access*.

One cannot over-emphasise that surgical drains should be large and preferably rigid: In case of peritonitis, drains may be used for antibiotic irrigation. The drain is removed when its production falls below 45–50 ml/day, and in any case within 72 hours.

Table 21.3
Incidence of maternal mortality

Authors	Year and location	Uterus	N°	N°	% of total
Kieser e Baskett	UK 2002	Scarred	18	1	6%
Flamm et al.	1994	Scarred	39	3	8%
Blanchette et al.	2001	Scarred	12	2	17%
Leung et al. *	1993	Scarred/Unscarred	99	19	19%
Yalda et al.	2009	Unscarred 64%	42	15	34%
Khan et al.	2003—Pakistan	Unscarred (85%)	34	16	35%
Gesessew et al.	2004—Ethiopia	Unscarred 92%	54	20	37%
Lema et al.	1991—Kenya	Scarred 57%	105	43	41%
Nkata	1996—Zambia	Unscarred 97%	32	14	47%
Diab	2005—Yemen	Unscarred 71%	60	33	55%
Hibbard et al.	2001	Scarred	10	6	60%
Mokgokong	1976—S. Africa	Scarred/Unscarred	335	261	78%

In the case of a highly septic abdominal cavity, primary skin closure is strongly contraindicated; apply three or four apposition sutures only.

As these are patients who could very easily develp peritonitis and paralytic ileus, it is advisable to insert, during surgery, a nasogastric tube to remain for at least two days.

It is essential that an indwelling urinary catheter remains for at least 14 days, as prophylaxis for urinary fistulas.

Abdominal compartment syndrome is to be kept in mind.

BIBLIOGRAPHY

1. Albrecht K, Gail L. Preterm spontaneous uterine rupture in a non labouring grand multipara, A case report. J Obst Gynaec Can. 2008;30(7):586-9.
2. Al Saleem MH, Makseed M, Ahmed MA, Gupta M. Rupture of the gravid uterus: experience of the Maternity Hospital Kuwait. Med Princ Pract. 2000;9(2):97-105.
3. Asakura H, Nakai A, Ishikawa G, Suzuki S, Araki T. Prediction of uterine dehiscence by measuring lower uterine segment thickness prior to the onset of labour: evaluation by transvaginal ultrasonography. Nippon Med Sch. 2000;67(5):352-6.
4. Blanchette H, Blanchette M, McCabe J, Vincent S. Is vaginal birth after cesarean safe? Experience at a community hospital. Am J Obstet Gynecol. 2001;184(7):1478-84; discussion 1484-7.
5. Chipangwi JD, Zamaere TP, Graham WJ, Duncan R, Kenyon R, Chinyama R. Maternal mortality in the Thyolo district of southern Malawi. East Afr Med J. 1992;69:675-9.
6. Chuni N. Analysis of uterine rupture in a tertiary Center in Eastern Nepal: lessons for obstetric care. J Obst Gynaec Research. 2006;32(6):574-9.
7. Diab AE. Uterine ruptures in Yemen. Saudi Med J. 2005; 26(2):264-9.
8. Ebeigbe Peter, Enabudoso Ehigha, Ande Adedapo. Ruptured uterus in a Nigerian community: a study of sociodemographic and obstetric risk factors. Acta Ostetrica et Ginecologica Scandinaviva. 2005;84;(12):1172-4(3).
9. Ekpo EE. Uterine rupture as seen in the University of Calabar Teaching Hospital, Nigeria: a five-year review. Journal of Obstetrics & Gynaecology. 2000;20(2):154-6.
10. Faleimu BL, Ogunniyi SO, Makinde OO. Rupture of gravid uterus in Ife-Ife, Nigeria. Tropical Doctor. 1990;20:188-9.
11. Flamm BL, Goings JR, Liu Y. Elective repeat cesarean delivery versus trial of labor: a prospective multicenter study. Obstet Gynecol. 1994;83(6):927-32.
12. Gardeil F, Daly S, Turner MJ. Uterine rupture in pregnancy reviewed. Eur J Obstet Gynecol Reprod Biol. 1994;56(2):107-10.
13. Gessessew A, Melese MM. Ruptured uterus, eight years retrospective analysis, causes and management outcome in Adigrat Hospital. Tigray Region Ethiopia. Eth J of health Development. 2002;16(3):241-5.
14. Golan A, Sandbank O, Rubin A. Rupture of the pregnant uterus. Obstet Gynecol. 1980;56(5):549-54.
15. Gotoh H, Masuzaki H, Yoshida A, et al. Predicting incomplete uterine rupture with vaginal sonography during the late second trimester in women with prior cesarean. Obstet Gynecol. 2000;95(4):596-600.
16. Hibbard JU, Ismail MA, Wang Y, et al. Failed vaginal birth after a cesarean section: how risky is it? I. Maternal morbidity. Am J Obstet. 2001;184(7):1365-71; discussion 1371-3.
17. Kelly J, Fekadu R, Lancashire J, Redito P. A follow-up of repair of ruptured uterus in Ethiopia. Journal of Obstetrics & Gynaecology. 1998;18(1);50-2.
18. Kieser KE, Baskett TF. A 10-year population-based study of uterine rupture. Obstet Gynecol. 2002;100(4):749-53.
19. Lawson JB, Harrison KA, Bergstrom S. Maternity Care in Developing Countries. RCOG Press. 2003. pp. 205-10.

20. Lema VM, Ojwang SB, Wanjala SH. Rupture of the gravid uterus: a review. East Afr Med J. 1991;68(6):430-41.
21. Leung AS, Leung EK, Paul RH. Uterine rupture after previous cesarean delivery: maternal and fetal consequences. Am J Obstet Gynecol. 1993;169(4):945-50.
22. Lydon-Rochelle M, Holt VL, Easterling TR, Martin DP. Risk of uterine rupture during labor among women with a prior cesarean delivery. N Engl J Med. 2001;345(1):3-8.
23. Miller DA, Goodwin TM, Gherman RB, Paul RH. Intrapartum rupture of the unscarred uterus. Obstet Gynecol. 1997;89 (5 Pt 1):671-3.
24. Mishra S, Morris N, Uprety D. Uterine rupture: Preventable obstetric tragedies? Aust N Zealand J of Obst and Gyn. 2006;46:541-5(KB 97).
25. Mokgokong ET, Marivate M. Treatment of the ruptured uterus. S Afr Med J. 1976;50(41):1621-4.
26. Nkata Mulumba. Rupture of the uterus: a review of 32 cases in a general hospital in Zambia. BMJ. 1996;312:1204-5.
27. Nkwabong E. Spontaneous Uterine Rupture during Pregnancy: Case Report and Review of Literature. African Journal of Reproductive Health. 2010.
28. Rodriguez MH, Masaki DI, Phelan JP, Diaz FG. Uterine rupture: are intrauterine pressure catheters useful in the diagnosis? Am J Obstet Gynecol. 1989;161(3):666-9.
29. Shipp TD, Zelop C, Repke JT. The association of maternal age and symptomatic uterine rupture during a trial of labor after prior cesarean delivery. Obstet Gynecol. 2002;99(4):585-8.
30. Schrinsky DC, Benson RC. Rupture of the pregnant uterus: a review. Obstet Gynecol Surv. 1978;33(4):217-32.
31. Silberstein T, Wiznitzer A, Katz M, Friger M, Mazor M. Routine revision of uterine scar after cesarean section: Has it ever been necessary? Eur J Obstetrics & Gynecology and Reproductive Biology. 1998;78:26-8.
32. Smith GC, White IR, Pell JP, Dobbie R. Predicting Cesarean Section and Uterine Rupture among Women Attempting Vaginal Birth after Prior Cesarean Section. Eur J of Obstetrics & Gynecology and Reproductive Biology 1998;78:29-32.
33. Sundari TK. The untold story: how the health care systems in developing countries contribute to maternal mortalità. Int J Health Serv. 1992;22:513-28.
34. Taylor MB, Cumming DC. Spontaneous rupture of a primigravid uterus. J Reprod Med. 1979;22:168.
35. Van der Merwe V, Ombelet WUAM. Rupture of the uterus: A changing picture. Archives ofr Gynaecology and Obst. 1987;240(3):251.
36. Veal DJH, Furman KI, Oliver DW. South African traditional herbal medicines used during pregnancy and childbirth. J Ethnopharmacol. 1992;36:185-91.
37. Walsh CA, O'Sullivan RJ, Foley ME. Unexplained prelabor uterine rupture in a term primigravida. Obst & Gyn. 2006;108(3).
38. Zelop CM, Shipp TD, Repke JT. Uterine rupture during induced or augmented labor in gravid women with one prior cesarean delivery. Am J Obstet Gynecol. 1999;181(4):882-6.

CHAPTER 22

Monitoring Caesarean Section: Postoperative Recovery

The postoperative recovery period is the time interval between completion of surgery and discharge of patient.

On admission to the ward, the patient is accepted by the unit doctor.

WARD DOCTOR

The doctor takes over responsibility for management of the patient; the instruments used are *observation* and *therapy*.

OBSERVATION

Quickly review the anaesthesia record and the clinical record, the kind of surgery and any instructions for postoperative recovery.

Check that the patient:
- Is awake and open her eyes
- Can raise her head
- Is breathing normally; shows no hypoxia
- Is not pale
- Is not hypotensive or hypertensive
- Is not shivering; is not hypothermic
- Is not complaining of pain
- That analgesia has been prescribed.

If *recovery from anaesthesia is not complete*, or if she is *restless*, have her lie in the left semiprone position (Fig. 22.1), check patency of the airways; if she vomits, have the vomit aspirated and *notify the anesthetist*.

Finally, check for:
- Contraction of the uterus
- Blood loss from the genitals
- Catheter is in position.

Having completed this first step, the physician accepts the patient to the ward and arranges that the patient is placed in a bed: In *supine decubitus* for 8 hours after spinal anaesthesia; In *left semiprone position* after general anaesthesia, if recovery from anaesthesia is incomplete.

The Foley catheter, its balloon filled with the number of ml reported on the extremity set into the urinary collection bag, runs along the *right genitofemoral fold*, not below the thigh, which would risk it, being compressed to, compromise emptying of the bladder, which being full, would in turn impede contraction of the uterus. The urinary collection bag is placed on the right-hand side of the bed as the physician, on a round, stands on the patient's right; the tube should always include a loop allowing any haematuria to be seen.

THERAPY

Check the prescription of, or prescribe:

Infusion Therapy

That re-stabilisation or maintenance of hydroelectrolyte balance is undertaken; with non-complicated C-section, two litres are enough (1000 ml 5% glucose solution +1000 ml Ringer's solution or isotonic saline); otherwise follow the guides of capillary refill time, skin elasticity and the quantity and concentration of urine.

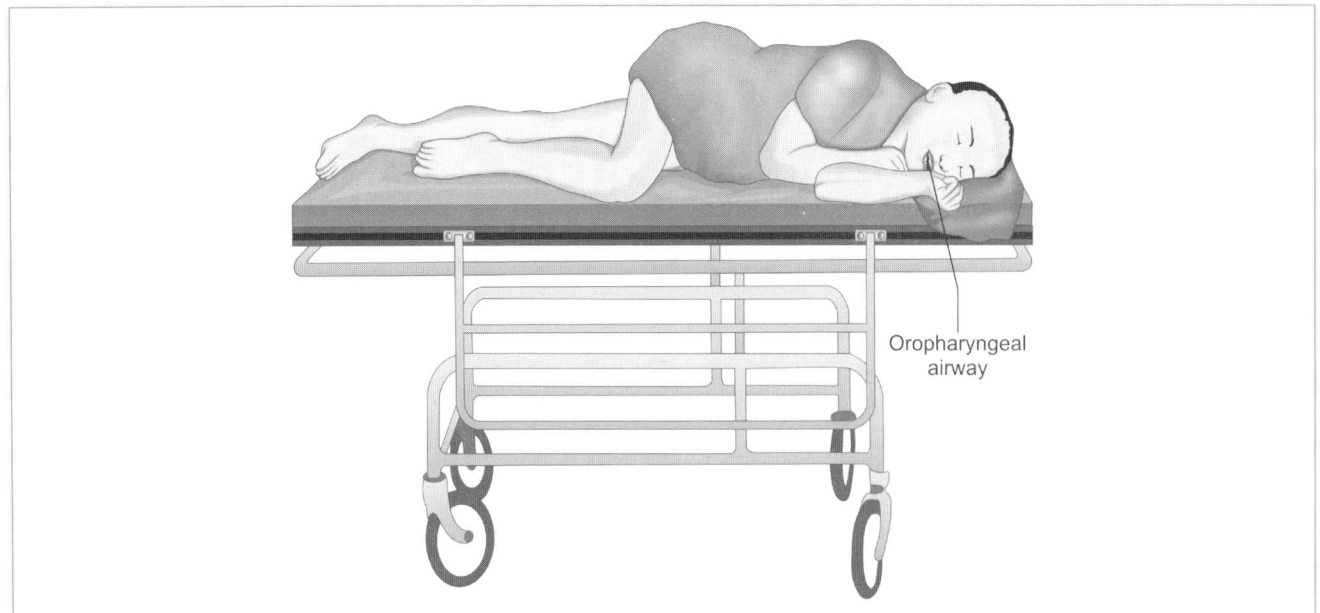

Fig. 22.1: Recovery from anaesthesia is not complete, the use of an oropharyngeal airway with the patient in the left semiprone position

Antibiotic Therapy

When prophylaxis alone is not considered enough (see Chapter on Preparing for Surgery), the recommended treatment consists of the intravenous association of three antibiotics (triple therapy): Metronidazole (500 mg × 3), ampicillin 1 g × 3 (if not available, penicillin 4 mega × 4), gentamicin (160 mg × 1).

Administration of Tetanus Toxoid (TT)

If the patient has never been vaccinated, or was not vaccinated during pregnancy, particularly if labour occurred in a village or in an outlying medical centre.

Postoperative Pain Management

Postoperative pain, along with infection and hydroelectrolytic imbalance, *is a complication of surgery whose adequate control will enable the patient to*:
- Breath better and more deeply (prophylaxis of lung infections)
- Get up sooner, with beneficial effects on the resumption of intestinal function
- Breast feed.

Some general principles apply:
- Patients who have undergone spinal anaesthesia require less postoperative analgesia
- A rational postoperative programme of pain prevention involves the administration of analgesics at set times or by continuous infusion, which can be supplemented if the base therapy proves insufficient
- Poly-pharmacotherapy is advantageous: Associating several drugs exploit their synergetic effects; drugs may be administered at lower dosages; this limits side effects
- Analgesics are more effective if administered before the onset of pain, or before it becomes significant
- Pain treatment by need only has little efficacy and should be proscribed.

Routinely used protocols are as follows:
- *Analgesia during the initial postoperative period*:
  - Pethidine 100 mg IM every 8 hours in three doses
  - Morphine 10 mg IM every 3–4 hours as requested; opiates should not be administered, or administered with great caution if Naloxone is not available on the ward; they can usefully be associated with antiemetics
  - Diclofenac 75 mg IM every 8 hours
  - Ketamine subcutaneous or intravenous
  - Demerol 50–75 mg IM every 3–4 hours
  - Vistaril 25–50 IM every 3–4 hours prn (pro re nata).
- *Follow-up analgesia*:
  - Ibuprofen 600 mg every 8 hours or as requested
  - Tylenol 1–2 mg PO every 6–8 hours as requested
  - Paracetamol associated with diclofenac
  - Paracetamol: 1g per os or IV every 6 hours, do not exceed 4g/24 hours)
  - Diclofenac: 50 mg per os every 8 hours, or 75 mg IM every 12 hours, or 100 mg given rectally every 18 hours; the oral route is to be preferred.

NSAIDs should be used with circumspection in patients:
- Whose kidney function is impaired (preeclampsia and eclampsia). NSAIDs require monitoring of renal function and diuresis throughout their period of use
- With peptic ulcers
- With NSAID-induced bronchospasm.

Correct analgesic therapy is assessed on the basis of:
- *Efficacy*, ability to *allay* pain adequately
- *Level of placation*, to prevent or to provide warning of respiratory depression due to pharmacological overdose
- *Assessment of efficacy* which is effected using pain measurement.

Measurement is the procedure by which descriptors or numbers are assigned to the factors under analysis (Bailey, 1986). In the case of pain, *evaluation scales* are used, which are:
a. *Validated*, i.e. they possess the characteristics:
   - *Validity*, the measure is proportionate to the phenomenon
   - *Reliability*, the precision of the measuring system is defined
   - *Sensitivity*, the instrument is able to trace variations in the event measured.
b. *Agreement*, the instrument offers readings that are objective and comparable to the patient's experience of suffering, which it proposes to recognise and speedily alleviate.

Every algometric scale originates from an assessment of pain through indicators that are translated into a numerical point score that can be correlated with severity.

Evaluation scales have to meet the following requirements:
- Validation (see above)
- Ease of comprehension
- Require little time for making a measurement
- Require little time for recording and processing data.

Algometric scales ought to become a working tool for nursing and medical personnel, and be included in the patient's graphic log.

Algometric scales may be:
- *Subjective* (self-report), based on a verbal or analogical description that the patient can give of their pain; constraints are imposed by cognitive and communicative capacity and by the patient's age. We may distinguish between:
   - Algometric (VDS, verbal description scale), Figure 22.2
   - Numerical algometric (NPIS, numeric pain intensity scale), Figure 22.3
   - Simple algometric scale (VAS, visual analogic scale) Figure 22.4, or mixed (visual analogic and descriptive, FRS- Face-rating scale).

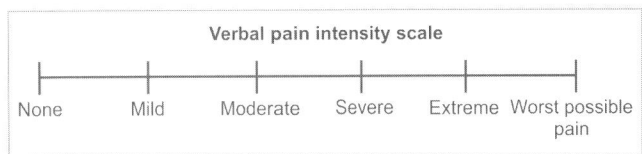

Fig. 22.2: Simple descriptive algometric scale

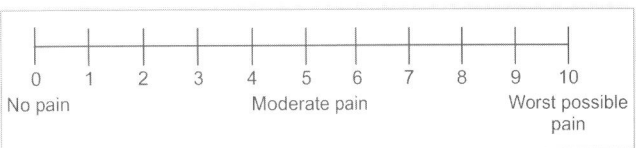

Fig. 22.3: Numerical pain intensity scale

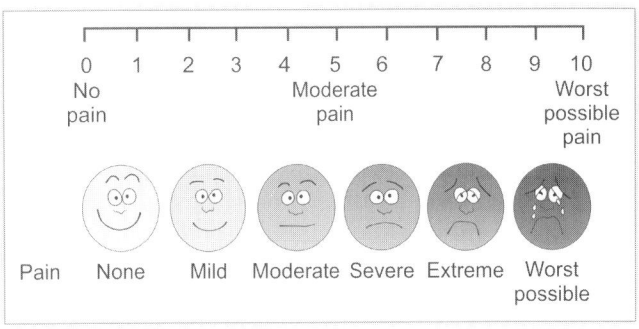

Fig. 22.4: Visual analogue pain rating scale

- *Objective*: To assess behavioural indices in response to a painful stimulus, deriving a score according to the intensity of the pain. These include:
- *Limitation of functional activity:* Functional activity scoring consists in inviting the patient to perform a movement that causes stress in the site of surgery, e.g. to cough or take a deep breath in the case of a C-section. A point score is then assigned: ABC
  A—No limitation in the movement
  B—Slight limitation
  C—Pronounced limitation, severe
- *Level of sedation:* The sedation index (Table. 22.1) is a more reliable indicator of depression than respiratory frequency. Opioids should be used with much circumspection if there is no naloxone available in the ward.

After 24 hours, the physician will review the pain score and adjust analgesia to it.

The duty ward sister or obstetrician

A. Fills in the bedside chart.
B. Fills in the chart of vital signs measured:
   - Every 15 minutes for the first hour
   - Every 4 hours for the subsequent 24 hours, and *arranges that the doctor is promptly notified if:*

Table 22.1
Level of sedation

Level of sedation	Response
0	Awake, attentive
1	Light sedation, responds promptly
1S	Sleep, wakes up promptly
2	Moderate sedation, unable to stay awake
3	Unresponsive

- Temperature is >38°C
- SBP is <90 mmHg or >140 mmHg
- DBP is >90 mmHg or <50 mmHg
- Heart rate is >130 or <60
- Respiratory frequency is >32 or <8
- Urine output is <60 cc over 2 hours or absent, compatibile with hypotension (insufficient renal perfusion pressure), dehydration or more simply obstruction of the catheter by a clot
- Algometric scale >8 (see section on pain)
- Sedation index ≥2 (in case of sedation with opiates, sedation index and respiratory frequency are measured every hour for first 12 hours, then every 2 hours for the subsequent 12 hours)
- Prepares form and receptacles for any laboratory tests.

C. *Commencing intravenous infusion therapy*

We recommend adoption of the general criterion that the normal patient (non-hyperpyretic and without abnormal fluid loss from drains or fistulas) requires approx. 1,500 ml daily per m² of body surface (see Table 6.8).

Should hyperthermia be present, a further 500 ml per day is administered for every °C of temperature above 37°. In case of dehydration, the amount of liquid to infuse will be indicated by the quantity and concentration of urine. It is advisable to keep the flow rate of solutions uniform throughout the period of therapy. In order to find the precise number of drops per minute required, the following calculation may be used:

a. The quantity of fluids prescribed is divided by 24 (hours) to obtain the hourly fluid intake.
b. The hourly quantity is divided by 60 (minutes) to obtain the amount per minute expressed in ml.
c. Administration sets are calibrated so that *20 drops correspond to 1 ml*. By multiplying the number of ml/min by 20, the number of drops per minute is obtained.

D. *Patient nutritional support*

Standard diet: The patient takes nothing by mouth for the first 8 postoperative hours (some authors encourage drinking water after 4 hours, if the operation, under spinal anaesthesia, was without incident). This is followed by the assumption of small amounts of water, at a frequency and quantity regulated by the patient herself. As intestinal function resumes, the patient begins a normal diet, progressing from liquids and semi-liquids onto solids.

The current orientation (Patolia, 2001; Mangesi-Hofmeyr - Cochrane Review - 2002; Adupa, 2003) is to favour an early solid diet (Early Solid Diet Protocol): The patient can start to feed herself with small amounts of solid food within the first eight postoperative hours. If tolerated, this diet leads to a more rapid resumption of intestinal function and cuts 24 hours off the period of hospitalisation.

E. *Mobilising the patient from bed at an early stage*

This should happen six hours after the operation, as an effective method for preventing thromboembolic complications.

F. *Prescribe and administer*

- Vitamin A
- Folic acid
- Iron sulphate
- Ergometrine
- TTB
- Immunise the neonate.

G. *Prescribe laboratory examinations for*

- Complete blood count or haemoglobin level
- Serology for syphilis
- HIV
- Blood group.

WARD EXAMINATION

The morning ward round is a thorough one; afternoon ward rounds are only for patients with particular problems or for admissions who have arrived since the morning round.

Clinical examination of the patient proceeds through the following steps:
- Examination of temperature and observation charts for postoperative recovery. Where fever is present without specific accompanying signs of wound infection, involvement of organs or systems, treat as for malaria or typhus (depending on the locally dominant pathology).

The physician stands on the patient's right-hand side and:
- Checks haematic crisis (colour of the mucosa, capillary refill time)
- Assesses the degree of hydration from skin elasticity, from the moistness or dryness of the tongue, from capillary refill time, from the quantity and concentration of the urine, (the urine drainage bag being situated on the right of the bed). If the patient is dehydrated, the treatment of choice is 5% glucose solution, which diffuses rapidly through the interstitial and intracellular spaces.

Daily fluid requirement is 1,500 ml per square meter of body surface, calculated using the Dubois body surface nomograph (Fig. 6.8). Any supplementation should be determined by the degree of dehydration, adding 500 ml for each degree of body temperature above 37°C.

Decide whether to remove the intravenous catheter and the Foley catheter; the latter is removed 24 hours after a normal C-section, and after 14 days (CBS—continuous bladder drainage), in the case of C-section indicated for cephalopelvic disproportion, obstructed labour or surgery involving an injury to the bladder.

Ascertain whether the following apply:
- The digestive tract is open to gas or faeces
- Urinary tract symptoms are present, indicative of:
- Urinary tract infection
- Stress incontinence is present in approx. 4% of patients following C-section
- Watery discharge (urine) from genitals resulting from injury to the urinary tract; (frequency following C-section is 0.1%)
- Continuous feeling of having a full bladder when the bladder is empty: Very often indicative of a *retrovesical haematoma* (bladder flap haematoma)—see below
- Complains of pain at the site of the wound or in the perineal region
- The presence of:
  - Haematic loss from the genitals, and its intensity. Irregular haematic loss during postoperative period has probably endometritis as a contributory factor rather than retained placental matter
  - Lochia discharge, note the characteristics (colour, odour, quantity).

Clinical Examination of Patient

- *Cardiorespiratory system*: Look for anaemic murmurs, pressure and heart rate. Women who have undergone C-section are at increased risk of thromboembolic disorders (deep-vein thrombosis and pulmonary embolism); for this reason particular attention should be paid to patients during postoperative recovery, complaining of symptoms in the chest (cough, or dyspnoea) or lower limbs (swollen, painful calves)
- *Abdomen*: Assess volume and tone of the abdominal walls; check intestinal sounds.

Paralytic ileus: Postoperative recovery following septic surgery (C-section with chorioamnionitis, uterine rupture, appendicitis or adnexa in pregnancy) is often complicated by ileus.

Intubation with a nasogastric tube is:
- A *prophylactic measure* during septic surgery, in which the development of an ileus is foreseen
- A *compulsory preliminary step* in any kind of intestinal surgery, especially when performed under emergency conditions.

In both cases, the tube has the function of freeing an extensive stretch of the gastrointestinal tract of its liquid and gaseous contents, by means of decompression. An anastomosis is more easily created in an unstretched intestine.

In the first case, the most commonly used nasogastric tubes are single-lumen (Levin) tubes in plastic or rubber. They are 76–125 cm in length and are sometimes fitted with radio-opaque tips for radiological identification.

This type of intubation has also been used in emergency intestinal surgery where Miller-Abbott tube GI tubes were unavailable.

Nasogastric Intubation

Nasogastric intubation may take place *intraoperatively* or with the *patient on the ward:*
- When applied *introperatively,* the surgeon will check correct positioning of the tube by palpation of the stomach
- *With the patient on the ward*, the application is very simple, here we note a few stratagems to facilitate the manoeuvre even under the most unfavourable conditions
- *Materials*: Nasogastric tube (ensure its patency with running water), a 50 ml syringe, a glass of water with a straw (or section of IV line), lubricants, (preferably watersoluble, as oil-based lubricants may create problems if the tube is introduced into the respiratory system).

It is always advisable to explain to the patient what is going to happen and to obtain the patient's consent. Always handle the patient gently, so that collaboration is encouraged, even where the manoeuvre fails on first attempt.

With the nasogastric tube in place, the patient may drink, as whatever is not absorbed will drain away.

Before intubating, **make a rough calculation of the depth to which the tube will be introduced**; this corresponds to the distance from the nose to the xiphoid process, to which 10 cm are added. If the tube can't be notched, apply a small piece of bandage at the calculated distance.

Intubation is performed with the patient supine or seated.
- Patient supine: The nurse stands by the patient's head and introduces the—adequately lubricated—tip of the tube into the nostril. Once this has been passed, they then, as best as possible, direct the tube end downward and anteriorly. Having reached the oropharynx, they

continue, while inviting the patient to swallow or to drink (so that the tube can ride the peristaltic waves as it passes down the oesophagus), or the patient breathes in.

When the measured distance has been covered, aspiration is performed using a syringe: If gastric contents are aspirated, the tube may be fixed; otherwise it should be inserted more deeply.

Another method is to place a stethoscope on the stomach and use the syringe to blow air down the tube: The sound of air bubbling into to the stomach will confirm correct intubation.

If the patient starts coughing or becomes cyanotic, the tube has most probably entered their airways and should be removed promptly.

- Patient seated: The same manoeuvre is performed, with the nurse facing the patient.

Over a short time period, considerable amounts of water and electrolytes can be lost through the tube. Their precise quantity should be noted, so that they can be replaced.

ABDOMINAL COMPARTMENT SYNDROME (ACS)

The abdominal cavity, bordered by the diaphragm, pelvis, retroperitoneum and abdominal wall, is a closed, partially rigid and partially extendable compartment and is comparable to an enclosed fluid. As such, it is subject to Pascal's Law, which states that "pressure applied to any point in an enclosed system of an incompressible fluid is distributed evenly across all other points in the fluid".

An increase in pressure inside an enclosed anatomical space alters the functioning of the organs and tissue contained therein. Such an alteration is referred to as *compartment syndrome*. When an increase in pressure affects the abdominal cavity, the set of ensuing changes is referred to as *abdominal compartment syndrome*. Abdominal compartment syndrome, the clinical phenomenon resulting from intra-abdominal hypertension, is characterised by changes not just in the functioning of the gastrointestinal tract and of other abdominal organs, but also by alterations to the cardiovascular, respiratory, renal and central nervous systems (Blasetti, Coletta, 2004). If not swiftly recognized and adequately treated, these alterations may develop into an irreversible multiple organ failure syndrome (Biffi, 2001).

We owe the nosological definition of this form to Kron (1984).

Aetiology

Intra-abdominal hypertension (IAH) has causes that are as follows:
- *Intrinsic*: Subdivided into acute and chronic
- *Acute intrinsic causes*, which are the kind we have to deal with here, are further subdivided into:

Primary, such as laparotomic surgery; according to Surgue (2005), approx. 33% of patients undergoing a laparotomy manifest IAH.

Secondary, due to an increase in intraperitoneal volume through
- *Ileus*, distension of the small or large intestine
- *Haemorrhagic or septic shock*: Endothelial damage leads to increased capillary permeability, which requires volemic expansion and a massive increase in extracellular volumes. This results in increased *intraperitoneal* volume, leading to oedema of the intestinal loops, as well as an increase in *extraperitoneal* volume from the resultant IAH. A similar mechanism is observed in post-ischaemic reperfusion of the mesenteric intestine with the release of free radicals of oxygen and vasoactive substances
- The presence of laparotomy packing gauze, left in situ to effect haemostasis
- Intraperitoneal haemorrhages
- *Closure of the abdominal fascia under tension*; plastic surgery for abdominal wall defects or for large hernias with reduction in the abdominal cavity of viscera that have lost their 'right of abode'
- Oedema of the abdominal wall with reduction in compliance.

Chronic intrinsic causes: Abdominal tumours.

Extrinsic causes:
- Flattening of the diaphragm and contraction of the abdominal wall muscles due to increased intrathoracic pressure through the presence of high quantities of fluid and/or gas (severe haemopneumothorax).

Quantification

Due to its high degree of compliance, the wall of the bladder acts in such a way that, when filled with between 50 and 100 ml of saline solution, it behaves like a passive diaphragm, thus ensuring that intra-vesical pressure corresponds precisely to intra-abdominal pressure. For this reason, measurement of the former is the method of choice for ascertaining intra-abdominal pressure: Ease of execution also speaks in favour of this method. We describe the method as originally proposed by Kron (1983), which is still in use today.
- Introduction of a Foley catheter (16–18 Fr); emptying of the bladder, which is rapidly re-filled (to avoid collapse of the bladder wall) with 50–100 cc isotonic solution. Clamping of catheter at collection end
- Superior to the clamping point, introduce a 16-gauge venous catheter connected to a pressure-sensing transducer or a water manometer, taking zero (0) to be the level of the pubic symphysis with the patient supine. According to Fusco (2001), this method leads to an overestimate of intravesical pressure of 3.8 +/- 0.29

mmHg compared to actual IAH over a range from 0 to 25 mmHg.

If a water manometer is used, H2O cm are converted into mmHg by dividing by 1.6 (specific weight of mercury). E.g. 25 cm H2O = 15.625 mmHg.

Reference values: There is no general consensus in the literature over which value of intra-abdominal pressure establishes ACS. The value varies between patients due to high degrees of anatomical-structural variation and the multiple factors influencing abdominal compliance. Meldrum (1997) proposed a graduated scale for abdominal hypertension:

Grade 1: 10–15 mmHg

Grade 2: 16–25 mmHg

Grade 3: 26–35 mmHg

Grade 4: >35 mmHg

Values of up to 10 mmHg are considered normal; the first cardiocirculatory and intestinal alterations manifest at values of >10 mmHg. Intra-abdominal pressure values of up to 25 mmHg are treated as IAH, which crosses over into ACS of varying degrees of gravity with values above 25 mmHg, until passing 35 mmHg.

Physiopathology of Intra-abdominal Hypertension

Initially, an increase in intra-abdominal pressure brings about changes in the respiratory and cardicirculatory systems, which aggravate the clinical picture (gastrointestinal, renal, endocrine and abdominal wall effects). These in turn affect the respiratory and cardiocirculatory systems, thus setting up a vicious circle.

Respiratory System

Raising of the diaphragm with resulting increase in pleural pressure, leads to:
- Decreases in compliance, in residual functional capacity and in lung volumes, with resulting hyoventilation and changes in the ventilation/perfusion ratio with ensuing hypercapnia and hypoxia
- The formation of areas of atelectasis, particularly in basal and/or dependant areas. Ventilatory and gas-exchange dysfunction bring about a deficit of oxygen intake and tissue hypoxia, with resulting metabolic acidosis and an increase in lactacidemia.

Cardiocirculatory System

Obstructed venous return, due to compression of the inferior vena cava, of the portal vein, and to increased intrathoracic pressure, which also obstructs venous return from the superior vena cava, leads to a reduction in preload.

A raised diaphragm and increased intrathoracic pressure often compromise ventricular compliance, with a decrease in the end-diastolic volume, due both to a reduction in preload and an increase in afterload through increased systemic vascular resistance.

These haemodynamic changes, amplified by hypervolemia, which is often present, are already evident at intra-abdominal pressure values of 20 mmHg, while at 30 mmHg, ventricular compliance is impaired.

Cardiocirculatory disorders are subdivided into *systemic*: Reduced cardiac output, hypotension, reduction in preload, increased afterload, and *regional*: Intestinal and hepatic hypoperfusion, reduced renal function and hyperglycaemia due to increased production of cortisol and catecholamine.

Gastrointestinal function: The reduction in arterial flows and hypoperfusion of the mucosa cause ischaemic damage to hollow and parenchymal organs. Values of 10 mmHg entail a reduction in hepatic and portal perfusion, which, if prolonged for 24 hours, is accompanied by the appearance of *petechiae* on the intestinal wall (Caldwell, 1987). Values of 20 mmHg lead to interrupted blood supply to the mucosa and to a 30% reduction in mesenteric arterial perfusion, which increases to as much as 70% if intra-abdominal pressure reaches 40 mmHg.

Ischaemic alterations to the intestinal mucosa cause deficits in the mucosal barrier responsible for bacterial transportation and for triggering the cytokine anti-inflammatory cascade, thereby activating SIRS (systemic inflammatory response syndrome) with development towards a multiple organ failure syndrome if a proportionate therapy is not initiated proactively.

Renal function: Kidney dysfunction comprises two components:
- *Pre-renal*: This component is essentially the effects of reduced renal perfusion resulting from the decrease in cardiac output (see below), with a resulting centralisation and redirection of circulation at the expense of the splanchnic circulation
- *Renal*, due to the direct compression on the renal parenchyma (renal compartment syndrome), with an increase in vascular resistance through compression of the veins and arterioles. A reduction in intrarenal perfusion, corticalmedullary shunt and venous stasis lead to further decreases in renal plasmatic flow and in glomerular filtration. Hormonal response takes the form of increased production of renin, ADH and aldosterone, which add to systemic and renal vascular resistance, reduce diuresis still further and worsen renal functional indices. Urine output starts to tail off at values of 15–20 mmHg, progressing to anuria at intraabdominal values of 30 mmHg.

Tissue damage: Intra-abdominal hypertension is responsible for ischaemia and oedema of the abdominal wall, whose reduced compliance contributes to increasing IAH. In particular, ischaemia of the fascia and muscles of the abdominal wall exposes them to risk of infection, including from anaerobes, with the development of *necrotizing fasciitis* or surgical complications, such as dehiscence and ventral hernia.

Diagnosis

The earliest sign of ACS is respiratory insufficiency. If the patient is under spontaneous ventilation, or shows PIP (intrapulmonary pressure) values above 35 mmHg under mechanical ventilation, haemodynamic changes will appear concomitantly with decreased indices of cardiac function, tachycardia and hypotension. Renal dysfunction appears later, as manifested by oliguria and anuria.

Therapy

The objectives are as follows:

a. *Ventilation target*, to implement a 'protective' ventilation strategy that will ensure adequate oxygenation and normal pH values. In the case of mechanical ventilation, avoid high intrathoracic pressures, which could aggravate intra-abdominal hypertension and at the same time cause high inhalation pressure in the airways.

b. *Haemodynamic target*: To maintain sufficient peripheral perfusion, an indispensable accompaniment to the ventilation strategy, to ensure adequate cellular oxygenation.

Under conditions of slight intra-abdominal hypertension up to 15 mmHg, normal blood-volume levels should be maintained. If intra-abdominal pressure exceeds 16 mmHg, or up to 25 mmHg, resuscitation with hypervolemia should be established to support circulation. Amines should be carefully titrated and deployed only where necessary: Under conditions of centralisation, vasoconstrictive pharmacological stimulants aggravate the unstable and precarious circulation via the splanchnic plexus, worsening lactoacidosis, often present in these circumstances. In Maxwell's (1997) volemic expansion therapy, preference is usefully given to colloids and plasma-expanders over crystalloids, to limit the loss of fluids from the so-called third space.

Examination of the Wound

- *Characteristics of dressing* (dry, haematic/purulent secretion): The dressing is removed at different points according to different schools of thought. In the West, this is done on the day after the operation; in low resourced countries, on the fifth post-operative day, although it may be renewed if need be in the meantime
- *Appearance of the laparotomic wound*: Look out for signs of infection, such as worsening pain, redness, exudate, superficial or deep dehiscence; when these are present, the physician should arrange for the wound to be dressed daily. Every second skin suture is removed on the seventh post-operative day, the remaining ones on the eighth day. Continuous suturing is not indicated in low resourced countries as, in the event of seroma or purulent exudate, the drain will very often compromise the entire suture. This does not happen with interrupted sutures, where only one stitch needs to be removed.

Monitoring Uterine Involution

The physician or obstetrician takes hold of the uterine fundus and realigns it—i.e. elevates it and compresses it gently against the pubic symphysis. For all its simplicity, this manoeuvre is of fundamental importance:

- *It stimulates contraction*
- *It corrects the physiological postpartum retroversion of the uterus*, due to the weight of the empty uterus bringing it into a posterior position against the concave sacral spine, where it is held by intra-abdominal pressure. This is accentuated when (as may happen in low-resourced countries) the mother returns early to physical activity.

Under these conditions, uterine involution of a retroverted uterus will lead to a stabilisation of the retroversion, one of the principal causes of the so-called 'one-child sterility' to be found in resource-poor countries.

Having realigned the uterus, one proceeds to:

- *Monitoring of uterine involution*: This consists in taking the umbilicus as a point of reference and indicating how many transverse fingerbreadths the uterine fundus is located above or below it, recording the finding on the daily chart.

  For example, a fundus located:
  - *Three fingerbreadths above the umbilicus* is recorded as follows: F = 3↑
  - *At umbilical level*: F = 0.

  This will make it very easy to monitor uterine involution.
- *Monitoring of the uterine borders:* If these are not well defined and very painful, it is a sign of impaired involution and inflammation
- *Uterine mobility*: Impaired uterine involution with very limited and painful lateral mobility is compatible with metritis/parametritis (puerperal infection), sometimes caused by a retrovesical haematoma that has transformed into an abscess and spread to the broad ligaments. If mobility is limited on one side only, and is not painful, there is reason to suspect haematoma of the broad ligament. This may be primitive, or secondary to the spread of a retrovesical haematoma to the site.

When presented with impaired involution associated with a constant feeling of a full bladder, even when the bladder is empty and the catheter removed, there is reason to suspect *retrovesical or bladder-flap haematoma*.

Retrovesical or 'Bladder Flap' Haematoma

This is a haematic accumulation in the vesicouterine space following uterine suturing with incomplete haemostasis, or originating from lesion of a vessel during surgical mobilisation of the bladder.

The first clinical description and classification of haematoma goes back to Munro Kerr (1926), who hypothesized that this complication was a result of lower-segment transverse hysterotomy.

The first ultrasound account goes back to Baker (1985), which has been followed by a long stream of reports (Tinelli, 2009).

Clinically, it is characterised by fever, falling haematocrit levels and a retropubic mass. The main complications are as follows:
- Spread to the broad ligament and to the retroperitoneal space
- Abscess formation, which may lead locally to a necrotizing lesion of the suture, requiring hysterectomy, and/or spread to the broad ligament, establishing a clinical picture of puerperal sepsis.

On ultrasound the haematoma has the appearance of an elliptical formation with major axis parallel to the uterine incision, measuring between 2 and 11 cm in breadth and from 2 cm to 6 cm thick, non-homogenous, where solid matter alternates with fluid areas. Constantly present is the 'inflammatory pattern' of the myometrium. It is difficult to differentiate between haematoma and abscess.

Treatment: The first indication for surgical treatment goes back to Munro Kerr, who, fearing, in the pre-antibiotic era, spread of inflammation to the abdominal cavity if the haematoma formed an abscess, drained it by the vaginal route, surgically mobilising the bladder from the cervix until accessing the accumulation. Many procedures for drainage are available when hysterectomy is not necessary: laparotomy, laparoscopy (Winset, 1986; Achonolu, Gemer, Tinelli, 2009) and percutaneous drainage.

Extraperitoneal drainage (Fig. 22.5) after Greenhill is, in our opinion, the preferred operation.

"A Gridiron incision is made above and parallel with Poupart's ligament and the fascia and muscles are split as in appendectomy. As soon as peritoneum is reached it is pushed toward the median line without being opened. The two index fingers are inserted in the wound and gradually spread to the broad ligament until the haematoma is reached and blood and clots will drain. A long curved clamp (Fig. 22.5) is directed toward the haematoma guided carefully by one or two fingers; after the insertion into the haematoma, the clamp is opened bearing in mind the proximity of the uterine suture. A Penrose drain (Fig. 22.6) is inserted and left in place until there is very little drainage. Layered closure of the abdominal wall".

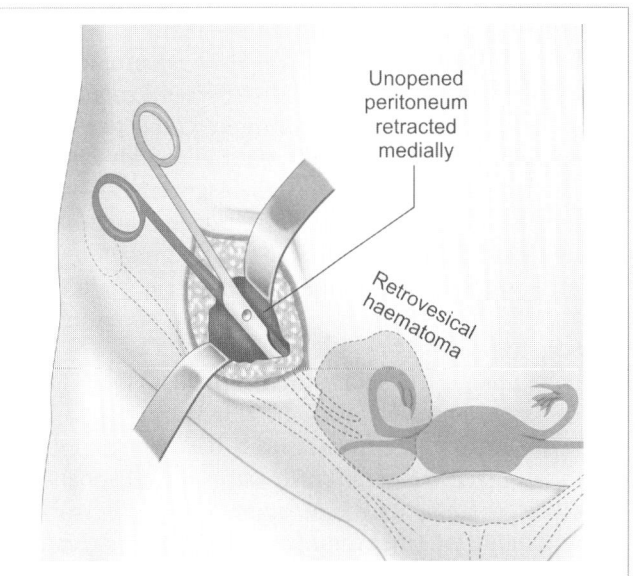

Fig. 22.5: Extraperitoneal drainage for a retrovesical haematoma McBurney incision; the peritoneum is not opened but displaced medially. Initial access to the accumulation is via digital separation, which is then enlarged using forceps

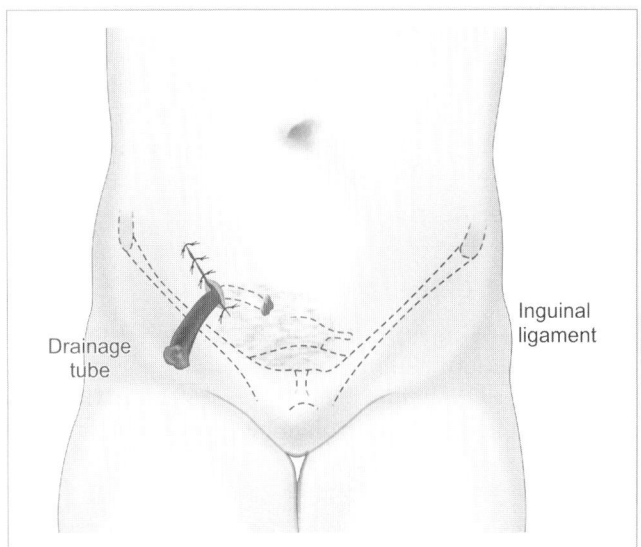

Fig. 22.6: Retrovesical haematoma; evacuation is complete, with a drain left in situ

The authors recollect of a haematoma/abscess that by good fortune made its own way almost all the way down, and whose vaginal drainage was very easily done; with hindsight, however, the authors suspected they had misdiagnosed cases of C-section followed by fever.

Urinary System

Urinary tract infections and stress incontinence occur in 4% of post C-section patients, while urinary tract lesions have an incidence of 0.1%.

Observation of the External Genitalia

- *Pronounced vulvar oedema*: This is referred to in Western Africa as 'Kanula syndrome' from *kanula*, which means 'to push'. It is very common with cephalopelvic disproportion or obstructed labour, especially when part of the labour takes place in the village or in an outlying medical centre. Oedema of the external genitalia are often associated with bruising and abrasions on the thighs from blows inflicted by local senior women, who blame the parturient for not pushing hard enough out of cowardice
- *Perineotomies*: These are often very deep and infected. It is expedient to dress them with water and diluted hypochlorite solutions in a sitting bath (the patient sits in a receptacle containing luke-warm water, hypochlorite or disinfectants, or even detergent powder, twice a day for 15 minutes). Once these wounds have been cleansed, they are easy to repair
- *Purulent secretions* are often observed following Csection; many years' experience suggest *uterine instillation*, which consists in irrigating the uterine cavity through a urinary catheter, using a commercially available bleach solution (hypochlorite) diluted in a ratio of 1:6 with lukewarm water (1 litre).
    - Blood loss from the genitals results from endometrial processes: The above remarks should prove applicable.
- *Bilateral compression of the inguinal ligament*, particularly in its inferior third. Any complaints of pain should be considered in relation to venous vessel thrombosis (Vecchietti's sign).

Examination of the Lower Limbs

Swollen and painful calf: The patient, in supine decubitus semiflexes the lower limb: Palpation will allow identification of an increase in volume or pain in the calf muscle (Homan's sign), indicative of thrombophlebitis.

Ulcers

Examination of the back to look for pressure ulcers, unconscious patients should be mobilised frequently.

Reassure the patient if she is finding, or will encounter, difficulties with breastfeeding, depression, post-traumatic stress, faecal incontinence and dyspareunia.

BIBLIOGRAPHY

1. Acholonu F, Minkoff H, Delke I. Percutaneous drainage of fluid collections in the bladder flap of febrile post-cesarean-section patients. A report of seven cases. J Reprod Med. 1987;32(2):140-3.
2. Adupa D, Wandabwa J, Kiondo P. A randomised controlled trial of early initiation of oral feeding after caesarean delivery in Mulago Hospital. Kampala, Uganda. East Afr Med J. 2003;80(7):345- 50.
3. Baker Me, Bowie JD, Killamn A. Sonography of post caesarean section bladder flap haematoma. Am J Rad. 1985;757-61.
4. Bamigboye AA, Hofmeyr GJ. Local anaesthetic wound infiltration and abdominal nerves block during caesarean section for postoperative pain relief. Cochrane Database of Systematic Reviews. 2009, Issue 3. Art. No.: CD006954. DOI: 10.1002/14651858.CD006954. pub2.
5. Bar Guy, SheinerEyal, LezeroviztAdi, Lazer Tal, Hallak. Mordechai Early Maternal Feeding Following Caesarean Delivery: A Prospective Randomized Study. Obstetrical and Gynecological Survey. 2008;63(6):352-4.
6. Biffi WL. Secondary abdominal compartment syndrome is highly lethal event. Am J Surgery. 2001;182:645-8.
7. Caldwell CB. Changes in visceral bloodflow with elevated intra-abdominal pressure. J Surg Res. 1987;43:14-20.
8. Fusco MA. Estimation of intra-abdominal pressure by bladder pressure measurement: validity and methodology. J Trauma. 2001;50:297-302.
9. Gemer O, Shenhav S, Segal S, Harari D, Segal O, Zohav E. Sonographically diagnosed pelvic hematomas and postcesarean febrile morbidity. Int J Gynaecol Obstet. 1999;65(1):7-9.
10. Kron L. The measurement of intra-abdominal pressare as a criterion for abdominal re-exploration. Ann Surg. 1984;199:28-30.
11. Malvasi A, Tinelli A, Tinelli R, Rahimi S, Resta L, Tinelli FG. The post-cesarean section symptomatic bladder flap hematoma: a modern reappraisal. J Matern Fetal Neonatal Med. 2007;20(10):709-14. Review.
12. Mangesi L, Hofmeyr GJ. Early compared with delayed oral fluids and food after caesarean section.Cochrane Database of Systematic Reviews 2002, Issue 3. Art. No.: CD003516. DOI: 10.1002/14651858. CD003516.
13. Maxwell RA. Secondary abdominal compartment syndrome: an un-derappreciated manifestation of severe hemorrhagic shock. J Trauma. 1999;47:995-9.
14. Meldrum DR, Moore FA, Moore EE. Prospective characterization and selective management of the abdominal compartment syndrome. Am J Surg. 1997;174:669.
15. Patolia DS, Hilliard RL, Toy EC, Baker B. Early feeding after cesarean: randomized trial. Obstet Gynecol. 2001;98(1):113-6.
16. Surgue M, Buist MD, Hourihan F. Studio prospetticosull'ipertensione intra-addominale e funzioner-enaledopolaparotomia. Br J Surg. 1995;82:235-8.
17. Tinelli A, Malvasi A, Vittori G. Laparoscopic treatment of post-cesarean section bladder flap hematoma: A feasible and safe approach. Minim Invasive Ther Allied Technol. 2009:1-5.
18. Winsett MZ, Fagan CJ, Bedi DG. Sonographic demonstration of bladder-flap hematoma. J Ultrasound Med. 1986;5(9):483-7.

CHAPTER 23

Complications of the Laparotomic Wound Suture

WOUND DEHISCENCE

Dehiscence of a laparotomic wound (burst abdomen) here refers to a postoperative, partial or total solution of continuity of all of the sutured layers of the laparotomic wound, with exposure of abdominal contents.

This represents a major complication of abdominal surgery and has an incidence of 0.2–1.2%. Carlson (1997) examines studies of this issue, conducted between 1900 and 1997. Dividing them into four groups, it was found:
- Before 1940; 12 studies (>71,000 incisions), incidence 0.4%, (range 0.24%–3.0%)
- From 1950 to 1984; 34 studies (>320,000 incisions), incidence 0.59% (range 0.24%–5.8%)
- From 1985 to 1996; 18 studies (>18,133 incisions), incidence 1.2%.

An interesting finding is that the incidence of wound dehiscence is now increasing; a role here is undoubtedly played by the growth in geriatric surgery (Spiliotis et al., 2009).

One of the most important studies in the field of obstetrics is that conducted by Mowatt (1971), who found 50 cases in a series of 2,175 patients: An incidence of 2.3%.

A grave complication is the mortality rate of 30%. But tragedy on this scale is avoidable, as dehiscence is generally incurred through the use of incorrect surgical technique in isolating and repairing the wound during laparotomic surgery, which is itself already replete with risk factors.

Aetiopathogenesis

Wound dehiscence is a consequence of the interaction between risk factors that are either mechanical or septic, or both in varying degrees, during the wound repair process.

This interaction may occur preoperatively (the individual), intraoperatively or postoperatively, and may work in isolation of or in association with other factors during the various phases of wound healing.

(Please refer to Chapter 19 for more on the physiology of wound healing).

Preoperative Risk Factors
(the surgical terrain)

Preoperative factors concern the general (preoperative) condition of the patient. Of relevance are the patient's sex (dehiscence is twice as common among males) and age (incidence grow with increasing age). Clearly, the former factor does not apply to caesarean sections, where instead significant conditions are malnutrition, protein deficiency (hypoalbuminaemia is a marker for malnutrition), deficiency of vitamin C and of zinc.

Vitamin C is important for the strength of healing tissue, and a deficiency disrupts normal healing processes, leading to an eight-fold increase in the incidence of wound dehiscence. This alone justifies the administration of vitamin C to malnourished surgical patients.

The role played by zinc in wound healing is not clearly understood, but it is a co-factor in many enzymatic and mitotic processes.

Intraoperative Risk Factors

These concern:
- *Characteristics of the surgery*: Here emergency is a risk factor
- *The type of laparotomy*: Vertical laparotomies are at greater risk of dehiscence than transverse laparotomies. In the former, the incision cuts transversely through aponeurotic fibres: In the latter, the incision runs parallel to them (Fig. 13.18). In Sloan's (1930) study population, the ratio between dehiscence in vertical laparotomies compared to transverse laparotomies was 30:1. This ratio falls to 8:1 in Mowatt's (1971) study
- *Correct surgical asepsis and isolation of the surgical field and of the incision*
- *Wound closure technique*: The resistance of catgut to tensile stress breaks down after the 10th postoperative day. Excluding cases in which catgut was used to repair the wound, it is rarely the suture that gives way; it is more frequently the fascia that proves unable to withstand the mechanical stress it is subjected to. This happens when an insufficient bite of fascia is included in the suture, or where the choice of suturing method does not meet the requirements of holding the surfaces in contact with each other *in both the transverse and longitudinal directions.*

Furthermore it is indispensable that the surgeon be aware that repairing the laparotomic wound in a septic operation requires a technique and material different to those used in nonseptic surgery.

a. *Single-layer closure (mass closure) or layered closure?* (Fig. 23.2). A multicentric analysis of 12, 249 patients with abdominal wounds, conducted in nine countries (Weiland et al., 1998), found that single-layer sutures had a slight advantage in terms of fewer dehiscences and ventral hernias, while they had a higher incidence of infection.

The same study concluded that *single-layer closure should be preferred for its safety, efficacy and speed.*

b. *Continuous suturing or interrupted sutures?* Conclusions are not uniform, but agree in finding a slight increase in dehiscence among wounds closed using interrupted sutures, (Fagniez et al., 1985, Whipple and Elliot, Jenkins 1976). This is because the function of suturing, to keep surfaces in contact, can break down with interrupted suturing between one suture and the next.

These authors conclude that *"continuous suturing is an adequate technique for its safety, efficacy and speed of execution".*

c. *Which type of interrupted sutures: Simple after Gallagher* (Fig. 23.1) *or the two Smead Jones variants* (Figs 19.6 and 19.7; Fig. 23.2B). Very few studies have been conducted on this question and the available data would not be significant.

d. *Width of stitch:* The 1-cm rule is held to be the ideal, (both for continuous and for interrupted suturing), that is: 1 cm in width of stitch and 1 cm interval between one stitch and the next, with a 4:1 ratio between length of suture thread and wound length. A ratio of less than 4:1 appears to be associated with an increased risk of abdominal wall dehiscence or ventral hernia (Israelsson, L.A. et al., 1996). Vershney et al. recommend the inclusion of muscle tissue to a depth of 1 cm in each bite; this is said to increase suture strength and results in a thread-length to wound-length ratio of 6:1.

e. *Suture material*: Van't Riet M, et al., (2002) carried out a meta-analysis of 15 studies (study populations not less than 100 patients), amounting to a total of 6,566 patients, looking at short-term and long-term outcomes of laparotomic wound repairs using various suture materials: Absorbable (polyglyconate: Maxon, and polydioxanone: PDS), and nonabsorbable (nylon: Ethicon and polypropylene: Polene). No difference whatsoever was observed between the two material types

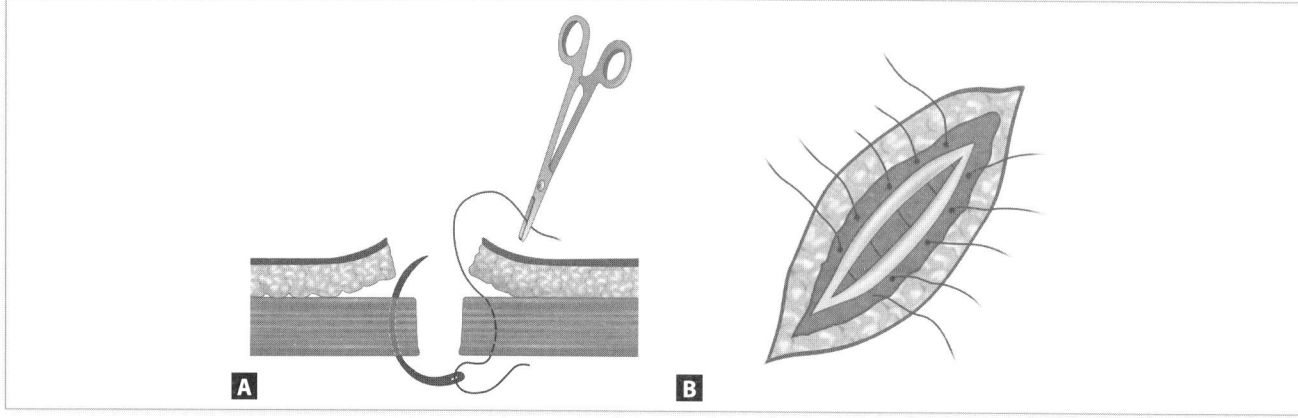

Fig. 23.1A and B: Single-layer closure using Gallagher sutures. (A) Transverse section highlighting how the suture should include fascia, muscle and peritoneum; (B) Anterior view

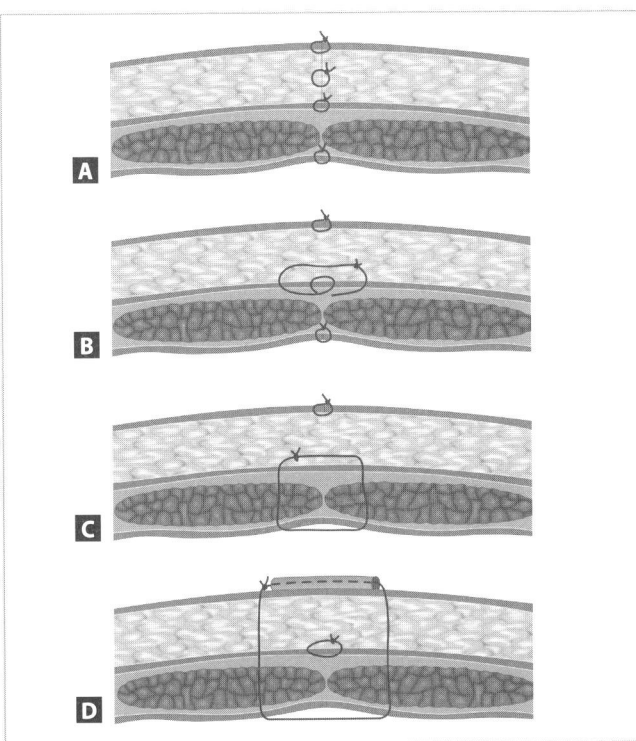

Fig. 23.2A to D: Techniques of abdominal wall closure. (A) Layered closure; (B) Modified Smead–Jones closure; (C) Mass closure; (D) Retention suture

over the short term, while there was a higher incidence of pain at the wound site and fistulous developments were noted with non-absorbable materials. The latter were, however, to be preferred when patients present multiple risk factors, for which a prolonged repair process may be considered (Israelsson et al., 1996).

f. *Thickness of suture material used*: It is obvious that a very fine suture material of equal strength will be more liable to tear the tissue to which it is applied.

g. *Suturing the skin during septic operations*: In these cases, the principle of the "delayed primary suture" should be followed. This consists in apposing the wound edges using three or four stitches, and proceeding with repair of the subcutis and cutis on the 3rd to 4th postoperative day, once inflammation has been brought under control.

Postoperative Risk Factors

A. *Septic causes:* These follow inadequate surgical asepsis and isolation of the operating area and laparotomic wound edges during septic operations, and include:
- *C-section with severe endocavity infections* combined with putrefaction, particularly following intrauterine foetal death, following obstructed labour, or with prolonged rupture of membranes
- *Repair of uterine ruptures*
- Pelviperitonitis, perforation in the case of typhoid fever, appendicitic abscess or other laparotomic surgery whose indication is an inflammatory process.

In some cases, as well as disrupting the healing process, infection causes a necrotising action on the fascia, which undergoes structural subversion, with separation of fibres leading to structural collapse, that is, *necrotising fasciitis*.

B. *Mechanical causes*: High intra-abdominal pressure with contribution by such 'instigators of dehiscence' as:
- Coughing
- Vomiting
- Paralytic ileus, which can lead to wound distension of up to 30% (Jenkins, 1971)
- Urine retention.

Symptomatology

The clinical picture has been reasonably well codified: We distinguish between:

a. *Prodromal stage:*
- Recovery of the patient's general condition does not show its usual rapidity: In general, an African woman is already on her feet the day after the operation
- Postoperative recovery is marked by fever
- Canalisation is slow
- Persistent and accentuated pain at the operation site
- One week on from surgery, the wound is still painful and red
- In 85% of cases, a salmon pink or brownish red serous secretion is present, which is often foul smelling
- Respiratory complications are common; the patient avoids coughing because of the pain at the site of surgery.

b. *Dehiscence* can occur:
- *Very early on*, spontaneously and without warning, becoming manifest on removal of the dressing (5th postoperative day) with knuckles of bowel or omentum presenting on inspection
- Or *between the 7th and 14th postoperative days*, generally preceded by an increase in intra-abdominal pressure; the patient feels a sensation of pulling strain and rupture.

Therapeutic Approach

This is dependent on the patient's condition:
- *Conservative therapy*: The patient's condition contraindicates surgery
- *Surgery is indicated*: The operation takes place immediately, proceeding through the following steps:
  - Cover the wound with sterile gauze soaked in isotonic solution
  - Carefully wash the area surrounding the wound using soap and water (washing powder will do fine) and eliminate all necrotic matter and suturing material

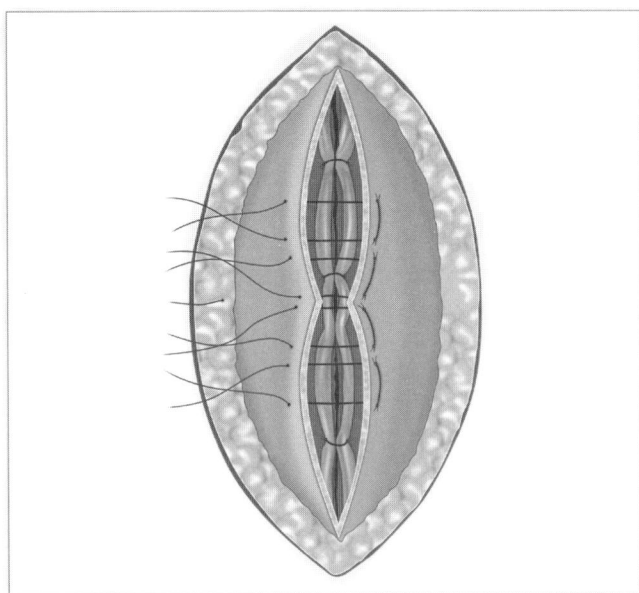

Fig. 23.3: Repair to the fascia with overlaid edges (imbrication), used where the fascia is particularly lax or in closure of septic operations with obese patients. Sutures are first applied along the whole length of the fascia. Knotting begins after they have been applied

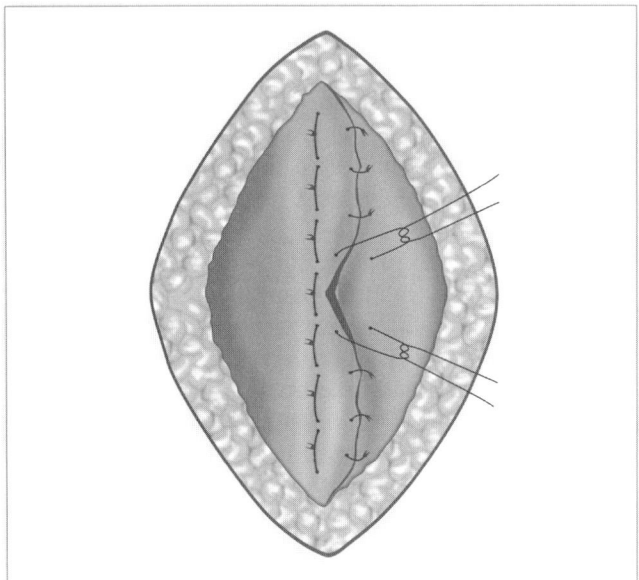

Fig. 23.4: On knotting the first layer, one starts laterally and works medially in alternating turns, completing in the centre of the wound. Suturing of the second layer; the free edge is overlapped (imbrication)

- Access to two veins, preferably with a large caliber intravenous cannula.
- *Rapid rehydration* of the patient with 5% glucose solution and normal saline in a ratio of 2:1
- *Antibiotics:* So-called triple therapy (ampicillin 1 g x 3, metronidazole 500 mg x 3, gentamicin 80 mg x 2) intravenously.

In the operating room, remove all cutaneous and fascial sutures and inspect the underlying layers. When faced with partial dehiscence, broaden the opening until reaching the original edges of the wound. Carefully remove adhering omentum and intestinal loops, remove from the wound edges any suturing material, fibrin and necrotic tissue. At this point access is open to the abdominal cavity: Exploration of surrounding tissue should be restrained to avoid spreading an otherwise localised infection throughout the abdomen. Cavity toilet using metronidazole or antibiotics in isotonic solution; it is expedient to leave the fluid in the cavity to be absorbed via the peritoneum and intestines.

- Preparation of two drains that should be away from the edges of the suture (external borders of the rectus abdominis muscles): One is placed on the left, draining the recto-uterine pouch (pouch of Douglas), the other subdiaphragmatic, on the right, as prophylaxis against an hepatic abscess or "Fitz Hugh Curtiss syndrome", to which the abdominal circulation of peritoneal fluid contributes.

Irrespective of which repair technique is used, it is essential that load easing or retention sutures be placed through all layers of the abdominal wall, including the skin and usually (although not always) the peritoneum. (Figs 19.9 to 12; 23.2D), all abdominal layers are held together without tension; the sutures take the tension off the wound edges. It is virtually impossible for dehiscence to occur while these sutures are in place because of the great amount of tissue they would have to disrupt in order to pull out. They are usually placed with a number 1, or greater, suture, and are especially useful in treating a wound that has already undergone dehiscence.

As the inflammatory process at the wound edge produces (Adamsons RJ et al., 1966) *collagenases* to help with removal of necrotic debris and the zone of *collagen degradation* extends for approximately 1.5 cm from the edge, being the fascia partially digested, sutures should be placed at least at 1.5 cm from the wound edge (Tera H et al., 1976). In patients at increased risk of wound disruption, sutures should be placed 2 cm from the edge.

- *Suturing of the abdominal wall,* can be performed as:
  a. *Single-layer closure (mass stitching),* effected by means of:
    » Interrupted sutures, using non-absorbable, nonporous suture material, in order to avoid capillary spread of serum and infections. Here Gallagher sutures (Fig. 23.1) or one of two Smead Jones variants (Figs 19.6 and 19.7) should be used
    » Continuous suturing is not recommended.

b. *Layered closure*: This is the method we prefer (see Chapter. 19); if particular weakness of the fascia is feared, we recommend double-layer suturing, imbricating the flaps of the fascia (Figs 23.3 and 23.4).

If dehiscence has resulted from an infective process, closure of the fascia of Camper is omitted and just a few appositional sutures are applied to the skin; iodine-soaked gauze is applied between skin and fascia. Having deferred the primary suture, closure is performed on the 3rd or 4th day.

ENTERIC FISTULAS

These are uncommon but dangerous complications, usually observed after accidental lesion of the intestine, which occur:

- During lysis of adhesions, particularly if performed bluntly (sharp dissection should always be preferred), when this is complicated by an intestinal injury that is not adequately repaired
- When intestine is included in the suturing, particularly in load easing or retention sutures
- Following an appendectomy executed concomitantly to a C-section (faecal fistula).

Symptomatology

Observation of the appearance of pus or intestinal contents, the passage of gas through the wound or drain, will confirm the presence of a fistula.

The severity of a fistula depends on:

- *Height*: The appearance of charcoal at the wound or drain within 15–20 minutes of its oral administration points towards a superior level communication, at the jejunum or ileum
- *Quantity*: An amount above 1,500 ml in 24 hours over more than three days.

Therapy

If adequately treated, fistulas tend to close by themselves spontaneously; treatment is therefore generally conservative, consisting in supplementation of the fluid and electrolytes lost through the fistula. To prevent cutaneous maceration, zinc oxide is spread on the skin around the fistula outlet—or better still, metacrylate-based adhesives.

Apply a colostomy bag. Antibiotic therapy; adequate nutrition.

When the fistula is high, or shows no sign of closing, or when outflow remains high, refer the patient to a specialist surgeon. We point out that fistula repair is a difficult operation and that there is a 70% mortality rate for fistulas with a capacity above 1,500 ml per day, and a mortality rate of 30% for low capacity fistulas.

BIBLIOGRAPHY

1. Fagniez PL, Hay JM, Lacaine F, et al. Archives of Surgery 1985;120:1351.
2. Israelsson LA, Jonsson T, Knutsson A. Suture Technique and Wound Healing in Midline Laparotomy Incisions. European Journal of Surgery. 1996;162:605-9.
3. MA. Acute Wound Failure. Surgical Clinics of North America. 1997;77:607-36.
4. Mowat James, Bonnar John. Abdominal Wound, Dehiscence after Caesarean Section. Br Med J. 1971;2:256-7.
5. Spiliotis J, Tsiveriotis K, Datsis A, Vaxevanidou A, Zacharis G, Giafis K, Kekelos S, Rogdakis A. Wound dehiscence: is still a problem in the 21th century: a retrospective study. World Journal of Emergency Surgery. 2009;4:1749.
6. Tera H, Aberg C. Tissue strength of structures involved in musculoaponeurotic layer sutures in laparotomy incisions. Acta Chit Scand. 1976;142:349.
7. Van't Riet M, Steyerberg EW, Nellensteyn J, Bonjer HJ, Jeekel J. Meta-analysis of techniques for closure of midline abdominal wape incisions. British Journal of Surgery. 2002; 89:1350-6.
8. Weiland DE, Bay RC, Del Sordi S. Choosing the Best Abdominal Closure by Meta-analysis. American journal of surgery. 1998;176:666-70.

CHAPTER 24

Postcaesarean Wound Dehiscence

Post caesarean section (C-section) hysterorrhaphy (uterine suturing) dehiscence may occur early or late.

EARLY UTERUS AND ABDOMINAL WALL SYNCHRONOUS DEHISCENCE

There are few references to this issue in the literature; we have located one only (Eke et al., 2005), which cites two cases. Here we contribute three cases, observed over five years, one of a patient operated on in our own unit and two others from neighbouring hospitals. We argue that uterine scar dehiscence is often misdiagnosed and poorly documented and occurs almost exclusively in outlying healthcare facilities, which fail to communicate with the local scientific bodies. The authors are aware of 5–6 further cases that occurred over the past 5–8 years in neighbouring facilities in the Horn of Africa.

Aetiology

A typical observation is in a primigravida on whom C-section was performed due to obstructed labour with foetal death 2 or 3 days previously

A constant feature is chorioamnionitis at the time of surgery, with extensive putrefaction. In our own case, and in those referred to us, and in those other cases we are aware of, access to the abdominal cavity was via a midline, suprapubic, subumbilical laparotomy, followed by a short vertical hysterotomy, which, in our case, did not reach the fundus. In the other two cases referred to us, the fundus was reached (classic C-section), and this most probably applies to the other cases as well.

The distinction is a pertinent one in that in so-called short C-sections, which do not reach the fundus, the percentage of uterine ruptures during later pregnancies is approximately 2.5%, compared to 7.5% for classic C-sections in which the fundus is reached by the hysterotomy. In the two cases reported in the literature, (from Nigeria), the hysterotomy was transverse on the LUS.

The cause of dehiscence is to be traced to sepsis that has disrupted the processes of wound healing.

Symptomatology

Dehiscence of the hysterorrhaphy, which is revealed by concomitant dehiscence of the laparotomic wound, generally occurs between the 5th and 7th postoperative days. It is preceded by the set of symptoms already described above for dehiscence of the abdominal wall suture: Fever, pain at the site of surgery, reddish, foul smelling secretion, and passing flatus delayed.

Diagnosis is made because the patient reports that "something has broken" or the discovery is made on dressing the wound during the 5th–7th postoperative days.

The laparotomy wound is dehiscent, incomplete involution of the uterus has occurred; the anterior wall is partially in contact with and adherent to the abdominal wall. The wound edges have thickened, have a lard-like appearance and are irregular where the sutures have become detached. The uterine cavity is brownish in colour, covered in a serous secretion, and foul smelling: The intestinal loops adhere to one another and to the lateral wall of the uterus.

Therapy

After two unsuccessful operations, in which lysis of the adhesions and resuturing of the wall was attempted, and having identified the impossibility of proceeding with a hysterectomy, and in the absence of any consensus in the literature, the technique we shall describe below was successfully attempted. Having met with success, the same technique was also used with similar satisfactory outcomes in two further cases.

The operational steps are as follows:
- Careful lavage of the abdominal wall and of the edges of the laparotomic wound using soap and water (washing detergent will do)
- Careful disinfection and isolation of the surgical field
- Lavage of the abdominal cavity, edges lysis of adhesions
- Meticulous surgical toilette of the wound with removal of necrotic tissue and refreshing of the edges, uterine cavity swabbing with tincture of iodine (or equivalents)
- Introduction into the uterine cavity of a drainage tube which passes externally through the cervix and vagina and is secured to the uterine cavity by means of an absorbable 2/0 suturing material. The edges of the uterine incision and of the abdominal wall are sutured together "the suture begins from the right or left edge of the laparotomy, runs through fascia, muscle and peritoneum, pierces the homolateral uterine wall, enters the uterine cavity and from inside the cavity makes the return journey towards the other wound edge. Four or five sutures suffice. In the interval between the most inferior suture and its immediately superior neighbour, a drain is left into the cavity; cutaneous approximation sutures follow
- Uterine instillation with clorhexidine wash or with sodium hypochlorite (bleach) solution may be performed via the abdominal or vaginal drain.

Improvement of clinical conditions and uterine involution are extremely rapid; the abdominal drain is removed on the 3rd–4th postoperative day; no residual utero-cutaneous fistulas; the vaginal drain is spontaneously expelled on the 5th to 6th postoperative day. In two cases we were able to verify outcomes 3 and 4 months later; in the 3rd month the endometrial stripe was clearly evident and in the 4th month spontaneous menstruation occurred.

The two cases reported in the literature refer to repairs to a low transverse hysterotomy.

Prophylaxis

Septic C-section; Gallagher sutures, uterine peritonealisation with inverting sutures.

LATE DEHISCENCE OF HYSTERORRHAPHY

This may be *symptomatic or asymptomatic*.

Symptomatic Late Dehiscence

This is also an uncommon occurrence, but better documented than the above (Larssen 1995, Nanda et al., 1997, Revlin, 2005, Tsuyoshi Baba, 2005, Wagner, 2006, Pollio et al., 2007). The largest survey of cases is that of Revlin, which is of 7 cases over five years.

Aetiology

Chorioamnionitis is present at the time of surgery in virtually all of the cases reported in the literature. With a high degree of frequency, the postoperative course is complicated by bladder flap haematoma. Chorioamnionitis is not reported in Nanda's (1997) two cases, where the indication for surgery was placenta previa.

Symptomatology

From the data reported in the literature, the clinical picture is dominated by profuse metrorrhagia, generally appearing (Rivlin et al., 2004) 3-4 weeks postoperatively. In just one case (Tsuyashi Baba) it appeared on the 11th postoperative day.

Uterine bleeding is constantly preceded by worsening to some degree of the patient's general condition, with abdominal distension and vesical tenesmus.

On *palpation* a tympanitic abdomen, distended and drum-like, with free fluid in the cavity, frequently with partial uterine involution, on deep palpation of the retropubic region, moderate pain. Lateral mobilisation of the uterus, exerted through the abdominal wall, is painful; occasionally pleural effusion is present.

Ultrasonography

Occasionally haematoma in the uterovesical pouch precedes the true clinical picture, which is characterised by distended intestinal loops and free fluid in the cavity; the uterus appears involute, sometimes with an inflammatory pattern of the anterior uterine wall. The sonographic appearance apart from necrosis and dehiscence of the suture is related to the time elapsed between surgery and assessment and shows the presence between the bladder and the usually enlarged post partum uterus of a purely anechoic hematoma or a septated cystic mass or a solid appearing haematoma with ill-defined margins. Some authors (Revlin, 2005) argue that MRI offers greater diagnostic accuracy, but this is obviously not relevant to resource-poor countries.

On vaginal examination, the anterior fornix is thickened (haematoma of the vesicouterine space); the uterine cervix, sometimes open, allows access to the cavity, where friable uterine wall discontinuity is detectable at the isthmus.

Diagnosis

The rarity of this clinical picture makes diagnosis difficult. The late onset of metrorrhagia in a patient who has undergone a C-section, the impaired uterine involution, the tenderness of lateral mobilisation of the uterus, the moderate pain on deep palpation of the vesicouterine space, the absence of endocavity material, the presence of a corpuscular accumulation in the vesicouterine space; the increased thickness of the anterior fornix and sometimes access to the cavity via a patent cervix together enable a diagnosis; but a definitive diagnosis will come on exploratory laparotomy, which is advisable, given metrorrhagia and anaemic state of the patient.

The data presented strongly advise against performing dilation and curettage of the uterine cavity in the presence of ultrasound evidence of a patent cavity.

On opening, a large area of necrosis is revealed at the site of surgery, with friable and bleeding edges and, in Tsuyoshi Baba's (2005) case, a purulent accumulation.

Treatment

Treatment has not yet been well codified and will vary with the clinical picture encountered. Conservative therapy may be implemented in 50–70% of cases. This consists in surgical toilet of the hysterotomy edges and their re-suturing in double-layer, using a slowly absorbable material, N° 1 (a finer suture thread would risk laceration of myometrium). The first layer suture is simple continuous; the second is external mattress suturing, followed by visceral peritoneal closure. An alternative is subtotal hysterectomy (Larssen, Nanda).

Asymptomatic Late Dehiscence

This is detected during a transvaginal ultrasound examination conducted on a patient following a C-section, who was complaining of recurrent pelvic pain and/or irregular menstruation and/or desire for another pregnancy.

The ultrasound reveals dehiscence of the scar, or thinning of the anterior uterine wall, incompatible with a further pregnancy.

In a series of 5 cases, Klemm et al. (2008) proceeded to excision of the scar tissue by the vaginal route using laparoscopic technique, and to reconstruction of the uterine wall.

Their finding was to recommend transvaginal ultrasound monitoring of the uterine scar during the postoperative course and subsequently, particularly in anticipation of future pregnancies.

BIBLIOGRAPHY

1. Asakura H, Nakai A, Ishikawa G, Suzuki S, Araki T. Prediction of uterine dehiscence by measuring lower uterine segment thickness. Prior to the onset of labour: evaluation by transvaginale ultrasonography. Nippon Med Sch. 2000;67(5):352-6.
2. Eke N, Jamabo RS. Case Report: Synchronous dehiscence of the abdominal and uterine wounds. Mary Slessor Journal of Medicine. 2005;5:(1).
3. Klemm P, Koehler C, Mangler M, Schneider A. Laparoscopic and vaginal repair of uterine scar dehiscence following cesarean section as detected by ultrasound. Journal of Clinical Ultrasound. 2008;36(6):381-3.
4. Larsen JV, Janowski K, Krolilowski A. Secondary post partum haemorrhage due to uterine wound dehiscence. Cent Afr J Med. 1995;41(9):294-6.
5. Nanda S, Singhal S, Sharma D, Sood M, Singhal SK. Non-union of uterine incision: a rare case of secondary post partum haemorrhage; a report of 2 cases. Aust N Z J Obstet Gynaecol. 1997;37(4):475-6.
6. Pollio F, Staibano S, De Falco M, Buonocore U, De Rosa G, Di Lieto A. Severe secondary postpartum hemorrhage 3 weeks after cesarean section: alternative etiologies of uterine scar non-union. J Obst and Gyn Research. 2007;33(3):360-2.
7. Rivlin ME, Carroll CS, Morrison JC. Conservative surgery for uterine incisional necrosis complicating caesarean delivery. Obstet Gynecol. 2004;103:1105.
8. Rivlin ME, Patel RB, Carroll CS, Morrison JC. Diagnostic imaging in uterine incisional necrosis/dehiscence complicating caesarean section. J Repr Med. 2005;50:928-32.
9. Tinelli Andrea, Malvasi Antonio, Tinelli Raffaele, Cavallotti Carlo, Tinelli Francesco. Conservative laparoscopic treatment of postcaesarean section bladder flap haematoma: two case reports. Gynecological Surgery. 2007;4(1)53-6.
10. Tsuyoshi Baba, Miyuki Morishita, Masami Nagata. Yasushi Yamakawa, Masahiro Mizunuma. Delayed postpartum hemorrhage due to caesarean scar dehiscence. Archives of Gynaecology and Obstetrics. 2005;272(1):82-3.
11. Wagner MS, Bédard MJ. Postpartum uterine wound dehiscence: a case report. J Obstet Gynaecol Can. 2006;28(8):713-5.

CHAPTER 25

Obstructed Labour Injury Complex

The obstructed labour injury complex refers here to the set of pressure-trauma injuries incurred in the pelvic soft tissue and nerves during cephalopelvic disproportion or obstructed labour, when these have not been promptly (within three hours) identified and adequately treated. This symptom complex involves the following:

- The *urinary system*: Stress incontinence, urethrovaginal fistula, urethral damage up to complete destruction, vesicovaginal fistula, uterovaginal fistula, chronic pyelonephritis, kidney failure and secondary hydronephrosis
- The *reproductive system*: Cervical laceration usually affecting the anterior lip only, but which may extend to complete destruction, vaginal stenosis, secondary pelvic inflammatory disease and secondary infertility, amenorrhea
- The *digestive system*: Faecal incontinence (anal sphincter) rectovaginal fistula, acquired rectal atresia
- The *skeletal system*: Osteitis pubis
- The *peripheral nervous system*: Drop foot (paralytic pes equinus), neurogenic bladder dysfunction
- The *integumentary system*: Maceration of the perineal skin and medial face of the thighs by urine and faeces
- The *foetus*: Foetal death is approximately 95%
- *Social relations*: Due to the foul smell coming from the patient: Social isolation, divorce and depression which can lead to suicide.

VESICOVAGINAL FISTULAS

The anterior vaginal wall (bladder, urethra) is at greater risk than the posterior wall; in fact, isolated vesicovaginal fistulas make up 85% of cases.

Vesicovaginal fistulas are more common among primigravidae than among multiparae. Among primigravidae, who are often very young and with an android pelvis, contributory factors are often cephalopelvic disproportion or deep transverse arrest. Among primigravidae, failed proprogression of the presenting part is often put down to cowardice on the young girl's part in not pushing hard enough; labour is more protracted, pressure has a longer duration and fistulas are more extensive.

Aetiopathogenesis

During labour, the bladder becomes an extrapelvic organ, apart from its base, neck and the urethra (Fig. 25.1).

When cephalopelvic disproportion or obstructed labour are not identified promptly and adequately treated, the foetal head exerts pressure on the:
- *Posterior face of the symphysis and the soft tissue lodged in between*: Bladder and anterior vaginal wall (Fig. 25.1), pressure that results in vascular lesions with widespread ischaemia and resulting tissue necrosis: Pressure necrosis → fistulas
- *Posterior vaginal wall and rectum*: Necrosis from pressure necrosis → rectovaginal fistulas
- *Lumbar and sacral nerves.*

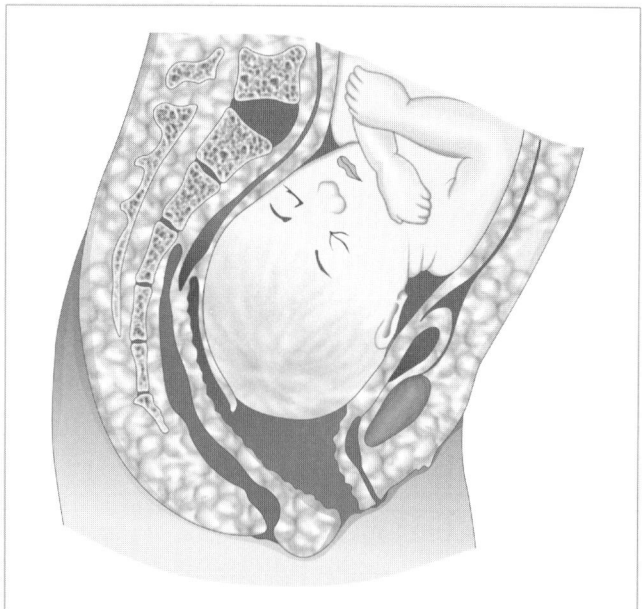

Fig. 25.1: The bladder becomes an extrapelvic organ during labour, apart from its base, neck and the urethra. With cephalopelvic disproportion and during obstructed labour, the soft tissue lodged between head and symphysis (highlighted in light grey), and the rectum, are subject to ischaemic pressure. This pressure also affects the sacral plexus and the sciatic nerve (Brian Hancock—Practical Obstetric Fistula Surgery)

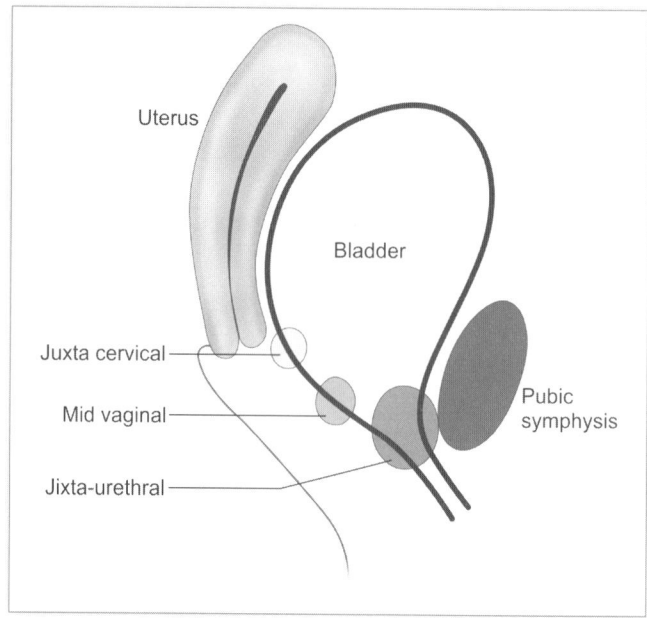

Fig. 25.2: The various position of ischemic injury and classification of vesicovaginal fistulas according to site: Juxta-cervical, midvaginal, Juxta-urethral (Brian Hancock—Practical Obstetric Fistula Surgery)

Responsibility for fistulas used to be attributed to the obstetric manoeuvre employed (C-section, forceps, suction cap, symphysiotomy, craniotomy) in removing the mechanical obstacle; but the fistula would have presented in any case, due to the above mechanism.

The number of fistula cases currently present in Africa is 1,500,000 with an increasing trend as populations grow.

Anatomical Classification

Fistulas used to be classified according to site, size and tissue quality.

A. Site: Proceeding caudally (Fig. 25.2):
- *Juxta cervical*: The fistula opens into the cervical canal (intracervical fistula) or into the anterior fornix, as it is close to the trigone, the ureteral openings are often located towards the border of the fistula (Fig. 25.5C). These are often found at sites where the majority of C-sections are performed; the characteristics of the fistula will indicate its origin: If caused by surgical error, the edges are clean with good quality of surrounding tissue; if the edges are irregular and scarred, it will have been caused by pressure necrosis, and would have occurred independently of surgery.
- *Mid-vaginal*: (Fig. 25.2) These are situated approximately 4 cm from the external urethral orifice; they may be small in size or they may extend cranially to involve the cervical canal or laterally to reach as far as the pubis
- *Juxta urethral*: (Fig. 25.2) This is at the level of the vesicourethral junction. An ischaemia of short duration will produce a simple fistula; if pressure is prolonged, it will produce a circumferential fault-line, separating the urethra from the bladder. It is generally observed after a prolonged expulsive phase and is frequent among patients who have undergone infibulation, particularly pharaonic circumcision.

B. Size
- Small: <2 cm
- Medium: 2–3 cm
- Large: 4–5 cm
- Extensive: ≥5–6 cm.

C. Difficulty of repair
 a. *Simple*: Easy access, trophic tissue, moderate size
 b. *Complicated*:
  » Difficult access
  » Extensive substance loss
  » Scarring and poor quality of surrounding tissue
  » Ureteral openings on the margins of the fistula
  » Destruction of urethra
  » Rectovaginal fistula
  » Ureterovaginal fistula.

Functional Classification

This is the classification currently used, as proposed by Kees Waaldijk (1994); it takes into account whether or not the *urine continence mechanisms* have been impaired; it covers an area roughly 5 cm in diameter, located distally to the external urethral orifice (Figs 25.3 and 25.4).

1. Not involving the closing mechanism.
2. Involving the closing mechanism
   A. Without (sub) total urethra involvement
      a. Without circumferential defect.
      b. With circumferential defect.
   B. With (sub) total urethra involvement
      a. Without circumferential defect.
      b. With circumferential defect.
3. **Miscellaneous:** Ureteric or other exceptional fistulas.

Documentation of Fistulas

Early documentation is essential, and should include the topography, morphology and dimensions of fistulas, which should be recorded on the treatment chart as shown in Figure 25.5.

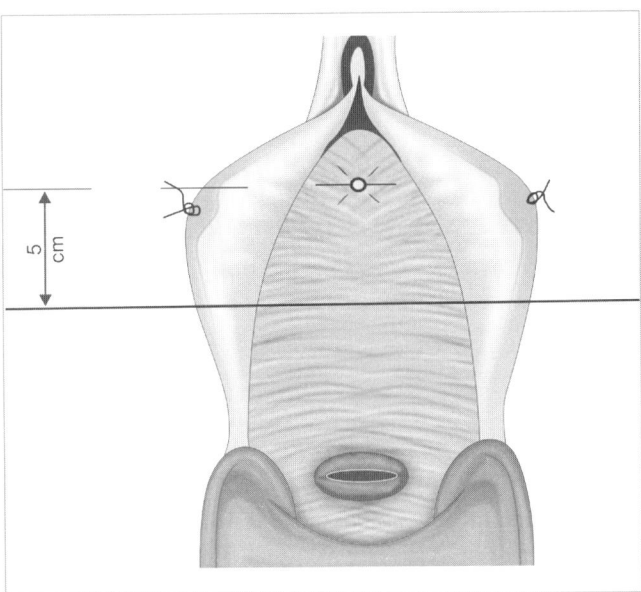

Fig. 25.3: Closing mechanism, frontal view (Kees Waaldijk—Step-by-step surgery of vesicovaginal fistulas)

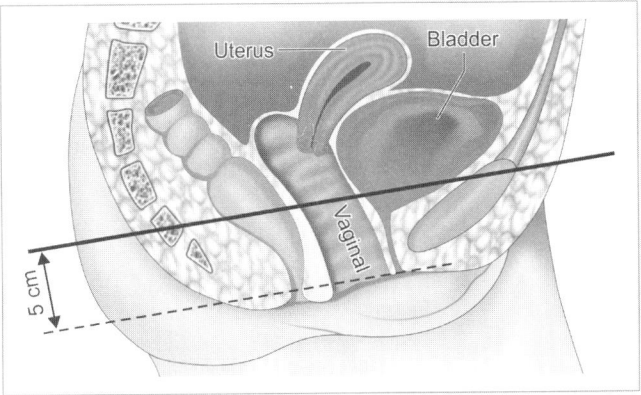

Fig. 25.4: Closing mechanism—Sagittal view—after Kees Waaldijk

ANATOMICAL FUNCTIONAL CLASSIFICATION OF RECTOVAGINAL FISTULAS

These are less frequent than the above: 15% of total fistulas. Their classification, also as proposed by Kees Waaldijk (1994), is as follows:

1. Proximal fistulas
   a. Without stenosis of the rectum.
   b. With stenosis.
   c. With circumferential fault line.
2. Distal fistulas
   a. Without involvement of the anal sphincter.
   b. With involvement of the anal sphincter.
3. Mixed, various fistulas.

Fistulas are further classified according to *size*.

Diagnosis

The medical record shows continuous, uncontrolled leakage of urine following delivery or laparotomic surgery; on physical examination of patient, presence of accretions on the perineal skin and leakage of urine.

The first step comprises a differential diagnosis between urinary stress incontinence (common after parturition with dystocia) and fistula. All you will need is to fill the bladder with 60–80 ml isotonic saline and invite the patient to

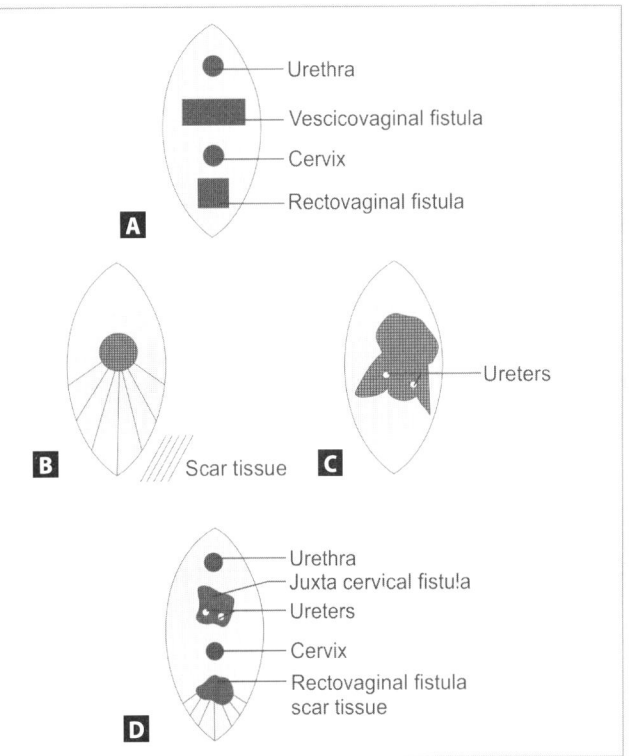

Fig. 25.5A to D: (A) Graphic representation of vesicovaginal fistula and rectovaginal fistula; (B) Scar tissue; (C) Ureteral openings on the edge of the fistula; (D) Juxtacervical fistula with ureteral openings on the margins of the fistula; rectovaginal fistula with scarring of the inferior margin

cough. If urine is extravated through the urethra even when pressure is applied to the neck of the bladder, this will prove indicative.

Sometimes it is necessary to diagnose differentially between a vesicovaginal fistula and an *ureterovaginal* fistula. Decisive here is the dye-test, which consists in introducing dry compresses into the vagina and then to inject into the bladder 50–60 ml of gentian violet or methylene blue; remove the catheter; apply pressure to the neck of the bladder and invite the patient to cough:
- If the gauze is soaked in urine, but not coloured, this is a sign of a *ureterovaginal* fistula
- If the gauze is stained with dye, the dye test is positive and the fistula is vesicovaginal.

Fistulas are often associated with:

Neurological Lesions

Trauma of the Sacral Plexus

The presenting part also exerts pressure on the lumbosacral plexus. Depending on the intensity and duration of this pressure, it will give rise to two kinds of phenomena which may present either in isolation or in association:
- Atonic bladder with overflow incontinence with leaking urine
- Minor or major stress incontinence with leaking urine
- Sphincter ani paralysis with stool_flatus incontinence
- Saddle anaesthesia of vulva perineum /buttocks with ulceration due to anaesthesia.

Sacral plexus trauma is regularly encountered immediately following obstructed labour delivery, it heals spontaneously and most patients have no complaints after 4-6 weeks.

Lesion of the Common Peroneal Nerve

The sciatic nerve (Fig. 25.6) is a mixed nerve, formed of fibres originating from all of the nerves of the sacral plexus (L4, L5, S1, S2 and S3). It is the most voluminous nerve in the plexus and is considered to be its terminal branch. The sciatic nerve comprises two components that run through it separately, and which separate near the popliteal fossa, giving rise to the *tibial nerve*, which is the direct continuation of the sciatic nerve, and the *common peroneal nerve*. Being the peroneal nerve part of the intrapelvic sciatic nerve, the compression of the lumbosacral plexus or of the sciatic nerve, may result in its (peroneal nerve) minor or total function loss and since it is serving the mm tibialis anterior, extensor hallucis longus, extensor hallucis brevis, extensor digitorum longus, extensor digitorum brevis, peroneus longus, peroneus brevis and peroneus brevis; a partial atrophy of these muscles with weakness or loss of

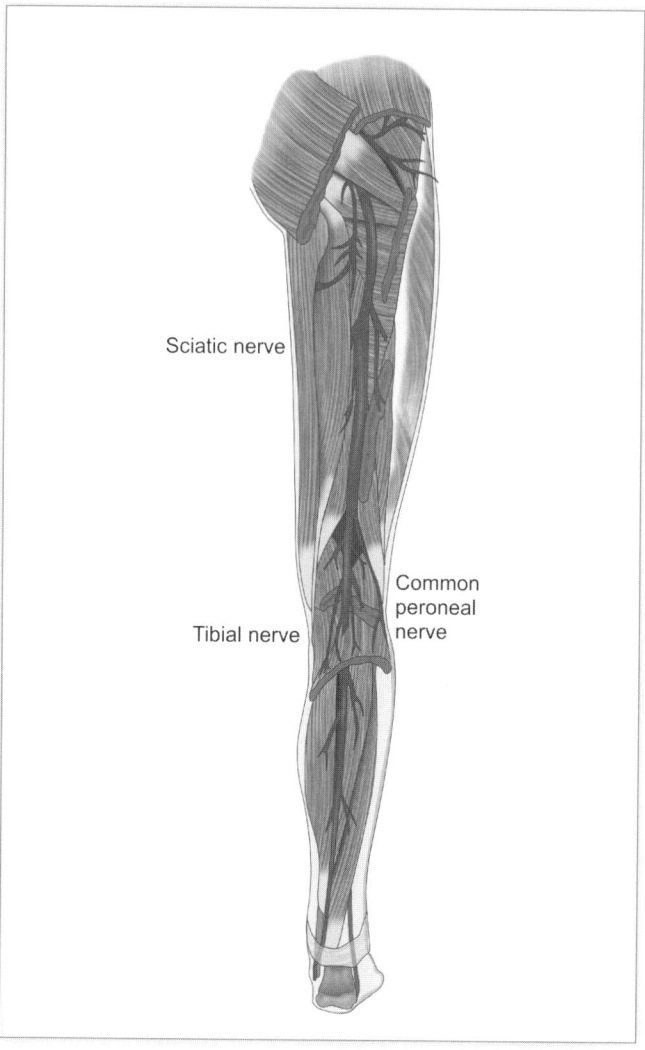

Fig. 25.6: Sciatic nerve

dorsiflexion and eversion of the foot will derive. One of the most frequent clinical manifestations is "drop foot, paralytic pes equinus" (a neuromuscular disorder characterised by difficulty in flexing the foot dorsally when walking). The incidence of peroneal nerve trauma in the obstetric fistula is high; since signs of it are found in over 85% of the patients who present within 3 months after childbirth, assessment of the degree of trauma should be a mandatory part of the routine examination.

The degree of trauma is estimated by voluntary muscle testing (VMT) according to the Medical Research Council or MRC scale 0–5 whereby:

Grade 0 = No muscle activity

Grade 1 = Slight muscle contraction

Grade 2 = Moderate muscle activity (active dorsiflexion of the big toe)

Grade 3 = Half of the dorsiflexion movement possible, when gravity is excluded

Grade 4 = Complete dorsiflexion, muscle weakness present

Grade 5 = Normal

Treatment consists in use of a plaster cast of the foot over four to five weeks.

Treatment of Vesicovaginal Fistulas

Timing of Surgery

It used to be thought that repair of a fistula should wait at least three months to allow "tissue vascular stabilisation". This concept is no longer current, having been replaced by the approach by which the earlier the repair is made, the more effective it is expected to be.

The size of a fistula will indicate which treatment pathway to follow:

a. *Fistulas of small dimensions:*
   - Apply immediately an indwelling urinary catheter (Foley, CH18), paying care that the bulb does not exert traction on the neck of the bladder, which could interfere with the healing process. This measure, of continuous bladder drainage over 4–6 weeks along with dressing of the fistula, will very often prove sufficient to encourage spontaneous closure of a small fistula.

   The use of a sitz bath for 15 minutes twice daily is expedient; where antiseptics (clorhexidine wash or similar) are not available, washing powder will suffice.
   - No antibiotic covering is necessary
   - Oral assumption of liquids: At least 6–8 litres of water per day, to produce from 4,000–6,000 ml of urine per day, this amount is necessary to prevent blockage of the catheter and urinary tract infections
   - Low-protein diet
   - Haematinics per os: Folic acid and iron sulphate.

b. *Large fistulas*: The above measures should be augmented by daily toilet of the fistula with excision of necrotic edges. As soon as the edges have been cleansed, and bleed easily, proceed with surgery.

Method

Successful repair of a fistula follows one simple rule (Sims–Emmet): "*after excising the course of the fistula, trophic tissue should be matched according to anatomical planes and without tension*".

Before the operation, prepare:
1. Lignocaine solution (known locally as "Jungle Juice"): 80 ml isotonic saline, 10 ml local anaesthetic without adrenaline, ½ ampule of adrenaline.
2. Dyestuff solution based on gentian violet or methylene blue, 200 ml.
3. Syringe (with wide cone), 60–80 ml gauge (for injecting the dyestuff).

Surgery

Type I	Only closure
Type IIAa	Closure and something has to be done about continence
Type II Ab	Circumferential repair by end-to-end vesicourethostomy
Type II Ba	+ Urethra reconstruction with urethra tissue
Type II Bb	+ Urethra reconstruction with other tissue (bladder)
Type III	Ureter rein plantation or something else

Operation: Apart from meticulous watertight closure of bladder and urethra (Type I)

- Spinal anaesthesia
- Patient in very accentuated lithotomy position; it is essential that the operating table is fitted with a back rest to stop patient from slipping. Some authors recommend placing patient in a prone position: This is not recommended, as it interferes with the patient's respiration
- Application of a weight valve: Auvard vaginal speculum, placing a piece of gauze between this and the anus
- The labia minora are tied back against the genitofemoral fold to enlarge the operating field
- Possible extension of the operating field by perineotomy, with an extension between a simple mediolateral episiotomy and a Schukhardt incision (that also includes the levator ani muscle)
- Through the course of the fistula, a Foley catheter is introduced into the bladder. The bulb is filled and traction on the catheter will cause the bulb to adhere to the fistula, whose edges, along with the surrounding tissue, will be under tension and adequately identified
- Using the lignocaine solution, the tissue surrounding the fistula is infiltrated. Generally 60–80 ml will be used; the infiltration has a double function: Haemostasis and separation of the planes, which will greatly facilitate surgical preparation
- *Separation and mobilisation of layers*: The plane of cleavage between the bladder and vagina is along Halban's fascia situated between bladder and vagina and constituted by fibro-connective tissue strips (pubo cervical fascia) between which there are large numbers of blood vessels and muscles and nerve endings and by a layer (lamina) of the vaginal wall that dissection isolated artificially; this "fascia" increases in thickness and firmness as we move laterally from the midline.

In normal tissue, the plane of cleavage between the vaginal wall and bladder is quite easy to find, but this becomes progressively more difficult as the fistula is approached. For this reason, separation begins from a point

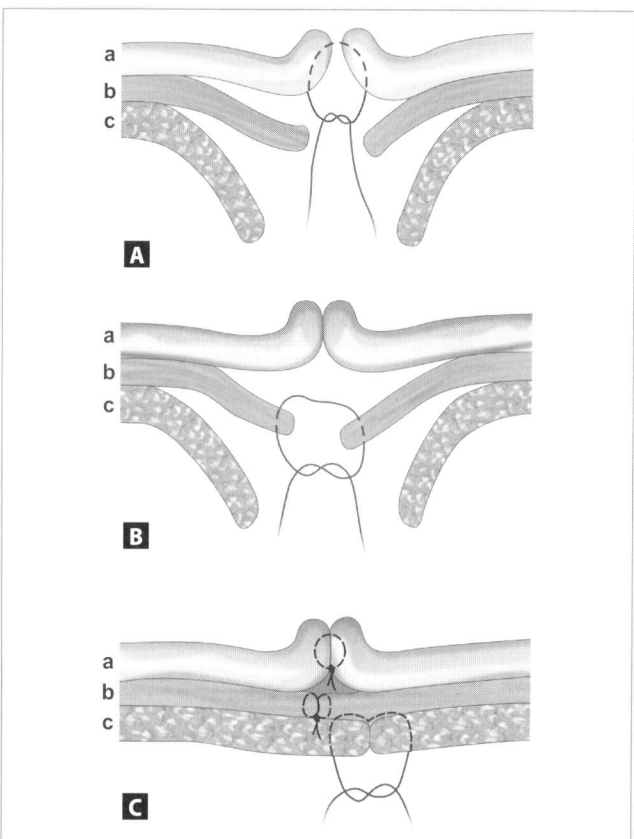

Fig. 25.7: Repair technique for vesicovaginal fistula: Repair follows the anatomical strata; (A) Repair of lesion using single inverting sutures that include the muscularis and a small part of the mucosa; (B) Closure of the fascia using everting sutures; (C) Closure of vagina; some authors recommend everting sutures

- Repair of the fistula, that happens in three layers employing Vycril 3/O or 4/O (or similar).
  a. *Suturing of the bladder* using inverting sutures that start from alternate ends to meet in the middle (Fig. 25.7A). Having completed the suturing, a Foley catheter is introduced into the bladder via the urethra. Inject 100 ml of dyestuff solution; clamp the catheter to prevent extravasation of the dyestuff. Invite the patient to cough to highlight any areas where apposition of the edges is not satisfactory. These are corrected by additional sutures.
  b. Repair of the fascia (Fig. 25.7B), using everting sutures.
  c. Suturing of the vaginal wall (Fig. 25.7C) with everting sutures.

Some authors argue that the greatest danger in a successful repair is the pressure exerted on the bladder neck by the bulb of a Foley catheter that has not been properly secured; to prevent this from happening they suggest securing the catheter (not Foley) in the bladder as shown in Figures 25.8 to 25.12.

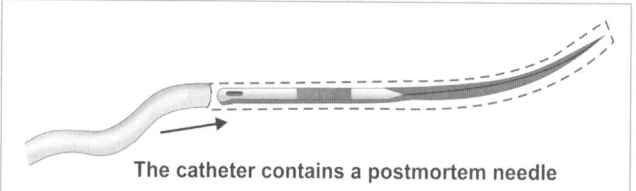

Fig. 25.8: Repair of the fistula is completed by inserting an indwelling urinary catheter, which should *not* bear down on the base of the bladder, or on the bladder neck. An alternative is to conjoin it to the dome of the bladder. A postmortem needle mounted with a 30 cm long folded (two ends) nonabsorbable thread is covered with a urinary catheter

reasonably distant from the fistula itself. Having completed infiltration and separation of the layers:
- The fistula is included in a line of section perpendicular to the longitudinal axis of the vagina. This line begins at the end of one labium minus and heads towards the fistula, doubling at 2–3 mm from it; it outlines the fistula and, having passed it, the two lines re-join to reach the end of the contralateral labium minus.

Detachment is expedited by Metzenbaum scissors, or even better Torek scissors, as used in ORL, whose angle greatly facilitates preparation of the layers for an extension that will enable tension-free closure of the bladder.

Removal of the Foley catheter used to exert traction on the edges of the fistula,
  - Refreshing of the edges of the fistula
  - If required, application of ureteric catheters to one or more openings of the ureters. This is done using ureteral catheters, introduced to a depth of approx. 8–10 cm, whose free ends are passed through the urethra (placing markers to distinguish the right catheter from the left one)

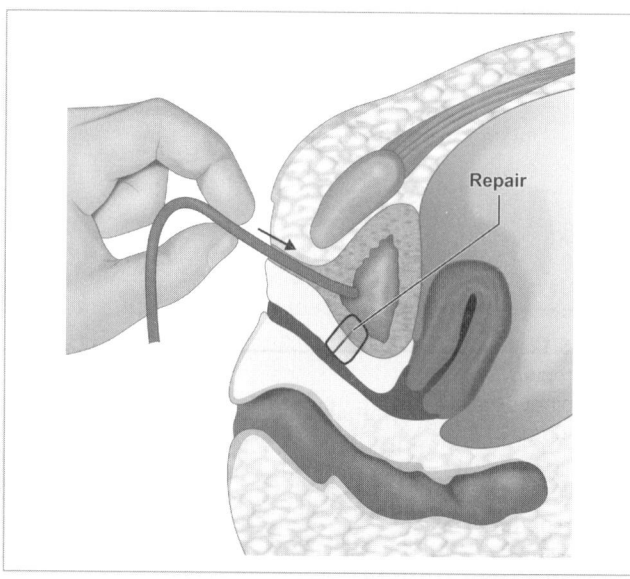

Fig. 25.9: The catheter is introduced into the bladder, its tip is directed towards the superior margin of the symphysis pubis

OBSTRUCTED LABOUR INJURY COMPLEX

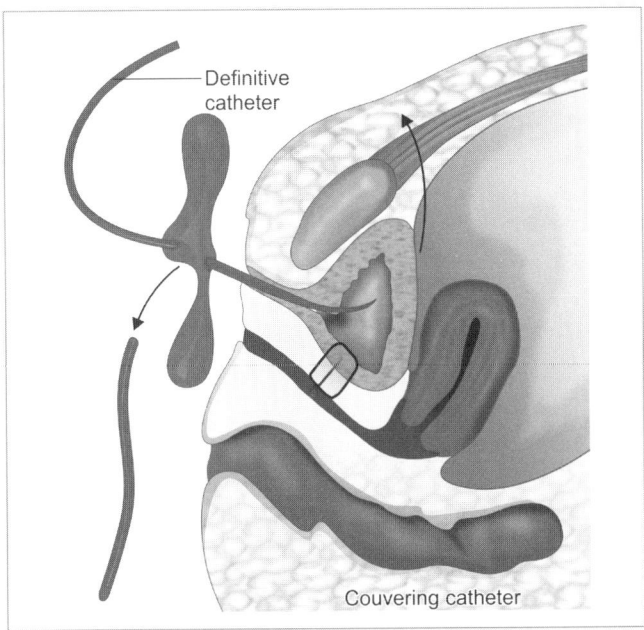

Fig. 25.10: The ensheating catheter is now removed and the definitive catheter is tied to the thread

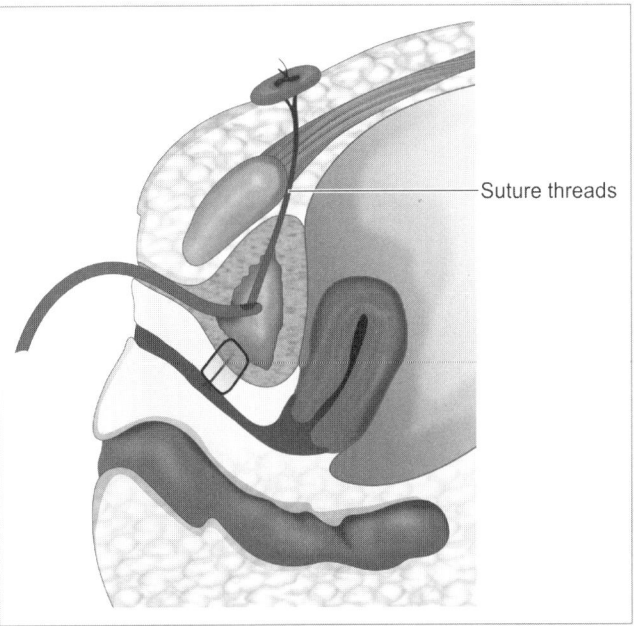

Fig. 25.12: The needle is extracted and the two strands are passed through a button and knotted; the draining catheter should be secured to the dome; a minor amount of mobility should be left. The site of fistula repair will not be subjected to stress

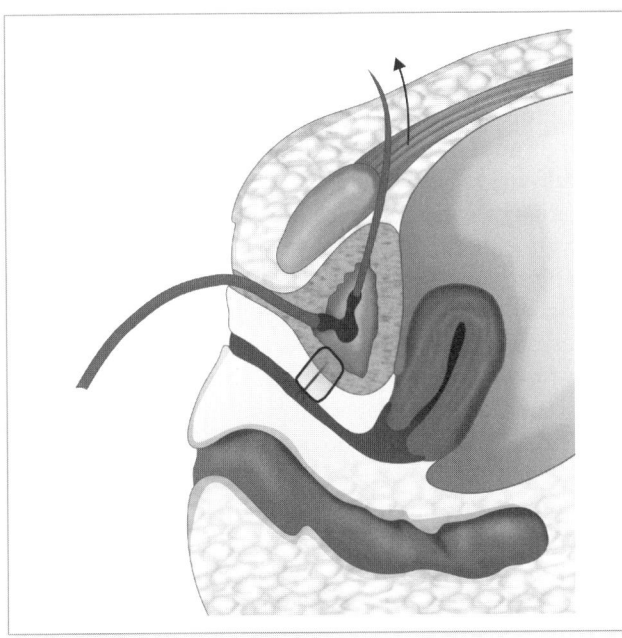

Fig. 25.11: Having as a reference point the superior margin of the symphysis pubis, the needle transfixes bladder, visceral and abdominal peritoneum and abdominal wall is pushed through the abdominal wall

The patient must drink at least 4–5 litres of water per day. The ureteric catheter(s) is (are) removed on the 2nd day. Removal of the urinary catheter takes place on the 12th day.

Having removed the catheter, the patient should continue to drink 4–6 litres of water per day in order to prevent or cure stress incontinence. Urinating every half an hour, micturition should be accompanied by Kegel exercises.

Kegel exercises are vesicoperineal muscle exercises that consist in interrupting the flow of urine several times and continuing with the same muscle movement ten times after each micturition.

BIBLIOGRAPHY

1. Hancock B. First steps in vescico-vaginal fistulas repair. The Royal Society of Medicine Press, 2005.
2. Kelly J. Repair of obstetric fistulae. Obstet Gynecol. 2002; 4:205-11.
3. Lawson JB. The management of genitourinary fistulae. Clin Obstet Gynecol. 1978;5:209-36.
4. Mahfouz BN. Urinary fistulae in women. J Obstet Gynaecol Br Emp. 1957;64:23-34.
5. Waaldijk, Kees. The immediate management of fresh obstetric fistuas. A J Obst Gyn. 2004;191:795-9.
6. Waaldijk K. Immediate indwelling bladder catheterization at postpartum urine leakage. Trop Doc. 1997;27:227-8.
7. Waaldijk K. Step by step surgery of the vesico vaginal fistulas. Campion Press, 1994 Edinburg.
8. Waaldijk K. The immediate surgical management of fresh obstetric fistulas with catheter and/or early closure. Int J Gynaecol Obstet. 1994;45:11-6.
9. Ward A. Genito-urinary fistulae: a report on 1789 cases. Proc 2nd Int Congress Obstet Gynecol in Lagos, 1980.
10. Zacharin RF. Obstetric fistula. Springer Verlag New York-Wien; 1988. p. 140-3.

CHAPTER 26

The Newborn

On delivery 5–10% of neonates require some kind of assistance (Saugstad, 1998) and between 1% and 10% of hospital-born neonates require respiratory assistance (Palme-Kilander, 1992). According to WHO data (1995), more than one million neonates die every year, with perinatal asphyxia accounting for 19% of cases. It has been argued that the adoption of simple resuscitation procedures would improve the survival chances of these one million cases.

It follows that anyone in charge of an obstetric unit in a low-resourced country should have a sound command of the fundamentals of neonatal resuscitation, as illustrated in this chapter, and should be able to impart these principles to their colleagues.

The guidelines here described reflect International Guidelines 2000 and 2005.

INTRODUCTORY REMARKS ON PHYSIOPATHOLOGY

Correct assistance to the newborn on delivery and during the first hours of extrauterine life require awareness of some of the mechanisms of the way the respiratory system adapts to its new environmental conditions.

In cephalic presentations, the thorax in its passage through the birth canal is subjected to pressures which reduce its circumference, the costovertebral angle and elongates the overall length of the thorax.

This mechanical process has two results:
- On *delivery of the head*, the superior airways—pharynx and mouth—are exposed to atmospheric pressure, which is lower than that within the thorax, still descending the birth canal. This pressure gradient is responsible for expulsion of mucous and amniotic fluid into the oropharynx, therefore necessitating *clearing of the upper airways, nose, pharynx and mouth*
- On *expulsion* of the trunk, the deformation imparted to the thorax by the birth canal is relieved; the ribs reacquire their primitive position (restitution of rib elasticity), and thereby negative pressure develops inside the lungs. This negative pressure enables opening of the alveoli and passage into the lungs of a certain amount of air, which will be retained as the *residual volume*. This passive deformation of the thorax and the subsequent restitution of its elasticity, referred to as *preparatory respiratory movements*, are normally followed by spontaneous respiration with the space of six seconds.

The first act of inspiration, short and powerful, generates a negative pressure of 40 cm H_2O that will further expand the alveoli. A contribution to this process is made by the presence of *surfactant,* which reduces the superficial tension of the fluid bathing the alveoli. After this first inspiration and with those that follow, the residual volume progressively increases.

The above series of events, present in neonates delivered vaginally in cephalic presentation, considerably aids respiratory assistance, should it be required. In neonates delivered by caesarean section or in breech presentation, clearing of the upper airways and the preparatory respiratory movements have first to be provided before true respiratory assistance can begin. Hence, the necessity to *adapt neonatal*

respiratory assistance according to the mode in which delivery has been expedited:
a. Vaginal delivery: Cephalic presentation.
b. Vaginal delivery: Breech presentation or C-section.

A second distinction follows this initial one: Whether or not meconium-contaminated amniotic fluid is present and has been aspirated perinatally.

MECONIUM ASPIRATION SYNDROME

Approximately 10% of neonates whose amniotic fluid is stained on birth with meconium will go on to develop meconium aspiration syndrome (MAS).

Meconium is a dark-green substance, 85–95% of which is water, the remainder comprised of epithelial cells, lanugo, mucous and intestinal secretions (bile) and contents of the foetal intestine. Under normal conditions, this is the first emission from the neonate's intestines in extrauterine life.

Innervation of the foetal intestine is completed from the 34th gestational week onwards. This means that from this stage on, the foetal intestine is sensitive to nervous stimulation, and that vagal stimulus, induced by a rise in foetal endocranial pressure, or by hypoxia through placental insufficiency, maternal hypertension, pre-eclampsia, oligohydramnios, smoking and drug dependency (cocaine), or umbilical cord compression, can promote peristalsis, relaxation of the sphincter and discharge of meconium; MAS may also be caused by maternal infection and chorioamnionitis.

The above explains two types of phenomena:

- That, before the 34th gestational week, even under the action of the stimuli mentioned above, meconium will not be discharged into the amniotic fluid
- That the presence of meconium-stained amniotic fluid is observed only among term or post-term neonates. The effects of meconium in the amniotic fluid have been well documented; meconium changes the amniotic fluid, reducing its antibacterial effects and therefore increasing the risk of prenatal bacterial infection. It also has an irritant effect on foetal skin, increasing the incidence of erythema toxicum neonatorum. Much more severe, however, are the effects of aspiration of meconium-stained amniotic fluid, either during labour or at delivery, through foetal distress and gasping respiration.

Aspiration initiates four clearly distinct mechanisms, all of which lead to *hypoxia*: Obstruction of the airway, changes in surfactant, chemical pneumonia and pulmonary hypertension. The resulting clinical picture, 'meconium aspiration syndrome' is more severe among post-term neonates, in that the lower amount of amniotic fluid concentrates the meconium content, with a greater likelihood of obstruction of the airways.

- *Obstruction of the airways*: This may be total or partial. Total obstruction brings about atelectasis of corresponding areas; partial obstruction leads to 'air trapping' and overdistension of the alveoli. The mechanism is as follows: During inspiration, enlargement of the airways promote the inrush of air, but air outflow on expiration is impeded by a reduction in the calibre of the airways through the presence of thick, viscous meconium. This leads to the formation of a valve action, responsible for incomplete emptying of the alveoli and their progressive overdilation and rupture, with escape of gasses into the pleura (pneumothorax), into the mediastinum (pneumomediastinum) or pericardially (pneumopericardium)
- *Alterations in the surfactant*: Some constituents of meconium, particularly palmitic, stearic and oleic acid, due to their lower surface tension, remove surfactant from the alveoli, with resulting atelectasis
- *Chemical pneumonia*: Enzymes, bile salts and fats contained in the meconium exert an irritating action on the airways and on the pulmonary parenchyma, liberating cytokines (including tumour necrosis factor, TNF), with resulting pneumonia, which develops after a few hours of the aspiration
- *Pulmonary hypertension.*

Meconium inhalation can also occur postpartum due to insufficient removal of meconium before the first inhalation, or through the use of positive-pressure ventilation.

Collateral, non-pulmonary signs of meconium inhalation and ingestion may appear within 24 hours of birth, and include greenish-coloured urine.

LABOUR ASSISTANCE AND ASSISTANCE TO THE NEWBORN

Differences in the respiratory mechanisms present at birth in the newborn delivered vaginally in cephalic presentation and the newborn delivered vaginally but in breech presentation, or the newborn delivered by C-section, leads to differences in the delivery assistance given to the newborn during the first hours of extrauterine life. For this reason, delivery assistance and immediate postnatal assistance to the newborn will be treated separately for:

1. Vertex presentation, vaginal delivery.
2. Breech presentation, vaginal delivery.
3. Delivery by caesarean section.

Delivery Assistance and Immediate Postnatal Assistance in Vertex Vaginal Delivery

a. Assistance during labour.
b. Postnatal assistance.

Assistance During Labour

On *delivery of the head*, the superior airways—pharynx and mouth—are exposed to atmospheric pressure, which is lower than that within the thorax, still progressing through the birth canal. This pressure gradient is responsible for expulsion of mucous and amniotic fluid into the oropharynx, necessitating *clearing of the upper airways, nose, pharynx and mouth*. The birth assistant completes this process, initially by clearing and then aspirating oropharynx, with a bulb syringe or suction catheter.

Simultaneously, the head will turn a bluish colour, which generally frightens the novice assistant into omitting these operations.

The novice forgets that *hypercapnia* is one of the stimuli that cause the respiratory centres to initiate the first breath, which spontaneously restores normal appearance to the head colour.

Having delivered the head and trunk, it is advisable to place the newborn onto a level below that of the mother, without hurrying to clamp the umbilical cord (delayed cord clamping). This will:

- Allow *blood flow* from the placenta to the foetus; flow may be promoted by milking the umbilical cord before it is cut. According to Barcroft (1940) and Sturgeon (1956), this manoeuvre will allow 75–80 ml of umbilical cord blood to be saved, a useful move in malarial areas in which maternal anaemia and malnutrition with resulting foetal anaemia are very widespread
- Increase foetal blood volume, expedient in the case of a depressed neonate. This step should be omitted with preterm neonates, where, due to deficient development of the cardiovascular system, it may lead to circulatory overload.

It should be clear that the common practice of placing the newborn with unclamped umbilical cord at a level above the placenta (on the mother's lap) is inadvisable as it promotes gravity-driven blood flow in the opposite direction, i.e. from foetus to mother.

A loop of umbilical cord, clamped at each end, may be conserved for blood-gas analysis; its internal blood values will remain unchanged for one hour.

Postnatal Assistance

The baby is considered born once the umbilical cord has been cut. Now calculation of the first physiological actions begins.

Having delivered the foetus and correctly placed it in supine decubitus with trunk and head sloping slightly downwards from the abdomen and a 4 cm thick soft pad below the base of its neck, so that its head is hyperextended. The neonate's general condition is assessed: Respiration, heart rate, muscle tone, colour, responses, (diagnostic index); presence of meconium in the amniotic fluid or on the skin, and gestational age—preterm or term.

Many indicators for assessment have been proposed and we attach the most commonly used one, the Apgar score, which bears the surname of the physician who invented it, but also serves as a mnemonic for the functions covered: Appearance, Pulse, Grimace, Activity and Respiration (Table 26.1).

It is recommended that measurements are taken at 3 and 5 minutes postpartum; the values for the various signs are added together. Apgar score: 10–7 normal newborn; 6–5 slight asphyxia; 4–3 severe asphyxia; 2–1 critical asphyxia.

Otherwise, more simply note the following:

- Presence/absence of meconium in the amniotic fluid or on the skin
- Weak or absent responses
- Persistent cyanosis
- Prematurity.

After this, assessment of the newborn is based on respiration, heart rate and skin colour.

As it is difficult to detect the central (neck) or peripheral (extremity) pulse in a neonate, (Gandy 1964, Theophilopoulos, 1998), heart rate is determined by auscultating the precordium with a stethoscope, or by assessing pulse at birth via the umbilical cord. The latter method should be preferred; as the pulse can be detected immediately before any resuscitation operations are required. If this is not possible, the stethoscope should be used. Foetal heart rate should remain stable at above 100 bpm; an increase will indicate improvement, a decrease worsening of the neonate's condition.

Assessment is followed by assistance (Flowchart 26.1), which will be conducted according to the neonate's general condition, and whether or not the amniotic fluid is stained with meconium:

Table 26.1

Apgar scoring system

	0	1	2	Index
Heart rate	Absent	Below 100	Above 100	
Respiration	Absent	Shallow, irregular, slow	Good	
Muscle tone	Flaccid	Some glexion of extremities	Active movement	
Cry responses	No response	Grimace, yes	Sneeze Energetic crying	
Colour	Blue or pale	Pink body, extremities cyanotic	Completely pink	

THE NEWBORN

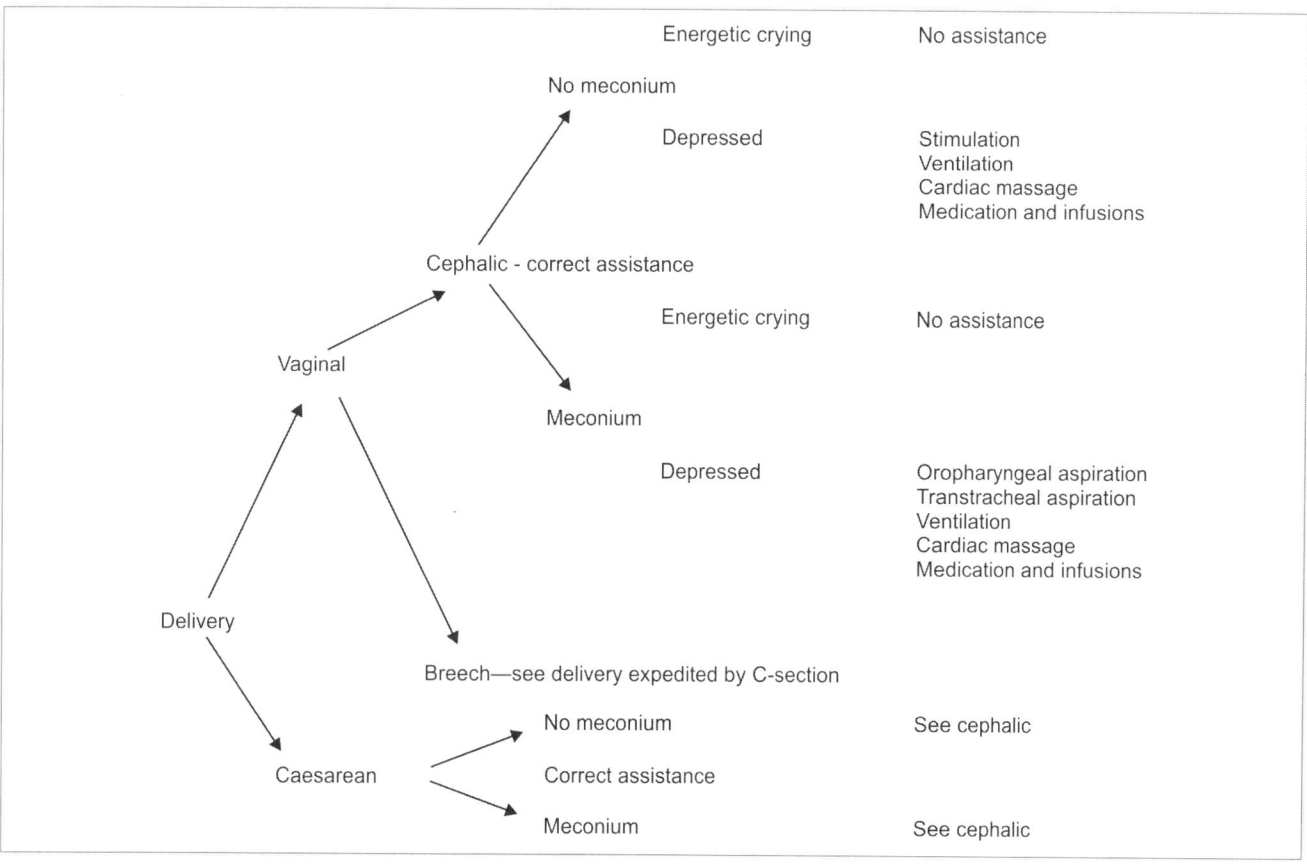

Flowchart 26.1: Algorithm of resuscitation in the newborn infant

- Toilet of the airways
- Tactile stimulation
- Assisted ventilation
- Cardiac massage
- Infusion of medication and fluids.

Amniotic Fluid not Stained with Meconium

a. *Clearing of the airways*: Clearing (possibly by aspiration) of the upper airways is not necessary if the newborn is crying and respiration has begun spontaneously (Estol PC, 1992).

b. *Tactile stimulation:* This involves the handling mentioned above and drying of the newborn, with additional rubbing of the back or tapping of the foot soles. In most cases, this is enough stimulation to trigger primary respiration in neonates still in primitive apnoea. If these measures are not promptly followed by effective respiratory effort, and if the heart rate is below 100 bpm, one is probably faced with secondary apnoea. Stimulation is now interrupted and ventilation should be started promptly in O_2 enriched atmosphere with positive pressure (Dawes, 1968).

c. *Assisted ventilation:* This is performed using a ventilation bag (Ambu bag) or by endotracheal intubation along with an Ambu bag.

In performing both operations (expansion and assisted ventilation) paediatric Ambu bags (or equivalent self inflating bags) are used, that must be fitted with a safety maximum pressure valve, allowing air to escape when pressure within the circuit exceeds 40 cm H_2O. Knowledge that a safety valve is fitted will help overcome the unfounded fear that excessive peak pressure can damage the alveoli, a fear which may otherwise impede correct expansion of the lungs.

The mask should be of the right size to cover nose and mouth, but should not cover the eyes or chin; a round mask will suffice for a premature newborn, while an anatomically formed mask is better suited for a term newborn. The edge of the mask should preferably be soft (air seal), to allow better adhesion of the mask without exerting excessive pressure (Palme 1985). There should not be more than 5 ml of dead space inside the mask.

Assisted ventilation acts in two ways:
- Expansion of the lungs

- Respiratory assistance, to ensure suitable breathing activity at a frequency and volume to meet the neonate's functional requirements.

Expansion of the alveoli is obtained after 5–6 ventilations (Vyas H, 1985, 1986), effected by prolonged and decisive pressure, close to maximum, in an oxygen-enriched atmosphere. Success is shown by expansion of the ribcage, after which assisted ventilation may begin at a rate of 30–40 respiratory acts per minute:
- The *rhythmical rising and sinking of the neonate's chest* at each breath indicates correctly assisted ventilation; if this is not present, ventilation pressure is insufficient or the mask is not held correctly against the neonate's face
- The *colour of the skin and mucosa* will provide a guide in deciding on the volume, inspiration pressure and respiratory rate.

Particularly in cases of respiratory depression, ventilation should aim to compensate for the neonate's respiratory acidosis by means of respiratory alkalosis.

The assessment of cardiac activity does not require a stethoscope; all that is needed is to grasp the umbilical cord between thumb and forefinger to detect the rate and intensity of the pulse. The heartbeat can also be felt through the chest wall.

Term Newborn with Birth Asphyxia

If breathing is absent at birth, muscle tone reduced and the heart rate below 100 bpm, a preliminary measure may be to apply gentle pressure to the thorax and then release it, in imitation of the effect of pressure in the birth canal; pharyngeal aspiration followed by tracheal intubation under guidance of a laryngoscope should be performed immediately.

A laryngoscope with a straight N° 0 spatula is used for premature neonates and a N° 1 spatula for term. The following rule should be followed to avoid intubating the main right bronchus (which is a direct continuation of the trachea): The depth to which the endotracheal tube should be introduced is 6 + *birthweight*:

E.g. if the newborn weighs 2.5 kg, the length of tube from the buccal fissure to the trachea will be 6 + 2.5 = 8.5 cm.

Correct intubation will show the following features:
- Symmetrical expansion of the chest with each breath
- Absence of inflation of the epigastric region (stomach)
- Emission of water vapour from the tube on expiration
- Respiratory noises can be heard with equal intensity at each armpit
- Respiratory (ventilation) noises cannot be detected at the stomach
- Improvement of the neonate's heart rate, of colour and muscle tone.

If after 30 seconds of endotracheal ventilation, the heart rate remains below 60 bpm, cardiac massage is indicated at a ratio of 3:1 to that of ventilation, making a total of 90 compressions and 30 ventilations per minute.

The neonate's head position should not be changed after intubation; any changes in position could lead to the tube coming out of the trachea, or to advancement of the tube into the main bronchus (usually the right bronchus).

Cardiac Massage

Cardiac massage here refers to the operation of compressing the heart between sternum and vertebrae;
- *Pressure is exerted on the lower third of the sternum* (Orlowski JP, 1986; Phillips GW, 1986)
- To be effective, the pressure should generate a *perceptible peripheral pulse*; this is generally obtained by reducing (through compression) the distance between sternum and vertebrae by 1/3. If necessary, the distance may be reduced by as much as half
- *Relaxation of compression should happen slowly*; keep the thumbs pressed against the sternum during the release phase; the compression/relaxation ratio should be slightly higher for relaxation, to promote the neonate's circulation (Dea et al., 1990)
- Compression may be exerted in two different ways (Thaler MM, 1963, Todres ID, 1975, David R, 1988)
- *Index and middle finger of one hand (two finger technique)*, exerting pressure on the inferior third of the sternum, while the other hands helps to support the back
- *Two thumbs placed on the inferior third of the sternum, while the palms and four fingers of both hands wrap around the trunk (two-thumb encircling hands technique)* (Fig. 26.1).

The latter technique is to be preferred to the former, as it can generate an effective systolic pressure and adequate perfusion of the coronary arteries (Thaler 1963; Toder 1975; David 1988; Menegazzi 1993; Houri 1997).

The massage-to-breathing ratio should be 3:1, giving a total of 90:30 (compressions/ventilations) per minute.

Cardiac massage should be continued until spontaneous heart rate is equal to or above 60 beats per minute.

Applying a Catheter or Cannula to the Umbilical Cord

Catheterisation of the umbilical cord is the procedure of accessing the neonate's cardiocirculatory system by inserting a catheter or cannula into an umbilical vessel (usually a vein) in order to administer medication or infusions, or to connect the newborn to measuring instruments.

Figure 26.2 shows the correct positioning of the newborn with, we think, sufficient clarity. It should go without saying that the procedure is to be carried out under strictly aseptic conditions.

THE NEWBORN

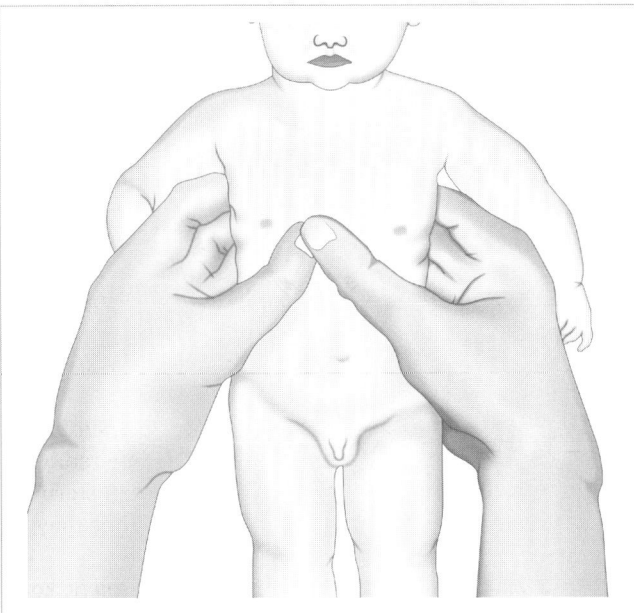

Fig. 26.1: Cardiac massage, two-thumbs, encircling hands technique: The neonate's trunk is held between the fingers and palms of both hands; from their anterior position, the thumbs exert pressure on the inferior third of the sternum

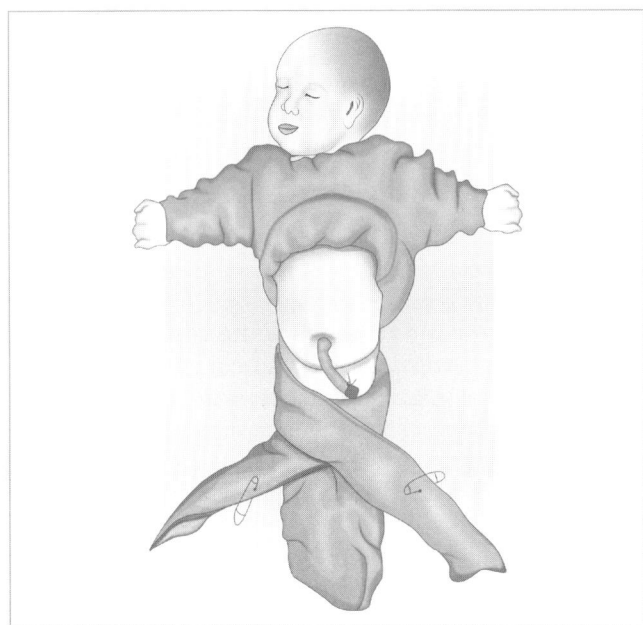

Fig. 26.2: Correct positioning of a newborn for catheterisation of the umbilical cord

The following equipment will be required:
- Peristaltic pump with discharge port (optional)
- Bottle of Ringer's or Hartmann's solution with infusion set
- 5 ml syringe filled with isotonic saline connected to:
  - Umbilical vein catheter, (not always available, but can be replaced by a nasogastric tube, as used in newborn nutrition N° 5–6; diameter 3.5 or 5F), applied to which, at 8–10 cm from the end, is a sleeve of adhesive plaster, 1 centimetre in height
  - A round of suture material N° 1 or 2
  - Sterile cloth with central opening, or alternatively a sterile glove wrapping liner, with a slot cut in its middle
  - Tincture of iodine
  - Scalpel blade
  - Small surgical pliers.

Method: The steps are as follows:
- Immobilisation of the newborn as in Figure 26.2
- Disinfection, using tincture of iodine, of the periumbilical skin and the distal part of the umbilical cord, which is passed through the slot in the sterile cloth or glove wrapping liner, and held in tension.
- Using chromic catgut or absorbable suture material (1 0 2), a ligature is applied to the base of the umbilical cord; the knot is made in two throws; the knot is tightened only lightly
- Segmental *resection of the umbilical cord* at a maximum distance of 2 cm from the skin, to avoid unnecessary convolutions; the cut should preferably be made at a bevel (Fig. 26.3) to increase the cut surface and thus, the visibility of the vessels.

Now one proceeds to
- *Catheterisation of the umbilical vein* (Fig. 26.4). If resection is made at the recommended distance of 2 cm, the umbilical vein should be located at 12 o'clock.

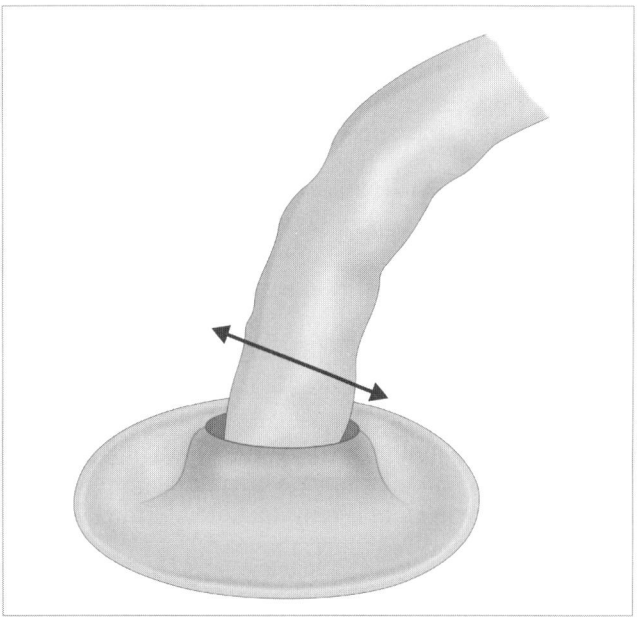

Fig. 26.3: Resection of the umbilical cord at approx. 1–2 cm from its insertion: The lower the gestational age, the greater the obliqueness of cut required to facilitate visualisation of the vessels

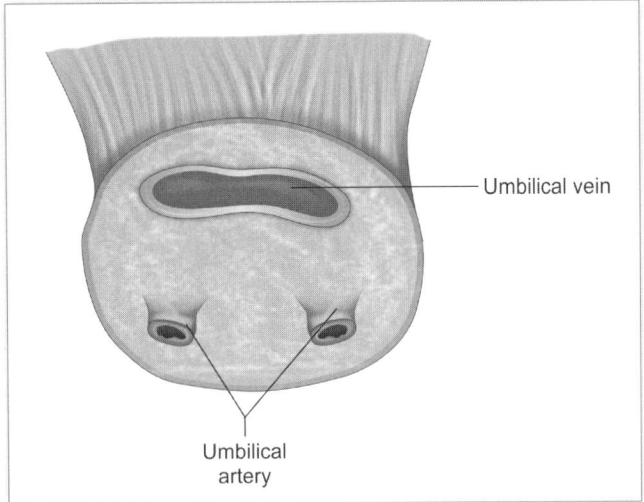

Fig. 26.4: When the cut is made 2 cm from the base, the vein is located at 12 o'clock (cranially) and appears wide, soft, gaping and fine-walled

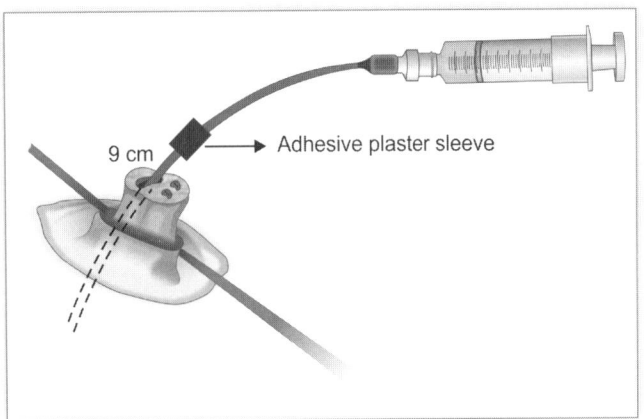

Fig. 26.5: Umbilical catheter with sleeve of adhesive plaster: The anchor sleeve is applied at a distance of 9 cm before introducing the catheter. It serves as a marker for assessing correct positioning of the tube. A stabilising suture is tied to this

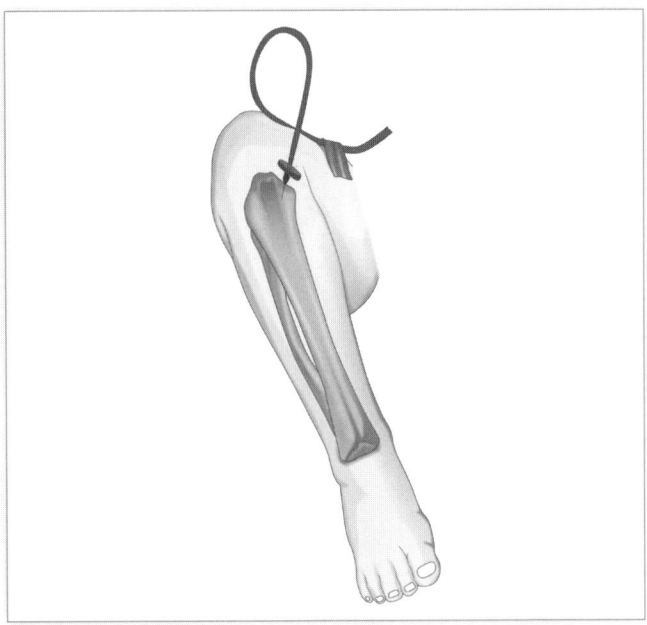

Fig. 26.6: Osseous venous access

The vein can be identified by its greater calibre and the thinness of its walls. On entering the abdomen, the umbilical vein soon directs cranially; this is the direction in which the catheter should be directed, up to a distance of 8–10 cm, where the ligature is attached to the adhesive plaster sleeve. Having introduced the catheter to a depth of 8–10 cm, aspiration on the syringe will confirm blood flow (Fig. 26.5). The knot is tightened and a second throw applied. The ligature is now anchored to the adhesive plaster sleeve, as described above.

If need be, the catheter may be connected to a manometer (Abbot and Pharmaseal), which is zeroed at the level of the mid-axillary line. This will give us an expression of central venous pressure, which can be used to guide infusion therapy.

When the umbilical vein or other direct venous access is not feasible, intraosseous access (Fig. 26.6) can be used as an alternative route for administering medication or fluids.

Arterial catheterisation lies beyond the scope of this work.

The risk should be borne in mind that umbilical catheters may function as carriers of *neonatal necrotizing enterocolitis.*

Administration of Medication and Fluids

- *Medication*: Adrenaline is an adrenergic stimulant of alpha and beta-receptors; it is used in asystolia, when the heart rate remains below 60 bpm after 30 seconds of ventilation and commensurate cardiac massage. With cardiac arrest, the vascular constriction induced by alpha adrenergic stimulation is its most important function (Zaritsky 1984). This is because vasoconstriction increases perfusion pressure during cardiac massage, thereby allowing oxygen to be given up to the heart and brain (Berkowitz 1991).

Other actions of adrenaline are to improve the heart's contractile power, stimulate spontaneous contractions and increase the heart rate.

Adrenaline is administered intravenously at a dosage of 0.01–0.03 mg/kg (0.1–0.3 ml/kg of a 1:10,000 solution). Doses can be repeated every 3–5 minutes, as required. Higher doses are not recommended. In animal experiments, the administration of higher doses was followed by reduced cardiac output, (Burchfield DJ, 1993; Berg et al., 1996). Furthermore, according to JF Pasternak (1983), hypotension followed by hypertension can lead to a risk of cerebral haemorrhage, especially among preterm babies.

- *Fluids*: Hypovolaemia should always be suspected in a newborn who fails to respond to resuscitation measures, particularly if there was blood loss on resection of the umbilical cord. Correction is effected by infusion of lactated Ringer's solution or of isotonic saline. The initial dose is 10 ml/kg, injected slowly over 5–10 minutes. This dose can be repeated after 10 minutes where adequate clinical assessment finds commensurate response to the infusion.

Some authors suggest higher doses, but the circulatory overload these may cause is not without complications, such as intracranial haemorrhage, which has been observed in both term and preterm neonates (Usher, 1965; Funato, 1992).

Albumin solutions to correct hypovolaemia are often unavailable, and are not indicated, due to the risk of infectious diseases and because they have been associated with an increase in mortality (Cochrane Injuries Group Albumin Reviewers, 1998).

The administration of O Rh negative blood may be indicated later, to replenish large-scale blood loss.

The administration of bicarbonate during neonatal resuscitation is still controversial and is currently contraindicated, because the hyperosmolarity and CO_2 release that result from its use may prove harmful to the functioning of the myocardium and nervous system (Papile et al., 1978; Kette et al., 1990; Kette et al. 1991).

AMNIOTIC FLUID STAINED WITH MECONIUM

According to (Wiswell, 1990) meconium is observed in the amniotic fluid in 12% of deliveries. When a delivery is accomplished vaginally, aspiration of the nose, mouth and oropharynx using a 12–14 (French) catheter (Locus, 1990) before expulsion of the trunk, considerably reduces the frequency of MAS (Carson, 1976).

The removal of meconium from the airways should precede any other form of assistance; this does not apply if the newborn is crying energetically, as endotracheal aspiration would then not be without complications (Linder, 1998; Wiswell, 2000) and long-term outcomes are not favourable. However, in a considerable number of cases (20–30%) meconium is observed in the trachea without respiratory acts. This finding is compatible with meconium aspiration during intrauterine life (Falciglia, 1988; Rossi, 1989), and confirms the advisability of endotracheal aspiration for all neonates with respiratory depression. If, at birth, the amniotic fluid contains meconium, breathing is absent, muscle tone reduced and the heart rate is below 100 bpm, pharyngeal aspiration of meconium followed by tracheal intubation under guidance of a laryngoscope should be performed immediately.

After intubation, aspiration through a second tube inserted into the endotracheal tube is not very effective due to the density and viscosity of meconium. It is recommended instead to apply suction a few times directly to the endotracheal tube—whose calibre will allow more effective aspiration. The tube is then removed, washed and replaced.

This measure is to be repeated until the residue of meconium is very small or absent (Wiswell, 1993; Greenough, 1995), or until heart rate indicates that resuscitation measures must proceed without delay. If the heart rate or respiration is strongly depressed, positive pressure ventilation should be implemented, even if residues of meconium- stained amniotic fluid remain, immediate expansion of the alveoli is necessary, using the method described above.

Gastric aspiration should be postponed until after initial resuscitation is complete, to avoid inspiration of meconium.

Assistance to the Newborn Delivered Vaginally in Breech Presentation

See the following section.

Assistance to the Newborn Delivered by Caesarean Section

An advisable precautionary measure is to conduct neonatal resuscitation within easy reach of the operating room.

In case of necessity, the obstetrician will be able to intervene rapidly, and ensure that no ill-advised resuscitation measures are performed.

Distinct stages may be identified in neonatal assessment and treatment.

Intraoperative steps, which conclude with detachment of the neonate from the mother.
- During amniotomy, the operator will assess the characteristics of the amniotic fluid, whether it is clear, meconium- stained, purulent, foul smelling, etc.
- Once extracted, the foetus is held by the feet at a level below that of the bed, enabling gravity to promote:
  a. *Drainage* of fluid and secretions from the upper airways and from the oropharyngeal spaces. This manoeuvre is to be completed *before the first respiratory act* with gentle clearing of the mouth and pharynx using gauze (assisted by suction where necessary).

If the amniotic fluid is clear, even where large volumes are present, aspiration is not necessary. Amniotic fluid is normally in contact with the tracheobronchial tree and will cause no damage if inhaled. Aspiration is indicated where the fluid has pathological characteristics.

If clearing is incomplete and the amniotic fluid is very liquid and only slightly stained with meconium, oropharyngeal and gastric aspiration is indicated, but only briefly, to avoid overstimulation of the vagus nerve. Cleansing is followed by compression of the foetal thorax against that of the surgeon clearing in imitation of the pressure normally encountered during progress through the birth canal.

b. *Blood flow from the placenta* to the foetus: We refer the reader to the section on assistance to the newborn during delivery.

At this point, the foetus is detached from the mother and assessment and assistance of the newborn is initiated, passing through the steps described in the opening sections of this chapter. Here one should bear in mind the different forms of assistance implemented for the vaginally delivered newborn, which depend on whether or not the amniotic fluid is stained by meconium.

Assessment, Diagnostic Score

Treatment

a. Antibiotic therapy: The septic risk scoring system (Table 26.2) will guide identification of cases in which antibiotic therapy should be instituted. A point score of ≥3 indicates that antibiotic therapy should be initiated.

b. *Convulsions due to hypoxic-ischemic encephalopathy:* Convulsions frequently appear following resuscitation manoeuvres. Where a paediatrician specialising in neonatology is unavailable, the most commonly used protocols for controlling convulsions are as follows:
   - *Diazepam 0.1–0.3 mg/kg* given rectally; repeat the dose after 20 minutes if the convulsions have not been brought under control; if they persist even after a second dosage, move on to phenobarbital
   - *Phenobarbital, 10 mg/kg IM*: Repeat the dose after 1 hour; then 5 mg per day orally for 5 days.

c. *Clinical Assessment*:
   - Apgar score
   - Neurobehavioural score: After delivery, the newborn presents one hour of wakefulness followed by a period of 3–4 hours of deep sleep and decreased response to stimuli; variations in the score reflect reductions in the period of wakefulness and in muscle tone.

Complications

In the course of particularly difficult deliveries, fractures of the clavicle, humerus or of the femur may occur. No treatment is required; these will heal on their own in a very short time.

BIBLIOGRAPHY

1. Berg RA, Otto CW, Kern KB, Hilwig RW, Sanders AB, Henry CP, Ewy GA. A randomized, blinded trial of high-dose epinephrine versus standard-dose epinephrine in a swine model of paediatric asphyxial cardiac arrest. Crit Care Med. 1996;24:1695-1700.
2. Berkowitz ID, Gervais H, Schleien CL, Koehler RC, Dean JM, Traystman RJ. Epinephrine dosage effects on cerebral and myocardial blood flow in an infant swine model of cardiopulmonary resuscitation. Anesthesiology. 1991;75:1041-50.
3. Borell N, Elmstroem I. The shape of the foetal chest during its passage through the birth canal. A Radiographic study. Acta Obst Gynaec Scand. 1962;41:213.
4. Burchfield DJ, Preziosi MP, Lucas VW, Fan J. Effect of graded doses of epinephrine during asphyxia-induced bradycardia in newborn lambs. Resuscitation. 1993;25:235-44.
5. Carson BS, Losey RW, Bowes WA Jr, Simmons MA. Combined obstetric and paediatric approach to prevent meconium aspiration syndrome. Am J Obstet Gynecol. 1976;126:712-5.
6. Cochrane Injuries Group Albumin Reviewers. Human albumin administration in critically ill patients: systematic review of randomized controlled trials. BMJ. 1998;317:235-40.
7. David R. Closed chest cardiac massage in the newborn infant. Pediatrics. 1988;81:552-4.
8. Dawes GF. Fetaland Neonatal Physiology: A Comparative Study of the Changes at Birth. Year Book Medical Publishers; 1968. pp. 149-51.
9. Dean JM, Koehler RC, Schleien CL, Berkowitz I, Michael JR, Atchison D, Rogers MC, Traystman RJ. Age-related effects of compression rate and duration in cardiopulmonary resuscitation. J Appl Physiol. 1990;68:554-60.
10. Estol PC, Piriz H, Basalo S, Simini F, Grela C. Oro-naso-pharyngeal suction at birth: effects on respiratory

Table 26.2

Septic risk scoring system

	0	1	2	Index
Duration of ROM*	<12 h	12–24 h	>24 h	
Maternal temp.	36.7–37.2	37.2–37.8	>37.8	
Apgar score at 5'	8–10	5–7	<5	
Appearance of AF	Clear	Stained with meconium or blood	Purulent or foul smelling	
Weight of foetus	>2500	1500–2500	<1500	

* ROM rupture of membranes

adaptation of normal term vaginally born infants. J Perinatal Med. 1992;20:297-305.
11. Falciglia HS. Failure to prevent meconium aspiration syndrome. Obstet Gynecol. 1988;71:349-53.
12. Funato M, Tamai H, Noma K. Clinical events in association with timing of intraventricular haemorrhage in preterm infants. J Pediatr. 1992;121:614-9.
13. Gandy GM, Adamson SK Jr, Cunningham N, Silverman WA, James LS. Thermal environment and acid-base homeostasis in human infants during the first few hours of life. J Clin Invest. 1964;43:751-8.
14. Greenough A. Meconium aspiration syndrome: prevention and treatment. Early Hum Dev. 1995;41:183-92.
15. Houri PK, Frank LR, Menegazzi JJ, Taylor R. A randomized, controlled trial of two-thumb vs. two-finger chest compression in a swine infant model of cardiac arrest. Prehosp Emerg Care. 1997;1:65-7.
16. International Guidelines for Neonatal Resuscitation: An Excerpt From the Guidelines 2000 for Cardiopulmonary Resuscitation and Emergency Cardiovascular. Pediatrics 2000;106(3):29.
17. Kette F, Weil MH, Gazmuri RJ. Buffer solutions may compromise cardiac resuscitation by reducing coronary perfusion pressure. JAMA. 1991;266:2121-6.
18. Kette F, Weil MH, von Planta M, Gazmuri RJ, Rackow EC. Buffer agents do not reverse intramyocardial acidosis during cardiac resuscitation. Circulation. 1990;81:1660-6.
19. Linder N, Aranda JV, Tsur M. Need for endotracheal intubation and suction in meconium-stained neonates. J Pediatr. 1988;112:613-5.
20. Locus P, Yeomans E, Crosby U. Efficacy of bulb versus DeLee suction at deliveries complicated by meconium stained amniotic fluid. Am J Perinatol. 1990;7:87-91.
21. Menegazzi JJ, Auble TE, Nicklas KA, Hosack GM, Rack L, Goode JS. Two-thumb versus two-finger chest compression during CPR in a swine infant model of cardiac arrest. Ann Emerg Med. 1993;22:240-3.
22. Orlowski JP. Optimum position for external cardiac compression in infants and young children. Ann Emerg Med. 1986;15:667-73.
23. Palme-Kilander C. Methods of resuscitation in low-Apgar-score newborn infants: a national survey. Acta Paediatr. 1992;81:739-44.
24. Papile LA, Burstein J, Burstein R, Koffler H, Koops B. Relationship of intravenous sodium bicarbonate infusions and cerebral intraventricular haemorrhage. J Pediatr. 1978;93:834-6.
25. Palme C, Nystrom B, Tunell R. An evaluation of the efficiency of face masks in the resuscitation of newborn infants. Lancet. 1985;1:207-10.
26. Parer JT, King TL. Electronic foetal monitoring and diagnosis of foetal asphyxia. In: Hughes SC, Levinson G, Rosen MA (Eds). Schnider and Levinson's Anaesthesia for Obstetrics. Lippincott Williams and Wilkins; 2002. p. 634.
27. Pasternak JF, Groothuis DR, Fischer JM, Fischer DP. Regional cerebral blood flow in the beagle puppy model of neonatal intraventricular haemorrhage: studies during systemic hypertension. Neurology. 1983;33:559-66.
28. Phillips GW, Zideman DA. Relation of infant heart to sternum: its significance in cardiopulmonary resuscitation. Lancet. 1986;1:1024-5.
29. Rossi EM, Philipson EH, Williams TG, Kalhan SC. Meconium aspiration syndrome: intrapartum and neonatal attributes. Am J Obstet Gynecol. 1989;161:1106-10.
30. Saugstad OD. Practical aspects of resuscitating asphyxiated newborn infants. Eur J Pediatr. 1998;157:S11-5.
31. Thaler MM, Stobie GHC. An improved technic of external cardiac compression in infants and young children. N Engl J Med. 1963;269:606-10.
32. Theophilopoulos DT, Burchfield DJ. Accuracy of different methods for heart rate determination during simulated neonatal resuscitations. J Perinatol. 1998;18:65-7.
33. Todres ID, Rogers MC. Methods of external cardiac massage in the newborn infant. J Pediatr. 1975;86:781-2.
34. Usher R, Lind J. Blood volume of the newborn premature infant. Acta Paediatr Scand. 1965;54:419-31.
35. Wiswell TE, Bent RC. Meconium staining and the meconium aspiration syndrome: unresolved issues. Pediatr Clin North Am. 1993;40:955-81.
36. Wiswell TE, Tuggle JM, Turner BS. Meconium aspiration syndrome: have we made a difference? Pediatrics. 1990; 85:715-21.
37. Wiswell TE. Meconium in the Delivery Room Trial Group: delivery room management of the apparently vigorous meconium-stained neonate: results of the multicenter collaborative trial. Pediatrics. 2000;105:1-7.
38. World Health Report. Geneva, Switzerland: World Health Organization; 1995.
39. Zaritsky A, Chernow B. Use of catecholamines in pediatrics. J Pediatr. 1984;105:341-50.

SECTION 4

Alternatives to Caesarean Section

- Version—Breech Presentation, Transverse and Oblique Lies
- Symphysiotomy–Vacuum Extraction (Foetus Alive–Head Engaged)
- Destructive Operations—A Vanishing Art in Modern Obstetrics (P Sikka, 2011)

CHAPTER 27

Version—Breech Presentation, Transverse and Oblique Lies

Version is an obstetric manoeuvre performed during pregnancy or labour by which a foetal unfavourable position, with reference to the mother, is changed to a more favourable one for delivery.

Version refers to corrective manoeuvres for three different clinical conditions each of which requires manoeuvres suited to gestation age and complexity:
- Breech presentation—longitudinal lie
- Transverse (shoulder) presentation—transverse lie
- Oblique lie.

Version can take place by *external manipulation* or by *combined external and internal manipulation*.

The *version* is termed *cephalic* or *podalic*, according to the pole of the foetus that is brought into presentation:
- *External cephalic version* employs external manipulation to convert breech presentation to a vertex
- *Internal combined podalic version* employs intrauterine manipulation with assistance by the external hand to convert a cephalic transverse presentation to a breech.

BREECH PRESENTATION

Longitudinal lie

Breech presentation refers to a longitudinal lie in which a foetal part caudal to its iliac crest plane is the presenting part, its incidence at term is approximately 4% (Cruikshank 1986).

Aetiology

Premature delivery: The foetus is breech presenting more frequently during the fifth and sixth months of gestation. Spontaneous *physiological cephalic version* generally occurs around the seventh month. This means that breech presentations will increase in frequency the earlier labour sets in.

The forces involved in physiological version are the hydrostatic thrust of the breech (the minor force) and gravity acting on the heavier cephalic pole.

Opposing these forces is resistance (friction) of the uterine walls:
- *Changes in the weight ratio between head and trunk*: These include hydrocephaly, anencephaly and tumours at the caudal end of the trunk that keep the now lighter cephalic pole at the fundus
- *Increased foetal motility,* as is observed with polyhydramnios or in a hypotonic multiparous uterus
- *Obstruction of normal foetal motility*, as is observed with oligoidramnios, bicornuate or supseptate uterus, placenta previa or in the presence of entanglement of the umbilical cord
- *Contracted pelvis*, which should always be suspected, particularly in primigravida; about half of all breech presentations occur with them
- *Multiple pregnancy*
- *In most cases, the aetiology is unclear.*

When compared with cephalic presentation, breech presentation represents an increased risk for the foetus as it is associated with a higher incidence of:
- *Premature rupture of membranes*, with the danger of ascending infections
- *Uncoordinated uterine contractions* resulting in prolonged labour
- *Compression of the umbilical cord* during the first and second stage
- *Prolapse of a foot, hand or of the umbilical cord*
- *Urge* in the mother *to push too early*
- *Operative obstetric delivery* (forceps on posterior head, symphysiotomy)
- *Moulding of the head,* not progressive as it occurs in cephalic presentation, this leads on vaginal delivery to a sudden increase and decrease of intracranial pressure with risk of cerebral haemorrhage:
  - *Vaginal and pelvic floor trauma*
  - *Birth asphyxia*
  - *Increased perinatal morbidity and mortality.*

In 2000, after a critical review and statistical analysis of a substantial number of publications on methods for expediting delivery in breech presentation (complete and frank breech), the International Term Breech Collaborative Group (Hannah et al.) concluded that "a planned caesarean delivery is a substantially better method of delivery for the foetus" and that the orientation towards of delivery of a single foetus by the vaginal route in cases of breech presentation should no longer be encouraged. In this they endorsed a 20-year-long trend in which the incidence of C-sections for breech presentation had grown from 14% in 1970 to the current rate of almost 100% (Stafford, 1990). In the United States, breech presentation represents the third major indication for C-section after prior C-section and cervical dystocia (Galay et al., 1994).

The only other alternative to C-section as a method of accomplishing delivery from breech presentation is *external cephalic version*. This was little used before 1975, when a publication by Saling highlighted the efficacy of tocolysis in aiding the manoeuvre. Since then, there has been a growing consensus in favour of version, due to its high percentage of success, the safety of the manoeuvre (see below), and (which should be added) to the avoidance of the adverse effects linked to caesarean section (Lede, 2006). Elective recourse to version has reduced the number of C-section indications for breech presentation by two thirds (Zhang et al., 1993; Hofmeyr et al., 2007).

ECV is a valuable management technique and, in a properly selected population, poses little risk to either the woman or the foetus. If successful, ECV provides a clear benefit to the woman by allowing her an opportunity for a successful vertex vaginal delivery» (Frellick, ACOG, 2016).

We distinguish two forms of version:
- External version
- *Version by postural management.*

External Version

- *Indications*: Breech presentation of a single foetus with intact membranes, gestational age between the 34th and 40th week of pregnancy
- *Contraindications*: These are subdivided into *absolute* and *relative*:
  - *Absolute contraindications*: Maternal cardiac pathology, third-trimester gestosis, placenta previa, third-trimester haemorrhage, anhydramnios and oligohydramnios, premature rupture of membranes, ultrasound-confirmed umbilical cord loops, intrauterine growth retardation, nonreassuring cardiotocography, foetal distress, foetal abnormalities, uterine malformation, withheld consent, pelvic anomaly, indication for C-section, multiple pregnancy
  - *Relative contraindications*: Prior C-section, hypertension, obesity, anomalies of foetal growth.

Conditions

- Adequate pelvis
- The abdominal wall must be sufficiently thin and tractable to permit an accurate diagnosis
- Mobility of the whole of the foetus; the presenting part must not be deeply engaged; the membranes must be intact or just recently ruptured and in the latter case no prolapsed limb should be present
- Predictive factors for successful *external* version: A recent critical review (Kok M, 2008) in which 53 articles and 10,149 gravidae were analysed, identified the following predictive factors for successful external version: Multiparity, maternal weight below 65 kg, relaxed uterus, membranes intact or only recently ruptured, breech not engaged and head clearly detectable. Gestational age and Fundal height had no predictive value
- Gestational age: As pregnancy progresses, the volume ratio between the uterine cavity and foetus changes in favour of the foetus. It is therefore clear that the earlier the version is conducted, the greater the chances of its success. Indeed, the statistical data suggest an 80% success rate in early pregnancy. However, the drawbacks of performing this manoeuvre at an early stage should complications arise, consist in reversion to the initial lie (16%) and iatrogenic prematurity
- Timing of ECV.

The universal consensus is that external version should preferably take place towards the 36–37th week (69.5%

success rate, with 7% reversion to breech presentation), a gestational age justified by the fact that premature rupture of membranes and preterm labour are more common in breech presentations. This choice of gestational age is currently undergoing critical review, with an earlier attempt at version in the 34–35th week (Kornman et al., 1995; Hutton et al., 2007), where success rates have been found to be higher, iatrogenic prematurity less severe and more time available to repeat the corrective manoeuvre (one week later) should the foetus spontaneously revert. A 9.5% reduction has been recorded in non-cephalic presentations at delivery, with a 7% reduction in C-sections. One current orientation is that attempts at version can and should be made even after the 36–37th week, and consideration given to attempts at version up to when labour is in progress, where the membranes are intact (Schifrin BS, 1985; Stine et al., 1985; Hofmeyr, 2007).

A recent series of studies demonstrates that when labour is arrested by the use of tocolytic medication, version is still possible with a high success rate. When vaginal breech delivery is unadvisable, the manoeuvre should be conducted in the operating room to facilitate a C-section if external manipulation does not meet with success.

Safety of the Mother

This aspect of external version has been investigated by Zhang et al. (1993) and by Hofmeyr and Kulier (2007). Although the data available from the literature did not suffice for quantification of maternal complications, they would appear to be rare.

Safety of the Foetus

Zhang et al. (1993) also investigated this aspect of version: Risks to the foetus of stretching or compression of the umbilical cord, placental abruption, rupture of membranes and of preterm delivery are minimal, with complications at 1–2%. Another study, (Phelan et al., 1984), analysed variations in FHR. These were found to be present in 39% of cases, but were transitory in character and had no impact on the eventual outcome. Four foetal deaths were reported before 1980 (Phelan et al., 1984); these followed version manoeuvres conducted under general anaesthesia. Since this period, the literature has reported two further foetal deaths (Hofmeyr, 1983), which occurred in Zimbabwe, when the manoeuvre was carried out on preterm foeti without monitoring foetal cardiac activity, and without verification by ultrasound.

Method

Preliminary steps:
- *The abdominal wall* must be sufficiently thin and tractable to permit an accurate diagnosis
- *Mobility of the whole foetus:* The presenting part must not be deeply engaged; the membranes must be intact or just recently ruptured, and if ruptured, no prolapsed or leading limb should be present
- *Preoperative examinations and possibility of rapid access to operating room*: When labour is under way and the possibility of delivery by the vaginal route is excluded, the manoeuvre should be conducted under tocolysis in the operating room;
  - *Ultrasonography to rule out umbilical cord loops about the neck* or the presence of placenta previa
  - *Non stress test*: The cardiotocogram (CTG) should show a reactive test result.
    Ultrasonography and cardiotocography are not always available in low-resourced countries
  - *Access to the cardiocirculatory system via a venous catheter*:
    » The *fractionated dose administration of a tocolytic* (Orciprenaline, Terbutaline, Isoxsuprine, Ritodrine) *must always precede, as far as possible, external version* (Hofmeyr GJ; Gyte G, 2007). If the maternal heart rate exceeds 120 beats/minute, administration of the medication is stopped
    » *The manoeuvre should not be conducted under anaesthesia* as this would not allow early warning of the threat of uterine rupture, or detection of actual uterine rupture
    » The *patient's trunk is turned 30–45°* onto the side on which the foetal back is located
    » *A slight Trendelenburg position would be ideal.*

The manoeuvre consists of the following steps (Ranney B, 1973).

a. *Extraction of the breech from the maternal pelvis*: This may be carried out transvaginally (we strongly advise against this) or by abdominal manipulation, which we describe here
   - The abdominal wall is covered in talcum; other authors suggest ultrasound gel (not recommended)
   - The operator stands on the side of the patient on which the foetal back is located, turns side-on to the patient, sinks eight fingers into the pelvis and extracts the breech. The operator sits down and holds one hand on the breech in this position for some moments.

b. *Direction of rotation*: The question now arises, in which direction to turn the foetus over; the general rule is "*the foetus is rotated face downwards to maintain flexion*". Version should always take place with the foetal face in a caudal direction, to maintain flexion and thereby reduce the volume of the rotating body.

c. *Rotation and compression of the foetal poles* (Fig. 27.1): Having established the direction of rotation, the hand on the breech initiates the rotation while simultaneously exerting compression, which is accompanied by similar

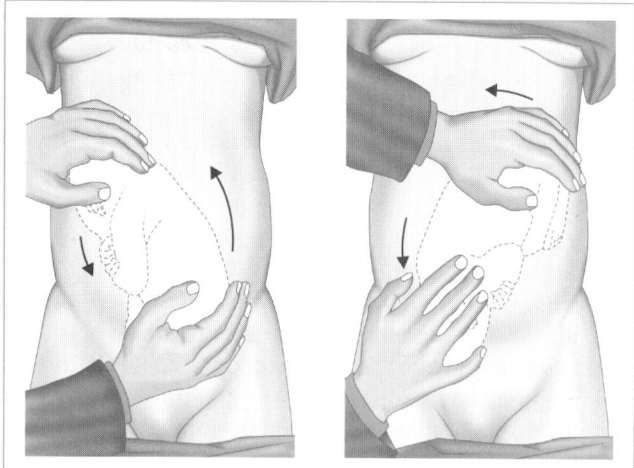

Fig. 27.1: Breech presentation—external version: Rotation is effected keeping the face always directed caudally, in order to maintain flexion of the trunk

   pressure exerted by the other hand on the cephalic pole. The purpose is to keep the head and trunk flexed, thereby facilitating the manoeuvre.
d. *At the slightest obstacle, discontinue the manoeuvre*, allow a few moments to pass, and then substitute the rotatory movement with one of oscillation (to and fro). Very often, this will overcome an obstacle incurred by a uterine contraction.
e. *Measure foetal heart activity* every 2 minutes.
f. *Manipulation must not last more than 5 minutes*, after which it is followed by a period of rest.
g. Following the manoeuvre, the FHR pattern will show poor reactivity for 15 minutes, but then recovers afterwards.

If the manoeuvre proves unsuccessful, therapeutic decubitus is used: This consists in having the mother lie on the side opposite that of the foetal back. In this way, the uterine fundus will sink down under the effect of gravity, and with it the head. Now version, still keeping the foetus facing in a caudal direction, will be greatly facilitated.

Stabilisation: In the past, after the desired lie or presentation had been attained, the foetal position was stabilized by means of:
- Applying bandages: Folded sheets were applied between the side previously occupied by the presenting part and the side onto which the foetal head has been deviated.
- Amniotomy, in order to promote engagement of the presenting part and to induce labour. We have reservations about this procedure because, if the head does not remain in the desired position, and if there is prolapse of the umbilical cord on amniotomy; there will be no further chance of using combined version, which requires full cervical dilatation.

We adopt the orientation indicated by Bergstrom (1992), which is to make no use of stabilising procedures, but to ask the mother to retain the therapeutic decubitus position (i.e. to lie on the side on which the foetal back is located). The mother is also instructed in how to maintain the new foetal lie, and is requested to visit the obstetric out-patient department on a weekly basis for monitoring.

Delivery Following External Version

Progress of labour following external version has been studied by Lau et al. (1997), who found an incidence of 16.9% for caesarean sections during labour due to foetal distress and uterine dystocia (dynamic and cervical) in the cephalic presentation group that had undergone external version. This was 2.5% higher than incidence in the control group.

Version by Postural Management

There is a current of thought (Elkin, 1982) which maintains that the adoption by the mother of specific positions (therapeutic decubitus) could promote or induce version; the positions cited are:
- The knee-chest or *genupectoral position* (Fig. 27.2), to be adopted for 15 minutes, every two hours, during the daytime for 5 days (Elkin's original protocol)
- The *genupectoral position* (Fig. 27.2), to be adopted for 10 minutes, three times per day, starting from the 34th week (Elkin's protocol modified)
- The *supine position* with the pelvis raised by a pillow (30 minutes, twice a day).

The efficacy of postural management in correcting breech presentation has been subjected to a critical review (Smith et al., 1999; Foulds, 2005; Hofmeyr et al., 2007). There are very few cases in the literature, most of which are anecdotal, and reliable conclusions cannot be drawn. Although Elkin's protocol may not facilitate version, it does

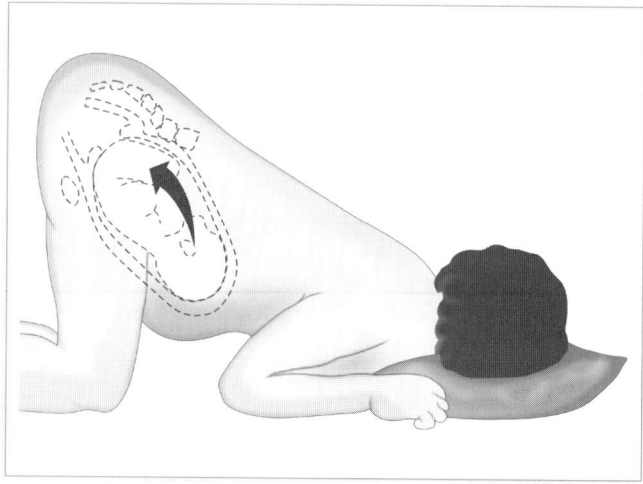

Fig. 27.2: Version by postural management

have beneficial effects on maternal psychological well-being, for which reason it should be recommended to all gravidae.

The Authors' View

We have reported the proposed protocols: The equipment listed is rarely available in peripheral hospitals in countries with limited resources, where sometimes no more than our hands, a stethoscope and a bed is available; but these will prove more than sufficient for conducting external version if the manoeuvre is preceded by careful clinical assessment of the gravid patient, of the uterus and pelvis, and is accompanied by careful auscultation of the foetal heartbeat during manipulation. In this we find comfort in the words of Lede (2006), who states that "External cephalic version (ECV) does not require very special conditions for its successful implementation; an examination table and a stethoscope are adequate".

Hofmeyr (2007) has tackled the problem of how to proceed under resource-poor conditions and concludes (and we agree) that in countries with limited resources, the priority is the mother's life, not that of the foetus. It is the mother who works the fields, carries water, gathers firewood, cooks for the children and feeds them. If she dies, the children will die.

All of the assembled statistical data agrees that, during external version, there is a (minimal) risk for the foetus, not for the mother. This contrasts sharply with the risks to the mother's life and well-being from a breech delivery with complications conducted in her village or in an outlying medical centre.

For this reason, we carry out external version as soon as the case comes to our attention (Kornman et al., 1995). This is often because, due to the long distances involved and safety considerations, it is not always possible for pregnant women to attend our out-patient obstetric clinic at the scheduled gestational stage.

TRANSVERSE LIE

Shoulder presentation

A transverse lie may involve:
- A single foetus, membranes intact
- A second twin.

These distinct clinical situations require different therapeutic approaches:

Single Foetus

(membranes intact or just recently ruptured)

In the past version during pregnancy or labour (Phelan et al., 1985) aimed to a cephalic or possibly at a podalic presentation. The current orientation is to bring the foetal head into presentation by the shortest possible route, and rules out breech presentation as a goal. A breech delivery is not without hazards for both mother and foetus, particularly if the birth assistant is not a very experienced one.
- *Contraindications and enabling conditions* are those described above
- *Gestational age:* The authors' orientation is that described in view of breech presentation. We intervene at an early stage, allowing ourselves a time frame in which the manoeuvre may be repeated (at weekly intervals). This is not always possible if one is assisting a term pregnancy or where labour is under way (although the manoeuvre is still attempted).

Method: This is a very simple manoeuvre. Having identified the head, one hand is placed flat upon it, one on the breech, and compressive pressure is exerted on the foetal poles (to make the foetus more compact). At the same time, the version manoeuvre is initiated, pushing the head (face) in a caudad direction. There are two recommendations:
- Do not execute this manoeuvre under anaesthesia
- The manoeuvre may prove unsuccessful—take note of this and do not persevere.

Second Twin

The time available before the cervix closes again is just 10 minutes; therefore a timely version is required. Before undertaking any manoeuvre, it is good practice to ensure that dilatation is complete; this is done by introducing the hand into the cervix and opening it, if the cervix allows itself to be opened as far as the pelvic wall, dilatation is complete.

If the second twin is in cephalic presentation, whether it is a mono- or bi-amniotic twin, rupture of any intact membrane will facilitate engagement and timings may be accelerated by using vacuum extraction.

If the second twin is in traverse lie, whether it is a monoor bi-amniotic twin, where membranes are still intact, external version should be attempted before amniotomy.

Should external version prove unsuccessful, timeliness of the following manoeuvre is essential (Tchabo, Tabai, 1992). In the past the delivery of the second twin or single foetus (transverse lie) by *internal podalic version* was considered the method of choice, actually there is consensus that this procedure should be reserved in cases in which the head cannot be caused to engage immediately and in which C-section is not feasible. Anyhow internal podalic version is here, for the sake of completeness, described.

The operator stands before the patient in a lithotomy position and, without crossing arms, puts a hand (Fig. 27.3) on each foetal pole (right hand on the right pole and similarly for the left); the hand resting on the breech is the *internal hand*.

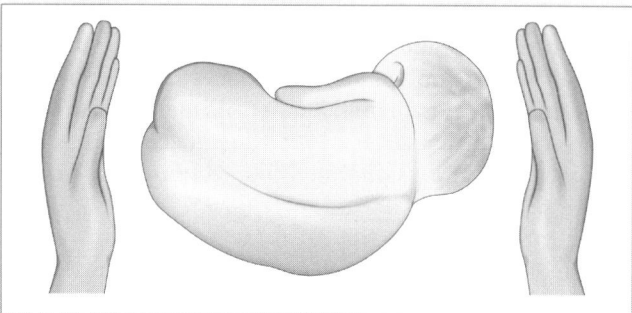

Fig. 27.3: Second twin—Left transverse lie: A left transverse lie that could not be corrected by external version. The operator, from in front of the patient, places one hand on each side of the abdomen; the hand on the foetal breech is the inside hand, which accesses the uterine cavity

Two manoeuvres are here described:
- First manoeuvre, consists of three steps:
  - *The first step: Converts the transverse lie into an oblique lie;* this is performed by combined action, pushing cranially, from the outside on the head and from the inside on the shoulders (Fig. 27.4)
- *Second step: Identify and grasp the limb or limbs on which traction will be exerted,* the following rule is applied:
  - In dorsoanterior presentation, traction is exerted on the inferior foot
  - In dorsoposterior presentation, traction is exerted on the superior foot or on both feet.

The reason for this is simple: The indicated foot is the most easily accessible one.

In dorsoposterior position, the manoeuvre is quite easy to perform. This is not the case with dorsoanterior lies, for which reason, proceed as follows: "the external hand presses the breech to bend the foetal trunk; this will allow the internal hand to insert itself between uterus and breech (Fig. 27.5). Sliding along the foetal thigh and leg, it will reach the foot (see Chapter 6 for differential identification of hand and foot).

Having identified and grasped a foot or feet, the foot or feet is/are lowered into the vagina and outside. Now follows the

- *Third step: Caudal traction and cranial push* (Fig. 27.6). Traction is exerted *not along the vaginal axis,* but obliquely to it.

If the cephalic pole is on the right, the operator moves to the right; if on the left, the operator stands on the left. Only in this way will it be possible for internal rotation to take place, which is achieved mainly through flexion of the foetal axis.

If all does not go to plan, we may try the following:
- Lowering the second foot. If traction has so far been exerted on one foot only, with the volume of one leg removed from the uterine cavity, may permit greater mobility of the foetal trunk
- *The Justine Siegemundin manoeuvre:* This author, now advanced in years, has carried out this manoeuvre once

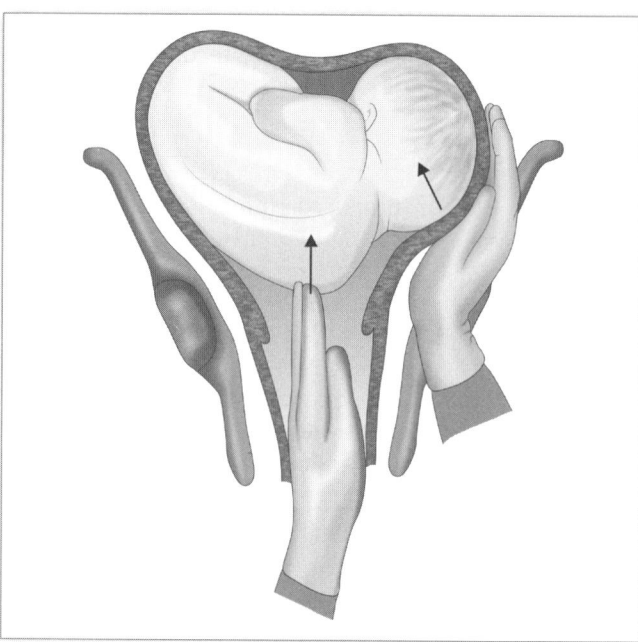

Fig. 27.4: First step: The left hand (with left traverse lie) accesses the uterine cavity and pushes the shoulders cranially; this is assisted by an external push in the same direction by the external hand acting on the head. This combined manoeuvre transforms the transverse lie into an oblique lie

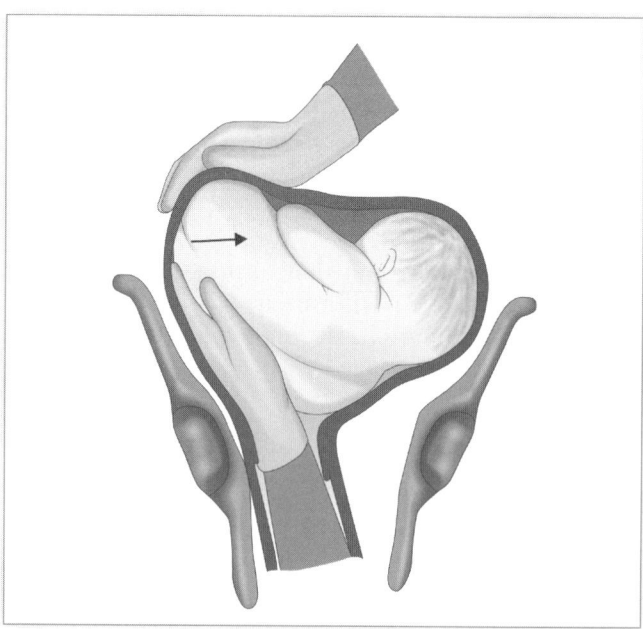

Fig. 27.5: Second step: The internal hand identifies and grasps the breech. The external hand increases foetal flexion to facilitate identification of the feet

only (and with success). It consists in applying to one foot a cord, which is held by the external hand (Fig. 27.7). Traction is exerted on the cord; counter-pressure is now exerted not externally, but internally by introducing the hand on the head-side into the vagina (Fig. 27.8).

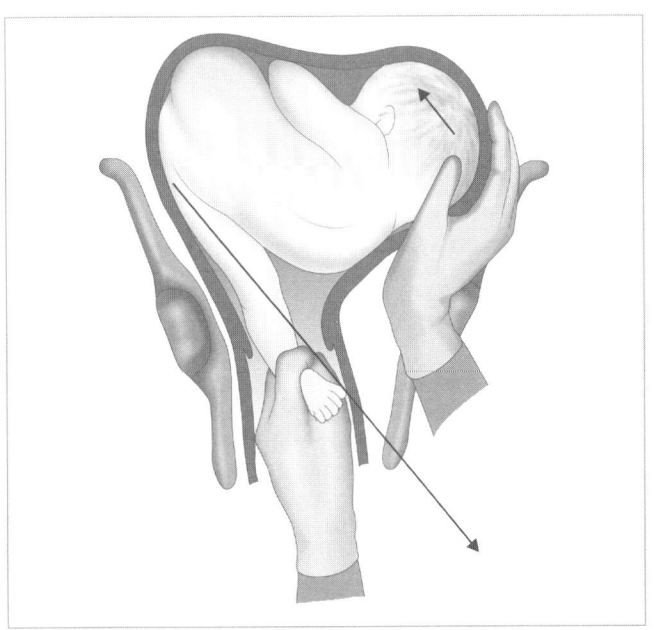

Fig. 27.6: Third step: The foot has been identified and grasped; the arrows indicate the direction in which traction/pushing should be exerted. Counter-pressure by the external hand is crucial in increasing the curvature of the foetal spine

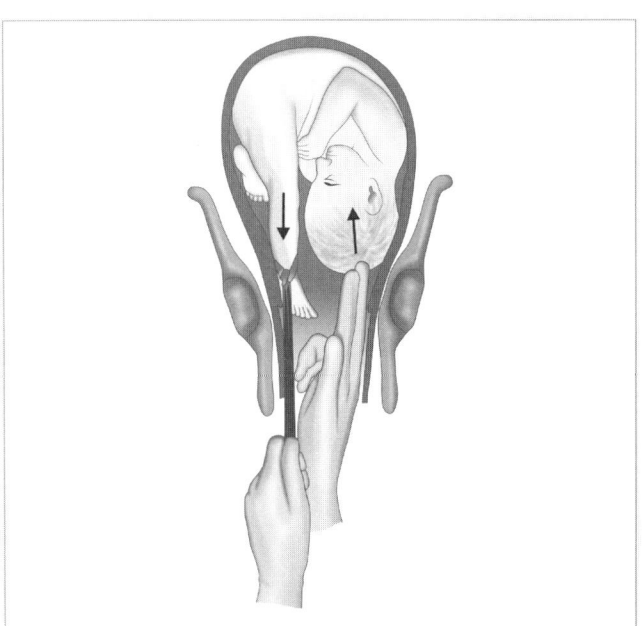

Fig. 27.8: The external hand exerts traction, while the internal hand, (the head-side hand is now internal), exerts counter-pressure on the foetal head from within

Method: Having identified the head, the hands are placed flat, one against each foetal pole. One hand impels the head in a caudal direction; the other hand imparts counter-pressure on the breech, acting in a cranial direction. Firm pressure is exerted on the two poles simultaneously in order to increase the curvature of the foetal spine, reduce the volume occupied by the foetus, and thus facilitate its movement of rotation.

Incision of the Cervix (the Duhrssen Incision)

Conditions may arise when life saving delivery is mandatory and the only obstacle to delivery is offered by the cervix, whose incision makes certain that the opening is adequate for delivery and accomplished within minutes and for more quickly than by C-section.

These conditions occur both in cephalic and breech presentation, where in case of a premature infant the incompletely dilated cervix accommodates the breech but not the larger unmolded head, which is trapped.

Conditions are:

In *vertex presentation, Duhrssen incisions* are safe only if the following condition is rigidly observed:
- The cervix must be partially effaced and dilated more than 6 cm
- The head must be engaged, accommodating only 1 finger above the brim or by vaginal examination at a station of no less than +3.

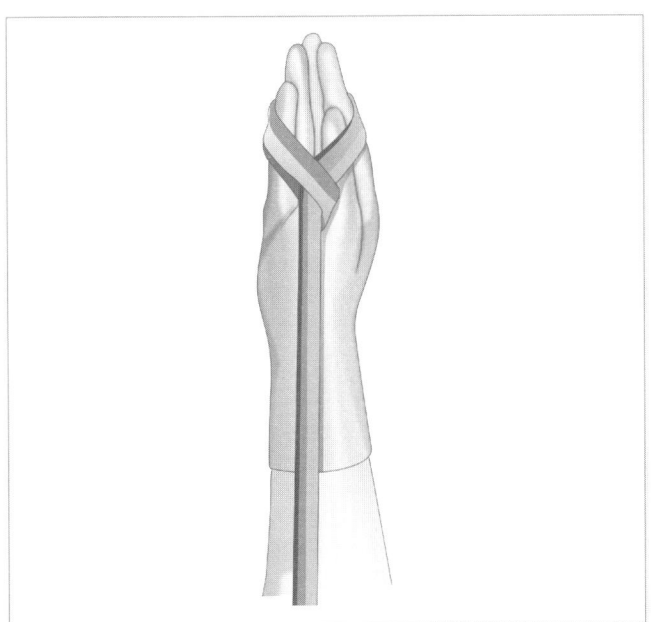

Fig. 27.7: Justine Siegemundin manoeuvre: The hand accessing the uterine cavity takes a cord with it, which is applied to the foot

Oblique Lie

Oblique lie is often associated with a pelvic anomaly, particularly among primigravidae. For this reason, any version manoeuvre must be preceded by careful assessment of the pelvis, and umbilical cord loops or placenta previa excluded.

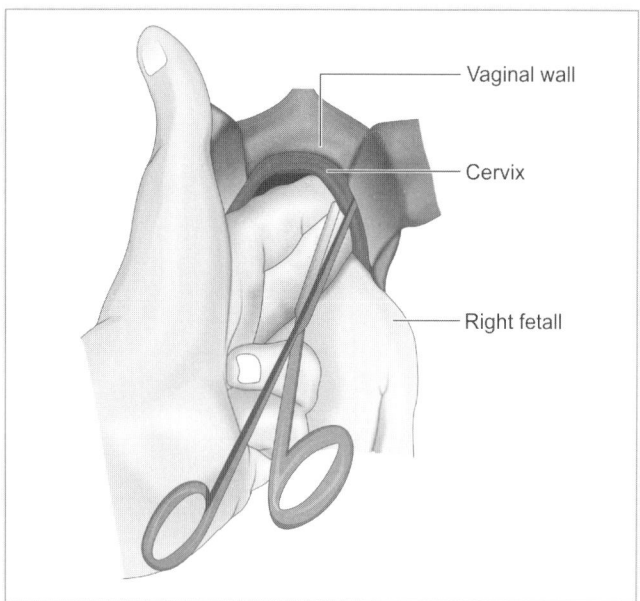

Fig. 27.9: Duhrssen incision

In *breech presentation* once the breech has been delivered the above conditions have already been met.

Procedure:

A middle finger is inserted into the cervix while the index is apposed and the external aspect; a bandage scissors is used, the blind incision should stop short of the vaginal reflection (Fig. 27.9).

In vertex presentation incision are made at 2. 6 and 10 o'clock, where the dilatation exceeds 6 cm, two incisions only will usually suffice: At 2, 6, or 3-9—at the site where spontaneous lacerations usually occur. *3 and 9 o'clock are too avoided* to prevent the upwards extension of the incision and tearing the uterine arteries.

In breech presentation only two incisions are possible.

BIBLIOGRAPHY

1. Bergstrom S. External cephalic version and daily post-versional maternal self-assessment of fetal presentation. A prospective study. Gynecol Obstet Invest. 1992;33:15-8.
2. Cruikshank DP. Breech presentation. Clin Obstet Gynecol. 1986;29:255-63.
3. Flamm BL, Fried MW, Lonky NM, Giles WS. External cephalic version after previous cesarean section. Am J Obstet Gynecol. 1991;165:370-2.
4. Founds S. Maternal Posture for Cephalic Version of Breech Presentation: A Review of the Evidence. Birth issues in perinatal care. 2005;32:137-44.
5. Frellick M. ACOG Issues Guidance on External Cephalic Version, February 03, 2016.
6. Gabay M, Wolfe SM, eds. Unnecessary caesarean sections: curing a national epidemic. Washington, D.C.: Public Citizen Health Research Group; 1994.
7. Gifford DS, Keeler E, Kahn KL. Reductions in cost and cesarean rate by routine use of external cephalic version: a decision analysis. Obstet Gynecol. 1995;85:930-6.
8. Hannah ME, Hannah WJ, Hewson SA, Hodnett ED, Saigal S, Willan AR. Planned caesarean section versus planned vaginal birth for breech presentation at term. Term Breech Trial Collaborative Group. The Lancet. 2000;356:1368-9.
9. Hofmeyr GJ, Kulier R. Cephalic version by postural management for breech presentation. Cochrane database of Systematic Reviews 2007, Issue 4, Art. n. CD000051. DOI10.1002/1461858.CD000051.
10. Hofmeyr GJ, Kulier R. External cephalic version for breech presentation at term. Cochrane Database of Systematic Reviews 2007, Issue 4. Art. n. CD000083, DOI: 10.1002/1461858. CD000083.
11. Hofmeyr GJ. Effect of external cephalic version in late pregnancy on breech presentation and caesarean section rate: a controlled trial. Br J Obstet Gynaecol. 1983;90:392-9.
12. Hutton EK, Hofmeyr GJ. External cephalic version for breech before term. Cochrane database of Systematic Reviews 2007, Issue 4, Art. n. CD000084.DOI:10.1002/1461858. CD000084. pub.2.
13. Kok M. Clinical factor can help predict outcome of external cephalic version. Am J Obst Gyn. 2008;199:631-7.
14. Kornman MT, Kimball KT, Reeves KO. Preterm external cephalic version in an outpatient environment. Am J Obstet Gynecol. 1995;172:1734-41.
15. Lau TK, Lo KW, Robers M. Pregnancy outcomes after successful external cephalic version for breech presentation at term. Am J Obstet Gynecol. 1997;176:218-23.
16. Lede R. External cephalic version for the management of breech presentation. RHL commentary (last revised 13 March 2006). The WHO Reproductive Health Library: Geneva.
17. Phelan JP, Stine LE, Edwards NB, Clark SL, Horenstein J. The role of external version in the intrapartum management of the transverse lie presentation. Am J Obstet Gynecol. 1985;151:724-6.
18. Phelan JP, Stine LE, Mueller E, McCart D, Yeh S. Observations of foetal heart rate characteristics related to external cephalic version and tocolysis. Am J Obstet Gynecol. 1984;149:658-61.
19. Ranney B. The gentle art of external cephalic version. Am J Obstet Gynecol. 1973;116:239-51.
20. Saling E, Muller-Holve W. External cephalic version under tocolysis. J Perinat Med. 1975;3(2):115-22.
21. Schifrin BS. Update on external cephalic version performed at term. Obstet Gynecol. 1985;65:642-6.
22. Smith C, Crowther C, Wilkinson C. Knee chest postural management for breech at term, a randomized, controlled trial. Birth issues in perinatal care. 1999;26:71-4.
23. Stafford RS. Recent trends in Caesarean section use in California. West J Med. 1990;153:511-4.
24. Stine LE, Phelan JP, Wallace R, Eglinton GS, van Dorsten JP, Schifrin BS. Update on external cephalic version performed at term". Obstet Gynecol. 1985;65:642-6.
25. Tchabo JG, Tomai BS. Selected intrapartum external cephalic version of the second twin. Obstet Gynecol. 1992; 79:421-3.
26. Van Dorsten JP, Schifrin BS, Wallace RL. Randomized control trial of external cephalic version with tocolysis in late pregnancy. Am J Obstet Gynecol. 1981;141:417-24.

CHAPTER 28

Symphysiotomy–Vacuum Extraction (Foetus Alive–Head Engaged)

SYMPHYSIOTOMY

Symphysiotomy is an obstetric procedure by which the diameters of a contracted pelvis are increased by partial surgical division of the ligaments of the symphysis.

The technique has fallen into disuse in the West, where it encounters dogged opposition among obstetricians who have never used it and who have no experience of obstetric practice in low-resourced countries.

The spread of, to obstructed labour, alternative approach—caesarean section—to low-resourced countries has not led to any lasting benefits in this respect. The following factors merit consideration:
- In *Primary Surgery* (1990), which has become a benchmark text for surgical problems in low-resourced countries, the author M King, dedicated extensive treatment to symphysiotomy (page 266)
- In the obstetric handbook for low-resourced countries, *Life-saving Skills, Manual for Midwives,* published by the American College of Nurse-Midwives (1991), symphysiotomy is given substantial treatment and is one of the procedures taught to midwives
- In 2002, Bjorklund conducted a review of 5,000 symphysiotomies carried out during the 20th century, describing them as "minimally invasive surgery for obstructed labour"
- In the *WHO Reproductive Health Library* 2008, symphysiotomy is indicated as an emergency procedure in cases of difficult extraction of the head.

Symphysiotomy should be carried out as an alternative to C-section in areas with high levels of perinatal mortality when:
- The operator is particularly experienced in conducting symphysiotomies
- The patient wishes to have more than four children
- There is little certainty that, on her next pregnancy, the patient will make her way to a hospital facility to undergo trial of labour or caesarean section.

Indications

Classic obstetrics included symphysiotomy among the methods for enabling engagement of the presenting part in cases of pelvic anomaly, while imposing the following limitations on its use: The true conjugate had to be equal or more than 8.5 cm in a uniformly contracted pelvis or equal to 8 cm in a flat pelvis. The operation also included section of the superior pubic ligament and of the interpubic disc, greatly compromising pelvic structural stability.

This approach has been completely revised: Symphysiotomy has a place in the relief of an *established obstruction* due to contracted pelvis and should never be employed to *anticipate it*.

Current indications are:
- Contracted pelvis
- Vertex presentation
- Prolonged second stage
- Failure to descend after proper augmentation

- Failure or anticipated failure of vacuum extraction alone
- Retention of head in breech presentation as recommended by WHO Reproductive Health Library "Vaginal breech delivery and symphysiotomy, 2008).

Conditions

Foetus is Alive

- Foetal weight between 2.3 and 3.5 kg or less than 4.000 g or fundal height less than 40 cm: See Chapter 6 for empirical assessment of foetal weight
- Cervix is fully dilated (no less than 8 cm)
- No over-riding of the head above the symphysis
- Head admitting no more than two fingers above the brim or at -2 station
- Caesarean section is not feasible or immediately available
- The provider is experienced and proficient in symphysiotomy.
  Foetus is dead: Craniotomy.

Contraindications

- Alteration of maternal body stability through obesity or hip pathology which, associated with a symphysiotomy, could lead to permanent disability
- Prior caesarean section
- Prior symphysiotomy
- Foetal weight over 4,000 grams; fundal height over 40 cm
- 3/5 of foetal head above the pubic symphysis after rupture of membranes
- Brow presentation
- Mentoposterior (chin posterior) face presentation.

Advantages

- Integrity of the birth canal is preserved
- Symphysiotomy, in contrast to a caesarean section, is safer for the mother, as it avoids a difficult delivery of the head and possible soft-tissue infections, which often follow difficult delivery of an impacted presenting part.

Anatomical and Theoretical Basis of Symphysiotomy

The ligaments (Fig. 28.1) associated with the symphysis pubica can be divided in two groups:

- *Rigid structures*: The interpubic disc is a cone-shaped layer of fibrocartilage which, laterally, adheres intimately to the layer of hyaline cartilage covering the symphysial surfaces and, at its superior and inferior margins, with the ligaments. This is the anatomical formation that is dissected during *symphysiotomy*
- *Elastic structures*: A fibrous periarticular sleeve, of which we can distinguish four ligaments:
  - *The anterior pubic ligament*, 5 mm thick, is closely connected with the fascial coverings of the muscles (pyramidalis, rectus abdominis, obliquus externus) arising from the conjoined rami of the pubis
  - *Posterior pubic ligament*, stretched between the two pubic bones; thin, membranous, it consists of the periosteum of the pelvis
  - *Superior pubic ligament:* This extends laterally along the crest of the pubis on each side to the pubic tubercle; it is a very thick fibrous mesh which, with the upper part of the anterior pubic ligament, limits the widening of the pubis and has, therefore, been defined as the "*frenum anatomicum chirurgicum superior*"!

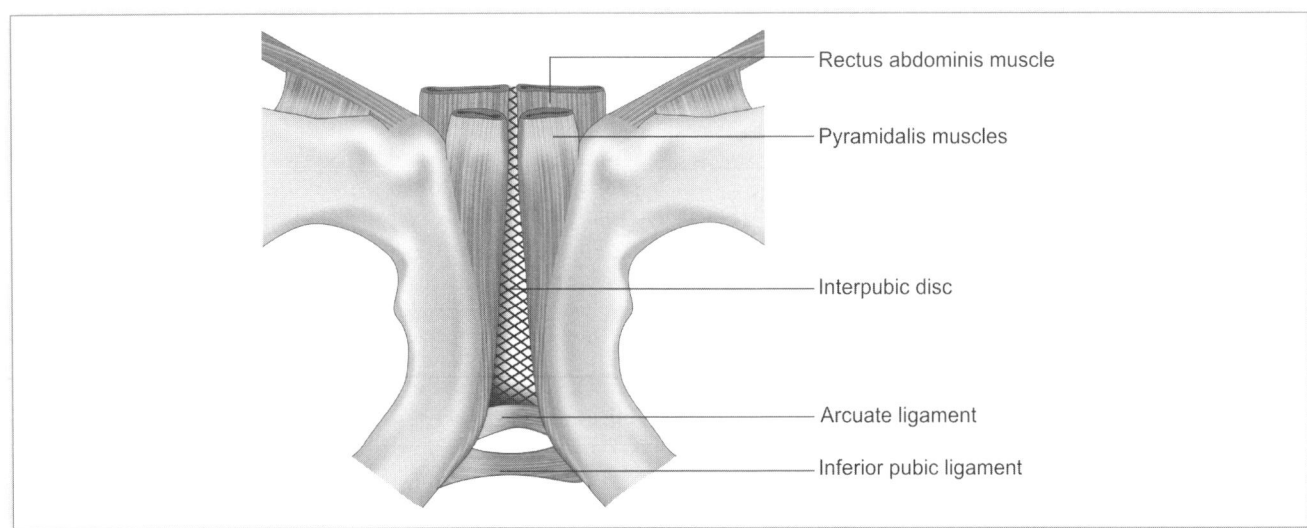

Fig. 28.1: Pubic symphysis, anterior view

- *Inferior pubic or arcuate ligament:* This is a thick, crescent-shaped band of closely connected fibres that fills the angle between the pubic rami, it has a height of 10 mm on the midline, a border adhering to the uppermost portion of the pubic arch and a free, sharp, very tough edge, against which the foetal head fixes and rotates in the course of delivery.

It was Zarate who first demonstrated that by cutting the interpubic disc, it was possible to make use of the elasticity of the superior and inferior pubic ligaments, thereby obtaining controlled dislocation of the two symphysis pubis articular surfaces and an increase in the dimensions of the bony ring during delivery (Fig. 28.2). Following delivery, the articular surfaces move back together, the solution of continuity heals and the pelvis regains its structural stability.

Each centimetre by which the two pubic bones are dislocated leads to an increase of 2 mm in the obstetric conjugate. Therefore, an average dislocation of 3 cm gains us 6 mm in the obstetric conjugate, to which 6–8 mm are added, gained by the exteriorising of the head into the interpubic space (Fig. 28.3), giving a total gain of 1.4 cm.

This may not seem like much, but its significance becomes clearer if we consider the resulting changes in the *circumference* and *surface area* of the pelvic inlet.

Circumference

The circumference of a circle is obtained by multiplying its diameter by 3.14: If we take the initial diameter to be 8.5 cm, the circumference will be: 8.5 cm x 3.14 = 26.8 cm as, following symphysiotomy, the diameter increases by 1.4 cm: 1.4 x 3.14 = 4.396 cm, the resulting circumference will increase by 4.4 (4.396) cm, taking it from 26.8 to 31.2 cm. This will be sufficient for a vertex presentation in which engagement follows the suboccipitobregmatic diameter (9.5 cm).

- In a bregma presentation, engagement follows the occipitofrontal diameter (12 cm) with a largest plane of progression of 34 cm
- In a brow presentation, engagement follows the occipitomental diameter (13.5 cm), which has a circumference of 35–36 cm
- In the face presentation, the circumference is 34 cm.

Surface Area

The surface of a circle is obtained by multiplying r^2 x 3.14.
  Initial surface area = 56.73 cm^2
  8.5 : 2 = 4.25 (radius); r^2 = 4.25^2 x 4.52 = 18.07
  18.07 x 3.14 = 56.73 cm^2
  Resulting surface area = 76.93 cm^2
  As, following symphysiotomy, the diameter increases by 1.4 cm: 8.5 cm x 1.4 = 9.9 cm
  9.9 : 2 = 4.95 (radius); r^2 = 4.95 x 4.95 = 24.50
  24.50 x 3.14 = 76.93 cm^2
  Therefore, the increase in surface area is 76.93 – 56.7 = 20.2 cm^2

A further increase in the available surface area is obtained through the resulting greater mobility of the sacroiliac joint, which promotes the movements of *nutation* and *counternutation* (see Chapter 2).

Procedure

The method we use is known as *subcutaneous partial symphysiotomy*; it consists in sectioning the interpubic disc of the pubic symphysis while preserving the integrity of the periarticular fibrous sheath. The steps are as follows:

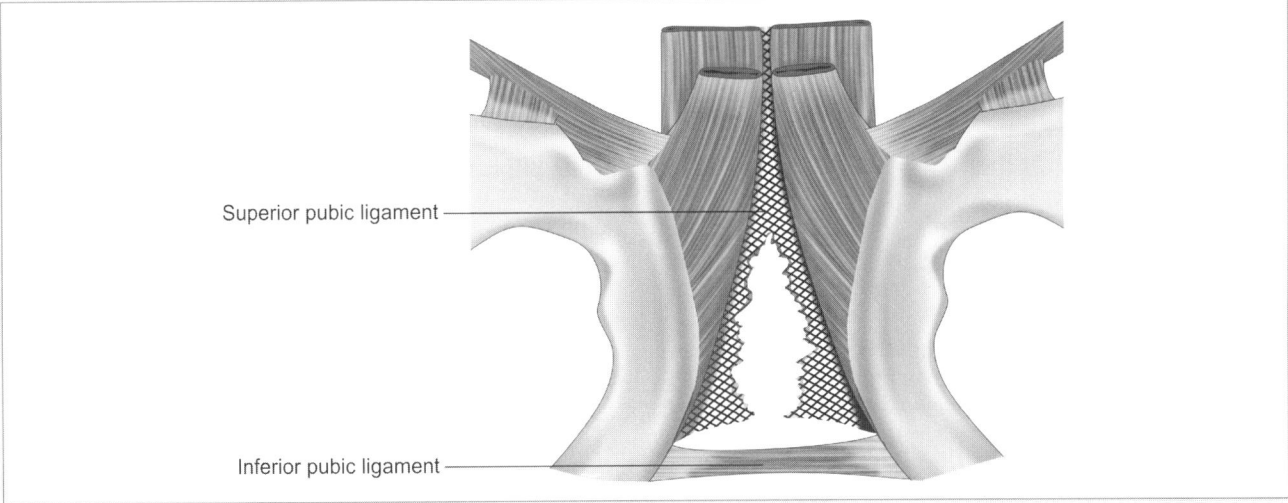

Fig. 28.2: Pubic symphysis after symphysiotomy, posterior view

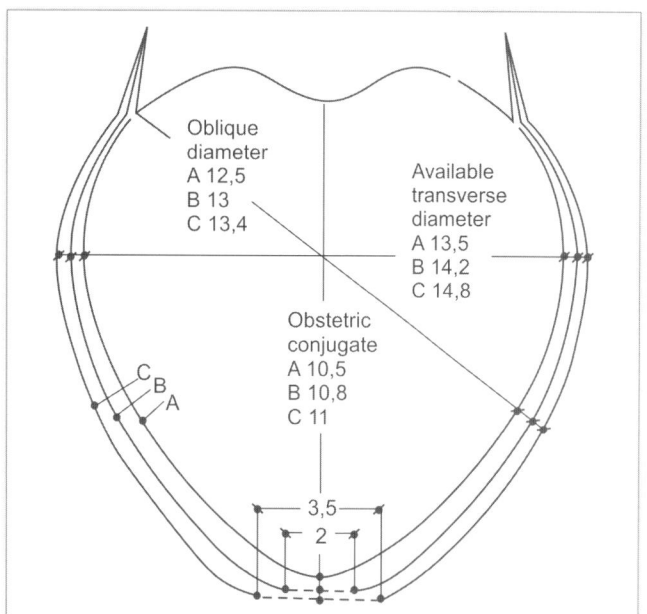

Fig. 28.3: Changes in diameters of the pelvic inlet following symphysiotomy: (A) Normal pelvis; (B) Diameters of the pelvic inlet after symphysiotomy with pubic diastasis of 2 cm; (C) Diameters of the pelvic inlet after symphysiotomy with pubic diastasis of 3.5 cm

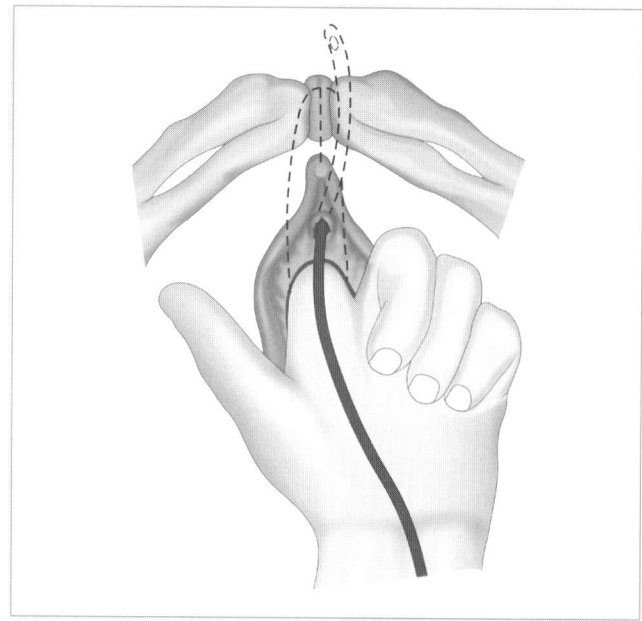

Fig. 28.5: A firm catheter inserted and displaced from the midline

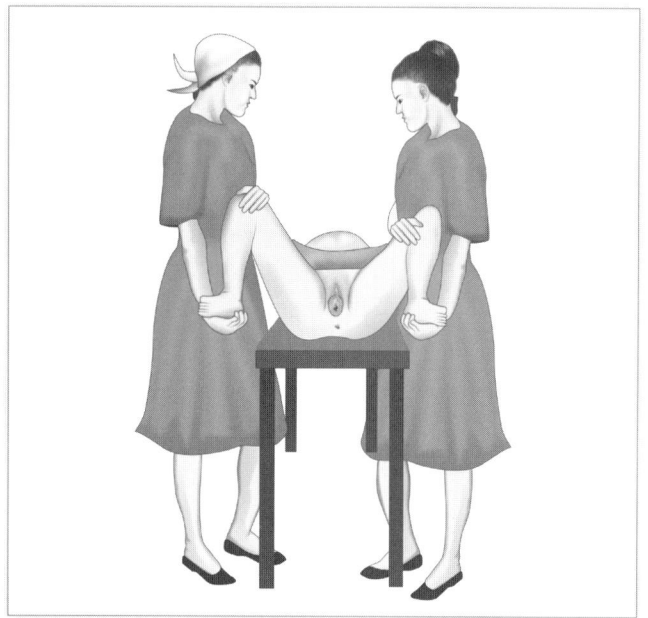

Fig. 28.4: The patient's feet are not resting on stirrups, but are held by two assistants, positioned one on each side to control the degree of abduction as determined by the operator, whose hand is placed on the pubic symphysis.

a. *The patient is put in lithotomy position* (Fig. 28.4); two assistants support the woman's legs with her thighs and knees flexed and exert a controlled abduction on the thighs; the abduction should not exceed 45° from the midline as an increase may cause tearing of the urethra, bladder and of the sacroiliac ligament (see Chapter 2). This procedure which is decisive for the *controlled dislocation* of the articular surfaces; success of the procedure could not occur if the patient had her legs held up in stirrups.

b. *Mediolateral episiotomy.*

c. *Apply antiseptic solution to the suprapubic skin.*
   – *Use local infiltration with lignocaine*
   – *Insert a firm catheter to identify the urethra.* Place an index finger in the vagina and push the catheter and with it the urethra, or index and middle fingers away from the midline (Fig. 28.5).

The volar aspect of the index and middle fingers of the operator's non-dominant hand are in contact with the posterior face of the pubic symphysis. These fingers, apart from displacing the urethra from the midline, serve to prevent the incision from going beyond the pubic symphysis. The fingers should preferably be wrapped in gauze, as the distinctive sound made by a scalpel on gauze will alert the operating surgeon.

d. *Using the needle* of a syringe containing 5–10 ml of local anaesthetic, the operator identifies the interpubic disc (by its reduced resistance) and leaves the needle in situ as a marker. 5 mm below the superior border of the symphysis a vertical stab incision is made. With the scalpel and using to-and-fro movements in a cranial-inferior direction, the interpubic disc is gradually cut through (Figs 28.6 to 28.8). It is essential that the cut

SYMPHYSIOTOMY–VACUUM EXTRACTION (FOETUS ALIVE–HEAD ENGAGED)

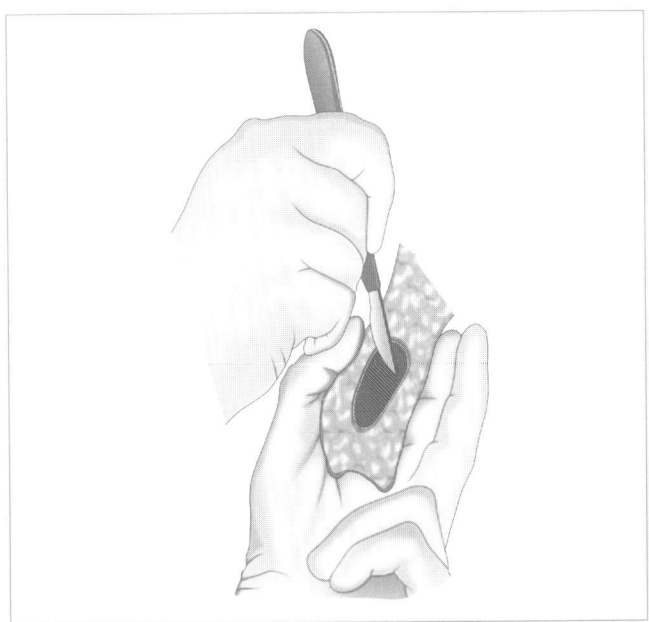

Fig. 28.6: The scalpel incises the interpubic disc 5 mm inferiorly to the superior border of the pubic symphysis

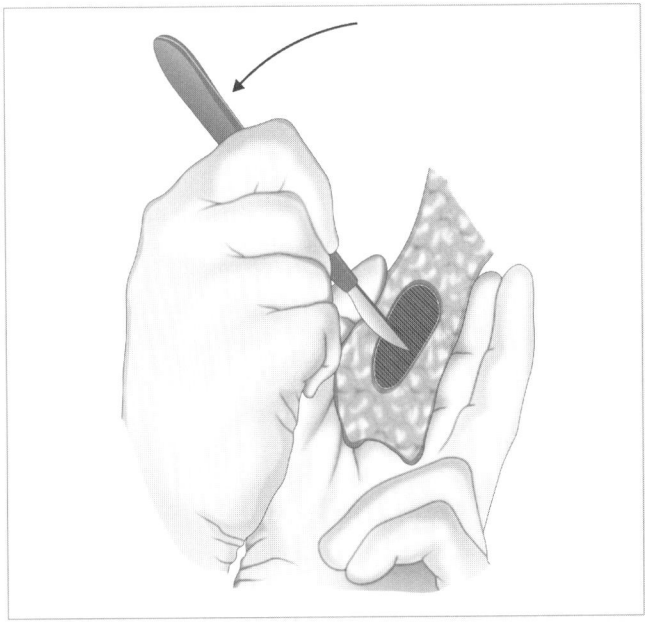

Fig. 28.7: Symphysiotomy—The scalpel proceeds with the section, moving in a cranial-to-inferior direction

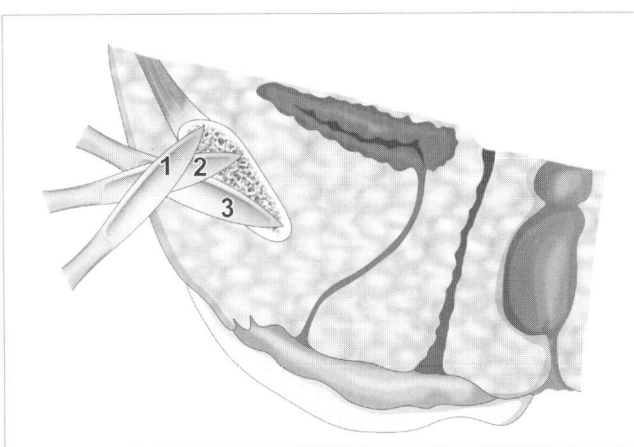

Fig. 28.8: Correct movement of the scalpel

keeps strictly to the midline in order to avoid damaging the joint cartilage, which would otherwise be subject to inflammation. Completion of the symphysiotomy is announced by a bony crepitation. The two assistants positioned at the sides will prevent dislocation of the joint ends from exceeding 2.5–3.5 cm, and the angle formed by the thighs from going beyond 80°. The operator's fingers, positioned in the vagina, monitor the extension of the enlargement. When the desired value has been reached, the patient's legs are placed on the stirrups.

Course of the Delivery

The symphysiotomy solves the problem of obstruction preventing the head's descent into the pelvis, but it does not solve the problem of delivery. Generally, a symphysiotomy is followed after a short time by resumption of contractions and rapid progress of *dilatation*, with similarly rapid accomplishment of the delivery. Sometimes the biggest hazard is a precipitous delivery, with lacerations incurred by the anterior vaginal wall.

At full cervical dilatation, if the head fails to descend further, fundal pressure by means of a Kristeller manoeuvre may be applied following episiotomy. As an alternative, whether dilatation is complete or not, vacuum extraction may be used (recommended).

Some doubts persist over the use of forceps, whether used with traction (Naegele, Simpson), or with rotation (Kielland). With the former, there is the fear that the blades may over-distend the vagina; with the latter, there is a suspicion that the unsupported bladder neck and urethra could easily be damaged.

On delivery, it is advisable to bring the thighs closer together, in order to prevent excessive dislocation of the symphysis.

Postpartum and Puerperium

Having accomplished the delivery and completed repair to the skin wound and to any solutions of continuity within the birth canal, the patient is placed in bed with her knees tied together and with an indwelling catheter. The patient should lie on her side. On the 3rd day she may sit up in bed; walking will be allowed from the 5th or 6th day postpartum, with the aid of crutches. By the 10th day, the patient should have a fair degree of independence. Heavy work should be avoided for one month.

There is often a residual stress incontinence, which will settle within two to three weeks.

Symphysiotomy is frequently followed by persisting diastasis of the pubic symphysis, which generally renders subsequent deliveries less problematic.

VACUUM EXTRACTION

The *vacuum extractor or ventouse* (Fig. 28.9) is an obstetric instrument designed to assist vaginal delivery by the application of traction to a suction cup attached to the foetal scalp. The cup's adhesion to the foetal scalp is obtained by means of a vacuum.

Mechanism of action: The diameter of the cup's lower rim is smaller than its internal diameter; when it is applied to the scalp, negative pressure developed inside the system causes the transudation of serum from the internal vessels to the surface of the scalp, forming a *caput succedaneum,* which adheres tenaciously to the cup's inside wall. The restriction at the cup's lower rim plays an important part, as it prevents the caput inside the cup, which has a larger diameter, from slipping out, as long as negative pressure is maintained.

Indications

Are subdivided into absolute and relative:
- *Absolute indications*: *Prolonged second stage of labour,* which usually results from a complex mix of poor or incoordinate uterine activity combined with subtle degrees of cranial deflection or other mild malpresentations and no bony outlet dystocia present. The definition of prolonged second stage depends on parity and epidural anaesthesia. In general, second stages of more than 2 hours without epidural anaesthesia and 3 hours with are the acceptable measures for nulliparas. One hour less in each category is the limit for multiparas.
- *Relative indications*:
  - Cardiopathy or pregnancy-induced hypertension, as these reduce the mother's physical strength
  - Scar from prior C-section or myomectomy: This reduces the amount of stress the uterus can withstand.

Contraindications

- Bony or soft parts (female genital mutilation) outlet dystocia
- Incomplete dilatation with prior C-section: This is because the lower segment scar site would now be subjected to a twofold stress: Cranially from normal contractive forces, and inferiorly from traction, possibly with scar dehiscence as the outcome.

Conditions

- *Fully dilated cervix,* 8 cm according to some author
- *No more than 1/5 of the head* should be above the pelvic brim
- *Normal uterine contractility:* 3-4 contractions every 10 minutes, lasting at least 30-40 seconds
- *Favourable abdominal pelvic score* (Knight, 1993) when the total point score for head fifths above the symphysis (Crichton) added to the score of skull moulding is ≤3. A total point score >3 is consistent with *cephalopelvic disproportion* and accomplishment of the delivery by the vaginal route is strongly discouraged.

Advantages

- It requires less training and less experience
- Randomised studies have shown that it causes fewer injuries to the birth canal than the forceps does
- Clear cut rules:
  - Favourable abdomino pelvic score
  - Three pulls rule
  - Unlike forceps the suction cup takes up no room in the pelvis.
- It can correct the degree of deflection
- Required rotation of the head occurs spontaneously
- No risk of excessive traction.

Disadvantages

The suction cup cannot be applied:
- To preterm delivery (intracranial haemorrhage)

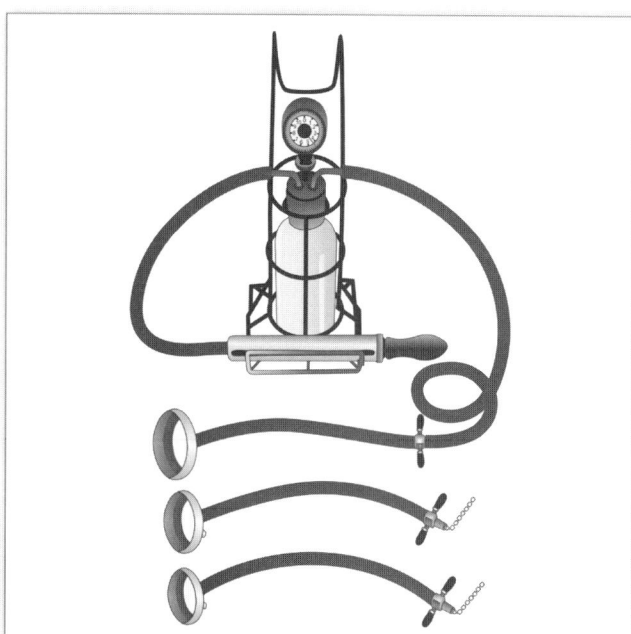

Fig. 28.9: Malmstrom's obstetric ventouse

- To face presentation
- To the aftercoming head in breech presentation (unlike forceps)
- When the mother is unable to assist the delivery with expulsive efforts.

Needs more complex equipment, subject to failure if not well maintained.

- It causes more trauma to the foetus (increase in intracranial pressure) than forceps does.

1. *Increase of intracranial pressure:* The caput succedaneum, the subcutaneous, serosanguinous, extra-periosteal fluid collection normally formed on the presenting portion of the scalp, which extends beyond the suture lines and usually associated with moulding of the skull bones, *is increased* by vacuum application: Artificial caput succedaneum which differs from cephal hematoma (Fig. 28.10).

Cephal hematoma: It is sub-periosteal Hg due to rupture of vein of Galen between the skull and periosteum. It is confined to suture lines, usually over parietal bones, the centre feels soft, it becomes visible on second or third day of life, it resolves over several weeks (8 weeks); when they are extensive can cause jaundice and anaemia. Occasionally associated with linear fracture of skull (5–20%), it requires no treatment, but treat infection, anaemia and jaundice. Aspiration of blood collection is *contraindicated as it will induce infection* (Table 28.1). This mass caput succedaneum is only partially absorbed by the skin's elasticity, it therefore depresses the cranial vault, reducing its surface area and thereby increasing intracranial pressure.

That such an increase occurs and that it is sizeable was elegantly demonstrated by De Boer's (1961) experiments, in which the ventouse was applied to very recently (a few minutes) deceased foeti. It was shown that following application, CSF pressure rose to 18 cm H_2O. That this increase reflects events in living foeti was demonstrated by the fact that it did not occur if the suction cup was applied some hours after death.

A suction cup has a surface of adhesion 5.55 cm in diameter, or 38 cm^2. The tractive force exerted will not generally exceed 10 kg, at which point the cup will slip out. This force can be resolved into two tangential vectors: T1 and T2 (Fig. 28.11), each one of which may be further resolved into two forces: A tangential force (tractive force) and a normal force, which has been quantified by Snoeck (1960), based on Malstrom's studies, to be 75 g/cm^2, the compressive component being equal to one half of the tractive force (Fig. 28.12). Sometimes it is necessary to combine simple traction with rotation. In terms of the physics, this is a combination of motions, in that a rolling friction has to be added to the sliding friction. This does not itself lead to an increase in intracranial pressure, but in requiring greater tractive force, it will increase the component of normal traction, responsible for the intracranial pressure.

It would seem clear that, following application of the suction cup, a further increase in pressure is added to the normal increase in intracranial pressure deriving from resistances within the birth canal. This further increase derives both from the mass of the caput formation, and the tractive force applied. It has been calculated that intracranial pressure during ventouse-assisted delivery is approximately twice that observed during a normal delivery.

2. *Physiological effects*: While this increase in intracranial pressure does not affect arterial blood flow, it does impede

Table 28.1

The caput is a mass interposed between the skin and the cranial vault

Caput succedaneum	Cephal haematoma
1. Present at birth on normal vaginal delivery	1. Appears within a few days after birth on normal or forceps delivery
2. May lie on suture, not well defined	2. Well defined by suture, gradually developing, hard edge
3. Soft, pits on pressure	3. Soft, elastic but does not pits on pressure
4. Skin ecchymotic	4. No skin change
5. Size largest at birth, gradually subsides within a day	5. Become largest after birth and then disappears within 6–8 weeks to few months
6. No underlying skull bone fracture	6. Underlying skull bone may fracture
7. No treatment required	7. No treatment required

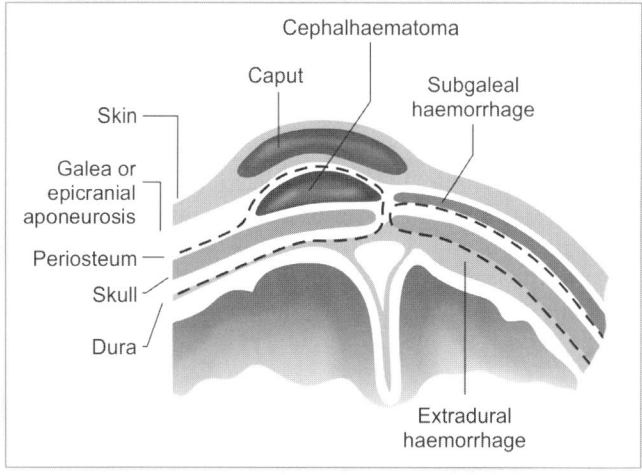

Fig. 28.10: Caput succedaneum, cephalhaematoma

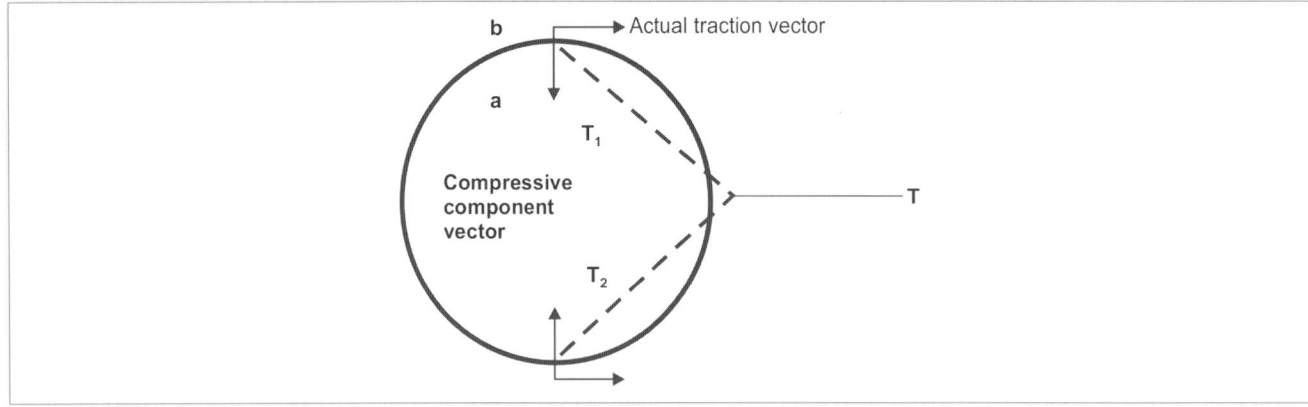

Fig. 28.11: Resolution of the tractive force exerted by the cup into two secondary forces which are in turn further resolved into two components: (a) Normal force—*the compressive* component; (b) Tangential force—*the actual traction*

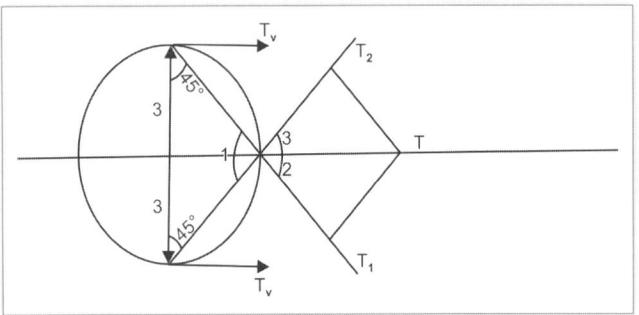

Fig. 28.12: Calculation of the forces acting on the foetal head during application of the suction cup: Compression (T_1) and traction (T_2): The compressive component is equal to one half of the tractive force

venous return: The outcome is cerebral congestion. The weak point of the vascular system is its capillary component. Even under normal conditions, capillaries are subject to lesions (presentation haemorrhages) and the increase in pressure will make them even more liable. Added to this is the action of vasoactive kinins, which form under conditions of acidemia.

Moreover, in cases of asynclitism, it is necessary to apply the cup to the leading part, thereby accentuating the asynclitism.

3. *Efficacy of forces applied*: It is evident that the use of traction to advance descent of the head through the birth canal is decidedly less efficacious than impulsion from above.

Awareness of the possible foetal damage that may derive from using vacuum extraction has led to strict codification of indications, methodologies and timings of traction, which are summarised in the 'three pulls' rule. This is described below in the section on the technique of applying traction.

Difficulties are to be expected if:

- Dilatation from 7 to 10 cm has taken more than three hours
- The symphysis-fundus distance is 40 cm or more (indicative of a large foetus).

Maternal complications:

- Vaginal lesions
- Cervical lesions are observed particularly when the cup is applied at less than complete cervical ripening. With dilatation of 7 cm, the cup diameter should not exceed 3-4 cm.

Lesions are related to: Cervical dilatation at the time of application, method of application, and the amount of tractive force exerted. In extreme cases, we may encounter annular detachment of the cervix, with cervicoisthmic insufficiency during subsequent pregnancies, or uterovaginal prolapse.

Procedure

- The labouring mother is comfortably seated in a 45° reclining position with her legs in lithotomy stirrups. Due to the effects of pelvic *nutation,* (rotation of the sacrum around the sacroiliac joint), this position will lead to *an increase in the anteroposterior diameter of the pelvic outlet*
- Ensure that the woman's bladder is empty, if a Foley catheter is in place, deflate the bulb
- Palpate the mother's abdomen just above the pubis bone to ensure that the baby's head is engaged in the pelvis, ideally no more than 1/5 of the head should be above the pelvic brim
- Perform the vaginal examination to ensure that the cervix is fully dilated and to ascertain the position of the head.

Select the cup:

- The cups may be soft or rigid; there is consensus that the soft bell cups should be considered for more straightforward occiput-anterior deliveries while the rigid M cups should be reserved for more complicated

deliveries, such as those involving larger infants, significant caput succedaneum (scalp oedema), occiputposterior presentation, or asynclitism. The soft bell cups are associated with fewer scalp injuries and no risk of maternal perineal injury
- Cups come in different sizes, which are to be selected according to the dimensions of the foetal head, and the amount of force to be exerted. It is incorrect obstetric practice to apply a cup to the head of a preterm baby
- On the cup's exterior is a lug, which should be oriented towards the occiput. Observing this lug's position when the cup has been applied will enable assessment of rotation by the presenting part.

Having selected the most suitable cup, press with two fingers on the perineum posteriorly to widen the vaginal opening, pass the cup through the vagina taking care to avoid touching the urethra or the clitoris.

Slide the cup along the baby's head so that it lies over the occiput, the correct point of application of the cup is the *flexion point which is 2–3 cm in front of the posterior fontanel or 6-cm posterior to the anterior fontanelle;* this point of application will promote flexion, descent and rotation of the head and ensures that the head remains flexed and that the smallest part of the head exits the birth canal first.

It seems clear that, with respect to the pelvis, *the site of insertion of the cup will vary according to whether the head is in occiputoanterior or in occipitoposterior position.*
- In the occipitoanterior position (Fig. 28.13), the cup will have to be pushed almost beneath the pubic symphysis
- In the occipitoposterior position; the lower rim of the cup is almost touching the sacral concavity (Fig. 28.14).

Run a finger around the perimeter of the cup to ensure that no maternal tissues are trapped under the cup.

Start creating negative pressure of 0.2 atm, increasing it to 0.6–0.8; traditionally, it has been recommended the pressure to be increased slowly in a stepwise procedure; some have advocated rapid increases in pressure as the rapid negative pressure application for vacuum assisted vaginal birth reduces the duration of the procedure whilst there is no evidence of differences in maternal and neonatal outcome (Suwannachat Bl et al., 2008).

During traction keep one finger on the edge of the cup and one on the foetal head for earlier sign of slippage of the cup can be detected and will enable to monitor descent of the presenting part.

Note that the line of traction should always be perpendicular to the plane of the cup, this reduces the risk of the cup slipping out of place.

Side-to-side or rotational movements may help progression.
- Invite the patient to indicate the onset and the end of each contraction, and to push while they last.

Apply constant steady traction during the contraction during which the mother will bear down.

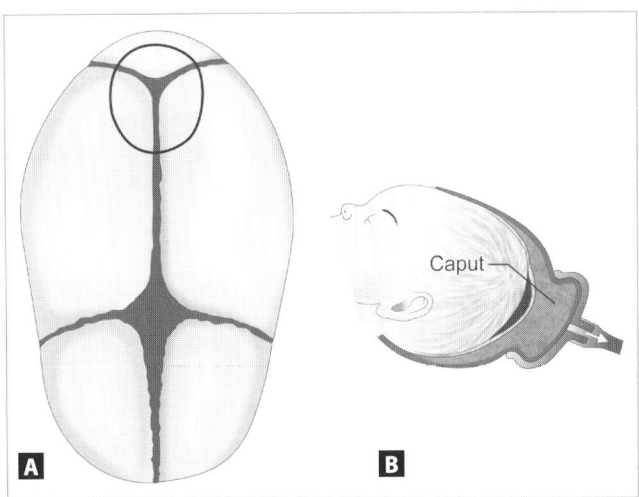

Fig. 28.13A and B: Correct application of the cup in the occipitoanterior position: (A) The centre of the cup should coincide with the pivot point (hypomoclion) located 1–3 cm anteriorly to the cup; (B) Caput formation

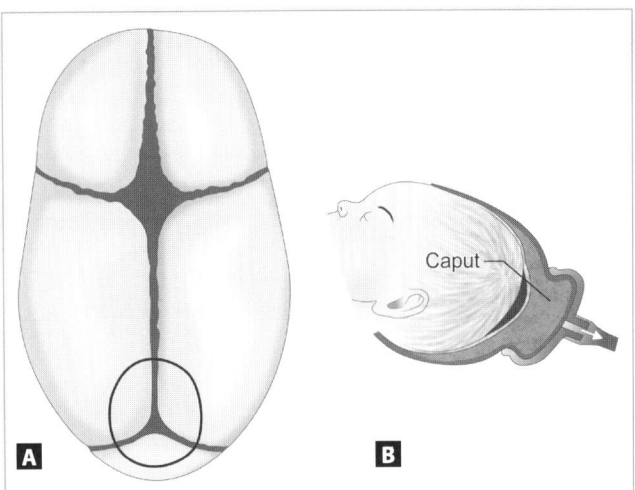

Fig. 28.14A and B: Correct application of the cup in the occipitoposterior position; (A) The cup is applied as posteriorly as possible, the lower rim almost touching the sacral concavity; (B) Caput succedaneum

Method and Direction of Traction

Direction of traction it varies according to position:

a. *Occipitoanterior position*: The traction is directed in line with the axis of the birth canal; that is initially downwards to bring the occiput below the symphysis, then progressively forward and finally upwards, in order to rotate the occiput around the symphysis; hence the saying "the operator start pulling in a *kneeling position*, then works *sitting* and ends up *standing*.

b. *Occipitoposterior position* (Fig. 28.15): The mechanism of delivery is as follows: An accentuated flexion of the head can be observed when the flexion point makes contact with the arcuate ligament. The flexion point or hypomoclion is located between the anterior fontanelle and the hairline. Rotation takes place around this point and expulsion is initially accompanied by a further flexion of the head, followed by deflection.

Expedition of delivery by vacuum extraction should reproduce this mechanism. For this reason, the cup is applied as far posteriorly as possible (Fig. 28.13A). Now follow traction in an anterior and upward direction (Fig. 28.15A), with the purpose of bringing the flexion point into

Table 28.2

Proposed classification for vacuum extraction procedures according to fetal Station and cranial position (modified from ACOG Practice Bulletin # 17, June, 2000)

Type of procedure	Description of classification
Outlet-vacuum operation	The fetal head is at or on the perineum; the scalp is visible at the introitus without separating the labia; the fetal skull has reached the pelvic floor. The sagittal suture is in the AP diameter (ROA, LOA, OA) or posterior (ROP, LOP, OP) position
Low-vacuum operation	The position/station of the fetal head does not fulfill the criterion for an outlet operation; the leading edge of the fetal skull is at station +2/5 cm, but has not reached the pelvic floor
Subdivisions	(a) Position is occiput anterior (OA, LOA, ROA) (b) Position is occiput posterior (OP, LOP, ROP) or transverse (LOT, ROT)
Midvacuum operation	Station
Subdivisions	(a) Position is occiput anterior (OA, LOA, ROA) (b) Position is occiput posterior (OP, LOP, ROP) or transverse (LOT, ROT)
Vacuum-assisted caesarean delivery	This includes all vacuum-assisted caesarean deliveries, unspecified technique
Special vacuum operations	This includes vacuum extraction operations not otherwise specified; full details are described in the dictated operative note
High-vacuum operation	Such procedures are not included in the classification

Abbreviation: OA, occipitoanterior; ROA, right occipitoanterior; LOA, left occipitoanterior; OP, occipitoposterior; LOP, left occipitoposterior; ROP, right occipitoposterior; LOT, left occipitotransverse; ROT, right occipitotransverse

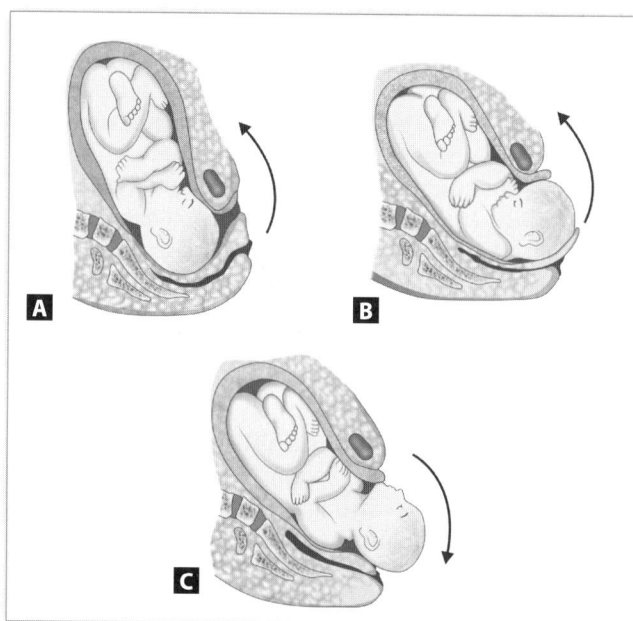

Fig. 28.15A to C: Mechanism of parturition in occipitoposterior position: The arrows indicate direction of traction

contact with the arcuate pubic ligament. Once this has been reached, cranial traction is increased (Fig. 28.15B) and, on crowning of the head, disengagement is effected by means of deflection (Fig. 28.15C).

To return to our previous remarks on the general theory of vacuum extraction, the 'three pull rule' should be strictly observed as a general rule (with exceptions where they are due), throughout the procedure. Randomised studies have shown this approach to be free of negative outcomes for the newborn.

- The first pull should mobilise the head from its point of impaction
- The second pull should bring the head to the pelvic floor
- The third pull should effect delivery or, at least, bring the head to the vulva, until the vulva crowns the head.

If one of these three pulls does not attain its set objective, stop the procedure and expedite delivery by a different technique: Symphysiotomy, caesarean section.

If, while observing this procedural protocol, the cup should detach twice, stop the procedure (Table 28.2).

The caput generally settles by itself within a few hours; the cephalhaematoma is normally reabsorbed over 3–4 weeks.

BIBLIOGRAPHY

Symphysiotomy
1. Crichton D, Seedat EK. The technique of symphysiotomy. South African Medical Journal. 1963;37:227.
2. Domini E. Il Forcipe Ostetrico. Verduci Edizioni Scientifiche Roma, 1978.

3. Duale S, et al. A follow-up study of pregnancy outcome in women with symphysiotomy versus caesarean section in Zaire. International Center for Research on Women, Washington DC. 1990.
4. Gaucherand J, Guarin P. Présentation du bregma; forceps après symphyséotomie à la Zarate. Soc Obst Gyn Lyon. 1950.
5. Gebbie DAM. Vacuum extraction and symphysiotomy in difficult vaginal delivery in a developing community. Brit Med J. 1966;2:1490.
6. Gebbie DAM. Symphysiotomy. Tropical Doctor. 1974;4:69.
7. Hartfield VJ. A comparison of the early and late effects of subcutaneous symphysiotomy and of lower segment cesarean section. J Obst and Gyn Br Cwlh. 1973;80:508-14.
8. King M, Bewes P, Cairms J, Thornton B. Primary Surgery. Oxford Medical Publications; p. 266-7.
9. Lasbrey AH. The symptomatic sequelae of symphysiotomy. S Afr Med J. 1963;37:231.
10. Maharaj D, Moodley J. Symphysiotomy and foetal destructive operations. Best Practice and Research Clinical Obstetrics and Gynaecology. 2002;16:117-31.
11. Marmey J, Lacroix A. Indications de la symphyséotomie de Zarate dans la pratique obstétricale marocaine d'après 56 observations. Semana Méd. 1953;60:676-85.
12. Marshal MA, Tebben Buffington S. Life saving skill manual for midwifes. American College of Nurse Midwifes Washington DC: USA. 1991.
13. Menticoglou SM. Symphysiotomy for the trapped aftercoming parts of the breech: a review of the literature and a plea for its use. Austr N Zealand J Obstetrics and Gynecology. 1990;30:1-9.
14. Myles MF. Textbook for midwives. Edinburgh: Churchill Livingstone. 1981;35:658.
15. Norman RJ. Six years experience of symphysiotomy in a teaching Hospital. South African Medical Journal. 1978;54:1121.
16. Nurse Clinician Training Modules Maternal and child health series. Ministry of Health, Maseru. 1984;5:72.
17. Philpott RH, et al. Obstetrics, Family planning and pediatrics. University of Natal Press, Pietermaritzburg. 1978;9:107.
18. Van Roosmalen J. Symphysiotomy as an alternate to cesarean section. Int J of Gynecology and Obstetrics. 1987;25:451-8.
19. Seedat EK, Crichton D. Symphysiotomy: technique, indications and limitations. Lancet. 1962. p. 555.
20. Suwannachat B, Lumbiganon P, Laopaiboon M. Rapid versus stepwise negative pressure application for vacuum extraction assisted vaginal delivery. Cochrane Database Syst Rev. 2008;16;(3):CD006636. doi: 10.1002/14651858.CD006636.pub2.
21. Zarate E. La symphyséotomie partielle ou bride sous-cutanée complete. Traité d'Obstétrique de Nubiola-Zarate, Barcelone. 1951;1:1104.
22. Zarate E. Symphyséotomie sous-cutanée partielle. Buenos-Aires. 1955.
23. WHO Reproductive Health Library 2008. Symphysiotomy for the trapped after coming head.

Vacuum extraction

24. Bird GC. Modification of Malmström's extractor. Br Med J. 1969;5:26.
25. Bird GC. The importance of flexion in vacuum extractor delivery. Br J Obst Gyn. 1976;83:194-200.
26. De Boer CH. The vacuum extractor or the forceps? III Weltkongress für Gynäekologie und Geburtshilfe. Wien. 1961. p. 83.
27. De Boer CH. Forceps or vacuum extractor? Lancet. 1964; II:875.
28. Malmström T. Vacuum extractoran obstetrical instrument. Acta Obst. Gynec. Scand. 1954;33:1-32.
29. Malmström T, Jansson I. Use of the vacuum extractor. Clin Obst Gyn. 1965;8:895-913.
30. Snoeck J. The vacuum extractor (ventouse) - an alternative to the obstetric forceps. Proc. Royal Soc Med. 1960;53:749.

CHAPTER 29

Destructive Operations—A Vanishing Art in Modern Obstetrics (P Sikka, 2011)

Destructive operations are a group of operations which aim at reducing the size of the head, shoulder girdle or trunk of the dead foetus to allow its vaginal delivery, thus maintaining integrity of the uterus and preventing from injuries to the genital tract; these procedures are as follows:
- Craniotomy
- Decapitation
- Cleidotomy
- Evisceration
- Spondylotomy.

Contraindications

- Living foetus, except in certain congenital anomalies incompatible with life as anencephaly which may be associated with large shoulder girdle. However, destruction of a living foetus for whatever the cause may not be accepted from the religious point of view
- Extreme degree of contracted pelvis, i.e. true conjugate <5.5 cm
- Impending rupture of the uterus
- Rupture of the uterus
- Partially dilated cervix
- Obstructing pelvic tumours
- Cancer of the cervix with pregnancy.

Complications

- Uterine rupture
- Injuries to the genital tract.

Destructive operations used in the past but now banned by Western obstetrics (Alfieri et al, 1936; Lorca C, 1948; Martius, 1948; Maggiora-Vergano, 1954; Merger et al., 1972) still find very specific indication in low-resoursed countries. There is an ample literature on the subject, including recent publications:

- Arora et al. (1999, Pondichery University Hospital, India) report 33 destructive operations from the period 1981–1991: 27 craniotomies, 2 decapitations, 4 eviscerations;
- Biswas (2001, University Hospital of Kolkata, India) reports 20 craniotomies and 23 eviscerations from the previous year
- Singhal et al. (2005, University Hospital of Haryana, India) reports 51 destructive operations from the previous 7 years: Craniotomies (69%), decapitations (19%)
- Adhikari et al. (2005, University Hospital of Kolkata, India) reports that during the 5 years between 1993 and 1998, foetal destructive operations were conducted for 36% of patients with obstructed labour. These included 67 craniotomies and 21 decapitations.

Statistically comparable results are to be found in Africa: Ozumba et al. (1991, Nigeria); Konje et al. (1992, Nigeria); Dafallah et al. (2003, Sudan).

We describe here the detailed techniques of craniotomy and decapitation, techniques culturally accepted in many low-resourced countries, which provide a reasonable—if sanguinary—alternative to caesarean section. In the above-mentioned circumstances, C-sections present two major drawbacks:

- In the short-term: Spread to the abdominal cavity of uterine inflammation, which is a constant presence with cephalopelvic disproportion or obstructed labour associated with a dead foetus. We point out that, following C-section due to dead foetus, maternal mortality may be as high as 70%
- In the long-term: C-sections compromise the patient's reproductive life due to the presence of a hysterotomic scar which may have been avoided.

Gupta and Chitra (1994, University Hospital of Delhi) studied outcomes in patients with obstructed labour, for the period 1985–1991, of destructive operations (56, either craniotomies or decapitations) compared to C-sections. They found that destructive operations were easier to perform and safer than C-section, and that maternal mortality was extremely low, if not absent, in the former. They therefore concluded that *"embryotomies play an important role in low-resourced countries"*. Similar conclusions were reached twelve years later by Parick (2006, India).

CRANIOTOMY

Craniotomy is a destructive operation that, in the case of an obstructed labour with a dead foetus and where other methods of delivery proved unsuccessful, effects for the purpose of facilitating the delivery, a decrease in size of the foetal head by puncture and evacuation of its content.

Classical obstetrics under the term of craniotomy comprises three different destructive operations:

Craniotomy: Perforation of the foetal head (cranium).

Cranioclasm: Crushing of the cranium.

Cephalotripsy: Crushing of the whole head including the base of the skull.

Indications

- Obstructed labour with a dead foetus. We remind the reader of the distinction between *cephalopelvic disproportion* and *obstructed labour*, in the former engagement did not occur, in the latter the engagement occurred but rotation and descent resulted in obstruction. We emphasise this distinction to prevent from performing, with the exception of hydrocephalus in cephalic presentation, craniotomy
- Impacted malpresented dead foetus as mento-posterior and brow presentation
- Hydrocephalus: Both in cephalic and podalic presentation
- Retained aftercoming head of a dead foetus.

Conditions

- Intact uterus
- Dead foetus, with the exception of hydrocephaly
- Cervix fully dilated, in any case not less than 7 cm
- Head deep in the pelvis, admitting no more than 2 fingers above the brim.

Instruments

- 4 Kocher forceps, straight, long and sturdy
- 1 strong pair of scissors for scalp incision; Dubois scissors are ideal (Fig. 29.1A and B)
- 1 perforator: Available models are the Smellie perforator (Fig. 29.2A) or the Simpson perforator (Fig. 29.2B). The latter features a transverse bar, which, apart from functioning as a return spring, is also a lock that has to be disengaged to permit opening of the instrument. With hydrocephalus, any kind of pointed instrument will suffice (e.g. Drew Smithe catheter)
- 1 Braun obstetric hook (Fig. 29.3).

Sites of Perforation

- *Vertex presentation*: The anterior fontanelle or in the parietal bone as near as to it
- *Brow*: The frontal bone
- *Face*: The orbit
- *Aftercoming head*:
  - The roof of the mouth
  - The foramen magnum
  - The occipital bone behind the mastoid
  - Through the spina bifida if present by a stiff catheter passed up to the spinal canal.

Procedure

As we noted in Chapter 11 in the section on preparing for surgery: "Patients exhausted by intense pain and lack of sleep can be anxious, fearful, hard to manage, presenting a

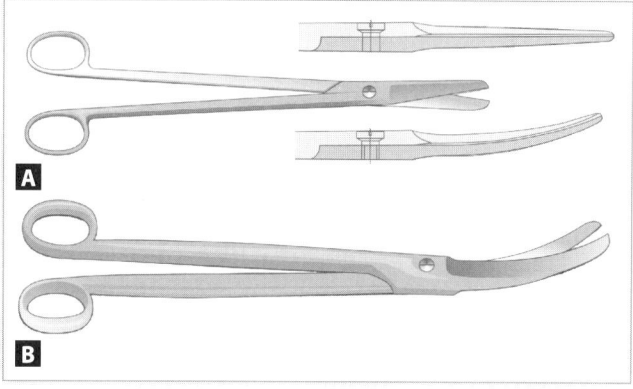

Fig. 29.1A and B: (A) Duval scissors; (B) Embriotomy scissors

270 THE CAESAREAN SECTION

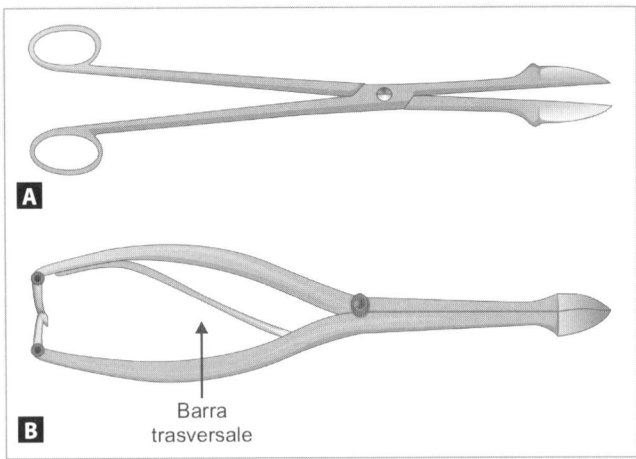

Fig. 29.2A and B: Perforators. (A) Smellie; (B) Simpson, fitted with transverse bar

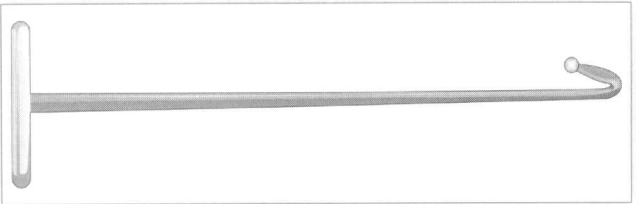

Fig. 29.3: Braun obstetric hook

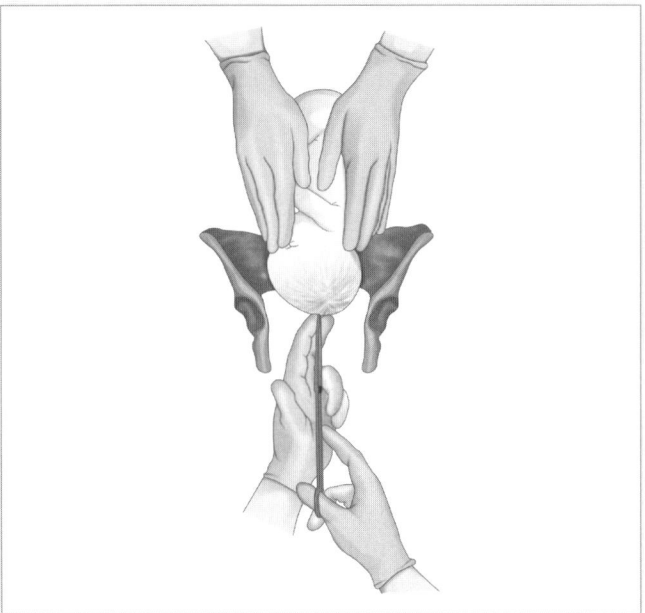

Fig. 29.4: Craniotomy: Note how the perforator is applied perpendicular to the head. The Kocher forceps have not been shown for the sake of clarity. The assistant should exert only moderate pressure on the foetal head

clinical picture generally described as 'maternal stress'. This condition is characterised by fluid imbalance, acid-base, electrolyte (hypernatremia) and caloric disorders and by infection of the birth canal."

Craniotomy should always be preceded by maternal resuscitation, drainage of the bladder and conducted under general anaesthesia.

Whichever instrument is utilised for perforation, it must be held *perprendicular to the surface*, to avoid the possibility of slippage and damage to nearby structures.

Any pressure exerted on the instrument must always be opposed by counter-pressure in the opposite direction. This can be effected by traction on the foetal scalp. Classic obstetrics recommends the association, by an assistant, of firm external pressure on the foetal head (Fig. 29.4). We disagree with this recommendation: The bladder may be distended and the lower uterine segment stretched even finer, leading thereby to traumatic injury. Moderate external pressure may, however, be applied.

The perforation site may be a suture, a fontanelle or a bony surface. Having identified the site, the scalp is grasped at two points 2 cm apart using two stout pairs of Kocher forceps. The forceps are pulled, tension is maintained and the incision is made in the fold of skin raised between them (Fig. 29.4). The Simpson's perforator is held closed in the operator's hand while its tip is protected by the fingers of the other hand which guide it through the birth canal up to the site of perforation and applied perpendicular to it.

The tip is forced into the site of perforation up to shoulders of the perforator (2–3 cm) which is then opened to produce a linear incision in the skull bones.

The blades are opened to a width of 3–4 cm by closing the handles. The instrument is then, turned 90° and the handles are opened and closed once more thus, producing a cruciate incision. Now insert the perforator deeper, up as far as its hinge, and open the blades to cut through the septi and brain matter, this will allow drainage of the CSF and brain matter. Once the cranial cavity has been evacuated, the two flaps of skin over the bone are grasped together using two or three sturdy Kocher forceps (Fig. 29.5).

This move has a dual function: It prevents sharp bone fragments from injuring the birth canal during descent of the head and facilitates descent through the traction on the forceps. It can sometimes prove necessary to further dismember the cranial vault; this can be done using sturdy Kocher forceps, or using a basiotribe (cranioclast), which is not always available in peripheral hospitals.

Classic obstetrics recommends craniotomy also in case of cephalopelvic disproportion; in such a case, the assistant should exert very firm pressure on the head, keeping it firmly impacted in the pelvic inlet, while the operator proceeds with the operation. This pressure is crucial, and justifies the remark that "it is not the operator holding the instrument who perforates the skull, but the person who presses the head".

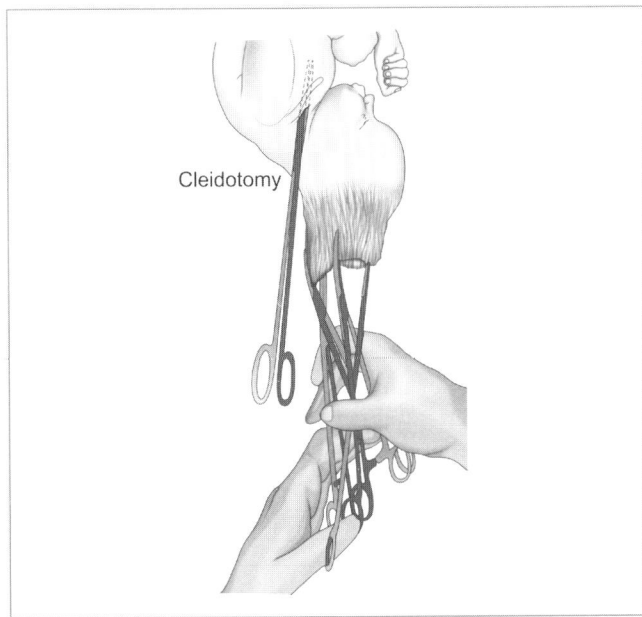

Fig. 29.5: Evacuation of the cranial contents has been completed; the flaps of skin are brought together using Kocher forceps. Where traction and rotation using the obstetric hook fail, section of the clavicle (cleidotomy) is performed

becomes the posterior one. Again apply a strip of gauze to the anterior axilla, pull downwards and extract the foetus.

Where this proves unsuccessful (foetal macrosomia), proceed to cleidotomy—mono or bilateral section of the clavicle (Fig. 29.5).

Craniotomy in Breech Presentation

The ideal site for a craniotomy is the occiput, but in order to avoid injury to the anterior vaginal wall, it is preferable to insert the perforator through a subcutaneous tunnel, leading to the occiput through the root of the foetal neck.

The method is as follows: The seventh cervical vertebra is identified and the overlying skin is grasped with Kocher forceps. Traction is applied and the fold of skin that forms is incised. Blunt scissors are then used to penetrate and open a tunnel until reaching the occiput. The same route is now used to insert the perforator; the manoeuvre described above is now performed. Once the septi have been cut through, traction will lead to expulsion of brain matter. Perforation should be preferred to excessive traction, which presents a concrete risk of posterior rupture of the lower uterine segment.

Extraction is often followed by uterine atony and profuse bleeding. This haemorrhage is controlled by:

- Immediate application of an indwelling urinary catheter
- Rehydration of patient and administration of glucose at the concentration available (5–50%)
- Intravenous administration of Ergometrine, followed by controlled traction on the umbilical cord:
- Putting on a long glove, enter uterus to check that no uterine ruptures have occurred
- If bleeding is profuse, perform manual control of haemorrhage (bimanual compression of the cervix) and in obstinate cases, transvaginal clamping of the descending branches of the uterine artery (Brigato-Guidi manoeuvre)
- Indwelling urinary catheter for at least two weeks (CBD—continuous bladder drainage)
- Sitz bath in antiseptic solution. Where antiseptic is not available, washing powder (commercially available brands) added to the bath will do fine.

If intervention is not prompt, craniotomy is often followed by complications, the most frequent of which are vesicovaginal or rectovaginal fistula and neurological complications through compression of the lumbosacral plexus (see the Chapter 25: "The obstructed labour injury complex").

Cleidotomy

Cleidotomy is division of one or both clavicles with an embryotomy scissors to reduce the biacromial diameter in shoulder dystocia with a dead foetus (Fig. 29.5).

While the elderly author (ED) has performed 8 craniotomies over the past 8 years on dead foeti with deeply impacted heads, he has never had to carry out a craniotomy on a floating head. This does not rule out the possibility of circumstances arising in which this is the only possible choice of technique.

In the case of hydrocephalus, collapsing of the foetal head and the resulting correction of cephalopelvic disproportion may be obtained by draining the cerebrospinal fluid through a spinal needle inserted through the abdominal wall, or vaginally using a Drew Smithe catheter, or by penetrating the sutures using any pointed instrument.

It is common for difficulties to arise with disengagement of the shoulders. This can be controlled using an obstetric hook (Fig. 29.3), which is inserted under an accessible axilla. If not already accessible, the axilla should be pulled into an anterior position by rotation and downward traction initiated from this position so that the shoulder engages under the symphysis.

Lack of an obstetric hook can be made up for by running some strong gauze under the armpit, tying the two strands together and pulling with this.

If descent is not obtained by hooking the anterior axilla, the following simple method, which has always proven successful, may be used.

Run some gauze under the anterior axilla and pull on the joined ends while simultaneously imparting a rotary movement to the trunk so that the anterior shoulder

Decapitation

Decapitation is severing of the foetal head from the trunk, it is one of the three methods used to deal with a dead foetus in transverse lie. The other two are as follows:
a. C-section. If neither trunk or head are available.
b. Evisceration, if the trunk is easily accessible.

Indications
- Neglected shoulder with a dead foetus
- Locked twins
- Double-headed monsters.

Conditions
- Intact uterus
- Dilatation greater than 8 cm
- Foetal head and neck are easily accessible.

Where these conditions are not met, conduct a lower segment vertical C-section, and decapitate the foetus *in utero*.

Instruments
- *Decapitation hook or a Braun Hook*
- *Stainless steel wire saw (Gigli) with handles* (Fig. 29.6). It is useful to have a spare one
- *Hooked metallic fingerstall* onto which the end of the wire saw is inserted; the fingerstall is worn on the operator's index or middle finger (Fig. 29.7A)
- Two rubber or plastic tubes (may be improvised using urinary catheters), through which the saw runs along two thirds of its length (Fig. 29.7 C). These function to prevent injuries to the vaginal wall during the saw's action
- *Stout scissors,* in the case of a small foetus.

Procedure
The procedure should be conducted in an operating room, preferably under general anaesthesia. The patient is placed in the lithotomy position.

Never resect a prolapsed arm. It is very useful for downward traction by an assistant and offers the operator control over the foetal trunk. If the arm is not prolapsed, proceed with disengagement.

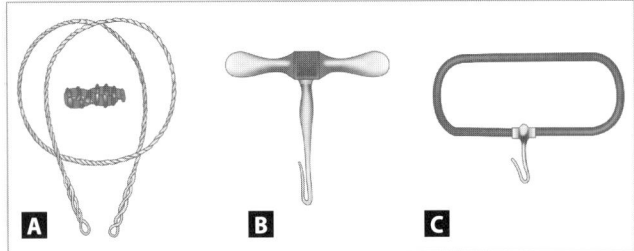

Fig. 29.6A to C: Gigli wire saw with handles. (A) Gigli wire saw; (B, C) handles

Either *decapitation hook* or *Gigli's wire saw* can be used.

The decapitation hook, protected by the palm of the left hand, is passed up over the child's shoulder and turned over the neck. If the hook is sharp, the neck is severed by sawing movement and if it is blunt rotate it to cause fracture dislocation of the cervical spines then the soft tissue is cut by an embryotomy scissors with a blunt tip.

Gigli's wire saw:
- Run the saw around the neck. There is a special fingerstall for this operation, which one connects to one end of the sawblade. If this is not available, attach the sawblade to a wire, which is passed around the neck (Fig. 29.7B). Traction on this wire will allow the sawblade to be applied to the desired point
- Alternatively, pass the sawblade over the neck and under an arm
- Pass the rubber or plastic sheaths over each end of the saw wire. They should cover two thirds of the saw's length (Fig. 29.7C)
- Attach the handles.

Hold the handles close together, to prevent injuries to the vagina.

A few firm strokes of the saw (three or four) will be enough to detach the head from the neck.

Having completed the cut, the assistant passes the arm to the operator, who exerts downward traction under control of the opposite hand, which is positioned in the vagina to prevent bony splinters from damaging the birth canal.

Disengagement of the head is effected as follows: Identify the head and turn the neck downwards. Grip this with two strong Kocher forceps (Fig. 29.7D), and exert traction. When the mouth is accessible, place one finger in the mouth to assist traction. Extraction will be easy.

EVISCERATION

Evisceration is the incision of the abdomen and/ or thorax to evacuate its viscera so reducing its size and allowing its vaginal delivery.

Indications
- Foetal ascites
- Thoracic or abdominal tumours.

Procedure
Under general anaesthesia, a large incision is made in the foetal abdomen with an embryotomy scissors then the viscera are evacuated manually.

If the thorax has to be incised first the abdominal viscera can be reached via the diaphragm.

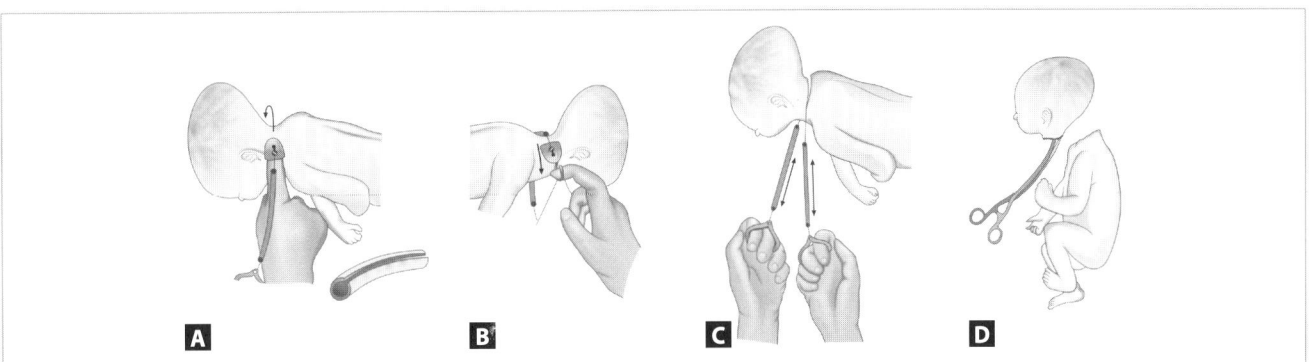

Fig. 29.7A to D: Some of the steps for decapitation: (A) Introduce two small sections of rubber tube, slit along their lengths, placing them over the sawblade; (B) Attach one end to the fingerstall, worn on the operator's index finger. The blade is passed right around the foetal neck and grasped by the operator; (C) Manipulating the handles, the operator cuts through the neck with a to-and-fro sawing movement; (D) The cut is complete. Throughout the procedure, an assistant exerts traction on the arm, which serves to hold the trunk immobile

Spondilotomy

Spondilotomy is division of the vertebral column.

Indications

Transverse impaction of a dead foetus when the neck cannot be reached.

In addition to evisceration when the foetus is large or pelvis is deformed.

Procedure

The vertebral column is divided by an embryotomy scissors. The foetus is delivered in 2 halves by traction on one arm to deliver a half and on a leg to deliver the other.

The birth canal should be explored after delivery.

BIBLIOGRAPHY

1. Adhikari S, Dasgupta M, Sanghmita M. Management of obstructed labour: a retrospective study. J Obstet Gynecol India. 2005;55:48-51.
2. Alfieri E, Bertino A, Clivio M. Vallardi, Milano. Trattato di Ostetricia. 1936.
3. Arora R, Rajaram P, Oumachigui A, et al. Destructive operations in modern obstetrics in a developing country at tertiary level. Br J Obstet Gynecol. 1993;100:967-8.
4. Biswas A, Chakraborty PS, Das HS, et al. Role of destructive operations in modern day obstetrics. J Indian Med Assoc. 2001;99:248-51.
5. Dafallah SE, Ambago J, El-Aguib F. Obstructed labour in a teaching hospital in Sudan. Saudi Med J. 2003;24:1102-4.
6. Gupta U, Chitra R. Destructive operations still have a place in developing countries. Int J Gyn Obstet. 1994;44:15-9.
7. Konje JC, Obisesan KA, Ladipo OA. Obstructed labour in Ibadan. Int J Gyn Obst. 1992;39:17-21.
8. Lawson JB. Obstetrics and Gynaecology in the Tropics. London: Edward Arnold (Publishers); 1974.
9. Lorca C. Tratado práctico de operaciones obstétricas. Ed. Ciéntifico- Médica, Madrid/Barcelona, 1948.
10. Maggiora-Vergano T. Lezioni di Clinica Ostetrica e Ginecologica tenute dal Prof. L. Cattaneo. Ed. Moderne, Roma, 1954/55.
11. Maharaj D, Moodley J. Symphysiotomy and foetal destructive operations. Best Practice and Research Clin Obst & Gynaec, 2002;16:117-31.
12. Martius H. Die Gerburtshilflichen Operationen. Thieme, Stuttgart, 1948.
13. Merger R, Lèvy J, Melchior J Ostetricia. UTET-Masson, Torino/Parigi, 1972.
14. Ozumba BC, Uchegbu H. Incidence and management of obstructed labour in eastern Nigeria. Aust NZJ Obstet Gynecol. 1991;31:213-6.
15. Parikh MN. Destructive operations in Obstetrics. J Obstet Gynaec India, 2006;56:113-4.
16. Sikka P. Destructive operations—a vanishing art in modern obstetrics. Arch Gynecol Obstet. 2011;283:929-33.
17. Singhal SR, Chaudhary P, Sangwan K, et al. Destructive operations in modem obstetrics. Arch Gynecol Obstet. 2005;273:107-9.

Index

Page numbers followed by *f* refer to figure and *t* refer to table.

A

Abdomen, clinical examination of 54
Abdominal cavity, lavage of 157
Abdominal compartment syndrome 216
Abdominal morphology 54
Abdominal palpation 206
Abdominal peritoneum 235*f*
Abdominal scores 73
Abdominal trauma, violent 198
Abdominal tumours 216
Abdominal wall 219, 235*f*
   anterior 128*f*, 129*f*
   closure 185
      techniques of 223*f*
   lateral 129*f*
   surgical anatomy of 128
   suturing of 224
   synchronous dehiscence 226
ACE inhibitors 93
Acetabulum 4
Acetylsalicylic acid 94
Adequate gestational age 196
Adrenaline 124
Airways
   clearing of 239
   obstruction of 237
Algometric scales 213
Ambu bag
   for adults 121
   for paediatric 121
Amniotic fluid
   not stained with meconium 239
   pathology 100
   stained with meconium 243
Amniotomy 110
Anaesthesia 121
   basic equipment 121
   basic medications 121
   data sheet 122*f*
   general 126
   intervention 123
   local 125
   monitoring 123
   premedication for 123
   types of 123
Analgesia 212
Analgesic effect 126
Android pelvis 17, 22, 35, 40
Antenatal monitoring form 46, 47
Antepartum risk assessment form 45
Anthropoid 21
   pelvis 17, 22, 35, 40, 71*f*
Anthropometric index 66
Antibiotic
   administration of 120
   therapy 212, 244
Anticonvulsant prophylaxis 95
Antihypertensive drugs used during pregnancy 93*t*
Anti-reflux function 179*f*
Apgar scoring system 238*t*
Arcuate ligament 11, 259
Arterial pressure 117
   control of 92
Artery 114
Assisted ventilation 239
   acts 239
Asymptomatic late dehiscence 228
Asynclitism 86
   anterior 37
   posterior 37
Atenolol 93
Atropinisation 125
Attacks, treatment of 95
Auvard vaginal speculum 233

B

Bandl's ring 30*f*
   of retraction 31*t*
Beta blockers 93
Birth asphyxia 250
Birth canal 4, 17, 17*f*
   abnormalities 142
   anomalies 99
   infection of 117
Bisacromial diameter 59
Bishop's score 72
Bitrochanteric diameter 61
Bladder 178*f*, 229
   and urethra, closure of 233
   dome, repair of 174
   flap haematoma 218
   injury 173, 204
      repair of 175*f*
   suturing of 234
   wall, posterior 174
Blind technique 177*f*
Blood
   flow 238
      from placenta to foetus 244
   group, determination of 120
   loss, control of 153
   pressure 81
Blunt expansion 149
B-Lynch technique 173*f*
   managing haemorrhages by 172
Body mass index 51
Bony pelvis 4
Boudeloque's conjugate 61
Braun obstetric hook 270*f*
Braxton-Hicks contractions 75
Breech from maternal pelvis, extraction of 251
Breech presentation 151, 249, 252*f*
   aetiology 249
Bumm pelvic line 139
Bupivacaine 124, 125
Burst abdomen 221

C

Caesarean section 89, 91
   alternatives to 247
   management 89
   monitoring 211
Calcium antagonists 93
Caldwell-Moloy pelvic classification 21
Calkin's methodology 76

Camper's fascia 139, 189, 193
Cannula to umbilical cord 240
Capillary refill 117
Caput succedaneum 74, 86, 263f
Cardiac arrest 196
　　operation 196
Cardiac massage 240, 241f
Cardiff counting system 50
Cardiocirculatory
　　disorders 217
　　system 195, 217
Cardiopathy 181
Cardiorespiratory aetiology 196
Central venous pressure 119, 242
Cephal hematoma 263
Cephalad extension 203f
Cephalhaematoma 263f
Cephalic circumference 69f
Cephalic presentations 32
Cephalic vein 114f
Cephalopelvic disproportion 86, 119, 163
　　sign of 81
Cervical canal, Foley balloon in 109
Cervical dilatation 78
Cervix
　　incision of 255
　　unfavourable 109
Cherney incision 138
Cherney low transverse laparotomy 138f
Chin posterior 258
Chronic intrinsic causes 216
Circulatory system 95
Cleidotomy 268, 271
Clinical obstetrics, diagnosis in 43
Coccyx 10
Collagen 25
Collateral measures 94
Collin's pelvimeter 48f
Common peroneal nerve 232
　　lesion of 232
Compartment syndrome 216
Compass method 66
Complete uterine rupture 207f
Celiotomy caudally, completing 134f
Connective tissue
　　component 27
　　composition of 25
Conservative management 207
Continuous suturing 188, 189
Contracted pelvis 249
Contractile activity 27
　　of myometrium 29
Contraction ring 31t
Cord
　　clamping 151
　　prolapse 103

Core ligaments 12
Corneal reflex 52
Correct application of tourniquet 113f
Correct scalpel grip 131f
Cotyloid cavity 4
Cranial vault 263t
Craniotomy 268, 269, 270f
　　in breech presentation 271
　　indications 269
　　procedure 269
Cranium of infant 39f
Crichton's hysterotomy technique 159
Cubital fossa 114f

D

Decapitation 268, 272
Deep tension sutures 192f
Dehydration 85, 115, 118
　　clinical manifestations of 117t
Delivery
　　course of 261
　　methods of expediting 105t
　　timing of 96
Destructive operations 268
Destructive surgery 208
Determining retropubic angle 71
Dextrose 124
Diabetes 181
Diagonal conjugate 16
Diazepam 99, 244
Dinoprostone 109
Distant ligaments 12
Diuresis 95, 98, 117
Dome of bladder 174
Dressing, characteristics of 218
Dubois body surface area nomograph 51
Duhrssen incision 255, 256f
Duval scissors 269f

E

Eclampsia 96
　　aetiopathogenesis 96
　　diagnose 97, 97t
　　sequence of symptoms 97
Elective extraperitoneal C-section 158
Electrolyte composition of plasma 118t
Electrolyte imbalance 116
Elkin's protocol modified 252
Ellipsoids 36f
Embriotomy scissors 269f
Emergency extraperitoneal C-section 159
Emmet's technique 187
Ensheating catheter 235f
Enter uterine cavity 172
Enteric fistulas 225
　　symptomatology 225
　　therapy 225

Evisceration 268, 272
External oblique muscle 129, 129f
Extraperitoneal drainage 219, 219f
Extraperitoneal transverse hysterotomies 157
Eye opening 52

F

Face presentation 32
Faecal incontinence 47
Fascia
　　closure of 188, 193
　　incision of 132f, 133f, 140f, 141f
　　　　superficial 132
　　superior edge of 142f
　　transverse section of 137f
Femoral vein 113
Fever 116
First layer seromuscular sutures 175f
First leopold manoeuvre 56f
Fish-shaped viscera retainer 187f
Fistula
　　documentation of 231
　　of small dimensions 233
　　repair of 234f
Fluid compartments of body 117f
Fluids, administration of 242
Foetal
　　adnexa, pathology of 99
　　anoxia 103
　　asphyxia 103
　　back 56f
　　distress 86
　　growth, retarded 94
　　heart rate 80
　　heartbeat 57f
　　　　auscultation of 60
　　indications 99
　　lie 103
　　　　unfavourable 103
　　mortality 200
　　　　incidence of 200t
　　motility
　　　　increased 249
　　　　obstruction of normal 249
　　parts, recognition of 72
　　pelvis 20f
　　poles, compression of 251
　　position 35t
　　skull
　　　　bones, moulding of 73
　　　　moulding of 81
　　symptomatology 205
　　well-being 79, 99, 195
Foetus 195
　　action on 126

alive 258
　delivery of 150
　safety of 251
　single 253
Forepelvis angle, width of 67

G

Gallagher sutures 222f, 227
Gardnerella vaginalis 43
Gastrointestinal function 217
Genitalia, observation of external 70, 220
Gestational age 253
Gestational hypertension 92
Gestational oedema 92
　proteinuria hypertension 92
　　classification 92
Gigli's wire 272
Glasgow coma scale 52t
Glover's sutures 175f
Gluteus maximus muscle 4
Gluteus medius muscle 4
Gluteus minimus muscle 4
Greenhill method 70
Gynecoid 21
　pelvis 22, 40, 71f

H

Haematocrit 138
Haemodynamic target 218
Haemoglobin 120
Haemorrhage 168, 171, 208
　control of 168
　surgical control of 169
Haemorrhagic shock 216
Haemostasis 185
Haemostatic procedures 169
Hand dorsal venous plexus 114f
Hartmann's solution 241
Head
　deflection of 103
　delivery of 236
　descent of 79
　disengagement of 150f
　flexion of 79
Heart rate 79, 81, 117
High semicircular hysterotomy 147f
Hodge's parallel planes 34f
Hodge's system 33
Homolateral round ligament 208
Hydration, preoperative 125
Hyperhydration 118
Hyperthermia 105
Hypertonic dehydration 119
Hypoalbuminaemia 221
Hypomoclion 40

Hypotension 124
Hypoxic-ischemic encephalopathy 244
Hysterorrhaphy 153
　late dehiscence of 227
Hysterotomy 144, 148, 159f
　breadth of 151
　choice, criteria of 146
　digital extension of 149f
　edges of 169
　extension and morphology of 149
　isolation of site for 142
　longitudinal 147f
　lower margin, central expansion of 169
　lower-segment 147f
　of corpus, vertical 163f
　repair, second layer 155f
　types of 107, 144, 147f
　vertical 162, 181
　wound edges of 168

I

Iliac spine
　anterior superior 6
　posterior inferior 6
Index finger on tendon 54f
Inferioriliac spine, anterior 6
Infiltration 125
Inflammation 185
　increased risk of 153
　prevent spread of 156
Infusion therapy 211
Interrupted sutures 189
Interstitial fluid, electrolyte composition of 118t
Intervillous space, infarction of 80, 102
Intra-abdominal hypertension 216
　physiopathology of 217
Intracellular fluid, electrolyte composition of 117t
Intracervical fistula 230
Intracranial haemorrhage 262
Intracranial pressure, increase of 263
Intramuscular administration 99
Intraoperative causes 202
Intraoperative complications, management of 168
Intrauterine growth retardation 162
Intravenous
　access 113
　administration 99
Ischaemic alterations 217
Ischaemic injury 230f
Ischial spine 6, 17
　characteristics of 71
Isobaric subarachnoid 124

J

Jarricot's reflex dermalgias 53f
Justine siegemundin manoeuvre 254, 255f
Juxta cervical 230
　fistula 231f
Juxtaurethral 230

K

Kehrer transverse hysterotomy 147f
Ketamine 126
Ketosis 85
Kocher forceps 187
Kreitzer's vascular stratum 27
Kustner laparotomy 138f

L

Labetalol 93
Labour
　actual 107
　assistance during 238
　elective induction of 108
　false 75
　indications for caesarean section
　　during 102
　　outside 91
　patterns of abnormal 75t
　progress of 78
　spontaneous onset of 108
　third stage of 153
　timing of 94
　trial of 106
　true 75
　with oxytocin, augmentation of 110
Laparotomic wound 218
　dehiscence of 221
　repair of 188f, 189f
　single-layer closure of 190f
　suture, complications of 221
Laparotomy 128, 130
　incorrect 132f
　lateral 130
　midline 130, 130f
　　subumbilical 131
　scar, characteristics of 107
　type of 174
　vertical 130, 130f
　wound, repair of vertical 186
Laplace's law 25
Lignocaine 125
　solution 124
Linea alba 132f
　edges of 140f
Ljubljana technique 177f
Low transverse hysterotomy 148f

Low transverse laparotomy 139*f*
   to pfannenstiel 137*f*
Lower limbs, examination of 220
Lower uterine segment
   injuries of 173
   rupture of 203*f*
Lumbosacral hinge, site of 69
Lumbosacral joint 10, 14
Lung disease 92, 181

M

Magnesium sulphate 99
Malaria, diagnose 97*t*
Malmstrom's obstetric ventouse 262*f*
Martin's pelvimeter 48*f*
Matany partograph 86
Maternal causes 181
Maternal complications 264
Maternal condition 81
Maternal distress 102
Maternal illness
   during pregnancy 91
   to pregnancy 92
Maternal indications 91, 105
Maternal intensive care 115
Maternal mortality 200
   incidence of 200*t*, 209*t*
Maternal perineal injury 265
Maternal prognosis 205
Maternal symptomatology 205
Maternal-foetal gas exchange 102
   compromise of 102
Maylard low transverse laparotomy 138*f*
Meconium aspiration syndrome 237
Medication, administration of 242
Mediolateral episiotomy 260
Membranes, characteristics of 72
Memory loss, short-term 126
Metabolic acidosis 116
Middle upper arm circumference 50
Midpelvis 65
Mid-vaginal 230
Mifepristone 109
Misoprostol 109
Monitoring diuresis 95
Morphology 19, 67
   of pure pelvic types 22*f*
Mother, safety of 251
Mucosa 117, 240
Mucus suction catheter 121
Müller ducts 27
Multiple pregnancy 249
Munro Kerr hysterotomy 147*f*
Muscle 141
   bellies, apposition of 187, 192
   component 26

   detachment of 141*f*
   fibre
      normal 25
      smooth 25
   layer
      intermediate 26*f*
      internal 26*f*
   tissue 192
Myomectomy 202
Myometrium 26, 26*f*

N

Nasogastric intubation 215
Nasogastric tube 121
Native uterus, rupture of 198
Neomyometrium 26, 26*f*
Neonate's chest 240
Nerve 114
Nervous system 117
Neurological lesions 232
Neuromuscular disorder 232
Newborn 236
   delivered by caesarean section 243
   delivered vaginally in breech
      presentation 243
   infant, resuscitation in 239*f*
   physiopathology 236
Nifedipine 93
Nose 238

O

Oblique muscle, internal 130
Obstetric conjugate 16, 62
Obstetric diameter, anteroposterior 16
Obstetric history
   chart 47
   past 44
   previous 43
Obstetric pelvic axis 17
Obstetric pelvis 19
Obstetric physical examination 54, 107
Obstructed labour 86, 119
   injury complex 229
Obturator foramen 4
Oliguria 98
One-centimetre rule 188
Operation, preparing for 113
Organs and systems 50
Osseous venous access 242*f*
Ovarian branch of uterine artery, ligation
   of 170*f*
Oxytocin infusion 85

P

Pain management, postoperative 212
Paleomyometrium 26*f*

Palpation 55
   starts 55
Paralytic ileus 215
Parietal peritoneum 186, 192
   posterior aspect 133*f*
Partial uterine rupture 204*f*
Partograph 75
   filling in 81
   structure of 78
Parturition 3
   anatomy of 1
   mechanism of 33, 35
   physiology of 1
   physiopathology of 33
Patellar reflex 54
Patient nutritional support 214
Pectineus muscle 6
Pelvic arrest 23, 24*f*
Pelvic axis 17*f*
Pelvic bone 4
Pelvic cavity 17
Pelvic clinical picture 205
Pelvic examination 69
Pelvic face 8*f*
Pelvic floor 18*f*, 19*f*
   trauma 250
Pelvic inlet 15, 61, 67
   diameters of 16*f*
Pelvic joints 11
Pelvic morphology 35
Pelvic outlet 17, 18*f*, 64*f*, 65
Pelvic pain, severe 205
Pelvic scores 73
Pelvic strait
   inferior 18*f*
   superior 16*f*, 33
Pelvic surface 10
Pelvic type 35*t*
Pelvic walls 71*f*
Pelvimeters 61
Pelvis 104
   altered inclination of 104
   anterior triangle of 136*f*
   assimilation 23, 24*f*, 40, 67
   evaluation of
      anterior 67
      posterior 68
   inclination of 23
   long 23, 36
   normal 36, 260*f*
   subdivision of 34*f*
   true 15
Perimortem caesarean delivery 195
Perimysium 141*f*
Peripheral venous pressure 120
Peritoneal closure 156

Peritoneal margin
  accessing lateral 187
  accessing superior 187
Peritoneum, closure of 187
Peroneal nerve 232
Pharynx and mouth 238
Phencyclidine, derivate of 126
Phenomena, types of 237
Physiological immaturity 201
Pigeaud's descent cylinder 35f
Placenta praevia 102
Placental abruption 102
Placental circulation, physiology of 28
Placental insufficiency 100
Plasmodium falciparum 102
Platipelloid pelvis 22
Platypelloid 21, 37
  android 37
  pelvis 19, 35, 40
    mixed 37
Pneumomediastinum 237
Pneumopericardium 237
Pneumothorax 237
Polydipsia 81
Polyuria 81
Pomeroy tubal sterilisation 183, 183f
Postcaesarean wound dehiscence 226
Posterior bladder wall, repair of 175
Posterior uterine segment, rupture of 203f
Postmortem caesarean delivery 195
Postnatal assistance 238
Postpartum clinical management 96
Potassium hydroxide 43
Predominantly lower-segment C-section 164, 163f
Preeclampsia 94
  classifications of
    moderate 94
    severe 94
    epidemiology 95
    monitoring for 95
    treatment of
      mild 95
      severe 95
Premature delivery 249
Preoperative hydration of non-dehydrated patient 120
Pronounced vulvar oedema 220
Prophylaxis 169, 174, 227
  against preeclampsia 94
  of bladder damage 133
Pubic arch, angle of 65
Pubic ligament
  anterior 11
  inferior 11, 259
  superior 11, 258

Pubic symphysis 11
  after symphysiotomy 259f
  anterior view 12f, 258f
Pubic-arch modelling 65
Pulmonary hypertension 237
Puncture fundus anteroposteriorly 172
Pyramidalis muscles 128, 133, 138f, 142f, 193f
  preparation of 141f

R

Recent obstetric history 47
Rectal administration 99
Rectovaginal fistula 231f
  anatomical functional classification of 231
Rectus abdominis 129
  muscles 128, 137, 137f, 187
  section of 129f
Rectus muscles 128, 136, 138f, 188f, 193f
  transection of 138f
Rectus sheath fascia, fibres of 135f
Reflexes 52
Reimplantation
  blind technique 177
  open technique 178
Renal function 217
Respiratory arrest 98
Respiratory depression 240
Respiratory effects 126
Respiratory rate 98, 117
Respiratory system 95, 196, 217
Retraction ring 30f
Retrovesical haematoma 219f
Right pelvic bone
  external view 5f
  internal view 6f
Ringer's solution 211

S

Sacral canal 10
Sacral cavity, assessment of 71
Sacral nerves 229
Sacral plexus, trauma of 232
Sacral promontory 15f
Sacral tuberous ligament 12
Sacroiliac joint 10, 12
  posterior view 14f
  right 13f
Sacroiliac ligaments
  anterior 12
  large 12
  posterior 12
  small 12
Sacrospinous ligament 7, 14

Sacrum 7
  left lateral aspect 11f
  superior view 9f
Scalp oedema 265
Scalpel dissection of fascia 141f
Scar tissue 231f
Scarpa's fascia 132
Scarred uterus 202
  rupture of 198
Scars, examination of 55
Sciatic nerve 232, 232f
Second leopold manoeuvre 56f
Sedation, level of 214t
Semicircular hysterotomy 148
Septic causes 223
Septic risk scoring system 244t
Septic shock 216
Single deep tension sutures 191f, 192f
Skin 190, 193, 263t
  colour of 240
  decubitus wounds, avoid 192f
  incision of 132f, 139f
  plane of 126f
Slightly mobile joint 11
Small pelvis, classifications of 20
Sodium hypochlorite 227
Soft tissue
  dystocia 99
  edema 74
  of birth canal, changes to 104
Spinal anaesthesia 124, 233
Spondilotomy 273
Strictly curvilinear 148
Subcutaneous partial symphysiotomy 259
Subcutaneous tissue 132f, 139, 139f, 189, 193
Subpubic arch 69f
Subpubic arch, assessing 71
Subpubic dead space 69f
Subumbilical laparotomy 130, 192
Superficial muscle layer 26f
Superficial veins 114f
  of forearm 114f
  of leg, anterior aspect 115f
  of thigh, anterior aspect 114f
Supine decubitus 211
Supine hypotensive syndrome 121
Suprapubic skin 260
Suturing material utilised, quality of 154
Symphysiotomy 257, 261f
  advantages 258
  anatomical basis of 258
  conditions 258
  indications 257
  theoretical basis of 258
Symphysiotomy-vacuum extraction 257
Symphysis-fundal distance, graph of 58

Symptomatic late dehiscence 227
   aetiology 227
   diagnosis 228
   symptomatology 227
   treatment 228
   ultrasonography 227
Symptomatology 204
Synclitism 36f

T

Tactile stimulation 239
Tendinous inscriptions 128
Tetanus toxoid, administration of 212
Therapeutic approach 117, 223
Third leopold manoeuvre 57f
Third trimester gestosis 92
Third trimester haemorrhage 99
Thoms classification 20t
Thumb on tendon 54f
Tibial nerve 232
Tissue damage 217
Transabdominal hysterotomy 91
Transversalis fascia 128
   and peritoneum 133, 141
Transverse diameters 16
Transverse hysterotomy 135, 147, 147f, 152
   lower-segment 147f
Transverse laparotomy
   techniques 136t
   wound, repair of 191
Transverse lie 253
Transverse transperitoneal hysterotomies 147
Transversus abdominis 130
   aponeurosis of 130
True pelvis, assessment of 60
Tubal sterilization 181, 182
   classic indications 181
   elective indications 182
   indications 181
   Madlener technique for 182
Tumefaction 206f
Turner classification 20t
Twin, second 253

U

Ulcers 220
Umbilical catheter 242f
Umbilical cord
   catheter to 240
   catheterisation of 241, 241f
   pathology 100, 103
   resection of 241f
Unscarred uterus 201
Upper airways 238
Ureter
   dorsal side of 177f, 180f
   implant 178f
   injuries to 176
   reimplantation of 177f
Ureteral reimplantation 176
   preliminary steps 176
Urethra 229
Urinary incontinence with postpartum onset 47
Urinary system 219
Urinary tract, injury to 173
Urine 81
   ketones test 81
Uterine artery 145
   ascending branch of 170
   forceps on 171
Uterine atony 168
Uterine bleeding, managing 172f, 173f
Uterine blood vessels 162
   hysterotomy affecting 170
   ligation of 170f
Uterine causes 181
Uterine cavity 226
   through posterior wall 172
Uterine cervix 27, 72, 207f
Uterine contractile activity 79
Uterine corpus, changes affecting 28f
Uterine devascularisation 170, 170f, 171, 171f
Uterine exteriorization 152, 152f
Uterine fundus 26f
Uterine haemorrhages 168
Uterine hyperkinesia 102
Uterine hyperstimulation 109
Uterine incision, repair of 173
Uterine inertia 85
Uterine involution, monitoring 218
Uterine morphology, changes in 104
Uterine peritonealisation 227
Uterine polarity with hyperkinesis, normal 30
Uterine rupture 103, 108, 144, 177f, 182, 198, 205
   complicated 204f
   diagnosis of 205
   during labour 199
      diagnosis of 205
   during pregnancy 198
   incomplete 206
Uterine scar dehiscence 198
Uterine segment, lower 27, 144, 145f, 147, 202
Uterine serosa 198
Uterine suturing 166f
   first layer of 155f, 165f
   second layer of 165f
Uterus 4, 25, 144, 145f
   early 226
   histology of 26
   mechanical functions of 25
   still intact 146

V

Vacuum extraction 262
   advantages 262
   conditions 262
   contraindications 262
   disadvantages 262
   indications 262
Vaginal deliveries, previous 107
Vaginal examination 227
Vaginal wall
   and rectum, posterior 229
   anterior 229
Vein 114
Vena cava syndrome, pathogenesis of inferior 122
Venous
   cut down 114
   pressure, mean 119
Ventilation 240
   target 218
Vertex presentation 32
Vertex vaginal delivery 237
Vertical caesarean section, lower-segment 164
Vesicolysis 177f
Vesicovaginal fistula 175, 229, 231f
   aetiopathogenesis 229
   classification of 230f
   repair technique for 234f
   treatment of 233
Visual analogue pain rating scale 213f
Volkman retractors 134f
Voluntary muscle testing 232
Vulvar fissure 70

W

Walcher's position 14
Ward doctor 211
Ward examination 214
Washing detergent 227
Washing powder 223
Water balance 118, 118t
   concept of 118
Water deficit 118
Wound dehiscence 221
Wound healing 185
Wound, examination of 218

Y

Youssef's syndrome 175

Z

Zangenmeister's manoeuvre 57, 58